ESSENTIALS OF MEDICAL PHARMACOLOGY

Dr. Aarushi Singh

ALLIED
HEALTH
PRESS

Essentials of Medical Pharmacology

Author: **Dr. Aarushi Singh**

Allied Health Press
4164 Lakeshore Road
Burlington ON L7L 1A4
Canada
www.alliedhealthpress.com
Email: orders@arclereducation.com

ISBN: 978-1-77956-817-5

ABOUT THE AUTHOR

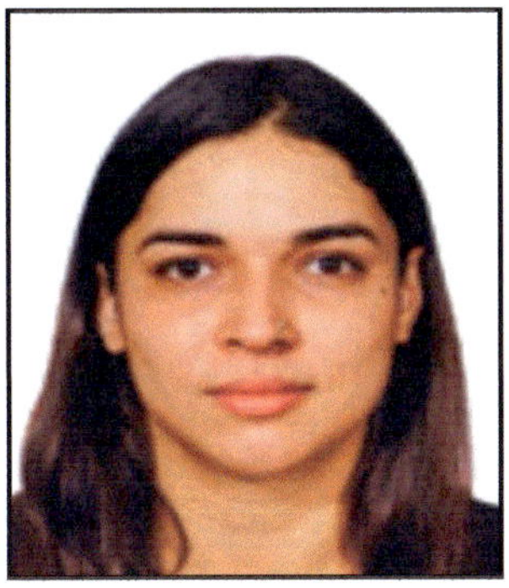

Dr. Aarushi Singh is an accomplished chemist currently serving as an Assistant Professor in the Department of Chemistry at Ramjas College, University of Delhi. She embarked on her academic journey with a B.Sc. in Chemistry from Ramjas College in 2011, followed by a Master's in Chemistry from the University of Delhi in 2013. Driven by a passion for research, Dr. Singh pursued her Ph.D. at the same institution, completing it in 2021. Her doctoral thesis, conducted under the mentorship of Prof. Ramesh Chandra and Dr. Rakeshwar Bandichhor, focused on the synthesis of biologically active Pyrazinoindoles and their mechanistic interaction studies.

Dr. Singh has accumulated significant research experience through various prestigious roles and projects. She worked as a Senior Research Fellow at the Indian Council of Medical Research (ICMR), where she developed inhalable nanomicelles for lung cancer treatment. She has also held positions as a Research Associate at the University of Alberta, Canada, focusing on the synthesis of Piperidinyl allylboronates, and at the Max Planck Institute for Multidisciplinary Sciences in Germany, where she synthesized magnetic resonance contrast agents.

Her international experience includes a stint as a Visiting Scientist at Humboldt Universität zu Berlin, Germany, and as a Ph.D. Exchange Student at the Japan Advanced Institute of Science and Technology (JAIST), where she studied the inhibition of protein aggregation by zwitterionic polymers. These experiences were supported by several prestigious fellowships, including the Shastri Research Student Fellowship and the JASSO Fellowship.

Dr. Singh's research interests are broad and interdisciplinary, encompassing multi-step organic synthesis, heterocyclic synthesis, and the development of biologically active compounds. Dr. Singh has authored one book and published over 15 original scientific research papers in internationally recognized journals. In addition to her research, Dr. Singh is dedicated to teaching and mentoring the next generation of chemists. Her diverse background and international collaborations enrich her teaching, providing students with a global perspective on chemical research and applications.

Dr. Aarushi Singh continues to contribute to the field of chemistry through her innovative research, dedicated teaching, and active participation in the scientific community. Her work aims to bridge the gap between advanced research and practical applications, making complex chemical concepts accessible and impactful.

Brief Table of Contents

Getting Started with This Book

Chapter Openers

A list of Chapter Outline is presented providing a brief Introduction to what will be covered in the chapter.

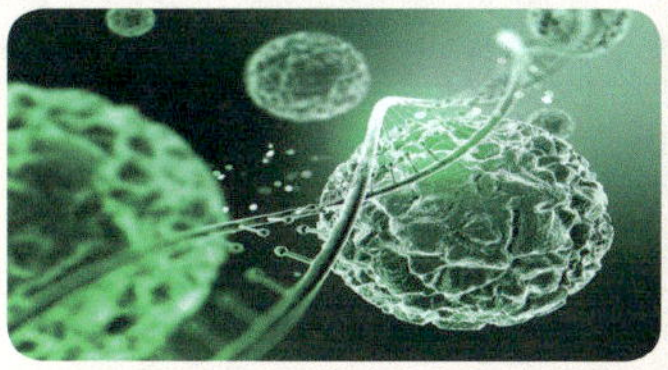

LEARNING OBJECTIVES

After studying this chapter, you will be able to:

1. Discuss the scientific method in biology;
2. Explain the cell theory;
3. Discuss the genetics and heredity;
4. Evolution and natural selection;
5. Focus on ecology and ecosystems;
6. Learn about human biology;
7. Evaluate the plant biology;
8. Explain the microbiology;
9. Focus on current trends in biology.

Introduction

Often referred to as the science of life, biology is a broad field of study aimed at comprehending the several kinds of life on Earth, from tiny creatures to sophisticated multicellular entities. Comprising several subfields, including molecular biology, ecology, and evolutionary biology, each of which advances our knowledge of living systems, this field clarifies the mechanisms controlling life events, including development, reproduction, and interaction with the surroundings, which is the central goal of biology. Moreover, biology fills in the void between the natural sciences and medicine by offering a necessary understanding of health, illness, and the interactions between organisms and their environments. Dealing with urgent global issues such as climate change, biodiversity loss, and new diseases depends on an awareness of these complex biological interactions, therefore highlighting the critical part biology plays in modern civilization. Fundamentally, biology explores and tests ideas about the living world using the scientific method. Through methodical observation and experimentation,

1.1. The Scientific Method in Biology

Learning Outcome

1. Describe the steps of the scientific method;
2. Focus on hypothesis formation;
3. Learn about experimental design.

Learning Outcomes

The beginning of each section of every chapter contains a set of Learning Outcomes that inform students of concepts they should understand. These outcomes help students understand what they should be able to do if they have mastered the material in that section.

Test Your Knowledge

Throughout each chapter, Test Your Knowledge cues you to note which topics have been covered and to self-test your understanding of the material presented.

Test Your Knowledge

1. Explain why correlation does not imply causation in scientific experiments.
2. How does the scientific method help reduce the influence of personal opinions in research?

Chapter Summary

The Summary Section appear at the end of each chapter and summarize main concepts covered throughout the chapter. These points provide key concepts in an engaging and meaningful way.

Summary

The investigation of biological principles highlights the importance of a comprehensive view of life by reflecting the intricate interactions that occur within living systems. The complexity of biology goes beyond individual species or systems, as this essay highlights; it also includes the interactions that mold ecosystems and affect biodiversity. Researchers can conduct in-depth analyses of metabolomic data using sophisticated technologies like MetaboAnalyst, which offer insights into the molecular mechanisms underlying these interactions. As demonstrated by the developments in MetaboAnalyst, for example, the integration of diverse omics data promotes a thorough understanding of metabolic pathways and helps identify important biological markers necessary for research on development and disease (Chong et al., 2018). Additionally, the phenomenon of ecological invasions is a key component of biological research and a vital field of study. The introduction of non-native species into unfamiliar habitats has significant ramifications and calls for multidisciplinary management strategies. Examining the origins and effects of these biological incursions, invasion science has become a crucial field that highlights the need to comprehend ecological dynamics and community interactions. As interest in biological invasions increases, new findings are emerging that put conventional ecological theories and practices to the test. The importance of incorporating various scientific viewpoints is shown by this developing discipline, which also highlights how invasive species shape ecosystems and advances our knowledge of ecological resilience (David et al., 2013). When taken as a whole, these discoveries from invasion science and metabolomics highlight the value of multidisciplinary biology research. Fostering cross-disciplinary collaboration and utilizing technological breakthroughs to improve our comprehension of intricate biological interactions are crucial as we look to the future of biological research. In addition to deepening our understanding of the complexities of life, this method lays the groundwork for tackling urgent environmental issues. Future studies can ensure the continued relevance of biology in a world that is constantly changing by acknowledging the interconnection of biological systems and opening the door to creative solutions that support sustainability and biodiversity conservation. We might imagine a thorough comprehension of life that serves both academia and society at large through ongoing investigation and integration of scientific knowledge.

Knowledge Assessment

The chapter includes material designed to review and reinforce each content. It includes Critical Thinking Questions to help test of your understanding of information presented in the chapter and Short answer Questions to review your understanding of the key concepts presented in the chapter.

Critical Thinking Questions

1. **Who is known as the "Father of Modern Biology"?**
   a. Aristotle
   b. Charles Darwin
   c. Gregor Mendel
   d. Louis Pasteur
2. **What is the basic unit of life?**
   a. Atom
   b. Molecule
   c. Cell
   d. Organism
3. **Which branch of biology studies the interaction of organisms with their environment?**
   a. Genetics
   b. Ecology
   c. Physiology
   d. Botany
4. **Which macromolecule is the main source of energy for living organisms?**
   a. Proteins
   b. Lipids
   c. Carbohydrates
   d. Nucleic acids
5. **DNA is primarily responsible for which function in living organisms?**
   a. Energy production
   b. Protein synthesis
   c. Storing genetic information
   d. Regulating body temperature

Short Answer Questions

1. What is biology, and why is it important to study biology?
2. What are the three main domains of life, and how are they different from one another?
3. Define homeostasis and give an example of how it works in living organisms.
4. What is the cell theory, and why is it fundamental to biology?
5. How do autotrophs and heterotrophs differ in the way they obtain energy?
6. What is the scientific method, and how is it applied in biological research?
7. Discuss how biology helps address global challenges such as climate change, disease, and food security.
8. Explain the levels of biological organization from the smallest unit to the largest. Provide examples at each level.
9. Describe the relationship between structure and function in biology, giving specific examples from cells or organs.
10. How has the discovery of genetics shaped our understanding of inheritance and variation among organisms?

Supplementary Materials

Key Terms: A list of key terms is given for quick reference

KEY TERMS FROM THIS CHAPTER

Annotation enrichment analysis	Biological structure	Cell
Cell theory	Cellular structure	Ecology
Ecosystems	Genetics	Human biology
Microbiology	Natural selection	Organism
Plant biology		

Further Resources: Recommendations for additional readings, websites, and multimedia resources.

References

1. Argelaguet, R., Velten, B., Arnol, D., Dietrich, S., Zenz, T., Marioni, J. C., Buettner, F., et al. (2018). Multi-omics factor analysis—A framework for unsupervised integration of multi-omics data sets. *Molecular Systems Biology, 14.* https://doi.org/10.15252/msb.20178124.
2. Bacher, S., Blackburn, T. M., Essl, F., & Genovesi, P. (2017). *Socio-Economic Impact Classification of Alien Taxa (SEICAT).* https://core.ac.uk/download/286567949.pdf (accessed on 8th March 2025).
3. Barnett, R., Brace, S., Cucchi, T., & Dobney, K. (2013). *Divergent Evolutionary Processes Associated with Colonization of Offshore Islands.* https://core.ac.uk/download/20664364.pdf (accessed on 8th March 2025).

Detailed Table of Contents

CHAPTER 5

Drugs Affecting the Cardiovascular System 155

CHAPTER 6

Drugs Affecting the Respiratory System 191

CHAPTER 7

Drugs Affecting the Central Nervous System 229

CHAPTER 8

Drugs Affecting the Gastrointestinal System 263

CHAPTER 14

Drug Development and Clinical Trials 487

CHAPTER 15

Pharmacology in Special Populations 523

LIST OF FIGURES

LIST OF ABBREVIATIONS

ACE	Angiotensin-Converting Enzyme
ACEi	Angiotensin-Converting Enzyme Inhibitors
AD	Alzheimer's Disease
ADHD	Attention Deficit/Hyperactivity Disorder
ADME	Absorption, Distribution, Metabolism, and Excretion
ADR	Adverse Drug Reaction
AgNP	Silver Nanoparticle
AMP	Antimicrobial Peptide
AMR	Antimicrobial Resistance
ANS	Autonomic Nervous System
ARB	Angiotensin Receptor Blocker
ASD	Autism Spectrum Disorder
ASM	Antiseizure Medication
BBB	Blood-Brain Barrier
BD	Bipolar Disorder
BDNF	Brain-Derived Neurotrophic Factor
CKD	Chronic Kidney Disease
CNS	Central Nervous System
COPD	Chronic Obstructive Pulmonary Disease
CVD	Cardiovascular Disease
DDI	Drug-Drug Interaction
DFU	Diabetic Foot Ulcer
DOAC	Direct Oral Anticoagulant
DPI	Dry Powder Inhaler
DRP	Drug-Related Problem
ECMO	Extracorporeal Membrane Oxygenation
ECT	Electrochemical Transistor

EDC	Endocrine-Disrupting Chemical
ENS	Enteric Nervous System
EPS	Extracellular Polymeric Substance
ERAS	Enhanced Recovery After Surgery
FDA	Food and Drug Administration
FFAR	Free Fatty Acid Receptor
GABA	Gamma-Aminobutyric Acid
GERD	Gastroesophageal Reflux Disease
GI	Gastrointestinal
GPCR	G Protein–Coupled Receptor
GR	Glucocorticoid Receptor
HDL	High-Density Lipoprotein
HIF	Hypoxia-Inducible Factor
HLA	Human Leukocyte Antigen
HPA	Hypothalamic-Pituitary-Adrenal
IBS	Irritable Bowel Syndrome
ICI	Immune-Checkpoint Inhibitor
LDL	Low-Density Lipoprotein
LDL-C	Low-Density Lipoprotein Cholesterol
MDR-TB	Multidrug-Resistant Tuberculosis
MMI	Metabolite Methimazole
MNP	Metal Nanoparticle
MRSA	Methicillin-Resistant *Staphylococcus aureus*
NPS	Novel Psychoactive Substance
NSAID	Nonsteroidal Anti-Inflammatory Drug
NSG	Next-Generation Sequencing
OSA	Obstructive Sleep Apnea
OST	Organic Solute Transporter
PAH	Pulmonary Arterial Hypertension
PBPK	Physiologically Based Pharmacokinetic
PCAB	Potassium-Competitive Acid Blocker
PCOS	Polycystic Ovary Syndrome
PD	Peritoneal Dialysis
PPI	Proton Pump Inhibitor
PRO	Patient-Reported Outcome
RAAS	Renin-Angiotensin-Aldosterone System

RSV	Respiratory Syncytial Virus
SCFA	Short-Chain Fatty Acid
SERD	Selective Estrogen Receptor Degrader
SNA	Sympathetic Nerve Activity
SNP	Single Nucleotide Polymorphism
SSI	Surgical Site Infection
SSRI	Selective Serotonin Reuptake Inhibitor
TAAR	Trace Amine-Associated Receptor
TDM	Therapeutic Drug Monitoring
TMDD	Target-Mediated Drug Disposition
TNF	Tumor Necrosis Factor
TSH	Thyroid-Stimulating Hormone
VNS	Vagus Nerve Stimulation

PREFACE

Pharmacology is the science of the interaction of chemical agents with living systems to cause changes in function. This science attempts to explain why drugs are effective, how the body processes drugs, and what affects their benefits and risks. The principles of knowing these are based on simple observations—why a specific compound eases pain, how it reaches the target, and why two individuals given the same dose react differently. These questions have motivated the scientific investigation of drug origins, mechanisms, and uses over the years, with more effective therapy and safer drugs being the outcome. By providing both basic principles and practical issues, this book provides a straightforward introduction to the subject, emphasizing the relationships between laboratory findings and clinical application.

Essentials of Medical Pharmacology condenses key concepts, the latest knowledge, and practical application into a single volume for students and clinicians. This text achieves a masterful balance of theoretical foundations—receptor theory and dose–response relations—with precise explanations of drug groups and their applications. Evidence-based clinical decision making is reinforced throughout, with inclusions of regulatory data from groups like the FDA and EMA. The broad coverage hinted at by the title is provided succinctly and succinctly so that readers may gain incrementally growing confidence as they read. The structure is one that fosters independent study with clear headings, summary tables, and case scenarios that show pharmacological principles shaping treatment decisions in day-to-day clinical practice.

The first three chapters provide the foundation for the rest. Chapter 1 defines what pharmacology is, from where it came in ancient herbal treatments to where it is now in drug discovery, and introduces subdisciplines like pharmacodynamics, pharmacokinetics, clinical pharmacology, and toxicology. Readers will find basic principles of drug action and interaction, an overview of the development pipeline and regulatory milestones. Chapter 2 addresses the next step in absorption, distribution, metabolism, and excretion—terms grouped as ADME—looking at bioavailability, first-pass effects, and the factors that predict how a compound travels through a body. The explanation of metabolism centers upon Phase I and Phase II reactions, the cytochrome P450 family, and genetic variability that affects drug clearance. Chapter 3 addresses pharmacodynamics: how drugs interact with receptors or other molecular targets, the dose–response relationship, potency and efficacy concepts, and the therapeutic index that distinguishes benefit from harm. Signal-transduction pathways and safety considerations provide the bridge between molecular events and clinical outcomes.

Chapters 4 through 12 build on those foundations to apply them to large organ systems and therapeutic classes. Chapter 4 introduces the autonomic nervous system in its two divisions—adrenergic and cholinergic—and analogous drug classes that mimic or block their actions and their clinical roles in hypertension and asthma. Chapter 5 introduces cardiovascular drugs, from diuretics and renin-angiotensin inhibitors to antiarrhythmics, lipid-altering drugs, and anticoagulants. Readers will observe how each class exerts its action, what side effects to watch for, and how to select between alternatives. Chapter 6 features respiratory drugs, from bronchodilators, anti-inflammatory drugs, and mucolytics, to other asthma and COPD drugs. Chapter 7 describes the central nervous system, with sedative–hypnotics, antidepressants, antipsychotics, antiepileptics, and analgesics, including anesthesia fundamentals. Chapter 8 on gastrointestinal pharmacology covers antacids, proton-pump inhibitors, laxatives, antiemetics, and drugs for inflammatory bowel disease. Antimicrobial agents in Chapter 9 focus on antibiotics, antifungals, antivirals, and antiparasitic drugs, with consideration of resistance mechanisms and stewardship measures. Endocrine pharmacology in Chapter 10 covers insulin, oral hypoglycemics, thyroid therapy, corticosteroids, reproductive hormones, and osteoporosis drugs. Chapter 11 introduces cancer chemotherapy, from traditional cytotoxic drugs to targeted drugs and immunotherapies, with discussion of managing toxicity and current trends. Chapter 12 then introduces toxicology and overdose treatment, with coverage of mechanisms of poisoning, antidotes for common drug overdose, chronic toxicity issues, and the effects of environmental toxins.

The final three chapters deal with specialized and novel topics. Chapter 13 discusses pharmacogenomics, how genetic heterogeneity affects drug selection and dosing, using examples from oncology, psychiatry, and cardiology, and discusses the ethical implications of genetic testing. Chapter 14 traces the evolution of drug development and the sequence of clinical trials, from preclinical research through Phase I to IV trials, submissions to regulatory bodies like the FDA and EMA, trial design issues, biostatistical approaches, and post-market surveillance. Chapter 15 considers the needs of the special populations: children, elderly, pregnant and lactating women, and patients with renal, hepatic, or other organ dysfunction. The subject identifies how physiological differences impact pharmacokinetics and pharmacodynamics and how to tailor therapy to maximize benefit and prevent harm in these population groups.

This book is for anyone seeking pharmacy and medicine careers, such as students, residents, nurse practitioners, physician assistants, and other healthcare professionals who must understand how drugs produce their effects, how to use them wisely, and how to anticipate and manage adverse effects. It also is a helpful resource for clinicians who must study for exams or who desire a rapid review of therapeutic options. Educators will find it suitable for inclusion in curricula, with clear educational goals and clinical case questions to support key concepts. By combining basic theoretical concepts with practical guidance, this book enables safe and effective patient care, permitting readers to make informed decisions and to adapt to new emerging treatment options.

PHARMACOLOGY

1

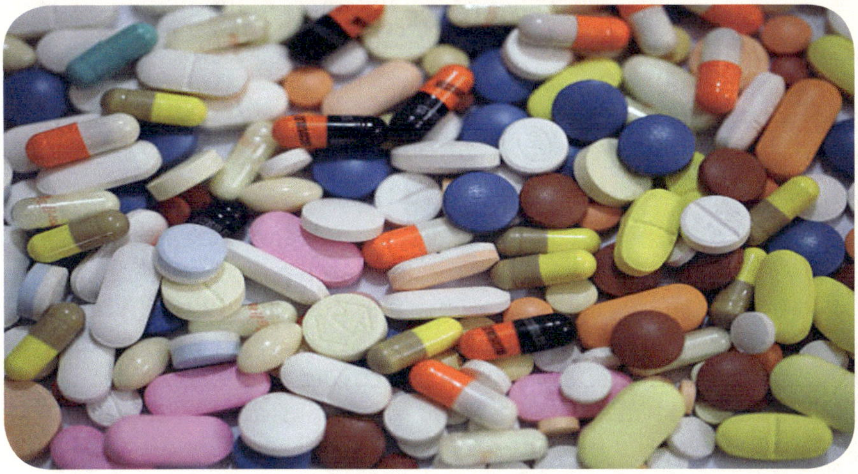

Introduction

The discovery of how different substances interact with living organisms, leading to therapeutic or toxic effects, has long fascinated scientific interest. This interest fuels pharmacology (Figure 1.1), a discipline committed to the study of drug mechanisms, action, and fate within biological systems. Pharmacology is a comprehensive science that encompasses drug composition, synthesis, biochemical and physiological actions, and medicinal use of chemicals in disease treatment. Through the systematic study of the effects of drugs on cellular functions and organ systems, pharmacology integrates knowledge from chemistry, biology, and medicine to maximize the efficacy of drugs and reduce side effects. This interdisciplinarity is critical to the creation of new medicines and the development of safety guidelines for drug application, reflecting the discipline's central position in modern healthcare and biomedical research (Simon et al., 2017). Although pharmacology has been interested in the interaction between drugs and the human organism in the past, its application is wider than mere treatment purposes.

LEARNING OBJECTIVES

After studying this chapter, you will be able to:

1. Describe drug classification
2. Discuss the pharmacokinetics
3. Define pharmacodynamics
4. Explore drug development and approval
5. Explain about adverse drug reactions (ADRs)
6. Identify the special populations in pharmacology

It is interested in the investigation of drug targets, such as receptors, enzymes, and ion channels, and their functions in health and disease. Contemporary pharmacology uses molecular and cellular biology methods to discover these targets and determine signal transduction pathways, consequently opening the door to precision medicine. Pharmacological studies also investigate the pharmacokinetics and pharmacodynamics of drugs—ranging from the body's substance absorption, distribution, metabolism, and excretion processes, to how these influence the action of drugs. This broad-based knowledge reflects the central position of pharmacology in drug discovery, formulation, and treatment strategies, consequently bridging basic science to clinical practice (Simon et al., 2017).

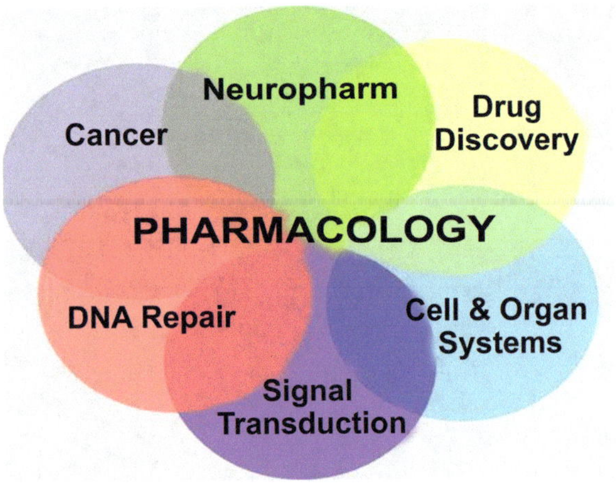

Figure 1.1. Pharmacology.

Source: KGRDCP (KGR Institute of Technology and Management) (2018). *Pharmacy-Related Infographic.* http://kgrdcp.com/wp-content/uploads/2018/05/13-1.png.

The influence of pharmacology is evident in its application to treating complex medical ailments, such as vascular cognitive impairment—a disorder induced by vascular etiology resulting in cognitive impairment. Pharmacological principles need to be known to comprehend the pathophysiological processes of these disorders to formulate effective interventions. Studies of neurovascular function and vascular risk factors have highlighted the promise of pharmacotherapy for prevention and treatment of vascular disease-related cognitive impairment. By the identification of the function of multiple risk markers and their drug modulation, pharmacology brings research into contact with clinical medicine. This unifying role highlights the general applicability of pharmacology to many areas of medicine and its improved capacity to address multifactorial disorders.

Explanation of Pharmacology as a Science

Pharmacology, as a science, serves as a bridge between chemistry and biology as it examines how chemical entities interact with living organisms in order to create therapeutic or toxic effects. Pharmacology covers the examination of drug actions and modes of action through which such substances affect physiological processes. Researchers within this discipline are interested in determining the absorption, distribution, metabolism, and elimination of drugs in the body, which is referred to as pharmacokinetics. Complementary is pharmacodynamics, the study of the biochemical and physiological impact of drugs and how they work at cellular and molecular levels. Through this dual aspect, scientists are able to produce safer and more efficient drugs, orienting the treatments to the condition and individual needs of the patient. Pharmacology builds medical progress through strict experimental methods and clinical research, improving the quality of healthcare results globally. Outside of drug-drug interactions, pharmacology broadens its investigation to dynamic drug-immune system interactions, as illustrated by sophisticated models of disease. The study has deciphered how some pharmacological responses are regulated by cellular stress pathways, including the endoplasmic reticulum stress reported in disseminated cancer cells. The revelation that the cellular milieu and immune monitoring have a critical role in dictating drug-disease interactions and treatment outcomes follows from this insight. These observations emphasize the need for cellular-level research in pharmacology to understand drug resistance and latency in disease progression in order to develop targeted therapeutic interventions. This complexity demonstrates pharmacology's intrinsic involvement in understanding disease states and precision medicine, emphasizing how molecular biology and immunology intersect in its scientific platform (Pommier et al., 2018). In addition, pharmacology is essential in maximizing clinical utility and providing effective patient care through concern with proper use of medications and devices. The science does not only involve drug development but also patient education and hands-on instruction on administration of medications. For example, the proper administration of metered dose inhalers in asthma treatment plays a significant role in therapeutic success since improper technique can result in inadequate delivery of drugs and less-than-optimal disease control. Pharmacology science analyzes such factors to enhance patient outcomes via educational interventions and device design refinements, underscoring the pragmatic significance of pharmacology in daily medical practice. In conclusion, pharmacology combines laboratory data with clinical necessity, exemplifying its crucial role in public health and patient-centered treatment plans (Mustafa et al., 2018).

Historical Development of Pharmacology

The path to contemporary pharmacology is rooted profoundly in ancient medicine that aimed at treating human illnesses with natural agents. Ancient societies, including Mesopotamia and Egypt, established the cornerstone of knowledge through recording the healing properties of plants and minerals, which represented the beginning of pharmacological thinking. These primitive experiences matured over the Greek and Roman periods, when systematic investigation into drug action was encouraged by eminent physicians such as Hippocrates and Galen. Their findings, though not strictly scientific, represented a significant movement away from mysticism towards empiricism. This development continued into the Renaissance, with the resurrection of classical texts and the beginning of new chemical methods, and culminated in more accurate preparation and delivery of drugs. This historical development represents a measured but revolutionary shift from anecdotal application to one more formal pharmacological science that laid the stage for modern therapy in medicine. Developments within experimental science over the seventeenth and eighteenth centuries played the critical role of shaping the scientific discipline of pharmacology. Employing the method of science facilitated the study of drug effects by scientists in highly controlled settings consistently. Early researchers like François Magendie and Claude Bernard laid the groundwork for experimental physiology principles that connected drug administration with quantifiable biological effects, thereby laying the foundations for pharmacodynamics and pharmacokinetics. These findings enabled the separation of therapeutic effects from toxicological effects, thus improving drug safety and efficacy. Also, the expansion of chemical synthesis during the nineteenth century allowed pure compounds to be synthesized, progressing from crude natural extracts to standardized drugs. The era highlighted experimental verification as central to pharmacology, its formation as a discrete scientific field governed by empirical proof and experimental acuity, qualities that continue to define the science today. The twentieth century saw a dramatic growth and institutionalization of pharmacology, with landmark scientific findings and formalization of teaching resources. The discovery of receptor theory revolutionized the comprehension of drug action at the molecular level, facilitating targeted drug design and tailored medicine. Progress in biochemistry and molecular biology further augmented pharmacological understanding, connecting genetic and cellular processes to therapeutic effects. Concurrently, the rise of regulatory bodies and peer-reviewed journals solidified pharmacology as a critical component of clinical practice and drug development. Clinical Pharmacology and Therapeutics exemplifies this era's dedication to rigorous evaluation and dissemination of novel therapeutic paradigms, underscoring the discipline's commitment to quality assurance through peer review (Terzic et al., 2017). Educational structures and materials, including graduate catalogs that detail pharmacological curricula, indicate the maturity of the discipline and its institutionalization within healthcare and academic communities (Cedarville University, 2016). All these developments emphasize the dynamic history of pharmacology evolving towards a science necessary to maximize human health (Figure 1.2).

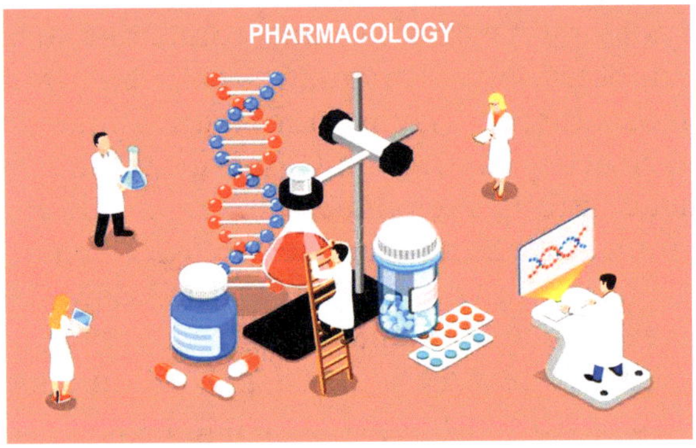

Figure 1.2. Development of pharmacology.

Source: Dreamstime (n.d.). *Isometric Flat Vector Conceptual Illustration: Pharmacology, Pharmaceutical Engineering, Drug Development.* https://thumbs.dreamstime.com/b/d-isometric-flat-vector-conceptual-illustration-pharmacology-pharmaceutical-engineering-drug-development-d-isometric-flat-208597703.jpg.

Importance of Pharmacology in Medicine and Healthcare

The history of medical therapies has been greatly influenced by the pharmacology science that provides a platform for understanding the interactions of drugs with biological systems to generate therapeutic responses (Figure 1.3). The absence of pharmacology would see the optimization and development of medicines devoid of scientific merit, thereby yielding less efficient or even unsafe interventions. By learning about the modes of action of drugs, pharmacology helps doctors forecast the outcomes of treatments, reduce toxic side effects, and customize drugs for the needs of individual patients.

Pharmacology is also an accelerator of new drug discovery, addressing unmet clinical needs and enhancing the quality of life for patients. Furthermore, pharmacological studies underpin evidence-based medicine so that therapeutic interventions are based on strong clinical data instead of anecdotal experience and therefore contribute to safer and more effective healthcare provision. In the clinical setting, pharmacology contributes significantly to improved diagnostic accuracy and the suitability of therapeutic regimens. An example is the treatment of multifaceted disorders like migraines illustrating the pivotal interface between pharmacological progress and patient care. Over the past few decades, rigorous studies of migraine pathophysiology have uncovered the importance of neurotransmitters such as serotonin (5-HT) and the creation of mechanism-based therapies, such as triptans and botulinum toxin therapies, that have greatly enhanced care for victims. Such advances are paradigmatic examples of how pharmacology connects fundamental research with clinical translation, taking discovery to meaningful impact on human health. In addition, the incorporation of pharmacological information into multidisciplinary healthcare teams facilitates more holistic patient management and minimizes the social cost of chronic diseases (Overy et al., 2014). The relevance of pharmacology transcends drug development and clinical practice to other areas of healthcare policy and public health. Knowledge of drug interactions, efficacy, and toxicity informs regulatory policies, such that medicines brought to market are subject to rigorous safety standards.

This surveillance safeguards populations from harmful drugs and encourages the logical use of therapeutics, obviating problems like drug resistance and polypharmacy. Pharmacology also supports health education, enabling providers and patients with information regarding medications to optimize compliance and preclude abuse. Facilitating these aspects, pharmacology not only improves individual patient care but also facilitates sustainable healthcare systems worldwide. Its interdisciplinary character brings to the fore the need for continuous research, training, and cooperation, as has been underscored in different academic studies of the discipline (Cochetti et al., 2009).

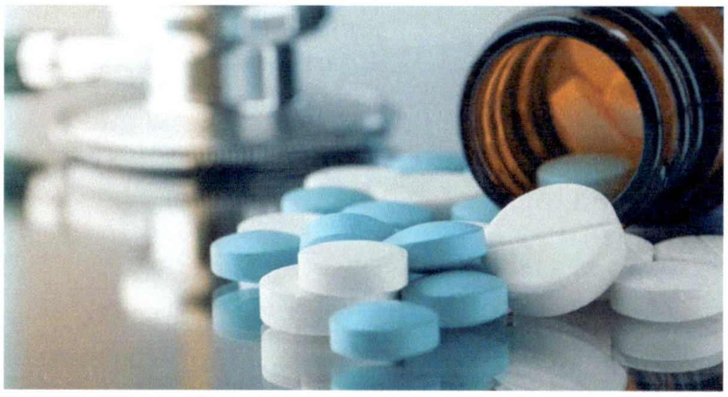

Figure 1.3. Pharmacology in medicine and healthcare.

Source: Pharm approach (2020). *Pharmacology.* https://www.pharmapproach.com/wp-content/uploads/2020/04/Pharmacology.jpg.

1.1. Drug Classification

Learning Outcome

1. Categories of Drugs Based on Therapeutic Use
2. Chemical Classification of Drugs
3. Mechanisms of Action in Drug Classification

Pharmacological agents classification into categories is pivotal to comprehending the drugs' therapeutic application and possible impact on human physiology. Classification systems of drugs are guides that enable easy identification and application of suitable medications according to their chemical profiles, mode of action, or clinical uses. For example, most of the classifications center around the drug's therapeutic effect and classify them as antibiotics, analgesics, or antineoplastics, thus bringing the treatment option into line with particular disease processes. This structured organization not only assists healthcare practitioners in prescribing the appropriate drug but also helps regulatory agencies in maintaining drug safety and efficacy standards. Furthermore, new technologies such as artificial intelligence portray promising functions in pharmacy education and decision-making and may revolutionize how drug classification information is utilized in clinical settings (Tiffany et al., 2023). The intricacy of drug classification is also brought to light when evidence-based medicine principles and pharmacoeconomics are taken into account, especially in chronic and systemic illnesses. In diseases such as rheumatoid arthritis, drug classification goes beyond therapeutic classes to encompass economic and epidemiological criteria that inform decisions on healthcare resource allocation. Methods like ABC and VEN analyses classify the drugs according to cost patterns and clinical need and thereby maximize the treatment regimens not only for effectiveness but also for cost effectiveness. This multi-faceted method synthesizes clinical pharmacology with financial viability so that critical medications remain accessible and adequately prioritized. For instance, immunomodulatory drugs, although costly, could be indispensable to patient results and therefore lie within classes that assure availability (Hayduchok et al., 2021). Drug classification systems also evolve to encompass new developments in pharmaceutical sciences as well as policies of regulatory control. With each new compound, classification is modified to fit new therapeutic targets and mechanisms. This requires ongoing education and flexibility among medical professionals, underscoring the need for precision and conciseness in drug naming and classification. Ensuring uniform classification methods also enables international standardization, making global communication and research collaboration possible. Finally, the validity of drug classification forms the foundation of successful pharmacotherapy, ensuring patient safety while enabling therapeutic advancement. The incorporation of cutting-edge technologies and pharmacoeconomic evaluations into these systems heralds an era where drug classification will be even more specific and patient-focused (Hayduchok et al., 2021; Tiffany et al., 2023) (Figure 1.4).

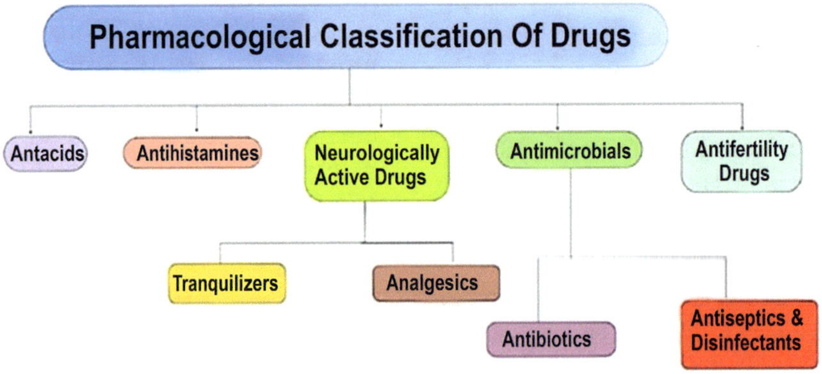

Figure 1.4. Pharmacological of drug classification.

Source: AnatomySystem. (n.d.). *Pharmacological Classification of Drugs.* https://anatomysystem.com/diagram/Pharmacological-Classification-Of-Drugs-scaled.jpg.

1.1.1. Categories of Drugs Based on Therapeutic Use

Pharmacology is a broad class of compounds, each having been formulated to affect particular pathological conditions or symptom relief, hence classifying drugs according to their therapeutic uses. Cardiovascular drugs are one major class, dealing with hypertension, heart failure, and arrhythmias. The drugs exert their action on varied physiological processes such as vascular tone control and contractility of the heart. Statins, for example, are ubiquitous lipid-lowering drugs of key importance in the prevention of atherosclerotic cardiovascular disease (CVD), as evident in clinical practice guidelines reflecting their proper use in therapy and risk stratification (François et al., 2019). Knowledge of these categories helps improve the clinician's skills to maximize treatment regimens by personalizing therapy according to both disease pathology and individual patient needs with reduced adverse effects through prudent pharmacological decision-making. In psychiatric and neurological disorders, therapeutic drug classification is no less important, motivated by the intricacy of the central nervous system (CNS) and the varied symptomatology of these diseases. Mood stabilizers, antipsychotics, anxiolytics, and antidepressants are important classes, each aimed at specific neurochemical pathways. Bipolar disorder (BD), for instance, illustrates this predicament and progress within this area; its management requires medications like lithium and anticonvulsants, which act on calcium signaling and neuronal excitability (Paul et al., 2017). Recent molecular and genetic findings highlight the relevance of calcium channel modulators in BD, and they provide a sophisticated picture of pharmacotherapy that goes beyond symptomatic treatment to molecularly targeted mechanisms. This drug class diversity is consonant with demands for precision medicines in psychiatry. Treatment of infectious disease provides another example of therapeutic drug classification, where antimicrobials are subclassified into antibacterials, antivirals, antifungals, and antiparasitics. Each drug group is distinguished by mechanisms acting in a selective, microbial-targeted manner that spare host cell safety. Such division optimizes the control of infection while avoiding induced resistance, becoming an increasingly emerging worldwide concern. Moreover, the therapeutic aims within this category extend beyond infection eradication to prophylaxis and symptom management, necessitating a comprehensive understanding of drug pharmacodynamics and pharmacokinetics. Thus, categorizing drugs by therapeutic use remains an essential framework in pharmacology, guiding rational drug selection and the development of novel therapeutic agents across medical disciplines.

1.1.2. Chemical Classification of Drugs

Knowledge of the chemical classification of drugs is vital to understanding how pharmacological agents are classified in terms of their molecular structure and chemical properties. This method of classification helps researchers and clinicians to predict the therapeutic and toxic effects of drugs as well as their mechanisms of action. Drugs having identical chemical structures tend to interact with biological targets in similar manners, allowing compounds to be grouped into classes like alkaloids, steroids, or beta-lactams. Improved cheminformatics and bioinformatics software have also improved the capability to thoroughly analyze and catalog these compounds. Tools such as PubChem enable access to large chemical information and structural data that underlie this drug classification and hence biomedical research and educational initiatives (Kim et al., 2018). Such molecular information promotes improved drug design, development, and personalized treatment through the association of chemical structure with biological action. This classification of drugs based on chemical structure is also substantiated by repositories such as DrugBank, which combine detailed molecular information and mechanism data. DrugBank not just offers chemical classifications but cross-links drugs to their biological targets and interaction profiles, showing the manner in which chemical features affect pharmacodynamics and pharmacokinetics (David et al., 2017). Such classifications cover various drug families like enzymes inhibitors, receptor antagonists, and ion channel modulators. Further, the inclusion of pharmacogenomic and metabolomics information facilitates an informed understanding of how chemical differences in drugs impact individual patient response. As such, chemical classification exceeds mere structural confines, integrating chemical identity with pharmacological application and safety profiles to reflect the ever-changing dynamics in pharmacological investigations and clinical utilization. Chemical classification is a prerequisite element that permits systematic research and communication in the field of pharmacology (Figure 1.5). By classifying drugs according to the central chemical moieties, scientists are better able to foresee drug behavior and enable more focused drug discovery pipelines and more informed clinical decision-making. The method also helps regulatory bodies standardize assessment metrics for drug approval and tracking side effects. As pharmacological agents become increasingly complicated, such as biologics and synthetic derivatives, chemical classification must keep pace with advances in technology. Resources such as PubChem and DrugBank are instrumental in this transformation, updating chemical information and offering interactive platforms for researchers globally (David et al., 2017; Kim et al., 2018). Ultimately, chemical classification enhances our understanding of drugs' molecular structure, allowing for safer, more efficient therapeutic approaches within the larger context of pharmacology.

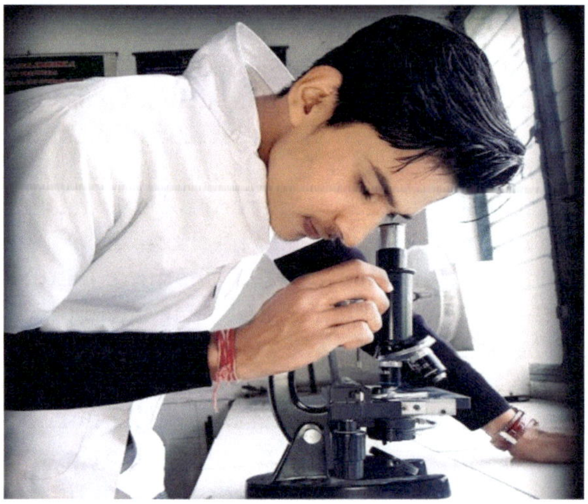

Figure 1.5. Chemical classification of drugs.

Source: Pharma Academias. (2024). *DMSCP. https*://www.pharmaacademias.com/wp-content/uploads/2024/01/cropped-dmscp.jpg.

1.1.3. Mechanisms of Action in Drug Classification

Knowledge of the intrinsic nature of drugs requires a full understanding of their mechanisms of action, which provide the basis of their classification. Drugs act on the body through specific interactions with biological targets such as enzymes, receptors, ion channels, or transport proteins. These interactions induce a cascade of biochemical and physiological responses that have a final impact on cellular functions. For instance, receptor agonists stimulate particular receptors to produce therapeutic effects, whereas antagonists block receptor activity to stop endogenous molecules from binding. Enzyme inhibitors, by contrast, reduce the catalytic activity of target enzymes and change metabolic pathways. Mechanisms of action thereby form a basis for classifying drugs into categories with comparable therapeutic effects and side-effect profiles, allowing clinical decision-making and drug development. The accuracy with which these mechanisms are grasped continues to improve, shaped by contemporary pharmacological studies and clinical recommendations (François et al., 2019). The intricacy of drug action goes beyond initial molecular interactions to encompass downstream signaling cascades and systemic responses. Most drugs exhibit selectivity not just for a particular target but also for receptor subtypes, affecting their efficacy and safety profiles. This selective activity is the basis for subclassifying drugs within larger categories, which is essential for personalized medicine strategies. In addition, certain drugs produce multiple mechanisms of action, either concomitantly or sequentially, leading to additive pharmacodynamic effects. These pleiotropic activities make classification more difficult but frequently increase therapeutic utility, as exemplified by multi-target drugs applied in cardiovascular and neurological disease. In clinical practice, knowledge of these subtle mechanisms helps to maximize pharmacotherapy by predicting possible drug interactions and side effects (Williams et al., 2018). The integration of knowledge of mechanisms of action into pharmacological recommendations guarantees that therapeutic approaches are evidence-based and patient-specific. For example, the categorization of lipid-lowering drugs or antihypertensives is largely dependent on their molecular targets and resulting physiological effect. Such frameworks help healthcare providers choose suitable drug regimens, modify dosages, and track efficacy and safety. Yet, although guidelines provide useful guidance, clinical judgment is still superior, recognizing patient-specific factors that may impact drug responsiveness. Therefore, mechanism of action-based systematic classification augments, but not supplants, individualized decisions on treatment, highlighting the continuous interaction between principles of pharmacology and empathic care (Williams et al., 2018; François et al., 2019).

Test Your Knowledge

1. What is mechanisms of action in drug classification?
2. Which of the following drug classes is based on chemical structure?

1.2. Pharmacokinetics

Learning Outcome

1. Absorption Processes of Drugs
2. Distribution of Drugs in the Body
3. Metabolism and Excretion of Drugs

Knowledge of the behavior of drugs in the body is essential to maximize therapeutic efficacy and minimize toxicity. Pharmacokinetics, an essential sub-science of pharmacology, examines the absorption, distribution, metabolism, and excretion (ADME) of drugs (Figure 1.6). This complex process establishes the concentration-time profile of a drug, which affects its pharmacological activity and safety profile. Variation among these processes can occur due to genetic variation, age, disease status, and environmental conditions, all of which influence drug exposure and response. Identification of these variables enables clinicians to tailor dosing regimens and enhance therapeutic efficacy. New developments in computer modeling have significantly improved the ability to predict such differences through incorporation of physiological and pharmacokinetic information, hence improving personalized medicine strategies and helping make drug development safer (Bailey et al., 2018). New developments in simulation and modeling technology have profoundly changed the field of pharmacokinetics by enabling scientists to forecast the behavior of drugs at various biological levels. Such platforms are capable of incorporating drug physicochemical properties in combination with species-specific physiological parameters to more precisely model drug dynamics. For instance, novel computational models have been created to analyze drug distribution and elimination pathways using in vitro information in conjunction with clinical data to provide better insights into interindividual variability. Such incorporation not only supports dose optimization within heterogeneous populations but also allows for the extrapolation of animal data to human beings, filling translational gaps in drug development. The capacity to model complex biological interactions allows researchers to initially investigate drug safety and efficacy prior to clinical trials, making the drug development process more efficient and improving patient safety (Bailey et al., 2018). Multilevel functional simulation techniques have broadened the domain of pharmacokinetics by placing this science within the context of integrative systems biology approaches.

One such advancement, which emanates from an international research project, is the development of complete physiological models that cover whole-organ functions to analyze drug action and risk comprehensively. For example, the development of a complete-heart model incorporated pharmacokinetics to evaluate the drug's proarrhythmic capability, merging the cardiac electrophysiology and drug absorption, and metabolism considerations. This multidisciplinary or multiscale solution offers a further mechanistic description of drug response and toxicity that links molecular drug interactions with responses at the level of organs and systems. Such developments not only enhance risk forecasting precision but also enable the optimization of regulatory assessments and targeted therapy plans by treating pharmacokinetic effects on intricate biological networks.

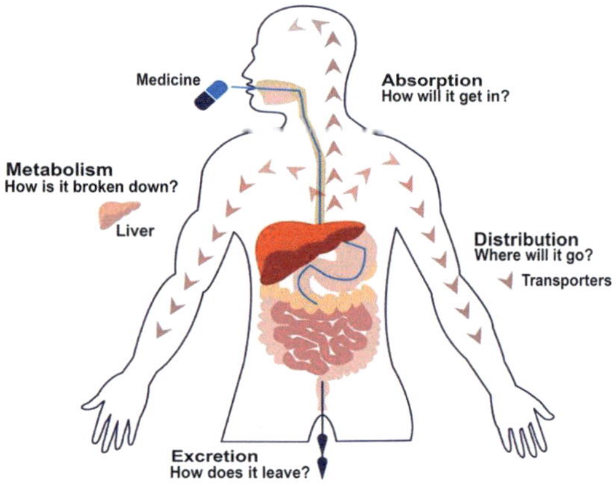

Figure 1.6. Pharmacokinetics and excretion (ADME).

Source: EUPATI (2020). *ADME*. EUPATI Toolbox. https://toolbox.eupati.eu/wp-content/uploads/sites/4/2020/07/ADME-v4_EN.png.

1.2.1. Absorption Processes of Drugs

The path of a drug in the human body starts with its absorption, an important pharmacokinetic process that eventually determines therapeutic effectiveness and safety. Drugs have to cross biological membranes first before they can enter systemic circulation, and the speed and extent of absorption are controlled by various factors including solubility, size of the molecules, and formulation. The major absorptive sites are the gastrointestinal (GI) tract and, depending on the route of entry, other mucosal surfaces. The most general mechanism is passive diffusion based on concentration gradients, and active transport and facilitated diffusion involve specific carrier proteins. Knowledge of these mechanisms is critical in maximizing drug design and delivery since they influence bioavailability, which is the proportion of the dose administered that enters systemic circulation. This fundamental understanding lays the ground for therapeutic drug monitoring (TDM), a process that takes into consideration individual patient response in dosing strategies (Ates et al., 2020). The drug absorption is made more complex by physiological factors like gastric pH, motility, and the availability of food or other drugs, which can all influence dissolution and permeation. For example, weakly acidic drugs are more easily absorbed in the acid environment of the stomach, while weak bases are better absorbed in the alkaline intestine. In addition, first-pass metabolism by the liver and gut wall enzymes can significantly decrease the extent of active drug that enters systemic circulation, requiring increased doses or different routes of administration. Developments in pharmacokinetics have highlighted the requirement for individualized dosing regimens based on the metabolic potential of an individual and interactions with drugs. These findings support the merit of incorporating absorption behavior into TDM approaches to maximize therapeutic efficacy and prevent toxicity (Ates et al., 2020). Clinical practice guidelines beyond the basic pharmacological concepts also stress the significance of monitoring drug levels to effectively control absorption variability. This is especially applicable for narrow therapeutic index drugs in which minimal changes in absorption may result in subtherapeutic or toxic effects. Methods like chromatography and sensor-based assays further enhance the accuracy of measuring drug levels with real-time observation of absorption kinetics. Personalized medicine strategies now more and more incorporate absorption profiles in combination with pharmacodynamic response to customize drug treatment, with emphasis on the emerging role of absorption studies in clinical pharmacology. Absorption processes are therefore not abstract theory but critical factors in determining rational use of drugs in patient therapy (Figure 1.7).

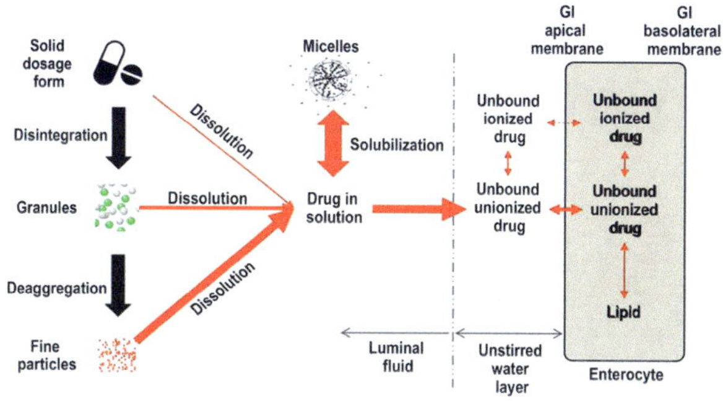

Figure 1.7. Absorption processes of drugs.

Source: ResearchGate. (n.d.). *Drug Absorption Process.* https://www.researchgate.net/publication/353214781/figure/fig2/AS:1056041961811969@1628791432742/Drug-absorption-process.ppm.

1.2.2. Distribution of Drugs in the Body

The drug's travel in the body continues beyond the first absorption, essentially including its delivery to organs and tissues throughout the body. When a drug has entered systemic circulation, it spreads based on variables like perfusion of the blood, tissue permeability, and the plasma protein affinity of the drug. Organ-rich, high-blood structures like the brain, kidneys, and liver normally experience greater early concentration because they are well-perfused. Additionally, drugs have differing extents of binding to plasma proteins like albumin, which is a reservoir that controls the free, pharmacologically active fraction of the drug. The equilibrium between bound and free drug has a very significant influence on therapeutic effectiveness and toxicity. It is such knowledge that explains why two drugs having equivalent plasma concentrations can have disparate clinical courses, highlighting the intricacy of drug action upon administration. This orchestration in delivery forms the basis for numerous pharmacodynamic effects and possible side reactions in clinical pharmacology. Physicochemical characteristics of drugs also govern their migration from blood vessels to tissues. Lipophilicity, molecular weight, and ionization status modulate a drug's movement through cellular membranes. Lipophilic drugs pass through membranes easily, reaching intracellular sites of action, whereas hydrophilic agents are confined to extracellular spaces until special transport mechanisms for their entry are available. Barriers like the blood-brain barrier (BBB) restrict distribution to the CNS selectively, providing neurological protection at the expense of making drug delivery more difficult for brain disorders. Drug accumulation in some tissues, either by physiological sequestration or active uptake, also affects therapeutic and adverse effects. To illustrate, certain macrolide antibiotics show specific selectivity towards pulmonary tissue, ensuring maximum effectiveness when applied in pneumonias uncovered through pharmacokinetic trials by gamithromycin (Croubels et al., 2012). These subtle distribution processes support the imperative need for specialized pharmacological treatment tailored according to drugs' characteristics as well as disease sites. aside from physical and chemical parameters, biological as well as behavioral attributes determine the dissemination of medication along with its aftermaths throughout the body. Genetic variation influencing transporter proteins and enzymatic metabolism has the potential to modify tissue distribution profiles, influencing drug responses between individuals. Moreover, disease conditions like inflammation change vascular permeability, which enhances drug penetration within the diseased tissue. Behavior patterns also meet drug distribution (Figure 1.8) as in description of addictive disorders where neuropharmacological changes modify drug bioavailability and receptor interaction (Ainslie et al., 2007). These observations highlight that distribution is not a fixed process but a dynamic interaction between the drug's characteristics, the physiological environment of the body, and even behavioral aspects. Understanding these layered influences is critical to maximizing dosing regimens and enhancing therapeutic outcomes in clinical pharmacology.

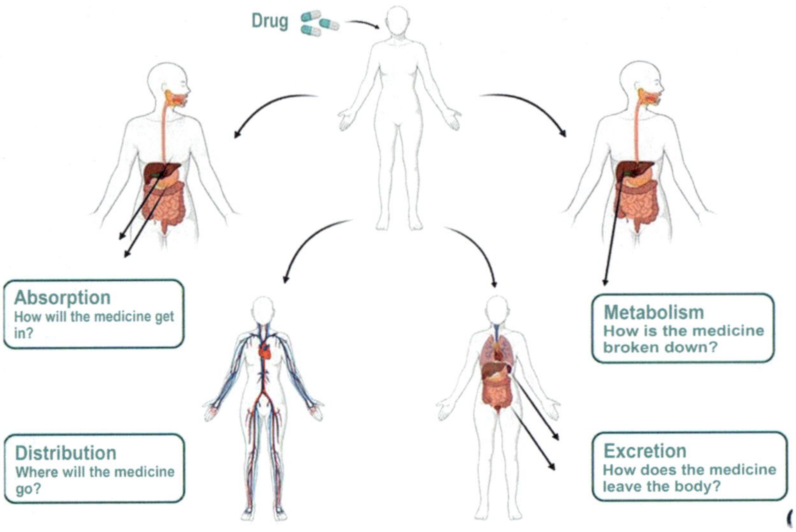

Figure 1.8. Distribution of drugs in the body.

Source: Creative Diagnostics. (n.d.). *Distribution of drugs.* https://qbd.creative-diagnostics.com/upload/image/distribution-of-drugs-1.jpg.

1.2.3. Metabolism and Excretion of Drugs

The drug-metabolizing capability of the human body is basic to the therapeutic efficacy and safety of pharmacologic interventions. Upon delivery, drugs are metabolized mainly in the liver, where enzymes conjugate and transform them into more water-soluble substances for excretion. Metabolic conversion generally takes place in two phases: Phase I reactions, where oxidation, reduction, or hydrolysis takes place, and Phase II reactions, where the drug is conjugated with endogenous substrates. Metabolic efficiency can be affected by age, genetic background, and physiological status, which modify enzymatic activity and thereby drug clearance. Appreciation of these complexities is essential for maximizing dosages and reducing toxicity, particularly in groups like the elderly, where modified metabolic rates can have a profound impact on drug disposition (Bertoncello et al., 2017). Excretion is the terminal phase in the elimination of drugs and frequently occurs via the kidneys, feces, or expired air. The kidneys are crucial by removing drugs or their metabolites from the blood through active secretion into the urine, depending on renal blood flow and glomerular filtration rate. Renal function decreases with age and some diseases, resulting in drug accumulation and increased risk of side effects. Other routes like biliary excretion into feces are involved for some compounds, particularly with greater molecular weights. Gender-specific physiological variations can also influence mechanisms of excretion, and evidence exists for differences in renal clearance and metabolism between the sexes, requiring sex-specific factors during drug development and therapy to maximize efficacy and safety (Chung et al., 2011). Age-related pharmacokinetic alterations profoundly affect drug metabolism and excretion, which present specific challenges in clinical practice. Elderly patients exhibit decreased hepatic metabolism because of reduced liver enzyme activity and diminished renal clearance, which requires careful monitoring and adjustment of doses. This is particularly pertinent when administering neuromuscular blockers and their antagonists in anesthesia, where incomplete removal can result in postoperative complications like respiratory distress. For example, sugammadex, a new agent employed to reverse amino steroid neuromuscular blockade, shows different pharmacokinetics in older persons, which emphasizes the need for age-based therapeutic approaches. Adding information regarding such physiological alterations contributes to improving the safety and treatment outcomes of the patient and reinforces the concept of personalized medicine for the pharmacologic management of aged populations (Bertoncello et al., 2017).

Test Your Knowledge

1. The main site of drug metabolism and excretion.
2. What is the role of plasma proteins in drug distribution?

1.3. Pharmacodynamics

Learning Outcome

1. Drug-Receptor Interactions
2. Dose-Response Relationships
3. Factors Affecting Drug Efficacy

Comprehending the relationship of drugs with the body is very important while studying how therapeutic agents cause their actions. Pharmacodynamics handles these interactions, mainly the correlation between drug concentration at the site of action and the effect produced (Figure 1.9). The receptor binding is the essence of pharmacodynamics, wherein drugs bind to certain cellular receptors to produce or suppress a physiological response. The binding affinity of a drug to its receptor and its intrinsic activity decide the strength and character of its effect. Dose-response relationships also give vital information regarding the size of drug action in proportion to dosage, finally leading to safe and effective therapeutic ranges. This understanding of drug effect is central to maximizing pain management and individualizing treatment regimens, as highlighted in clinical practice guidelines for opioid prescribing (Dowell et al., 2022). The pharmacodynamics mechanisms also include the idea of drug efficacy and potency, which direct clinicians toward choosing right medications. The term efficacy describes the highest effect that a drug can have, while potency is the dose that produces an effect. Patient-to-patient variability in these parameters can affect responses to treatment, underlining the necessity of monitoring and modifying therapy. Further, drug-receptor interactions can be through agonists, which stimulate the receptor, or through antagonists, which block them, thus regulating physiological processes either positively or negatively. Such interactions not only result in therapeutic effects but also lead to possible adverse effects, which again requires careful balancing in clinical decision-making. These factors are supported by guidelines for careful opioid starting and dose titration to counteract risks including overdose and dependence (Dowell et al., 2022). In addition to receptor pharmacodynamics, pharmacodynamics complements pharmacokinetics to maximize antimicrobial therapy, especially in critically ill patients such as sepsis treatment. Knowledge of time-dependent or concentration-dependent killing behavior of antibiotics refines dosage regimens to have adequate antimicrobial effect without causing undue toxicity. The value of such customized pharmacodynamic approaches is reflected in current sepsis guidelines, which suggest that dosing be optimized according to pharmacokinetic and pharmacodynamic factors to enhance patient outcomes. This incorporation highlights the continuous transformation of clinical practice, wherein an intricate understanding of drug action mechanisms guides evidence-based treatments across various medical conditions, further establishing pharmacodynamics as a central component in current pharmacology.

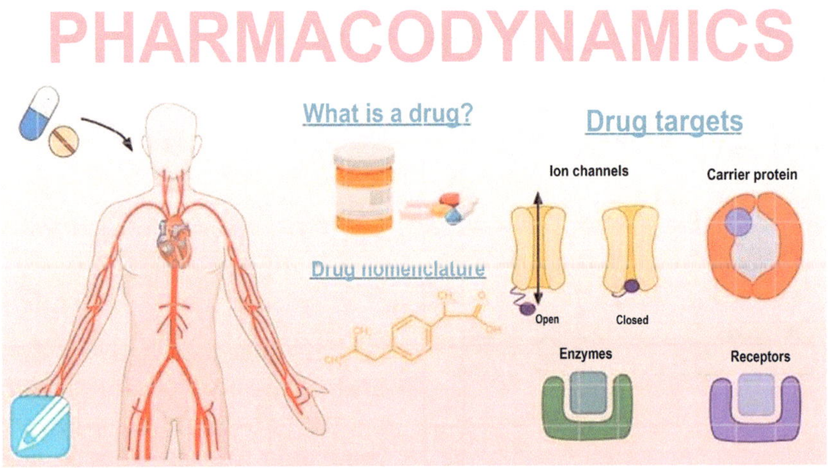

Figure 1.9. Pharmacodynamics.

Source: YouTube. (n.d.). *Thumbnail image for video K-R0LGZYlJY.* https://i.ytimg.com/vi/K-R0LGZYlJY/hq720.jpg?sqp=-oaymwEhCK4FEIIDSFryq4qpAxMIARUAAAAAGAElAADIQj0AgKJD&rs=AOn4CLAHI-ItvB48B-Xdvznn05hpawjvLA.

1.3.1. Drug-Receptor Interactions

Appreciation of the intricate dynamics of drug-receptor interaction is crucial in the practice of pharmacology since such interactions are the basis of drug efficacy as well as specificity. Drugs act by binding specifically to their receptors—proteins usually found on the cell surface or within cells—acting as biological targets of mediating signals inside the body. This process of binding is highly discriminate, with the interaction between a drug and its receptor determining the degree and duration of the drug's activity. Receptor subtypes further complicate these interactions, enabling differential response based on which receptor subtype the drug binds to. This specificity is what underlies therapeutic action of drugs as well as the phenomenon of side effects, when off-target receptors are erroneously activated or blocked. This interaction between agonists and antagonists depicts how complex drug-receptor interactions can be. The agonists can bind to and activate receptors as they replicate the natural endogenous compounds to effect a physiological effect. On the other hand, antagonists inhibit receptor activation by competing with agonists or irreversibly binding and thereby blocking the drugs or body's own chemical action. For instance, tramadol, a multi-receptor drug, illustrates affinity for multiple receptor systems, such as being a μ1 opioid receptor agonist while also inhibiting monoamine reuptake and some ligand-gated ion channels. These shared mechanisms account for both its analgesic effectiveness and variation of clinical action, which require cautious attention toward dosage and possible toxicity (Doostmohammadi et al., 2020). Drug-receptor interaction pharmacology, as advocated by drug guidelines such as those of professional organizations, highlights the relevance of drug-receptor interaction not just for optimal therapeutic gains but also for the management of side effects and drug interactions. Although these guidelines make evidence-based suggestions, they also emphasize the clinician's role in individualizing treatment plans according to individual receptor profiles and patient-specific variables. This is important, considering the complexity of receptor-mediated effects and the potential for receptor desensitization or modified response through genetic and environmental factors. Since healthcare professionals understand the importance of applying receptor information in clinical practice, they make sure that patients get drug regimens that are tailored for safety as well as efficacy (François et al., 2019).

1.3.2. Dose-Response Relationships

To understand the action of drugs in biological systems involves an awareness of the degree of variability across populations. It directly affects how different individuals may respond to an equivalent dose of a drug to yield variable therapeutic and adverse responses. The conditions like genetic factor, age, state of disease, and environment all have effects on pharmacokinetic factors like ADME. Sophisticated modeling and simulation techniques have since been created to combine these variables, based on data for drug physicochemical properties as well as individual physiological parameters. Such methods allow the prediction and assessment of dose-exposure-response relations in various populations, increasing the capacity to design pharmacological treatment optimally. This convergence is essential to guarantee both the safety and effectiveness of drugs, particularly in veterinary and human medicine in which heterogeneity of population is considerable (Bailey et al., 2018). The interaction between drug dose and the resultant pharmacological action is frequently measured by exposure-response studies, which assess how dosing regimens vary to affect efficacy and adverse effects (Figure 1.10). A good example is given by dasatinib, a tyrosine kinase inhibitor for the treatment of chronic myeloid leukemia. By population pharmacokinetic analysis of several clinical trials, it was shown that significant cytogenetic response was positively correlated with mean plasma drug concentration, whereas some adverse effects, like pleural effusion, were related to trough concentrations. Notably, dose optimization trials showed that a 100 mg once-daily dose regimen reduced adverse effects without sacrificing therapeutic activity, exemplifying the need for appreciation of pharmacodynamics with respect to pharmacokinetics in refining dosing strategies (Chen et al., 2013). These observations serve to emphasize the central position occupied by dose-response relationships in the optimization of drug therapy. By scrutinizing closely how dose changes affect both positive and negative effects, clinicians and researchers can more effectively navigate the fine line of maximizing treatment effects while minimizing risk. Optimization is particularly crucial when treating chronic diseases that necessitate prolonged drug exposure over time. The integrated application of modeling, clinical trial data, and close monitoring of therapeutic windows guarantees that personalized medicine remains dynamic, factoring in the significant influence of population variability on drug response. This holistic approach ultimately enhances patient care by promoting safer, more effective pharmacological regimens (Bailey et al., 2018; Chen et al., 2013).

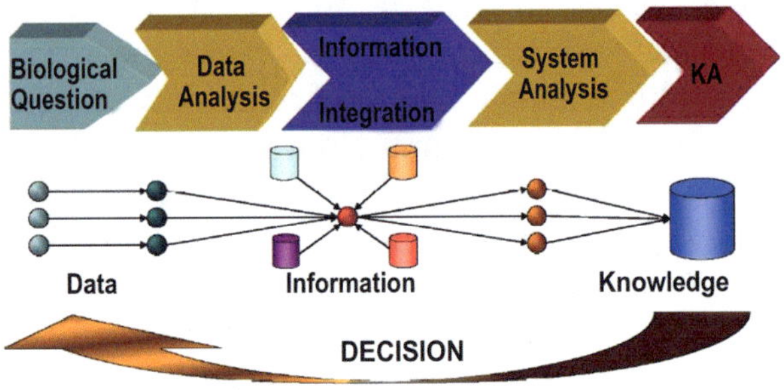

Figure 1.10. Dose-response relationships how drugs interact with biological systems.

Source: https://www.ddw-online.com/media/32/3a-figure-5.jpg.

1.3.3. Factors Affecting Drug Efficacy

Drug variability is frequently the result of differences in pharmacokinetics, which include ADME of drugs. Organ function, age, and genetic composition are important patient-specific variables that affect these processes, leading to changes in drug plasma concentrations and therapeutic outcomes (Figure 1.11). Hepatic impairment, for instance, decreases drug metabolism with resulting prolonged action or toxicity of drugs. Food consumption is another factor affecting drug absorption; certain drugs need to be taken with or without food to maximize bioavailability. Furthermore, drug-drug interactions (DDIs) can activate or inhibit metabolic enzymes, further complicating dose-response relationships. The example of Zanubrutinib, a Bruton's tyrosine kinase inhibitor, demonstrates how pharmacokinetic characteristics such as extended target occupancy in addition to reduced off-target activity are responsible for enhanced therapeutic effects and decreased adverse reactions, underlining the significance of pharmacokinetic aspects in therapeutic efficacy (Tam et al., 2021). Immunological and disease conditions also have critical roles in affecting drug action. Chronic conditions like type 2 diabetes mellitus may affect drug pharmacodynamics by changing receptor sensitivity or downstream signaling events.

The new pharmacology of diabetes drugs, such as oral semaglutide and weekly insulin, shows how patients' own physiological conditions and expectations as a population dictate therapeutic effectiveness. Social and economic determinants also indirectly influence efficacy by controlling access to treatment and compliance. Research measuring willingness to pay provides important information regarding how cost and patient preference influence treatment initiation and long-term use, highlighting that pharmacological effectiveness is closely entwined with extrinsic patient-oriented factors (Vaidya et al., 2024). Lastly, dosing regimens and formulation are part of optimizing clinical benefit with minimal adverse effects. Sustained therapeutic exposure, made possible by customized dosing regimens and optimized drug development, guarantees stable plasma levels within the therapeutic range. For example, the flexibility in dosing of Zanubrutinib—daily or twice daily—improves patient adherence and sustains efficacious drug concentrations, thus ensuring durable clinical responses. Such pharmacodynamic and pharmacokinetic accuracy becomes very important, particularly in multifaceted treatments such as cancer or advanced diabetes therapy, where variability among individuals requires stringent control. Finally, an in-depth understanding of inherent patient considerations, disease condition, and drug-related characteristics is required in forecasting and maximizing drug efficacy in clinical practice (Tam et al., 2021; Vaidya et al., 2024).

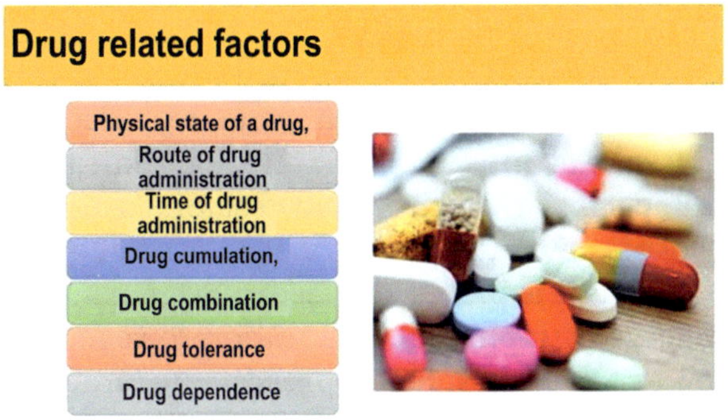

Figure 1.11. Factors affecting drug efficacy.

Source: Slideshare (2022). *Factors Affecting Drug Action in Pharmacology.* https://image.slidesharecdn.com/factorsaffectingdrugaction-200730092738/85/factors-affecting-drug-action-in-pharmacology-4-638.jpg?cb=1666357496.

Test Your Knowledge

1. What factor most significantly impacts how much active drug reaches its target tissue?
2. Explain dose-response relationships in biological systems?

1.4. Drug Development and Approval

Learning Outcome

1. Stages of Drug Discovery
2. Clinical Trials and Their Significance
3. Regulatory Agencies and Drug Approval Processes

The process from drug discovery to approval is a complicated and highly regulated procedure aimed at providing efficacy and safety for the patient (Figure 1.12). Drug candidates initially face intense preclinical testing involving lab and animal trials to assess pharmacodynamics and toxicity levels. Upon achieving promising results, the candidate progresses into clinical trials undertaken in phased steps on human subjects. Phase I trials are largely testing safety and dose in a small cohort of healthy volunteers, whereas Phase II extends testing to efficacy and adverse effects in those afflicted with the disease condition being targeted. Phase III trials also confirm efficacy and track side effects in larger cohorts. Reviewing compiled data in depth, regulatory agencies eventually provide final approval, weighing therapeutic gain against possible risk. This multilayered strategy serves to counteract uncertainties associated with drug development and puts patient well-being first in the course of therapeutic deployment (François et al., 2019). Advances in scientific knowledge regularly inform the pipeline of drug development by revealing new molecular targets and therapeutic avenues. For example, advances in technologies like regenerative medicine and molecular biology create new horizons for pharmacological interventions that were before inaccessible. The investigation of signaling pathways, organ regeneration mechanisms, and cellular progenitors is of special interest in cases such as androgenetic alopecia, for which there has been limited approval of conventional treatments by the FDA. New research explores methods of prolonging follicular growth phases or of stimulating regeneration of follicles, thus targeting underlying pathological mechanisms instead of treating symptoms. These novel approaches illustrate how drug development is increasingly guided by state-of-the-art biological knowledge and seek to deliver more effective and long-lasting treatments in regions of unmet clinical need (Alain et al., 2019). Even with these advances in science, the process of development and approval must also navigate rigorous ethical, legal, and regulatory frameworks to uphold public confidence and guarantee therapeutic dependability. Guidelines and recommendations from prominent clinical organizations help to normalize best practices but do not replace individual clinical judgement needed by medical professionals. The doctor has to consolidate revised official guidelines with patient-specific factors to maximize outcomes of treatment, in addition to regulatory requirements that cover prescribing practices. This balance highlights the central importance of regulatory control in ensuring healthcare standards, offering systematic channels for drug availability, and supporting evidence-based therapeutic choices. Generally, the dynamic interaction between innovation, regulation, and clinical use is central to the proper introduction of new drugs into the market (François et al., 2019).

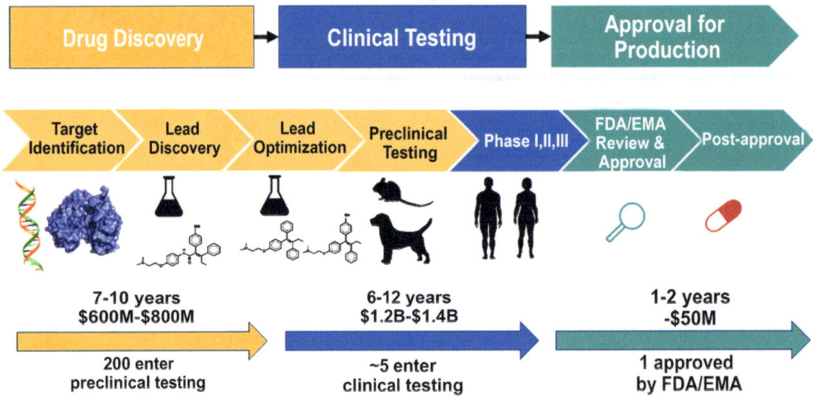

Figure 1.12. Drug development and approval.

Source: https://pub.mdpi-res.com/ijms/ijms-23-13568/article_deploy/html/images/ijms-23-13568-g001.png?1667899871.

1.4.1. Stages of Drug Discovery

The development of new pharmacologic agents starts many years before a drug becomes available to patients in a complex and multifaceted process called drug discovery. It starts with researchers who find possible biological targets for a disease, a process needing an in-depth knowledge of pathophysiology and molecular pharmacology. Following target identification, high-throughput screening techniques are employed to evaluate thousands of chemical compounds for those that affect the selected target, serving as lead candidates. At this stage, optimization drives modifications to enhance potency, selectivity, and pharmacokinetic properties, ensuring that the molecules possess desirable ADME profiles. Problems solved in structural biology, depicted by new inhibitors like CNP520 against BACE-1 for Alzheimer's disease (AD), are testaments to the ways in which specific understanding of binding sites and enzyme structure shapes lead optimization and specificity, all as a testimony to the paramount position of rational drug design within contemporary discovery science (Neumann et al., 2018). One of the most important stages in drug discovery is preclinical development, in which lead compounds are thoroughly tested *in vitro* and *in vivo* to determine their safety, efficacy, and pharmacodynamics. Preclinical development evaluates possible toxicity profiles, therapeutic windows, and side effects prior to the initiation of human trials. Traditionally, deficiencies such as off-target effects, lack of brain penetration, or toxicity have stalled drug candidates, emphasizing the significance of rigorous selection and optimization. For example, preclinical characterization of CNP520 responded to concerns observed in previous BACE-1 inhibitors, such as off-target inhibition of cathepsin D and hair depigmentation attributable to BACE-2 activity, by providing evidence of a good safety profile and high selectivity. Such caution guarantees fewer issues during clinical stages and underscores the important function of pharmacology in converting biochemical potency to successful and safe therapeutics (Neumann et al., 2018). After passing preclinical tests, investigational drugs proceed to the clinical trial phases, which systematically test safety, dosing, efficacy, and long-term effects in humans. Clinical development usually involves Phase I studies to establish safety and pharmacokinetics in healthy volunteers, Phase II to evaluate therapeutic effectiveness and dose-ranging in patients, and Phase III involving larger population studies to validate benefits and track adverse reactions. Regulatory guidelines and evidence-based practices, as outlined by professional organizations in cardiovascular medicine, demonstrate the stringent criteria for assessing new therapy. These guidelines guarantee that each step is based on systematic review of evidence, weighing risk and benefit to maximize patient care and guide regulatory decisions. Such formal development represents a continuum from laboratory discovery to effective, guideline-driven management and therapy.

1.4.2. Clinical Trials and Their Significance

The scientific advances in pharmacology are based to a large extent on the systematic testing of therapeutic interventions, which clinical trials strictly facilitate (Figure 1.13). By examining drug safety and efficacy through controlled settings, clinical trials confirm the validity of newly developed drugs prior to their extensive use in medicine. This approach ensures that therapeutic suggestions are supported by scientifically proven facts instead of anecdotal reports or theoretical postulates. In addition, well-designed clinical trials allow for the determination of proper dosages, possible side effects, and best patient populations, increasing the accuracy of treatment regimens. In an area where patient outcomes depend on the effectiveness of pharmacologic agents, the capacity to examine these parameters through clinical trials maintains the ethical requirement to do no harm and enhance health care quality in general. The designed format of clinical trials provides a systematic analysis of disparate therapeutic regimens against various disease states. For example, in conditions with complicated pathophysiology such as irritable bowel syndrome (IBS), clinical trials play a critical role in assessing the efficacy of different pharmacologic and non-pharmacologic therapies, including dietary and microbiota modification. These trials use randomized controlled designs to avoid bias, such that resultant outcomes can be guaranteed to be due to the intervention itself and not some extraneous factor (Alexander et al., 2018). It is particularly important in pharmacology, where patient heterogeneity and disease heterogeneity frequently make treatment regimens difficult. By combining evidence from several clinical trials, clinical practice guidelines can be developed, resulting in uniform treatment protocols that are based on the best evidence. Clinical trials also have a central role to play in shaping regulatory guidelines and healthcare policy, thus impacting the overall healthcare environment. For instance, recommendations generated by regulatory organizations depend heavily on evidence collected from clinical trials to determine standards of the administration of cardiovascular drugs (François et al., 2019).

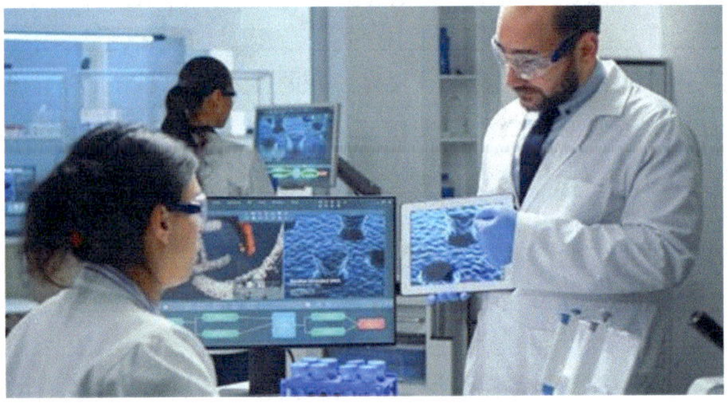

Figure 1.13. Clinical trials and their significance in pharmacology.

Source: https://external-content.duckduckgo.com/iu/?u=https%3A%2F%2Ftse3.mm.bing.net%2Fth%3Fid%3DOIP.riJ-74t7nP9r6Tb2-2aLLAHaD_%26pid%3DApi&f=1&ipt=c67ad4fef0f4df2873b5828466d15abdbfcdbd308f3eecb858691d3c42d2042b.

Not only do such recommendations guide clinical judgment among doctors but also guarantee that therapeutic choices comply with science-based strategies while respecting patients' individual needs. In addition, clinical trials supply the critical evidence base for post marketing surveillance to monitor real-world drug safety over prolonged periods. Consequently, the ongoing cycle of clinical investigation and revision of guidelines creates an adaptive pharmacological platform ready to integrate new therapies and maximize patient care in all medical disciplines.

1.4.3. Regulatory Agencies and Drug Approval Processes

The process from drug discovery to clinical application is regulated by a sophisticated regulatory system aimed at assuring the safety, efficacy, and quality of pharmaceutical products. A drug must go through a strict approval process under the oversight of regulatory authorities like the U.S. Food and Drug Administration (FDA) and the European Medicines Agency (EMA) before it is available on the market. These agencies review preclinical information, clinical trial data, manufacturing guidelines, and labeling data to ascertain whether a drug would be approved for public use. Their work goes beyond just approval; they on a continuous basis assess post-market safety and efficacy via pharmacovigilance mechanisms. Regulatory control is essential in maintaining public health, reducing adverse drug reactions (ADRs), and ensuring that therapeutic approaches rest on scientific fact. Within the regulatory approval process, clinical trials represent a pillar in confirming a drug's therapeutic value and safety profile. These trials are phase-dependent, with each phase set up to answer particular questions. Phase I trials test safety and dosage in a small number of healthy volunteers. Phase II trials test efficacy and side effects in a larger population of patients, and Phase III trials validate effectiveness and track adverse reactions in an even larger group of patients. Strong, well-controlled clinical information is what regulatory bodies need to make well-informed decisions regarding drug approval. Expert committee recommendations made in guidelines, even though they are not legally enforceable, become vitally important frameworks for these trials and for future medical practice. These recommendations underscore that health practitioners need to balance formal advice with personal clinical judgment to maximize patient care (Cosentino et al., 2019; François et al., 2019). The ever-evolving nature of drug research requires regulators continuously to review policymaking and approval procedures to respond to new scientific information and therapeutic breakthroughs. Regulatory agencies continually modify their procedures to incorporate advances like customized medicine, biologics, and new delivery systems. In addition, unifying global regulatory standards continues to be a worldwide challenge that affects drug availability and safety across the globe. Finally, although regulatory bodies offer a disciplined framework for drug approval, they also protect unique patient considerations by enabling healthcare providers to implement such guidelines in a wise and judicious manner. Such equipoise between institutionalized control and clinical prudence is necessary to further improve pharmacological science while maintaining therapeutic decision-making tailored to patients (Cosentino et al., 2019; François et al., 2019).

Test Your Knowledge

1. Which of the regulatory agencies and drug approval processes?
2. Explain about the Clinical Trials and Their Significance?

1.5. Adverse Drug Reactions (ADRs)

Learning Outcome

1. Types of Adverse Drug Reactions
2. Mechanisms Behind Adverse Effects
3. Strategies for Minimizing Adverse Reactions

In the clinical setting, the frequency of ADRs tends to complicate the therapeutic care of patients, especially among susceptible groups like the elderly (Figure 1.14). The reactions could be due to inappropriate use of medication or multifaceted drug–drug interactions, which may worsen the severity of health outcomes. A retrospective analysis of pharmacovigilance data revealed that over 30% of ADR reports in elderly patients involved potentially inappropriate medications, with common culprits including aspirin and diclofenac. This study also identified GI bleeding as the predominant severe clinical manifestation linked to these high-risk drugs. The results highlight the fact that increasing age, polypharmacy, and comorbidities like hypertension and coronary heart disease notably increase the risk of ADRs, highlighting the need for attentive drug review and monitoring to avoid harmful effects (Jiang et al., 2025). Pharmacotherapy of chronic diseases demands caution with respect to the nature and possible risks of ADRs for various drug classes. For example, during therapy of Primary Open Angle Glaucoma, changing patterns of prescription from beta-blockers to prostaglandin analogues indicate attempts to maximize therapeutic benefit at the expense of reducing adverse effects. Despite these changes, topical drugs remain the gold standard for therapy of glaucoma, with significant frequency of local ADRs like ocular dryness and burning, especially with agents such as timolol. These local side effects, though frequently mild, can affect patient compliance and overall treatment efficacy. Systemic ADRs are relatively infrequent but still need to be recognized in thorough pharmacological evaluations (Pandey et al., 2025). The intricacy of ADRs is also further increased due to the pharmacodynamic and pharmacokinetic interactions that often result in patients on multiple drugs. Analysis shows that regimens like aspirin-clopidogrel and aspirin-heparin are frequent causes of drug–drug interactions responsible for increased bleeding risk via additive pharmacodynamic action. Independent predictors of these interactions are the number of medications prescribed, ADR severity, and concurrent diseases such as diabetes and stroke. Consequently, clinical guidelines should give utmost importance to rational drug usage, especially in environments with polypharmacy, in order to avoid avoidable ADRs. Prescribers and health care systems have a fundamental responsibility to incorporate evidence-based methods of improving medication safety and efficacy among various patient populations (Jiang et al., 2025).

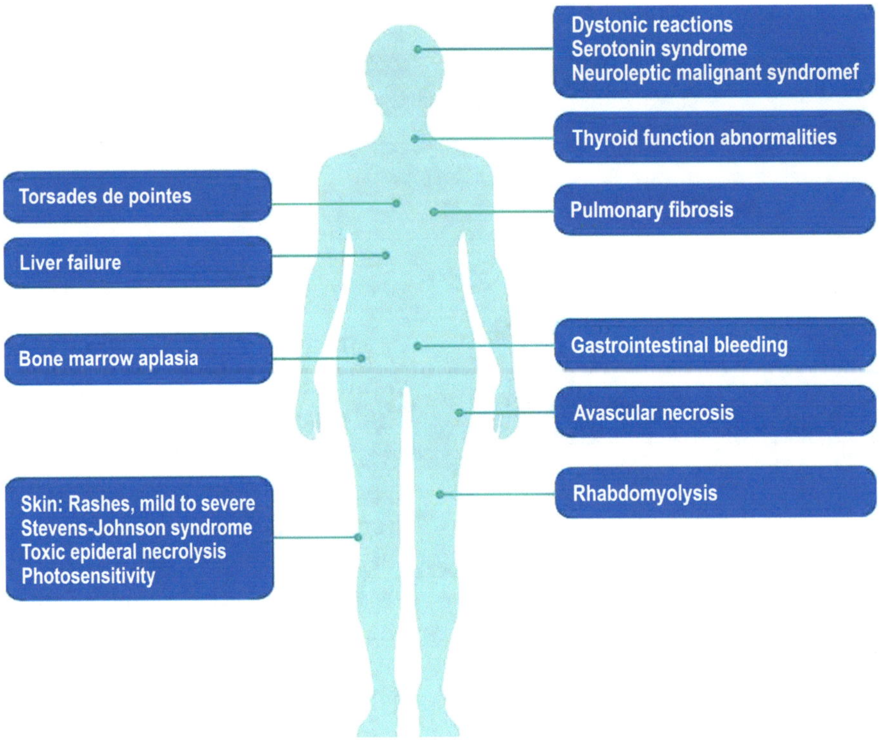

Figure 1.14. Adverse drug reactions (ADRs).

Source: BMJ (2018). *Adverse Drug Reactions (ADRs).*

1.5.1. Types of Adverse Drug Reactions

ADRs cover a wide range of unintended effects which can occur after the administration of pharmacologic agents. These reactions are usually divided into two major categories: Type A and Type B (Figure 1.15). Type A reactions are expected and dose-related, which are usually the result of the drug's well-known pharmacologic effects. These responses are most frequent and may have side effects like antihypertensive drugs-induced hypotension or insulin-induced hypoglycemia. Since Type A reactions are closely associated with the mechanism of action of the drug, they can often be managed by adjustment of dosage or withdrawal. Type B reactions, however, are unpredictable, nondose-dependent, and more often involve immune-mediated or idiosyncratic reactions. An appreciation for this duality is a fundamental basis for clinical decision-making and risk prevention during pharmacotherapy (François et al., 2019). Additional classification of ADRs continues on through Types C, D, E, and F, reflecting drug safety monitoring complexities. Type C reactions describe reactions that are brought about by prolonged use and result in cumulative toxicities, i.e., osteoporosis resulting from corticosteroid treatment. Type D reactions are delayed responses that sometimes do not manifest until well after exposure, such as carcinogenicity seen with some chemotherapeutic drugs. Type E reactions, or withdrawal reactions, are seen when a drug is discontinued, which can lead to rebound symptoms such as rebound hypertension. Finally, Type F reactions are failure of therapy, wherein the drug fails to produce its desired effect, possibly through drug-drug or patient-related interactions. Understanding these categories allows for an integrated strategy in pharmacovigilance and patient care (Williams et al., 2018). The therapeutic significance of distinguishing among types of ADRs is immense, as it determines risk evaluation, patient education, and treatment.

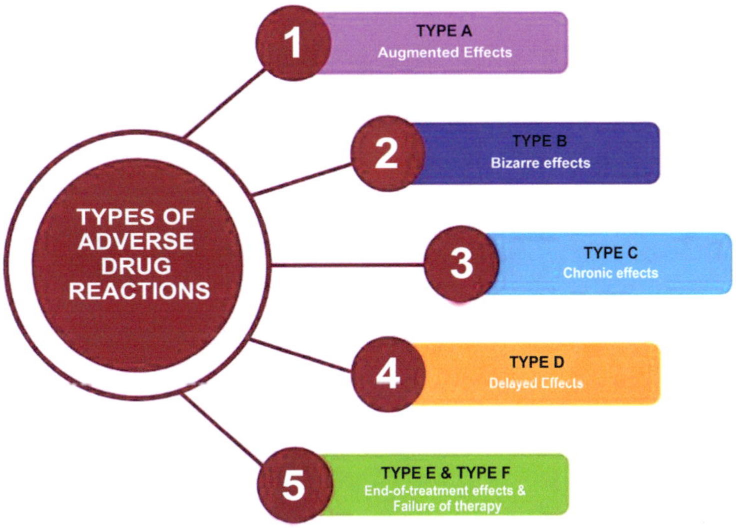

Figure 1.15. Types of adverse drug reactions (ADRs).

Source: https://lh5.googleusercontent.com/u_xvKgpYqMmEyFb4Oi0T_13-mz-keUHVyVxpwKCvos4GU2Z71I6FsddZ8v73as--86rzjEuYKCzKtAAYJtpQyF0PMZUhxIhLmKnAn9J2gK5zn8yoxvRoW1gW0Jnn_9s1R2LB4j_8gGR9Ue0R-w=s1600.

For example, being cognizant of dose-related Type A reactions leads to the adjustment of dosages carefully by healthcare providers so that toxicity is kept to a minimum without compromising efficacy. On the other hand, the unpredictability of Type B reactions requires care for early hypersensitivity or anaphylaxis signals, frequently necessitating drug discontinuation immediately. Furthermore, Types C and D reactions requiring long-term monitoring necessitate continual evaluation outside the boundaries of immediate treatment, further imposing the necessity for interdisciplinary patient care. Finally, the incorporation of ADR type knowledge into pharmacological practice maximizes drug safety and promotes optimal therapeutic effects in a wide range of clinical scenarios (François et al., 2019; Williams et al., 2018).

1.5.2. Mechanisms Behind Adverse Effects

Knowledge of how drugs work within the body is basic to understanding the processes of adverse effects (Figure 1.16). Pharmacokinetics, including drug ADME, is important in determining drug concentration within systemic circulation. Changes in these processes may increase or decrease the desired pharmacologic effect, and in some instances, produce toxicity or therapeutic failure. For instance, after bariatric surgery, the deranged GI anatomy unpredictably influences oral drug absorption, leading to enhanced drug exposure and increased risk of side effects. Specific drugs like lithium, levothyroxine, and immediate-release morphine have been reported to be of important safety concern under these physiological alterations.

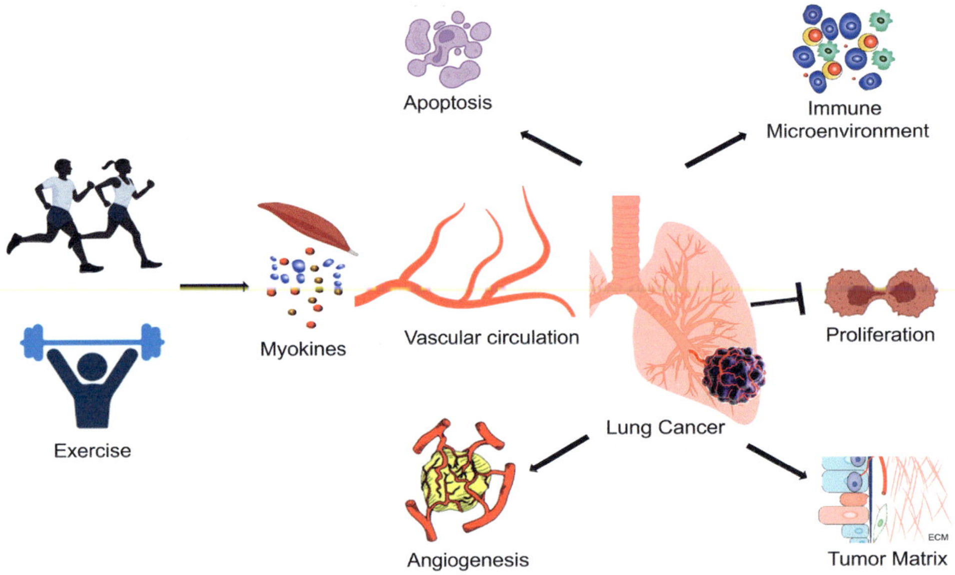

Figure 1.16. Mechanisms behind adverse effects.

Source: https://www.frontiersin.org/files/Articles/1244764/fimmu-14-1244764-HTML/image_m/fimmu-14-1244764-g001.jpg.

Therefore, disruption of usual pharmacokinetics may be a primary mechanism for ADRs, which requires careful clinical monitoring and dose adjustment to prevent harm and maximize therapy (Porat et al., 2025). On a cellular basis, adverse events frequently occur due to unforeseen interactions between medications and particular molecular targets. Certain pharmacologic agents interact non-selectively or modulate closely related subtypes of receptors, leading to off-target activity. For example, bisphosphonates, employed largely to suppress osteoclastic bone resorption, can cause undesirable skeletal or renal side effects because they accumulate in bone tissue and cause local cellular toxicity. Their mechanism of action is interference with metabolic enzymes and signaling pathways controlling bone turnover, but these interactions could elicit undesirable immune reactions or tissue injury when deregulated. Knowledge of these molecular processes explains why some drugs have a potential for side effects and highlights the need for careful therapeutic monitoring to achieve efficacy and safety (Mikosi et al., 2025). Beyond drug-specific characteristics, patient-specific factors like genetic heterogeneity and comorbidities play a major role in adverse effect profiles. Genetic polymorphism of drug-metabolizing enzymes can cause a changed rate of biotransformation, leading to increased risk of toxicity or failure of therapy. Other comorbidities like liver or kidney dysfunction change drug clearance, further increasing the risk of accumulation and adverse effects. Environmental influences and DDIs create additional complexity in these interactions. The complexity of such mechanisms underlines the need for patient-tailored pharmacotherapy strategies involving patient history, genetic testing, and strict clinical monitoring to predict and counteract adverse drug effects effectively. Such a shift in paradigm promises not only better therapeutic outcomes but also reduction in risks related to modified pharmacokinetics and pharmacodynamics (Mikosi et al., 2025; Porat et al., 2025).

1.5.3. Strategies for Minimizing Adverse Reactions

Successful management of drug therapy requires a holistic strategy to reduce adverse effects, and this starts with accurate patient assessment (Figure 1.17). Age, genetic factors, co-morbid diseases, and other drugs taken concurrently can dramatically influence drug metabolism and response. Customizing pharmacological treatment taking these differences into account reduces the risk of toxicity and hypersensitivity reactions. Additionally, clinicians ought to make evidence-based guidelines and protocols that reflect the current clinical evidence a priority in order to maximize drug choice and dosing. For example, guidelines based on international consensus panels provide important information for enhancing patient safety using adaptive treatment approaches, particularly in complicated cases like critical illness (Alhazzani et al., 2020). By combining patient-related factors with well-defined clinical models, healthcare professionals can significantly improve the therapeutic effect and reduce the rate and severity of ADRs. Along with individualized patient assessment, careful monitoring during pharmacotherapy is essential for timely detection and prevention of adverse effects. Repeated laboratory monitoring, clinical observation, and patient counseling enable healthcare professionals and patients to recognize early warning signals and respond timely. The utilization of biomarkers and diagnostic equipment intended for monitoring drug-related toxicities allows for preemptive adaptation of treatment protocols, preventing complications. In addition, maintenance of authoritative guidelines guarantees therapeutic choices factoring in revised risk-benefit analyses to protect patients from avoidable harm (François et al., 2019). Multidisciplinary team communication and patient communication support informed consent and active involvement, which are crucial to early detection of adverse reactions. Systematic pharmacovigilance and documentation lead to a cycle of ongoing improvement in drug safety practices. Of equal importance is the use of risk reduction strategies through education and technology support. Educating clinicians and patients regarding possible drug interactions, contraindications, and symptom identification can substantially minimize adverse outcomes. Incorporating electronic prescribing systems with decision support tools enables real-time alerts regarding dosing errors and dangerous drug combinations. These technologies enable safer prescribing practices, especially in polypharmacy situations prevalent among elderly and critically ill patients. Furthermore, continuous professional development commensurate with the latest clinical guidelines supports best practice in pharmacotherapy (Alhazzani et al., 2020; François et al., 2019). In summary, the convergence of education, technology, and evidence-based recommendations creates a strong platform for the avoidance of adverse reactions and enhancing overall patient safety in pharmacology.

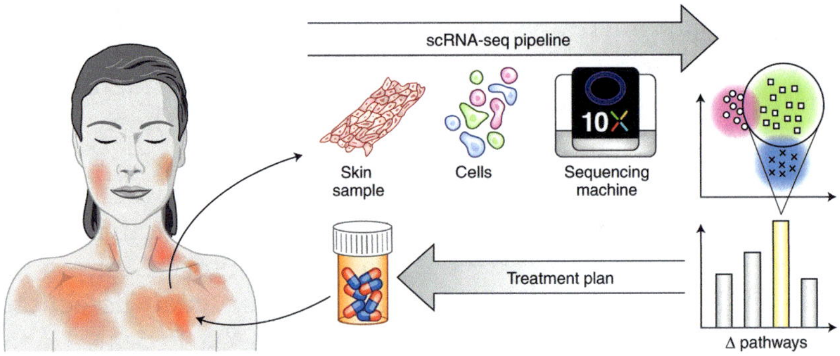

Figure 1.17. Strategies for minimizing adverse reactions.

Source: https://media.springernature.com/full/springer-static/image/art%3A10.1038%2Fs41591-020-0756-0/MediaObjects/41591_2020_756_Fig1_HTML.png.

Test Your Knowledge

1. What is drugs mechanisms behind adverse effects body?
2. The types of adverse drug reactions?

1.6. Special Populations in Pharmacology

Learning Outcome

1. Pharmacology in Pediatrics
2. Pharmacology in Geriatrics
3. Considerations for Pregnant and Lactating Women

In clinical pharmacology, the intricacy of drug therapy increases dramatically when dealing with special populations, including pediatrics, geriatrics, pregnant women, and comorbid patients. These populations tend to exhibit changed pharmacokinetics and pharmacodynamics, requiring meticulous attention in dosing and drug choice to maximize therapeutic effectiveness while avoiding adverse effects. For instance, elderly and neonatal patients experience physiological alterations that modulate drug ADME, complicating conventional dosing regimens. Furthermore, limited availability of systematic clinical studies within these subjects results in labeling limitations and a dearth of instructions for practitioners to use medication effectively and safely. Special consideration is needed in oncology, in which several chemotherapeutic drugs have out-of-date prescribing guidelines, necessitating regulatory efforts to revise drug labeling to capture new clinical evidence and enhance patient care (Balogh et al., 2019). Additionally, managing health disparities in various populations needs an interdisciplinary research infrastructure that accommodates inclusive clinical trials and translational research. Initiatives like the Mountain West Clinical Translational Research Infrastructure Network (MW CTR-IN) demonstrate how partnerships among several institutions can augment research capacity in far-reaching and heterogeneous geographic areas. Spanning large parts of underrepresented areas, this network fosters health disparity research addressing specific population needs, such as indigenous populations and rural populations. By providing pilot funding opportunities, it spurs cutting-edge research in pharmacology and corresponding health sciences aimed at unveiling differential drug responses and care barriers. Such inter-disciplinary and locally concentrated research is critical for the adaptation of pharmacological interventions to special populations, with a final outcome that enhances fair delivery of healthcare and maximizing therapeutic interventions (Kumar et al., 2019). The confluence of pharmacogenomics and personalized medicine highlights further the importance of identifying special populations in pharmacology. Individual differences in genetic variation affect drug metabolism, effectiveness, and toxicity, making it essential to tailor therapeutic regimens. Special populations typically introduce other genetic and environmental factors influencing pharmacologic effects, including ethnic group and socioeconomic factors. These are considerations that require advances in clinical research paradigms that include genetic screening and patient-specific information to optimize drug therapy. Integrating improved drug labeling initiatives with large-scale collaborative studies and individualized strategies, pharmacology can be developed to improve the lot of vulnerable populations, optimizing medication safety and effectiveness throughout the gamut of patient diversity (Balogh et al., 2019; Kumar et al., 2019).

1.6.1. Pharmacology in Pediatrics

Pediatric pharmacology is characterized by special challenges different from adult medicine, primarily as a result of physiological differences intrinsic to growth and development. Developmental maturation of organ systems, enzymatic pathways, and receptor sensitivities profoundly affect drug ADME in children. Such differences require judicious dose titration and attentive monitoring to achieve optimal therapeutic benefit with minimal side effects. Pediatric patients, unlike adults, experience dynamic physiological alterations that can shift pharmacokinetic parameters in an unpredictable manner over time. Further, the pediatric populations' heterogeneity—from neonates to adolescents—makes standardization of dosing regimens more difficult. As a result, empirical extrapolation of data from adults falls short to anticipate drug effectiveness or safety in children. This makes it imperative to have focused pediatric pharmacological studies to provide evidence-based medication protocols specific to pediatric patients' distinct metabolic and growth characteristics. A significant feature of pediatric pharmacotherapy is the special susceptibility of forming organ systems to drug toxicity. For instance, mitochondrial function, which plays a key role in energy metabolism, can be harmed by pharmacological agents and influence organ function at periods of peak growth. Recent research efforts have identified molecular targets like mitochondrial proteases that affect cellular homeostasis, with therapeutic modulation that is both promising and potentially mitigating pediatric disease progression (Bai et al., 2023). These findings underscore the imperative to understand drug interactions in the context of pediatric cellular biology to engineer treatments that maintain organ function while maximizing disease management. The incorporation of pediatric therapeutics of molecular pharmacology has large prospects for more exact interventions that avoid long-term morbidity caused by chronic childhood ailments. Some new developments in pediatric pharmacology involve the use of human-derived models for translation as a basis of drug evaluation concerning efficacy and safety, most relevantly with regards to neurodevelopmental diseases. Stem cell innovations have been key to creating the human neuronal model that models disease phenotypes typical of childhood illnesses, hence directed pharmacologic screening. This strategy has discovered compounds that have the potential to reverse particular pathogenic processes involved in pediatric neurological disorders and raised expectations for effective clinical treatments (Cleber et al., 2020). Having the potential to screen drug candidates in such biologically relevant platforms overcomes the ethical and practical constraints of pediatric clinical trials. As pediatric pharmacology continues to grow, it more and more integrates new methodologies that close the gap between bench research and clinical use, working to reverse the traditional lack of approved children's medications and provide greater therapeutic specificity for this at-risk population.

1.6.2. Pharmacology in Geriatrics

The process of aging involves complex changes in physiology that have a profound effect on pharmacokinetics and pharmacodynamics in the elderly population (Figure 1.18). Changes in GI absorption, decreased hepatic metabolism, and decreased renal clearance all alter the bioavailability and elimination of most drugs. For instance, reduced hepatic enzyme activity can extend drug half-life, leading to an increased risk of toxicity. In addition, alterations at the cellular and mitochondrial level, including impaired mitochondrial respiration and energy metabolism, are important in the changed pharmacological responses seen in the elderly (Ac Rín-Pérez et al., 2020). Knowledge of these mechanistic bases is critical for the optimization of therapeutic regimens, reduction of ADRs, and adaptation of dosage forms appropriate for this vulnerable population. Pharmacological treatment in geriatrics thus requires a sensitive understanding of these systemic adaptations to maximize efficacy while protecting patient safety. Polypharmacy, which is also prevalent among geriatric patients, adds to the complexity of pharmacotherapy because of the increased likelihood of DDIs and cumulative toxicity. The loss of physiological reserve that comes with aging tends to compound the vulnerability to such interactions, requiring careful medication reconciliation and monitoring. Recent findings highlight the use of personalized medicine strategies that take into account the changed mitochondrial function and metabolic potential typical of aging cells, as illustrated by recent research investigating mitochondrial oxygen consumption in frozen biological samples (Ac Rín-Pérez et al., 2020). These observations promote enhanced predictive modeling of drug response to inform clinical practice. Further, the combination of comprehensive geriatric assessment with pharmacological profiling benefits clinicians in weighing therapeutic gain against the threat of polypharmacy complications so that total outcomes in geriatric care are enhanced. Clinical practice guidelines and perioperative pathways increasingly capture the necessity of meeting pharmacological considerations due to age so that recovery is improved and morbidity minimized in the elderly patient. Improved Recovery After Surgery (ERAS) protocols, for example, include measures that reduce pharmacokinetic variability and drug-related adverse effects by maximizing perioperative drug management. Such evidence-based guidelines emphasize the need to modify drug regimens based on age-related metabolic alterations and the decrease in organ function. By linking therapeutic interventions with the physiological setting of the elderly, clinicians can optimize the maintenance of functional status and foster resilience. The interactive relationship between geriatric physiology and pharmacology highlights the need to continually revise clinical practice in response to new research, thereby improving patient-centered care specific to the elderly population.

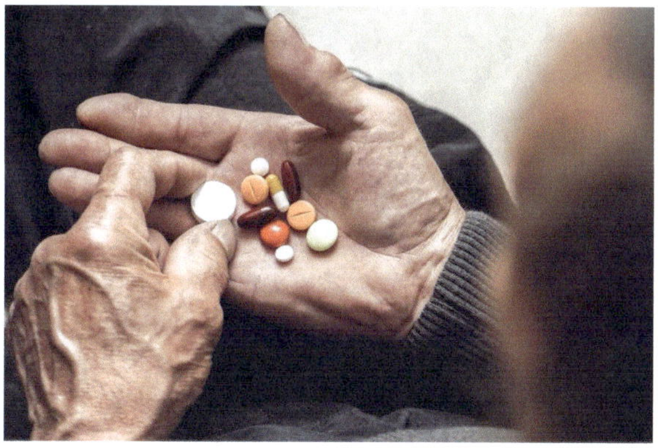

Figure 1.18. Pharmacology in geriatrics.

Source: https://d2jx2rerrg6sh3.cloudfront.net/images/Article_Images/ImageForArticle_24525_17065207532171781.jpg.

1.6.3. Considerations for Pregnant and Lactating Women

The physiological changes that take place during pregnancy significantly affect drug metabolism, distribution, and elimination, and thus require special attention in pharmacological management (Figure 1.19). Changes in hepatic enzyme activity, expansion of plasma volume, and modification of renal clearance can together affect the pharmacokinetics of drugs, possibly altering their efficacy and safety profiles. Even with these developments, widely accepted pregnancy-specific dosing recommendations are still lacking for most drugs, creating challenges for clinicians working to maximize therapeutic benefit. The latest advances in pharmacokinetic modeling offer promising paths to predict suitable antenatal dosing, including the intricate maternal-fetal dynamics. Notably, pregnant women and healthcare providers both demonstrate a strong interest in using such model-based doses, if clear explanations and transparent evidence on the rationale and safety are made available. This acceptance highlights the importance of greater integration and communication of pharmacological information specific to pregnancy to enhance quality of care (Ceulemans et al., 2024). The taking of complementary and alternative medicines (CAMs) by lactating women further complicates pharmacological considerations. Data show that a large percentage of breastfeeding mothers use herbal supplements and other CAMs, frequently in response to counsel from midwives or cultural custom. Yet, safety and effectiveness of most CAM products during lactation are still poorly investigated, leaving both mother and infant at risk. Interestingly, women with pregnancy loss history exhibit increased likelihood to use CAMs while breastfeeding, possibly due to increased anxiety and the search for perceived natural interventions. This trend emphasizes the need for healthcare practitioners to have open discussions, being aware of emotional considerations while providing evidence-based advice. Closing these gaps can prevent risks of unsupervised use of CAM and promote informed decision-making at this vulnerable time (Bettiol et al., 2018). The safe pharmacological management of pregnant and lactating women demands a multidisciplinary approach that integrates both biomedical information and psychosocial aspects. Caregivers need to ensure education that empowers women to engage actively in treatment decisions through clearly communicating benefits, risks, and the science underlying dosing strategies. Defying social stigmas, especially regarding pregnancy loss, is part of constructing supportive environments for open discussion regarding medication use and related concerns. In addition, institution-wide training of health care professionals regarding the specific pharmacodynamic and pharmacokinetic alterations with pregnancy and lactation would improve prescribing confidence and safety for patients. Blending new modeling technologies with patient-focused communication ultimately promotes the best therapeutic approaches, optimizing efficacy against mother's and child's well-being (Bettiol et al., 2018; Ceulemans et al., 2024).

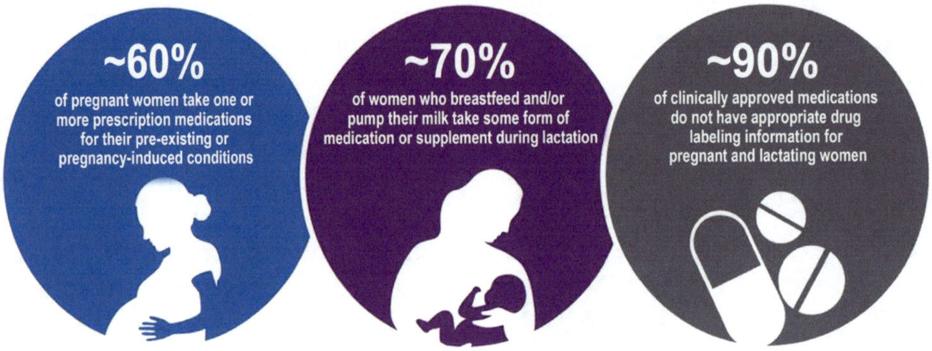

Figure 1.19. Considerations for pregnant and lactating women.

Source: https://i0.wp.com/obgynkey.com/wp-content/uploads/2021/07/gr1-2.jpg?fit=1200%2C422&ssl=1.

Test Your Knowledge

1. Discuss the pharmacology in geriatrics?
2. Which of the special populations in pharmacology?

SUMMARY

The complex interaction between drug characteristics and their biological actions reflects the complexity of pharmacology as a science. Appreciation of this interaction allows healthcare providers to make informed choices that maximize therapeutic benefits while reducing side effects. The dynamic evolution of pharmacological research necessitates ongoing learning and adjustment, as new drug categories and delivery methods become available. Due to the increasing understanding of drug interaction at the molecular level, pharmacology is an anchor science connecting laboratory findings and clinical use. This convergence is necessary for making personalized medicine approaches, which account for individual heterogeneity in response to drugs and ultimately improve patient care and safety. Additionally, compliance with set guidelines and clinical judgment continues to be paramount in addressing therapeutic challenges so that treatments both capture scientific progress and live up to ethical standards (François et al., 2019). Technological and materials science advances have played a great role in altering pharmacological development, especially by way of developments such as nanoparticles. Nanoscale materials have their own set of unique properties that can transform drug delivery and targeting, enhancing the effectiveness and selectivity of pharmacological treatments. The incorporation of nanoparticles in pharmaceutical preparations is an example of the enrichment of pharmacology by interdisciplinary collaboration that combines chemistry, engineering, and medicine to address clinical issues. Still, the environmental and health effects of these materials also require careful assessment to avert unintended effects. The physical and chemical behavior of the materials, including toxicity potential, are important to understand when developing these technologies into therapy. Therefore, contemporary pharmacology has to walk a tightrope between innovation and prudence with sound, sustainable implementation of innovative materials in patient treatment (Khan et al., 2017). In summary, pharmacology is an irreplaceable discipline that keeps advancing following scientific breakthroughs and technological developments. Its place does not only involve drug development but also optimizing patient treatment schedules, risk management, and enhancing health outcomes globally. The ethical and judicious application of pharmacological knowledge placed on health professionals underscores the imperative for continuous education and evidence-based practice (François et al., 2019). As the pharmacology landscape becomes increasingly complex with technologies such as nanoparticle applications, an in-depth understanding of drug mechanisms and societal implications is important. This holistic vision guarantees that pharmacology will remain a necessary science, growing in importance as a contributor to medicine and public health.

Future Directions in Pharmacological Research

The continuous evolution of pharmacological research is propelled by the imperative to address complex and multifaceted health conditions inadequately managed by current therapies. Recent developments have particularly emphasized targeted treatments that modulate specific biological pathways, offering promising improvements in efficacy and safety profiles. For instance, the pharmacologic investigation of the trigeminovascular system in migraine treatment demonstrates a paradigm shift wherein comprehensive pathophysiologic understanding guides innovative drug development beyond symptomatic relief to mechanism-based treatment. New pharmacologic modalities such as cannabinoids, hormonal regulators, and metabolic-targeted agents represent a more pervasive strategy to leverage multiple biological targets for improved patient outcomes. These developments highlight the importance of intense clinical research to establish these innovations as trustworthy and reliable, to show their translational value in actual clinical environments. This strategic targeting of pharmacologic targets highlights a path towards personalized medicine, which may reshape therapeutic scopes for many disorders (Pellesi et al., 2024). Frontier science increasingly identifies the complex interaction of pharmacologic agents with the human microbiome, especially the gut-x axis, as an exciting frontier in the development of new drugs. Immunological and biochemical interfaces of the GI tract represent key regulators of drug activity and toxicity and provide a need for new solutions for mycotoxin-induced disease and other forms of environmental stress. Natural agents with high content of bioactive compounds like polysaccharides and polyphenols have promising therapeutic benefits through maintaining intestinal integrity and inflammatory modulation. Such findings encourage forthcoming pharmacological innovation focused on tapping into microbiome modulation to boost drug safety and immunomodulatory efficacy. Additionally, combination therapy using natural-derived agents in concert with conventional pharmacotherapy may prove synergistic with fewer adverse effects and enhanced treatment options for intricate systemic disease (Li et al., 2024). Future pharmacological research will need to adopt multi-disciplinary approaches integrating molecular biology, systems pharmacology, and bioinformatics to expedite drug discovery as well as enhance therapeutic accuracy. The use of innovative computational modeling along with high-throughput screening will enable the identification of new drug candidates and their ability to interact within intricate biological networks. In addition, the use of biomarkers and genetic profiling can aid in the individualization of pharmacotherapy, targeting optimal doses and treatment regimens based on individual patient profiles. All these technological advances will also speed up testing of long-term safety and efficacy, filling the gaps in current knowledge. Finally, this integrated strategy holds the promise of changing pharmacology from a largely empirical discipline to a more predictive and preventive science, able to provide safer, more effective treatments for a wide range of diseases.

KEY TERMS FROM THIS CHAPTER

- Contemporary pharmacology
- Chemical classification
- Therapeutic drug monitoring (TDM)
- Clinical decision-making
- Genetic polymorphism
- Pharmacology
- Biological systems
- Forensic odontologists
- Adverse drug reactions (ADRs)
- International research
- Pharmacokinetics
- Drug classification
- Colecular
- Biological targets
- Forensic anthropologists
- Manner of Death

CRITICAL THINKING QUESTIONS

1. **Which of the following routes of drug administration has the fastest onset of action?**
   a. Oral
   b. Intramuscular
   c. Intravenous
   d. Subcutaneous
2. **Which of the following is a Phase I reaction in drug metabolism?**
   a. Glucuronidation
   b. Sulfation
   c. Oxidation
   d. Acetylation
3. **The therapeutic index of a drug is defined as?**
   a. ED50/LD50
   b. LD50/ED50
   c. TD50/ED50
   d. ED50/TD50
4. **Which receptor type is activated by adrenaline in the heart?**
   a. α1
   b. β1
   c. β2
   d. α2
5. **Which class of drugs is commonly used to treat hypertension?**
   a. Beta-blockers
   b. Antihistamines
   c. Proton pump inhibitors
   d. Antifungals

Short Answer Questions

1. What are the classification of drug?
2. Explain about the pharmacokinetics?
3. What is pharmacodynamics?
4. Which of drug development and approval?
5. What do you understand by adverse drug reactions (ADRs)?

Answer to Critical Thinking Questions

1. (c) 2 (c) 3. (b) 4. (b) 5. (a)

REFERENCES

1. Acín-Pérez, R., Benador, I. Y., Petcherski, A., Veliova, M., Benavides, G. A., Lagarrigue, S., Caudal, A., et al. (2020). A novel approach to measure mitochondrial respiration in frozen biological samples. *The EMBO Journal, 39*. https://doi.org/10.15252/embj.2019104073.
2. Ainslie, G., Atkinson, J., Tasnádi, A., Baldwin, M., Baron-Cohen, S., Becker, J., Becker, K., et al. (2007). *A Theory of Natural Addiction*. https://core.ac.uk/download/12354872.pdf (accessed on 9 May 2025).
3. Alhazzani, W., Møller, M. H., Arabi, Y. M., Loeb, M., Gong, M. N., Fan, E., Oczkowski, S., et al. (2020). Surviving Sepsis Campaign: Guidelines on the management of critically ill adults with Coronavirus Disease 2019 (COVID-19). *Intensive Care Medicine, 46*, 854–887. https://doi.org/10.1007/s00134-020-06022-5.
4. Ates, H. C., Roberts, J., Lipman, J., Cass, A. E. G., Urban, G., & Dincer, C. (2020). On-site therapeutic drug monitoring. *Trends in Biotechnology, 38*, 1262–1277. https://doi.org/10.1016/j.tibtech.2020.03.001.
5. Bai, M., Wu, M., Jiang, M., He, J., Deng, X., Xu, S., Fan, J., et al. (2023). *LONP1* targets *HMGCS2* to protect mitochondrial function and attenuate chronic kidney disease. *EMBO Molecular Medicine, 15*. https://doi.org/10.15252/emmm.202216581.
6. Bailey, A., Bon, C., Cox, E., Darwich, A., Dorey, A., Duwal, S., Ette, E., et al. (2018). Population variability in animal health: Influence on dose-exposure-response relationships: Part II: Modelling and simulation. https://core.ac.uk/download/159992803.pdf (accessed on 9 May 2025).
7. Balogh, E. P., Bindman, A. B., Eckhardt, S. G., Halabi, S., et al. (2019). Challenges and opportunities to updating prescribing information for longstanding oncology drugs. *The Oncologist, 25*(3), e405–e411. https://doi.org/10.1634/theoncologist.2019-0698.
8. Bertoncello, F., Carron, M., & Ieppariello, G. (2017). Profile of sugammadex for reversal of neuromuscular blockade in the elderly: Current perspectives. *Clinical Interventions in Aging, 13*, 13–24. https://doi.org/10.2147/CIA.S134108.
9. Bettiol, A., Bonaiuti, R., Crescioli, G., Firenzuoli, F., et al. (2018). The impact of previous pregnancy loss on lactating behaviors and use of herbal medicines during breastfeeding: A post hoc analysis of the herbal supplements in breastfeeding investigation (HaBIT). *Evidence-Based Complementary and Alternative Medicine, 2018*, Article ID 1035875, 7 pages. https://core.ac.uk/download/326839907.pdf (accessed on 9 May 2025).
10. Cedarville University. (2016). *2016–2017 Graduate Academic Catalog*. https://core.ac.uk/download/301490693.pdf (accessed on 9 May 2025).
11. Ceulemans, M., De Vries, L. C., De Wildt, S. N., Dibbets, R., et al. (2024). Willingness-to-use and preferences for model-informed antenatal doses: A cross-sectional study among European healthcare practitioners and pregnant women. *Frontiers in Pharmacology, 15*, 1403747. https://core.ac.uk/download/618291298.pdf (accessed on 9 May 2025).
12. Chen, T. T., Hochhaus, A., Kantarjian, H. M., Roy, A., et al. (2013). Differential effects of dosing regimen on the safety and efficacy of dasatinib: Retrospective exposure-response analysis of a Phase III study. *Clinical Pharmacology: Advances and Applications, 5*, 85–97. https://doi.org/10.2147/CPAA.S42796.

13. Chung, S. H., Mattison, D. R., & Soldin, O. P. (2011). Sex differences in drug disposition. *Journal of Biomedicine and Biotechnology, 2011*, Article ID 187103. https://doi.org/10.1155/2011/187103.

14. Cochetti, C. S. (2009). *Integrating 'Traditional' And 'Scientific' Medicine in Contemporary Cuba.* https://core.ac.uk/download/74352.pdf (accessed on 9 May 2025).

15. Cosentino, F., Grant, P. J., Aboyans, V., Bailey, C. J., Ceriello, A., Delgado, V., Federici, M., et al. (2019). 2019 ESC guidelines on diabetes, pre-diabetes, and cardiovascular diseases developed in collaboration with the EASD. *European Heart Journal, 41*, 255–323. https://doi.org/10.1093/eurheartj/ehz486.

16. Croubels, S., De Backer, P., De Baere, S., Meyer, E., et al. (2012). Pharmacokinetics of dexamethasone in pigs. https://core.ac.uk/download/55870214.pdf (accessed on 9 May 2025).

17. Doostmohammadi, M., & Rahimi, H. R. (2020). ADME and toxicity considerations for tramadol: From basic research to clinical implications. *Expert Opinion on Drug Metabolism & Toxicology, 16*, 627–640. https://doi.org/10.1080/17425255.2020.1776700.

18. Dowell, D., Ragan, K., Jones, C. M., Baldwin, G., & Chou, R. (2022). CDC clinical practice guideline for prescribing opioids for pain—United States, 2022. *MMWR Recommendations and Reports, 71*, 1–95. https://doi.org/10.15585/mmwr.rr7103a1.

19. Evans, L., Rhodes, A., Alhazzani, W., Antonelli, M., Coopersmith, C. M., French, C., Ribeiro Machado, F., et al. (2021). Surviving Sepsis Campaign: International guidelines for management of sepsis and septic shock 2021. *Critical Care Medicine, 49*, e1063–e1143. https://doi.org/10.1097/ccm.0000000000005337.

20. Ford, A. C., Moayyedi, P., Chey, W. D., Harris, L. A., Lacy, B. E., Saito, Y. A., & Quigley, E. M. M. (2018). American College of Gastroenterology monograph on management of irritable bowel syndrome. *The American Journal of Gastroenterology, 113*, 1–18. https://doi.org/10.1038/s41395-018-0084-x.

21. Furutani, K., Kurachi, Y., & Tsumoto, K. (2017). HD Physiology Project—Japanese efforts to promote multilevel integrative systems biology and physiome research. *NPJ Systems Biology and Applications, 3*(1). https://doi.org/10.1038/s41540-016-0001-0.

22. Gorelick, P. B., Scuteri, A., Black, S. E., DeCarli, C., Greenberg, S. M., Iadecola, C., Launer, L. J., et al. (2011). Vascular contributions to cognitive impairment and dementia. *Stroke, 42*, 2672–2713. https://doi.org/10.1161/str.0b013e3182299496.

23. Gustafsson, U., Scott, M. J., Hübner, M., Nygren, J., Demartines, N., Francis, N., Rockall, T., et al. (2018). Guidelines for perioperative care in elective colorectal surgery: Enhanced Recovery After Surgery (ERAS®) Society recommendations: 2018. *World Journal of Surgery, 43*, 659–695. https://doi.org/10.1007/s00268-018-4844-y.

24. Harding, S. D., Sharman, J. L., Faccenda, E., Southan, C., Pawson, A. J., Ireland, S. M., Gray, A. J. G., et al. (2017). The IUPHAR/BPS Guide to PHARMACOLOGY in 2018: Updates and expansion to encompass the new guide to IMMUNOPHARMACOLOGY. *Nucleic Acids Research, 46*, D1091–D1106. https://doi.org/10.1093/nar/gkx1121.

25. Harrison, P. J., Geddes, J., & Tunbridge, E. M. (2017). The emerging neurobiology of bipolar disorder. *Trends in Neurosciences, 41*, 18–30. https://doi.org/10.1016/j.tins.2017.10.006.

26. Hayduchok, I., Шаповалова, В., Ishcheikin, K. Ye., Chopyak, V., Шаповалов, В. В., & Шаповалов, В. В. (2021). Pharmacoeconomic approaches for pharmacotherapy of rheumatoid arthritis. *Likarska Sprava,* (1, 2), 70–79. https://doi.org/10.31640/jvd.1-2.2021(11).

27. Jiang, H., Lin, Y., Ren, W., Lu, L., Tan, X., Lv, X., & Zhang, N. (2025). Potential inappropriate medications and drug–drug interactions in adverse drug reactions in the elderly: A retrospective study in a pharmacovigilance database. *Frontiers in Pharmacology, 16,* 1546012. https://www.semanticscholar.org/paper/bfebce55c1c92f2eefeba65b1870e2f881df85eb (accessed on 9 May 2025).

28. Khan, I., Saeed, K., & Khan, I. (2017). Nanoparticles: Properties, applications and toxicities. *Arabian Journal of Chemistry, 12,* 908–931. https://doi.org/10.1016/j.arabjc.2017.05.011.

29. Kim, S., Chen, J., Cheng, T., Gindulytė, A., He, J., He, S., Li, Q., et al. (2018). PubChem 2019 update: Improved access to chemical data. *Nucleic Acids Research, 47,* D1102–D1109. https://doi.org/10.1093/nar/gky1033.

30. Kumar, P. (2019). Mountain West Clinical Translational Research-Infrastructure Network: Introduction. *Journal of Health Disparities Research and Practice, 12*(5), Article 1. https://digitalscholarship.unlv.edu/cgi/viewcontent.cgi?article=1987&context=jhdrp (accessed on 9 May 2025).

31. Kung, T. H., Cheatham, M., Medenilla, A., Sillos, C., De Leon, L., Elepaño, C., Madriaga, M., et al. (2023). Performance of ChatGPT on USMLE: Potential for AI-assisted medical education using large language models. *PLOS Digital Health, 2,* e0000198–e0000198. https://doi.org/10.1371/journal.pdig.0000198.

32. Li, K., Wang, S., Qu, W., Ahmed, A. A., Enneb, W., Obeidat, M. D., Liu, H. Y., et al. (2024). Natural products for Gut-X axis: Pharmacology, toxicology and microbiology in mycotoxin-caused diseases. *Frontiers in Pharmacology, 15,* 1419844. https://www.semanticscholar.org/paper/ec730da9b74e564b91b232b153104b189c91081e (accessed on 9 May 2025).

33. Mach, F., Baigent, C., Catapano, A. L., Koskinas, K. C., Casula, M., Badimón, L., Chapman, M. J., et al. (2019). 2019 ESC/EAS guidelines for the management of dyslipidaemias: Lipid modification to reduce cardiovascular risk. *European Heart Journal, 41,* 111–188. https://doi.org/10.1093/eurheartj/ehz455.

34. Mikosińska, A., Litwin, M., Parys, J., Kałuziak, P., Witek, A., Kaźmierczak, M., Jesionek, S., et al. (2025). Therapeutic potential of bisphosphonates–Review of medical indications, mechanism of action, interactions and adverse effects. *Journal of Education, Health and Sport, 77,* 57219. https://www.semanticscholar.org/paper/7914b214c8d262972343122d52fb3db24de41414 (accessed on 9 May 2025).

35. Mustafa, H. E., Rokza, M. S. A., & Elfaki, B. A. (2018). Knowledge and practice of asthmatic patients regarding the use of meter dose inhalers. *International Journal of Life-Sciences Scientific Research.* https://www.semanticscholar.org/paper/ae3820eae958039d1e6e2fc36555007c4d6fa461 (accessed on 9 May 2025).

36. Neumann, U., Ufer, M., Jacobson, L. H., Rouzade-Dominguez, M.-L., Huledal, G., Kolly, C., Lüönd, R. M., et al. (2018). The BACE-1 inhibitor CNP520 for prevention trials in Alzheimer's disease. *EMBO Molecular Medicine, 10.* https://doi.org/10.15252/emmm.201809316.

37. Overy, C., & Tansey, E. M. (2014). Migraine: Diagnosis, treatment and understanding c1960-2010. https://core.ac.uk/download/30696936.pdf (accessed on 9 May 2025).

38. Pandey, N., Kumar, S., Kumar, V. B., & Thakur, R. (2025). Study of drug utilization and adverse drug reaction pattern of anti-glaucoma drugs in patients with primary open angle glaucoma attending the glaucoma clinic at a tertiary care institute in Bihar, India: A cross-sectional study.

Journal of Clinical and Diagnostic Research, 19(4), FC08–FC12. https://www.semanticscholar.org/paper/b5c8883affeb6b1a07a1a27877ad4612468fd64a (accessed on 9 May 2025).

39. Pellesi, L., Do, T. P., & Hougaard, A. (2024). Pharmacological management of migraine: Current strategies and future directions. *Expert Opinion on Pharmacotherapy, 25*, 673–683. https://www.semanticscholar.org/paper/b2f855b018f7aa7b415a48b1b26cfa12fcbc178f (accessed on 9 May 2025).

40. Pommier, A., Anaparthy, N., Memos, N. K., Kelley, Z. L., Gouronnec, A., Yan, R., et al. (2018). Unresolved endoplasmic reticulum stress engenders immune-resistant, latent pancreatic cancer metastases. *Science, 360*. https://www.semanticscholar.org/paper/d0f08546e8bcac53b4a8a4081652491208c7a800 (accessed on 9 May 2025).

41. Porat, D., & Dahan, A. (2025). Pharmacokinetics after bariatric surgery: Adverse effects and drug safety issues in bariatric patients. *Expert Review of Clinical Pharmacology, 18*(3), 101–108. https://www.semanticscholar.org/paper/6d376bb695e54f90f4cc36fb9f0f5bfaed64d314 (accessed on 9 May 2025).

42. Tam, C., Ou, Y., Trotman, J., & Opat, S. S. (2021). Clinical pharmacology and PK/PD translation of the second-generation Bruton's tyrosine kinase inhibitor, Zanubrutinib. *Expert Review of Clinical Pharmacology, 14*, 1329–1344. https://www.semanticscholar.org/paper/2a627714ba5e05d14d23d1db443d8d5c7781d189 (accessed on 9 May 2025).

43. Terzic, A. M., & Waldman, S. A. (2017). Peer review certifies quality and innovation in clinical pharmacology & therapeutics. *Department of Pharmacology and Experimental Therapeutics Faculty Papers*, (85). https://core.ac.uk/download/129191658.pdf (accessed on 9 May 2025).

44. Trujillo, C. A., Adams, J. W., Negraes, P. D., Carromeu, C., Tejwani, L., Acab, A., Tsuda, B., et al. (2020). Pharmacological reversal of synaptic and network pathology in human *MECP2*-KO neurons and cortical organoids. *EMBO Molecular Medicine, 13*. https://doi.org/10.15252/emmm.202012523.

45. Vaidya, S., Atal, S., & Joshi, R. (2024). Willingness to pay (WTP) for newer treatment options for diabetes: A study among patients at a tertiary care center. *Cures, 16*(3), e56103. https://www.semanticscholar.org/paper/ef51f66f2612a2c23ea2558f9609b75b38c190ce (accessed on 9 May 2025).

46. Vasserot, A. P., Geyfman, M., & Poloso, N. J. (2019). Androgenetic alopecia: Combing the hair follicle signaling pathways for new therapeutic targets and more effective treatment options. *Expert Opinion on Therapeutic Targets, 23*, 755–771. https://doi.org/10.1080/14728222.2019.1659779.

47. Whelton, P. K., Carey, R. M., Aronow, W. S., Casey, D. E., Collins, K. J., Dennison Himmelfarb, C., DePalma, S. M., et al. (2017). 2017 ACC/AHA/AAPA/ABC/ACPM/AGS/APhA/ASH/ASPC/NMA/PCNA guideline for the prevention, detection, evaluation, and management of high blood pressure in adults: A report of the American College of Cardiology/American Heart Association Task Force on Clinical Practice Guidelines. *Hypertension, 71*. https://doi.org/10.1161/hyp.0000000000000065.

48. Williams, B., Mancia, G., Spiering, W., Agabiti Rosei, E., Azizi, M., Burnier, M., Clement, D. L., et al. (2018). 2018 ESC/ESH Guidelines for the management of arterial hypertension. *European Heart Journal, 39*, 3021–3104. https://doi.org/10.1093/eurheartj/ehy339.

PHARMACOKINETICS

2

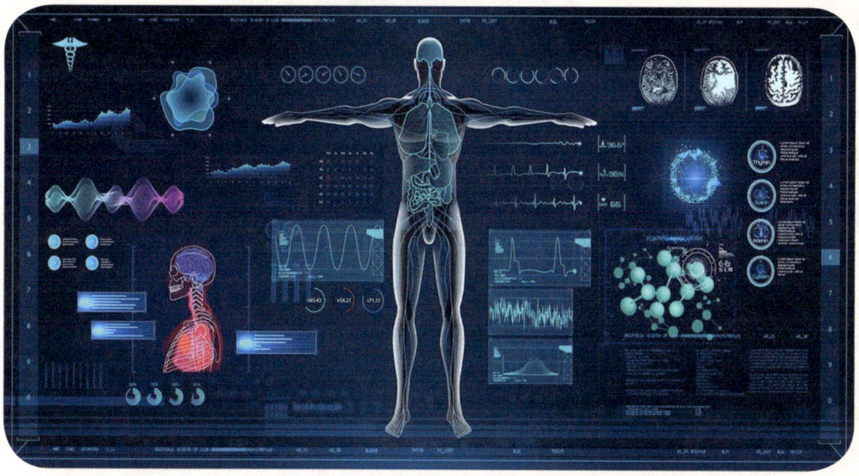

LEARNING OBJECTIVES

After studying this chapter, you will be able to:

1. Define of the Absorption
2. Which of Distribution
3. Discuss the Metabolism
4. Define Excretion
5. Pharmacokinetic Models
6. Explain The Clinical Applications of Pharmacokinetics

Introduction

The introduction of drugs into the human body triggers a complicated series of physiological phenomena that ultimately define the drug's final effects. Pharmacokinetics, a basic principle of pharmacology, examines these processes through an investigation of how drugs are absorbed, distributed, metabolized, and eliminated (Figure 2.1). Knowledge of these mechanisms is vital since they have a direct bearing on the concentration of a drug at its site of action and, in turn, its therapeutic effectiveness and toxicity. Specific clinical situations, like the application of extracorporeal membrane oxygenation (ECMO) therapy, reflect the dynamic concept of pharmacokinetics. ECMO distorts regular physiological functions and leads to profound alterations in drug pharmacokinetics, which can cause reduced drug effectiveness or greater side effects. The alterations are drug dependent, which emphasizes the importance of individualized dosing programs and rigorous pharmacokinetic monitoring in specific patient groups (Aebi et al., 2017). Pharmacokinetic modeling has emerged as a central tool for forecasting drug behavior in various populations and environmental settings. One of the leading methods is through physiologically based pharmacokinetic (PBPK) models, which combine biological and chemical information to model the absorption, distribution, metabolism, and excretion (ADME) of compounds. These generic models are complemented with parameter databases and quantitative structure-activity relationship (QSAR) modules to predict inter-individual variability and provide insights into the determinants of differential susceptibility in different demographic groups. Sophisticated statistical methods like

Markov chain Monte Carlo methods and multilevel population analyses further streamline the refinement of these models to facilitate Bayesian calibration, thus improving their precision and reliability. This combination of computational modeling and empirical data is a major step towards more complex pharmacokinetic phenomena (Bois et al., 2010). The basis of pharmacokinetics is that drug efficacy and safety do not only rely on the inherent properties of the drug but on how it is metabolized by the body. As drugs pass through the body, their concentrations vary as a function of organ status, age, genetic polymorphism, and disease states. These factors render the investigation of pharmacokinetics an integral component of targeted medicine, as dosing schedules must frequently be adjusted for the unique patient profile to maximize therapeutic effectiveness.

urthermore, situations involving disturbed physiology such as critical care with ECMO complicate the determination of precise dosages. Therefore, clinicians and researchers alike have to bank on empirical evidence as well as advanced pharmacokinetic models to inform drug therapy, promoting efficacy and safety in intricate clinical settings (Aebi et al., 2017; Bois et al., 2010).

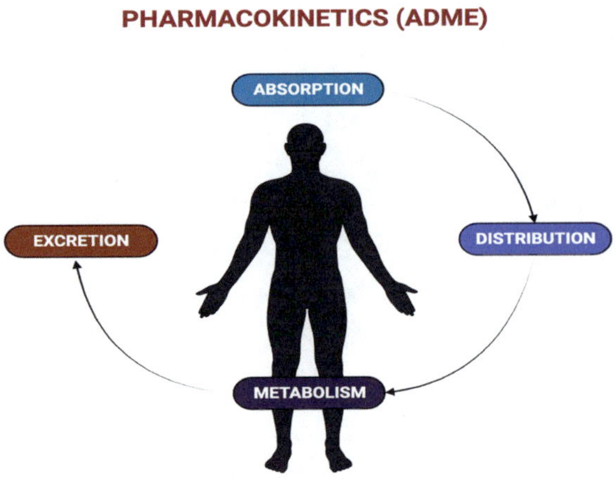

Figure 2.1. Pharmacokinetics.

Source: Pharmacology Mentor (2023). ADME (Absorption, Distribution, Metabolism, Excretion). https://pharmacologymentor.com/wp-content/uploads/2023/04/ADME-1.png.

Definition and Importance

Investigation of the mechanisms through which drugs act within the body provides significant information regarding their therapeutic effectiveness and safety. Pharmacokinetics, a discipline within pharmacology, is essentially concerned with the ADME of drugs. Through explaining these dynamic processes, pharmacokinetics offers a model that dictates dosing regimens and makes predictions about drug concentration profiles with time. This understanding is essential, especially when considering complex treatments such as chemotherapy or immunosuppressive therapy, where fine-tuning drug levels can significantly impact patient outcomes. Without precise knowledge of pharmacokinetic behavior, clinicians risk underdosing, leading to therapeutic failure, or overdosing, resulting in toxicity. Thus, the field not only brings together drug administration and therapeutic action but also constitutes a pillar in the optimization of patient-specific therapeutic approaches, establishing its deep relevance to the facilitation of personalized medicine. Beyond the simple task of drug monitoring, the importance of pharmacokinetics lies in the personalized individualization of therapy based on variability. Aspects of genetic polymorphisms, age, organ function, and comorbidities can radically affect pharmacokinetic variables, determining absorption rates, metabolism, and clearance of drugs. For instance, the application of pharmacogenetics is best seen in dosing of tacrolimus, an immunosuppressive drug that necessitates meticulous therapeutic drug monitoring (TDM) to prevent rejection or toxicity. Genetic differences in CYP3A5 have a significant impact on tacrolimus dose and therapeutic response, highlighting how pharmacokinetic evaluation comes together with genetic data to tailor treatment regimens.

These developments reflect the shift from broad dosing to precision medicine, wherein pharmacokinetics serves as a key instrument in maximizing efficacy while reducing toxicity, thereby improving both cure rates and patient safety (Brunet et al., 2019). Besides tailored dosing, pharmacokinetics has come to play a key role in the creation and enhancement of new therapeutic modalities. Emerging advances like nanomedicine take advantage of pharmacokinetic principles to deliver drugs more effectively. Copper ionophore-based anticancer therapies, for example, use targeted pharmacokinetic approaches to enhance tumor targeting and half-life, hence optimizing anticancer effect with minimal systemic toxicity. The modulation of copper homeostasis and the induction of cuproptosis by such nanomedicines are promising directions that illustrate the translational significance of pharmacokinetics in oncology. By enhancing drug targeting and pharmacokinetic properties, these developments illustrate how a thorough understanding of drug dynamics helps formulate complex therapies with greater specificity and therapeutic effectiveness (Noh et al., 2024).

2.1. Absorption

Learning Outcome

1. Mechanisms of Drug Absorption
2. Factors Affecting Absorption
3. Routes of Administration

The mechanism of a drug entering systemic circulation is a basic pharmacokinetic phenomenon, with direct implications on its therapeutic activity. After administration, the absorption of a drug is greatly dependent on its capacity to dissolve within bodily fluids and penetrate biological membranes. Low water solubility is a major challenge for most drugs, inhibiting the maximum concentration that can be absorbed and therefore diminishing bioavailability. In order to meet this, novel approaches using polymer nanocomposites have been developed with the use of biodegradable and bioactive polymers that improve solubility and permeability. Apart from helping in oral bioavailability improvement, these new materials provide controlled release functions, thus maximizing drug absorption and therapeutic efficacy (Figure 2.2). The incorporation of such materials into drug delivery systems emphasizes the changing sophistication of absorption mechanisms and their importance in drug development and design (Sharma et al., 2021). The absorption process is also made more complex when handling engineered drug delivery systems like liposomes, extended-release products, and antibody-drug conjugates. These systems alter the conventional pharmacokinetic pathways by manipulating the release and uptake profiles of active ingredients. Pharmacokinetic and pharmacodynamic modeling is a key method to illuminate these intricate processes, differentiating drug-specific and carrier-specific parameters for further insight. Modeling allows scientists to model and anticipate the absorption patterns and tailor formulations to maximize efficacy. This approach is especially useful in augmenting the creation of new drug delivery platforms, assisting in crossing the gap between clinical use and molecular design while making sure absorption rates are commensurate with therapeutic objectives (Zou et al., 2020). Intrinsic physiological processes, such as enzyme activity, gastrointestinal (GI) pH, and membrane permeability, are also critical in absorption. These factors do not only impact the dissolution of the drug but also stability and transport through intestinal barriers. Besides, extraneous factors like food or other drugs can modify the absorption kinetics and further complicate the pharmacokinetic profile. It is vital to comprehend such complex interactions particularly when formulating drugs with small therapeutic windows or targeted delivery requirements. Therefore, designing drug formulations to maximize absorption across different physiological conditions is still a central challenge. This ever-changing field continues to advance, embracing developments in polymer science and modeling methods to maximize drug absorption effectiveness and patient benefits (Sharma et al., 2021; Zou et al., 2020).

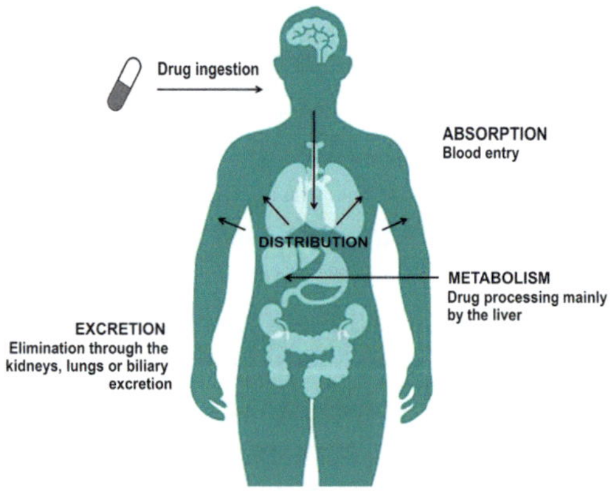

Figure 2.2. Absorption.

Source: https://static.wixstatic.com/media/160a9f_e46c0d673cd24d1d825e8c14b075d2f8~mv2.jpeg/v1/fill/w_1000,h_752,al_c,q_85,usm_0.66_1.00_0.01/160a9f_e46c0d673cd24d1d825e8c14b075d2f8~mv2.jpeg.

2.1.1. Mechanisms of Drug Absorption

One of the most important steps in evaluating a drug's effectiveness therapeutically is its absorption into systemic circulation, a phenomenon that is intricately mediated by the physicochemical nature of the drug and the biologic environment. The process of absorption mainly takes place in the intestinal tract, wherein the drug has to move through the epithelial barrier before it enters the bloodstream. Such movement can take place through passive diffusion, facilitated diffusion, active transport, or endocytosis. The interaction between these mechanisms determines drug entry rate and extent, influencing bioavailability (Figure 2.3) directly. Also, first-pass metabolism in the intestinal wall and liver can severely diminish the concentration of active drug entering systemic circulation, furthering the complexity of absorption. Elucidation of these complex processes is necessary for maximizing drug formulation and delivery to optimize pharmacokinetic profiles and ultimately the therapeutic outcomes of pharmacotherapy (N/A, 2022). The function of drug transporters and metabolizing enzymes in drug absorption is increasingly established as a factor in interindividual variation in pharmacokinetics. Transport proteins like P-glycoprotein are capable of actively effluxing drugs back into the intestinal lumen, restricting absorption and diminishing bioavailability. At the same time, metabolizing enzymes such as cytochrome P450 isoforms trigger biotransformation during absorption, modifying the chemical structure of the drug prior to systemic entry. Such interactions are reversible and are susceptible to modulation by a variety of factors such as genetic polymorphisms, disease states, and concurrent drug use. Improved recent developments regarding the transcriptional and posttranscriptional regulation of such proteins have diversified the possibility of predicting absorption profiles and tailoring therapy.

The clarification of molecular mechanisms controlling drug transport and metabolism is thus still crucial in responding to variability in pharmacokinetics (Abduljalil et al., 2019). Advances in *in vitro*, *in situ*, and *in silico* methods have transformed the characterization of drug absorption mechanisms by giving more precise predictive models. Such techniques enable systematic analysis of intestinal permeability and transporter interactions, thereby improving the ability to predict *in vivo* absorption and bioavailability. Computational modeling also combines physiological parameters with drug attributes to simulate absorption behavior in different conditions. Such models are of most use in surmounting poor solubility or high first-pass metabolism barriers by assisting in the development of new drug delivery systems and formulation approaches. Finally, marrying mechanistic knowledge with new technologies enhances a better appreciation of drug absorption, leading to the development of more efficacious pharmaceuticals (N/A, 2022).

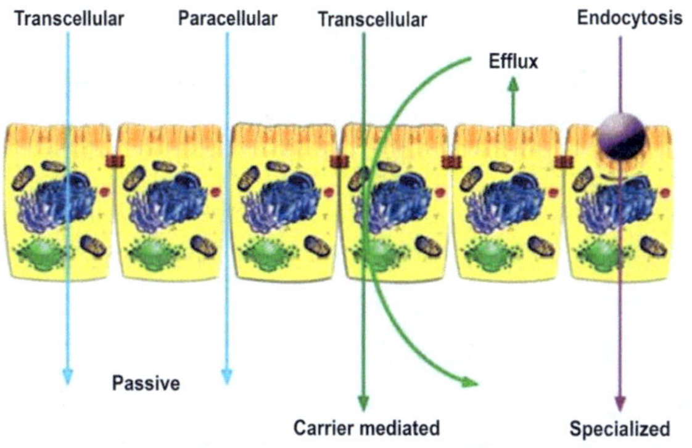

Figure 2.3. Mechanisms of drug absorption.

Source: https://i.ytimg.com/vi/3936mhQ9mEk/maxresdefault.jpg.

2.1.2. Factors Affecting Absorption

Absorption of a drug is affected by a multifaceted relationship of physical, chemical, and biological events (Figure 2.4) that together decide how quickly and in what manner the active ingredient comes into systemic circulation. Solubility of the drug in bodily fluids is one key factor which has a direct influence on its dissolution and subsequent absorption; solubility problems tend to hinder the bioavailability of the drug, especially for pulmonary products. For example, studies on inhaled budesonide formulations have shown that differences in pulmonary solubility and absorption rate constants have important effects on therapeutic responses. Nanocrystal suspensions and microparticle-embedded drugs exhibit different absorption characteristics mainly because of these factors, demonstrating the critical role of formulation design in maximizing drug delivery to target tissues (Cun et al., 2021). Additionally, physical form of drug, particle size, and the presence of excipients also influence absorption by influencing drug dispersion and interaction with biological membranes. Site of administration is also a critical variable that controls absorption by controlling drug exposure to enzymatic and transport systems. For instance, intraperitoneal delivery in peritoneal dialysis (PD) patients offers unique pharmacokinetic challenges as a result of varied absorption kinetics across peritoneal membranes. Since vancomycin dosing regimens for such patients are usually based on continuous ambulatory PD models, the absence of individualized pharmacokinetic data makes optimal therapeutic levels more difficult to achieve. The varied peritoneal membrane properties, fluid dynamics, and dialysis modalities all have the potential to change the absorption profile of intraperitoneally administered medications, making these factors important considerations when developing dosage regimens (Kraft et al., 2020). This emphasizes that absorption is not a homogeneous process but highly context-dependent. Physiological and pathological states also affect drug absorption by altering the environment where absorption takes place. Changes in GI pH, motility, enzyme activity, and regional blood flow can have a profound effect on the dissolution and transit time of orally administered drugs, thus impacting their overall bioavailability. As with pulmonary absorption, local solubility and rate constants may affect it, as illustrated in various inhaled drug products where drug release rates modulate absorption kinetics (Cun et al., 2021). Disease conditions like inflammation or fibrosis also tend to alter membrane permeability or the functionality of transport proteins, introducing additional complexity into the absorption process. Identifying and taking into account these complex factors are critical in pharmacokinetics to properly forecast drug behavior and maximize therapeutic effects.

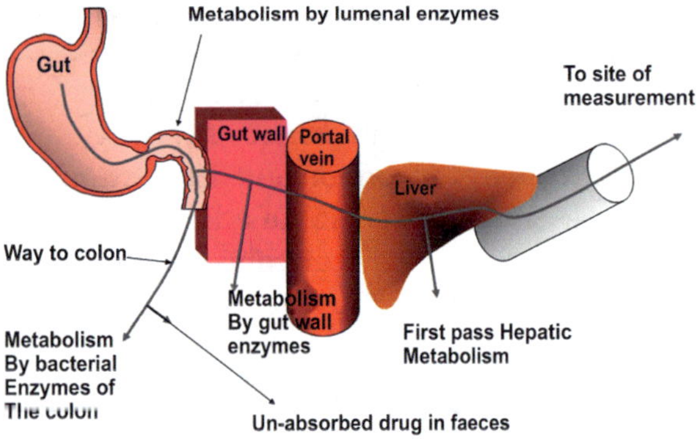

Figure 2.4. Factors affecting absorption.

Source: https://blogger.googleusercontent.com/img/b/R29vZ2xl/AVvXsEiMsx_dfy5cn0AIYP8dGygCIDxxzE7RQcS17HnJvFL6IE2WbCVXB_bFyCFi5SMvgtfzoH1JHfX6T1aRFzKOhvKWrgmKR0wkomVoqUEbN0tzTb-spu0bxu43T05IXjzETi0jUMx7bTKPcFag/s1600/absorption.png.

2.1.3. Routes of Administration

The route through which a drug is administered clearly affects its absorption, distribution, metabolism, and excretion (ADME), thus its overall pharmacokinetic profile. One of the most prevalent routes, oral administration, is subject to the intricate processes of GI absorption and first-pass metabolism in the liver, which may lower its bioavailability. Studies with synthetic genistein nanoparticles demonstrate that oral gavage in animal models yields significantly lower bioavailability than parenteral administration, as indicated by decreased maximum serum levels and area under the curve (AUC) values following irradiation exposure. In contrast, subcutaneous and intramuscular injections avoid much of the first-pass effect, yielding greater systemic exposure and increased therapeutic efficacy in radiation mitigation models. These variations highlight the significance of dosing route in drug design therapy, especially when treating compromised physiological conditions like post-irradiation injury where drug exposure could be changed (Salem et al., 2022).

Intravenous administration provides immediate and total bioavailability by introducing drugs directly into systemic circulation, bypassing absorption barriers. Nonetheless, other parenteral routes such as subcutaneous or intramuscular injections not only deliver sustained drug release but may also be more convenient in some clinical situations. Zebrafish embryo studies illustrate the pharmacokinetic significance of differing methods of administration, pointing out that microinjection into targeted body compartments can deliver more uniform and predictable distribution throughout the whole organism than the use of immersion methods. This differential exposure demonstrates how routes of administration influence tissue distribution and systemic exposure, impacting the pharmacodynamic effects. Moreover, molecular properties like lipophilicity impact the uptake and retention of substances in the organism, meaning that both physicochemical drug properties and route of administration synergistically determine pharmacokinetics (Guarin et al., 2021). With translational pharmacokinetics in perspective, awareness of species-related differences and dosing scaling from one animal model to another is also important to achieving optimal routes of therapy. These include consideration of clearance, tissue penetration, and bioavailability varying not only across administration routes but also due to anatomical and physiological differences among species. Allometric scaling using pharmacokinetic parameters estimated in animal data has predictive capacity in terms of dosing regimen in humans. For instance, murine and non-human primate model analyses treated by oral or parenteral administration illustrate minimal alterations in drug exposure under physiological stressors such as total-body irradiation, supporting the consistency of parenteral administration to achieve optimal drug exposure. Therefore, the administration route of choice (Figure 2.5) should be customized to both the drug's pharmacokinetic characteristics and the experimental or clinical situation in order to provide maximum therapeutic effectiveness (Salem et al., 2022).

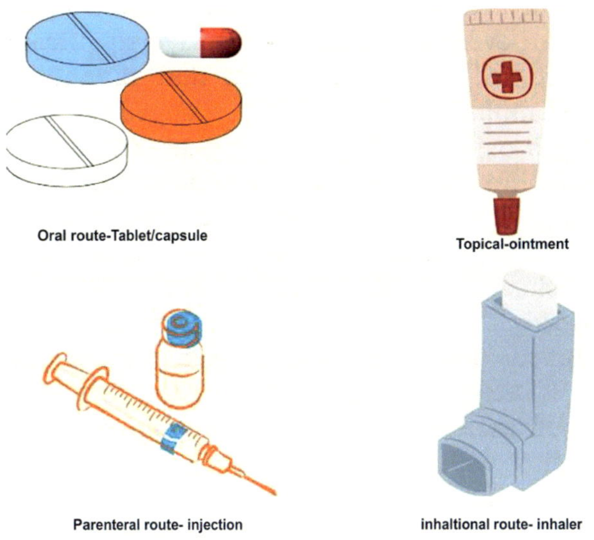

Figure 2.5. Routes of administration.

Source: Pharma Careers. (2023). *Routes of Administration.* https://www.pharmacareers.in/wp-content/uploads/2023/12/routes-of-administration-1024x1024.jpg.

Test Your Knowledge

1. What is routes of administration?
2. Which factors affecting absorption in relationship of physical?

2.2. Distribution

Learning Outcome

1. Volume of Distribution
2. Protein Binding
3. Blood-Brain Barrier (BBB)

Drug distribution is a process complicated by several physiological and biochemical variables that will dictate the magnitude and rate with which a drug spreads throughout compartments of the body. Following absorption, drugs must cross the circulation and penetrate into tissues, where it is regulated by blood perfusion, permeability of the tissues, as well as how drugs bind to plasma proteins or tissue constituents. For example, well-perfused organs such as the liver, kidney, and brain absorb drugs quickly, while distribution to fat or muscle tissue is delayed. Furthermore, drugs that bind to plasma proteins like albumin can greatly change their free concentration, impacting both efficacy and clearance. Knowledge of these subtleties is essential in optimizing treatment regimens, particularly since changes in distribution can produce either less-than-optimal levels at the site of action or higher toxicity at off-target sites. Development and aging have significant effects on drug distribution that cannot be overemphasized since body changes through stages of life strongly affect pharmacokinetic endpoints. In fetal and neonatal stages, body composition includes increased proportion of total body water and decreased fat content, which alters drug solubility and volume of distribution. In addition, organ maturity impacts plasma protein concentrations and BBB integrity, changing drug affinity and penetration in tissues. Such changes necessitate caution when drug administration is carried out in children since extrapolated doses from adults can be inappropriate and even harmful. Maturation of enzymatic and transport systems also interacts with distribution, thereby adding to the complexity of pharmacokinetics in early developmental stages (Wildt et al., 2001). In geriatric patients, the pharmacokinetic profile undergoes dramatic changes essentially because of reduced cardiac output and changes in body composition. Decreased total body water and increased fat content affect the volume of distribution, hydrophilic drugs having smaller distribution volumes and lipophilic drugs having extended retention. In addition, reduced plasma protein concentrations, including albumin, can increase the free fraction of protein-bound drugs, increasing their pharmacologic activity or toxicity. Impaired organ perfusion, especially in the liver and kidneys, not only affects drug excretion and metabolism but also indirectly impacts distribution by changing drug delivery to tissues. These age-related changes require close dose adjustments in older patients to prevent adverse reactions and maximize therapeutic benefit (Vitezi et al., 2013).

2.2.1. Volume of Distribution

The degree to which a drug redistributes in the body significantly determines its therapeutic activity and safety profile. At the center of such a notion lies the volume of distribution (Vd), which is a theoretical volume that calculates the amount of drug in the body in comparison to its concentration in plasma (Figure 2.6). Vd gives information about how much a drug distributes between plasma and tissue, not only the physicochemical properties of the drug but also patient-related factors such as body composition and plasma protein binding. Drugs with a high Vd will distribute into tissue and stay there for a long time, tending to have prolonged effects, whereas drugs with a low Vd will be found primarily in the plasma compartment. Recognizing these dynamics is of essence in TDM, where minute dosing increments guarantee effectiveness without toxicity. Current analytical technologies, such as chromatography and sensor-based technology, are becoming increasingly used to quantitate free drug levels precisely, which helps to improve Vd estimates and customized dosing plans (Ates et al., 2020). Clinical pharmacokinetics relies on computing the volume of distribution to assist in establishing effective loading doses for medications, especially drugs with low therapeutic windows. Vd is affected by factors like tissue permeability, plasma protein binding affinity to albumin, and fat solubility. For example, lipophilic drugs can have a disproportionately high Vd because of extensive sequestration in fat tissue, making their pharmacokinetic profiles difficult. Additionally, disease states like edema, obesity, or hypoalbuminemia can change drug distribution, and thus careful consideration must be taken during dosing. The interaction of these factors highlights the need to incorporate pharmacokinetic principles into practice. Improved measurement technology, as detailed in guidelines for different drug therapies such as anticoagulants, emphasizes the requirement for TDM to tailor treatment regimens by considering individual differences in Vd (Steffel et al., 2018). Correct estimation of volume of distribution is also crucial in the setting of drug-drug interactions (DDIs) and alterations in physiological conditions that alter pharmacokinetic behavior. A changed Vd can impact plasma drug levels, resulting in subtherapeutic action or toxicity, particularly with agents that need to be precisely titrated. Methods like liquid chromatography with mass spectrometry have enhanced drug quantification in biological matrices, both specificity and sensitivity, thus increasing our knowledge of Vd *in vivo*. Sensor technologies also hold the potential to deliver on-site, real-time drug monitoring at the bedside, finally bridging that gap between laboratory tests and bedside decisions. With the aid of these advances, clinicians can more effectively scale dosing regimens to changes in volume of distribution, further affirming the core position of Vd in individualized medicine and TDM (Ates et al., 2020).

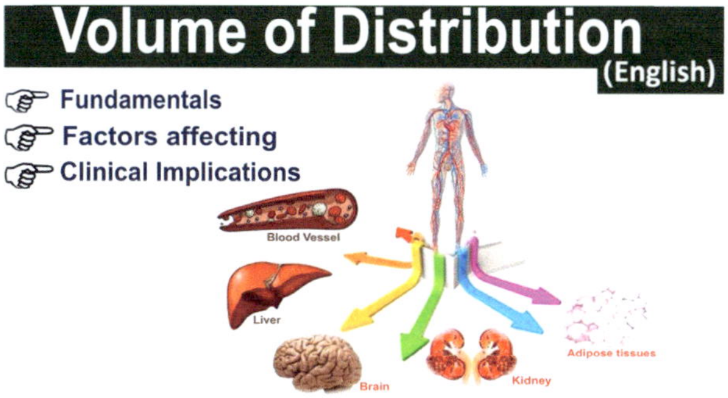

Figure 2.6. Volume of distribution.

Source: https://i.ytimg.com/vi/epjcbNdlvHw/maxresdefault.jpg.

2.2.2. Protein Binding

The fate of drugs in the body is seriously controlled by how they interact with plasma proteins, which is the driving factor for defining pharmacokinetics. The portion of the drug that interacts with plasma proteins like albumin or alpha-1-acid glycoprotein becomes only the unbound or free fraction pharmacologically active to reach tissues to exert its action and be subject to elimination mechanisms. Such a binding equilibrium has the ability to alter both the volume of distribution and clearance and influence drug effectiveness as well as toxicity profiles. Additionally, protein binding can extend in a tremendous range depending upon the chemical characteristic of the drug and pathophysiologic condition of the patient. In regulatory science, especially for modalities such as siRNA therapeutics, plasma protein binding analyses are incorporated in preclinical studies to more accurately predict pharmacokinetic and pharmacodynamic correlations, highlighting the importance of these analyses to inform dosing and safety considerations in drug development (Sara et al., 2022). Human pharmacokinetic prediction in drug discovery entails a combination of various pieces of data, such as protein binding properties. Protein binding influences not only drug distribution but also impacts metabolic clearance by modifying availability of the free drug for enzymatic reactions in the liver and other organs. Quantitation of protein binding data *in vitro* to *in vivo* pharmacokinetic predictions needs careful mechanistic understanding and modeling approaches, including PBPK modeling, for proper prediction of systemic exposure. Industry initiatives have focused on integrating protein binding profiles with other ADME information for improving human PK predictions and thereby the chances for clinical success. Such predictive approaches play a key role in streamlining drug candidates with desirable human PK profiles, which demonstrates how protein binding information informs decision-making in early development (Davies et al., 2020). The pharmacokinetic interplay between drug molecules and plasma proteins also involves the potential DDIs that can alter pharmacokinetic effects. Co-administered drugs or disease conditions can alter protein binding and cause a shift in the free to bound balance of the drug, having the effect of augmented pharmacologic effects or toxicity while the total plasma concentration remains unchanged. This complexity demands advanced *in vitro* and *in silico* approaches for the evaluation of plasma protein binding as part of integrated drug interaction risk assessments. The regulatory agency and industry policy emphasize the utility of protein binding studies not only for small molecule drugs but for new modalities as well to enable safer and more effective therapeutics development. Finally, knowledge of protein binding reaches beyond pharmacokinetics to include pharmacodynamics and toxicology, mirroring its central place in translational science (Davies et al., 2020; Sara et al., 2022).

2.2.3. Blood-Brain Barrier (BBB)

The targeting of therapeutic agents to the central nervous system (CNS) has been a long-standing problem because the body contains biological barriers which tightly control the diffusion of substances between blood and brain. One major barrier here is the BBB (Figure 2.7), a most selective semipermeable border composed of endothelial cells held together in tight junctions. This barrier shields the brain from toxic substances and pathogens while ensuring homeostasis. The same protective role, however, limits many drugs from entering neuronal tissues in therapeutic concentrations, making it difficult to treat CNS-related diseases. Recent advances in pharmacokinetics have attempted to take advantage of nanoscale drug delivery systems, including micro- and nanoparticles, that enhance bioavailability and enable targeted transport through the BBB. These advancements promise to optimize therapeutic effects through improving drug solubility, decreasing systemic toxicity, and achieving optimal localization at diseased sites (Evgeniy et al., 2022). The ability of a drug to permeate the BBB will greatly determine its pharmacokinetic profile, such as ADME. The physiological properties of this barrier, i.e., enzymatic function and selective expression of transporters, actively regulate penetration and clearance from the CNS. As an example, lipophilicity, molecule size, and charge influence passive diffusion, whereas active drug transport is controlled by efflux transporters such as P-glycoprotein and receptor-mediated transcytosis pathways. Studies on differential permeability of drug metabolites are significant in the development of advanced pharmacotherapy approaches. A recent comparison between doxapram and its metabolite ketodoxapram showed high differences in brain-to-plasma ratios of concentrations, indicating the significance of BBB penetrability in the therapeutic effectiveness of atrial fibrillation medications. Ketodoxapram's significantly decreased BBB crossing indicates a pharmacokinetic benefit by reducing central nervous side effects, with peripheral therapeutic effect preserved (Kraft et al., 2022). The comprehension and control of BBB permeability are critical to maximize drug delivery to brain tissues without impairing the protective functions of the barrier. New approaches, such as engineering nanoparticles for micro- and nanoencapsulation, are being developed as promising methods to improve pharmacodynamics and selectively address pathological foci in the CNS.

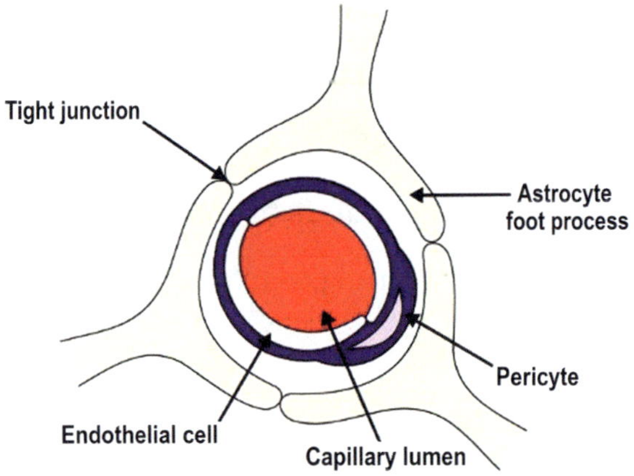

Figure 2.7. Blood-brain barrier (BBB).

Source: Medbullets. (n.d.). *Blood-Brain Barrier.* https://upload.medbullets.com/topic/113003/images/bbb%20-%20moises%20dominguez.jpg.

These approaches not only permit extended durations of drug action but also unlock opportunities for diagnostic imaging and targeted treatment of neurological disorders, cardiovascular defects, and inflammatory diseases. By unlocking the intricate interaction between the BBB and drug pharmacokinetics, scientists are able to create therapies with enhanced safety profiles and greater efficacy, marking the beginning of a new era of targeted pharmacotherapy that avoids the old constraints placed by the BBB (Evgeniy et al., 2022).

Test Your Knowledge

1. What is Blood-Brain Barrier (BBB)?
2. Which of drug redistributes in volume of distribution?

2.3. Metabolism

Learning Outcome

1. Phase I and Phase II Reactions
2. Role of the Liver
3. Genetic Factors Influencing Metabolism

Knowledge of the complex processes involved in drug metabolism is necessary to understand the drug's total pharmacokinetics. Metabolism is mostly used to describe chemical alteration of drugs in the body, usually taking place in the liver, where cytochrome P450 enzymes alter drugs to make it easier for the drugs to be removed (Figure 2.8). This alteration could either activate prodrugs to their drug form or inactivate active drugs, making them easier to be excreted. Metabolism rate affects plasma concentration of a drug, influencing both efficacy and toxicity. As metabolic routes can differ considerably between individuals because of genetic or environmental influences, the metabolic rate can account for a substantial proportion of interpatient variation in drug response. Metabolism is therefore an essential determinant in pharmacokinetics, guiding dosage regimens and monitoring to maximize clinical outcomes (David et al., 1974). Yet another crucial factor determining drug metabolism is the action of cellular transporters, influencing intracellular accessibility of substances and metabolites. Cellular transporters are either influx or efflux types and transport drugs across cell membranes actively in ATP-dependent processes. They can facilitate or hinder drug absorption and distribution and hence modulate metabolic reactions. To illustrate, organic solute transporters (OSTs) on the epithelial cell surface are main mediators for drug disposition, particularly in the intestine, facilitating bile acid uptake. These OSTs activity have the potential to cause non-linear pharmacokinetics by modifying the rates of elimination and bioavailability of drugs and making it increasingly difficult to forecast metabolism and whole-body drug disposal (Ahad et al., 2019). Such interaction highlights the requirement to take transport interactions into consideration during drug formulation and dosing. Metabolism also occurs in interaction with other pharmacokinetic phases including absorption and elimination, creating a network that broadly controls drug distribution. Metabolism may, in some instances, occur as a parallel activity to drug distribution, where the drug is transferred to metabolizing tissues, and elimination, in which metabolite products are disposed of via the renal or the biliary tracts. The concurrent existence of these unit processes demonstrates the intricacy of pharmacokinetics and underscores the need for combined models to describe drug kinetics precisely. Additionally, the metabolic capacity may become saturated at high concentrations of drugs, producing capacity-limited kinetics, which is different from mere first-order kinetics and changes drug clearance rates. Understanding these kinetic patterns is vital for anticipating drug accumulation and potential toxicity, ensuring safer and more effective therapeutic regimens (David et al., 1974).

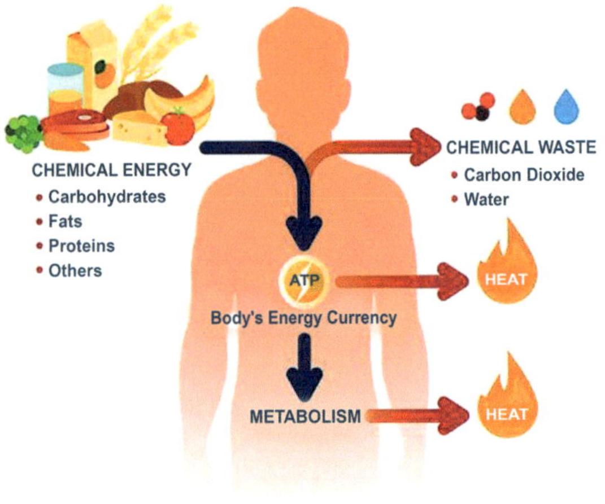

Figure 2.8. Metabolism.

Source: Lybrate. (n.d.). *Metabolism.* https://assets.lybrate.com/imgs/tic/enadp/image-of-the-metabolism.jpg.

2.3.1. Phase I and Phase II Reactions

Biotransformation is an essential process that facilitates the elimination of xenobiotics and endogenous compounds by converting lipophilic molecules into more hydrophilic forms. This transformation mainly occurs in the liver, involving a series of complex enzymatic reactions categorized into Phase I and Phase II metabolic pathways (Figure 2.9). Phase I reactions primarily introduce or expose functional groups through oxidation, reduction, or hydrolysis. These alterations are likely to enhance the polarity of the compounds but sometimes produce reactive intermediates that might need further alteration. For example, phytochemical compounds such as those in *Salvia miltiorrhiza* and *Ligusticum chuanxiong* have extensive Phase I reactions including methylation, oxidation, hydrogenation, dehydration, and hydroxylation, and they play an important role in increasing their bioavailability and pharmacological activity (Pang et al., 2025). Knowledge of the complexity of Phase I metabolism is important because it sets the stage for subsequent conjugation reactions in Phase II. After Phase I, Phase II reactions add to the hydrophilicity of metabolites by adding endogenous polar groups, thereby making them easier to excrete via renal or biliary routes. Such conjugation reactions involve acetylation, glucuronidation, glycosylation, and sulfation, which generally make the compounds less pharmacologically active. The synergistic action of Phase I and Phase II reactions effectively detoxifies and removes xenobiotics while influencing drug efficacy and toxicity. This is most pronounced in drug metabolism, where substances like traditional herbal remedies or synthetic inhibitors are subjected to such processes. Glucuronidation and acetylation, for instance, play a pivotal role in the metabolism of phenolic acids and phthalides in herbal products employed against cerebral ischemia, highlighting Phase II pathway clinical importance (Pang et al., 2025). Such metabolic processes are indicative of the body's capacity to achieve chemical homeostasis via coordinated enzymatic action. The action of cytochrome P450 enzymes, which are mainly engaged in Phase I metabolism, cannot be emphasized enough in the context of pharmacokinetics and drug interaction. These enzymes catalyze hydroxylation and desaturation reactions essential for the biotransformation of compounds such as synthetic protease inhibitors for viral infections. For instance, SARS-CoV-2 papain-like protease inhibitors show Phase I metabolism that is mainly catalyzed by CYP3A4, CYP3A5, and CYP2D6 isoforms, which catalyze hydroxylation at specific molecular positions. In addition, such metabolic processes can lead to DDIs based on the inhibition of major CYP enzymes, thereby altering the pharmacokinetics of co-administered medication. The Phase II metabolism that follows amplifies the excretion of these substances, making it important to understand both phases in order to maximize therapeutic regimens and reduce adverse effects.

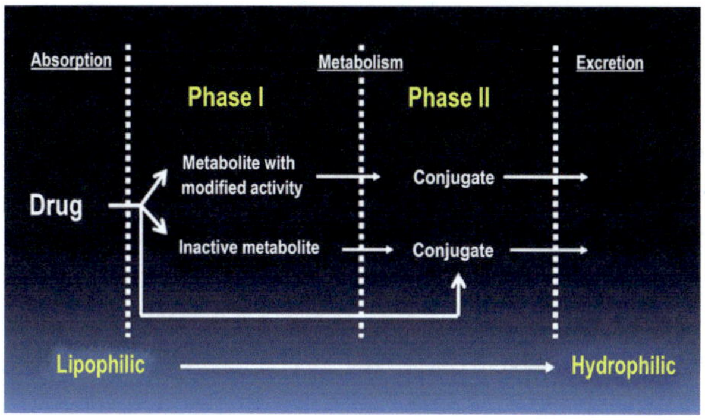

Figure 2.9. Phase I and phase II reactions.

Source: SlideServe. (n.d.). *Phase I and Phase II Metabolic Reactions.* https://image2.slideserve.com/3762537/phase-i-and-phase-ii-metabolic-reactions-l.jpg.

2.3.2. Role of the Liver

The drug metabolism in the human organism is a delicate, intricately regulated process in which enzymatic activity is of crucial importance. The central organ for this metabolic conversion is the liver, which contains a diverse set of drug-metabolizing enzymes tasked with converting lipophilic drugs into more hydrophilic compounds to ease excretion. The bio-transformation's involved are Phase I reaction, mainly oxidation and reduction, and Phase II reactions like conjugation. Modulation of these enzymes by genetic determinants, disease conditions, and foreign substances profoundly influences the pharmacokinetic profile of drugs, affecting both their efficacy and toxicity. The enzymatic systems of the liver, particularly those involving cytochrome P450 enzymes, continue to play a central role in explaining the variability of drug response between different individuals and the planning of individualized pharmacotherapy regimens. Recent developments have emphasized the function of xenobiotic receptors and noncoding RNAs in controlling these metabolic pathways, shedding new light on the liver's central position in drug metabolism (Abduljalil et al., 2019). Aside from metabolism, the liver is an irreplaceable location for drug clearance, with its double blood supply allowing efficient processing of substances taken up via the GI tract. Drugs passing into the liver through the portal vein are subjected to first-pass metabolism, and their bioavailability is greatly decreased thereby affecting dosing regimens. The ability of this organ to transport and eliminate metabolites either into the bile or into the systemic circulation reiterates its central role in pharmacokinetics. In addition, the interaction of hepatic transporters and metabolizing enzymes can lead to herb-drug interactions, in which the herbal compounds modulate the function of these proteins, consequently modifying the pharmacokinetic profile of traditional drugs. These interactions call for caution when herbal preparations are administered concomitantly with drugs since the liver-mediated changes may result in drug failure or toxicity (Horie et al., 2015). Disease progression and liver-related pathological states add complexity to its role in pharmacokinetics by modifying the expression and function of drug-metabolizing enzymes and transporters. Chronic liver disease, for example, can decrease enzymatic function, causing drug metabolism impairment and accumulation, which translates into dose titrations and careful monitoring. Progress in modeling approaches, such as PBPK models and gene-editing animal models, has improved the potential to forecast these changes and fine-tune pharmacotherapy based on this. It is thus important to understand the dynamic profile of the liver's enzymatic landscape during health and disease in predicting drug disposition and reducing adverse drug reactions (ADRs). These observations open the way to more targeted medicine strategies, combining hepatic function into broader pharmacokinetic assessments (Abduljalil et al., 2019).

2.3.3. Genetic Factors Influencing Metabolism

Drug metabolism variability frequently results from underlying genetic variations that influence enzyme function, with a profound effect on pharmacokinetics (Figure 2.10). The cytochrome P450 enzymes, especially the CYP3A and CYP2B6 isoforms, are key to metabolizing numerous drugs, and genetic polymorphisms in these genes have the potential to modify enzymatic performance, resulting in extreme inter-individual variability. For example, CYP3A5 mutations affect the metabolism of tacrolimus, an important immunosuppressant drug, such that expressor alleles can increase enzymatic activity and thereby enhance drug clearance. This type of genetic heterogeneity results in the need for individualized dosing regimens to maximize efficacy and minimize toxicity. Additionally, polymorphisms in genes that encode drug transporters, such as P-glycoprotein, affect drug absorption and distribution, also impacting systemic exposure to drugs. Along with demographic parameters like ethnicity and body composition, these genetic differences establish intricate pharmacokinetic profiles that require careful attention in clinical practice and drug discovery (M. S. et al., 2024). The influence of genetic variability on pharmacokinetics is clearly demonstrated through contrast studies between populations with varying allele frequencies.

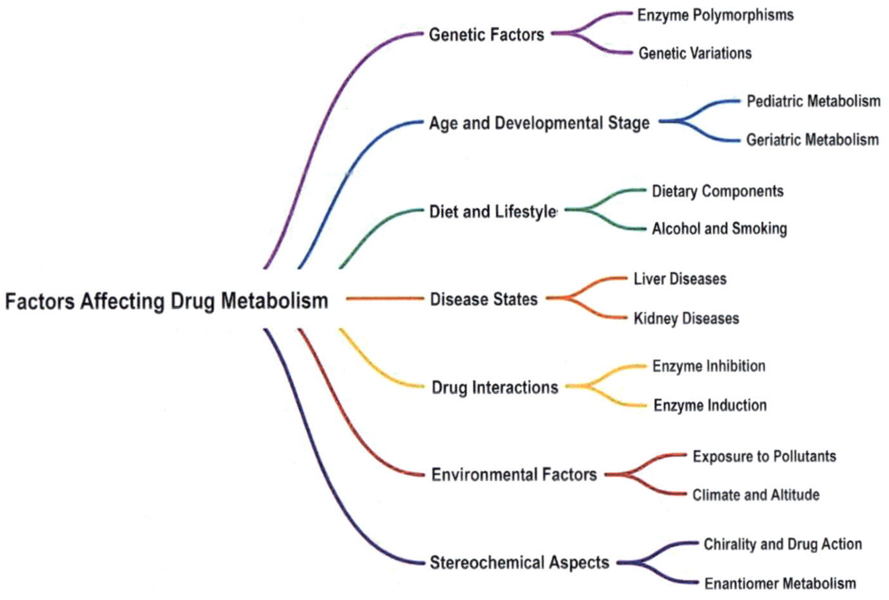

Figure 2.10. Genetic factors influencing metabolism.

Source: https://static.wixstatic.com/media/c7082f_c16f34f9095847cb8965c9753deaeb85~mv2.png/v1/fill/w_1000,h_666,al_c,q_90,usm_0.66_1.00_0.01/c7082f_c16f34f9095847cb8965c9753deaeb85~mv2.png.

Studies investigating efavirenz metabolism in African individuals found substantial heterogeneity in plasma drug levels that correlated with CYP2B6 and ABCB1 gene polymorphisms. The drug concentrations were influenced by these genetic differences, and so was the degree of auto-induction, where the drug alters its own metabolism with increasing time. Interestingly, Tanzanian patients had higher plasma efavirenz concentrations and greater decline over treatment weeks compared to Ethiopian counterparts, even when receiving the same regimens. This indicates that differential pharmacokinetics due to genetic factors combined with ethnicity result in variation in effects of therapy as well as risk of toxicity. Knowledge of these ethnically specific genetic determinants is crucial to maximize antiretroviral treatment and underscores the need for incorporating pharmacogenetic information into clinical practice (Habtewold et al., 2013).

In addition to enzymatic polymorphisms, interaction between genetic variations and physiological and environmental factors further increases the complexity of drug metabolism processes. For instance, physiological changes occurring during pregnancy influence absorption and clearance processes, which, when coupled with the patient's genotype, may require dynamic dosing modification. In addition, the interaction of genetic components with age and body composition affects drug distribution and metabolism, with obesity modifying CYP3A activity and thus rates of drug clearance.

These intricacies highlight that genetic influences on metabolism are not single-bodied but interactive with extrinsic variables, reaffirming the importance of a holistic approach in pharmacokinetic modeling. This in-depth knowledge makes personalized medicine possible, allowing clinicians to customize drug regimens that account for the individual patient's own genetic profile along with demographic and physiologic factors, ultimately maximizing therapeutic effectiveness and safety (M. S. et al., 2024).

Test Your Knowledge

1. The drug metabolism genetic factors influencing?
2. Which enzyme family is most critical for Phase I drug metabolism in the liver?

2.4. Excretion

Learning Outcome

1. Renal Excretion
2. Biliary Excretion
3. Factors Influencing Excretion

The elimination phase of the life of a drug within the body critically relies on efficient processes of excretion, the main avenues of the elimination of pharmacologically active drug substances and metabolites. Renal excretion, specifically, is the prevalent route, taking the form of glomerular filtration, tubular secretion, and reabsorption. The effectiveness of the process directly affects drug plasma concentration and action time, ultimately affecting therapeutic efficacy and potential for toxicity. Furthermore, conditions such as renal impairment may significantly impact rates of excretion, with the need to adjust dosing accordingly. Certain medications such as bilastine are examples of favorable pharmacokinetics because of their low level of metabolism and prevalent renal excretion, limiting the occurrence of DDIs by metabolic enzymes and highlighting the role of renal function in safe clearance of drugs (Leceta et al., 2017). Accordingly, awareness of the renal status of individual patients is critical in predicting efficacy of drugs as well as risk of accumulation. Complexity of excretion is further exemplified by the complex interaction of genetic, physiological, and environmental determinants of renal clearance processes. Excretion of uric acid illustrates this complexity, wherein decreased transporter function or glomerular filtration impairment may result in pathological accumulation, as in gout. This state is further compounded by metabolic and dietary factors, i.e., higher purine or fructose intake, which impair uric acid transporter function leading to defective excretion and inducing hyperuricemia (Anders, 2016). Moreover, the uricase expression context of humans is diametrically different from other organisms, highlighting species-specific profiles of excretion that modulate drug as well as metabolite clearance. Appreciation of these subtleties adds to a more refined pharmacokinetic model and guides clinical decision-making about patient-specific risk and individualized therapeutic regimens. Excretion also includes biliary and pulmonary routes, in addition to renal pathways, although renal clearance is the most important for most drugs. The interaction between drug excretion and metabolism is apparent, with some metabolites being subject to active secretion or reabsorption that can be pH-, transporter-, and co-medicament-dependent. Pharmacokinetic investigations elucidating such interactions, such as those examining bilastine, demonstrate minimal interaction with cytochrome P450 enzymes, suggesting minimal metabolic conversion and dependence on renal pathways for excretion (Leceta et al., 2017). Such profiles minimize concerns regarding metabolic inhibition or induction, simplifying predictions of drug clearance. In spite of this, in clinical experience, renal disease or co-administered nephrotoxic drugs can modulate excretion, thus influencing pharmacokinetics and requiring the use of attentive monitoring and strategies for dose adjustments to ensure therapeutic effectiveness and to avoid adverse effects.

2.4.1. Renal Excretion

Renal excretion is important to the elimination stage of pharmacokinetics, extensively determining the drugs duration and level of effect (Figure 2.11). Following systemic distribution and absorption, most drugs filter through the glomerulus then either passively reabsorbed or actively secreted into the renal tubules. Such action controls the concentration of the drug in the plasma and the tissues, providing therapeutic effects uniquely suited. For example, bilastine, a sedation-free H1-antihistamine, is mainly cleared through renal excretion with minimal metabolism, resulting in fairly predictable clearance and decreased chance of DDIs involving hepatic enzymes. This renal elimination provides a benefit in hepatically impaired individuals but requires careful administration in patients with impaired kidney function since decreased clearance can change drug exposure. Such pharmacokinetic profiles require clinicians to consider renal function carefully when dosing to maintain efficacy and prevent toxicity (Leceta et al., 2017). The complexity of renal excretion extends beyond simple filtration, involving tubular secretion and reabsorption, mechanisms that can saturate at higher drug concentrations. Emepronium, a quaternary ammonium compound, exemplifies this through its renal secretion characteristics, which demonstrate a low capacity and rapid saturation at elevated plasma levels. In anesthetized dogs, renal clearance contributed to approximately 30% of overall plasma clearance at moderate drug concentrations, suggesting the relative limited role of renal elimination in comparison to metabolic and biliary excretion routes. Such dynamic interactions of the various elimination channels emphasize the requirement to appreciate renal function in the perspective of total drug clearance. In addition, saturation of tubular secretion may result in nonlinear pharmacokinetics, which makes dosing regimens more complex and requires intensive therapeutic monitoring (Hallén et al.,

2009). Pharmacokinetic variability caused by renal excretion requires a tailored therapeutic strategy, especially in patients with impaired renal function, for example, the elderly or chronic kidney disease (CKD) patients. Drugs that are greatly dependent on renal elimination, such as bilastine, need dose adjustment to avoid accumulation and side effects. Yet, intricacies of renal handling, such as active transport and saturable kinetics, can add to the complication of drug clearance predictions in dysfunctional kidneys. Practically, this requires thorough evaluation through renal function biomarkers and knowledge of drug-specific pathways of elimination. Furthermore, the clinical question regarding bilastine safety in renal impairment identifies evidence gaps, underlining a necessity for further research to further define dose recommendations and maximize patient outcomes (Leceta et al., 2017).

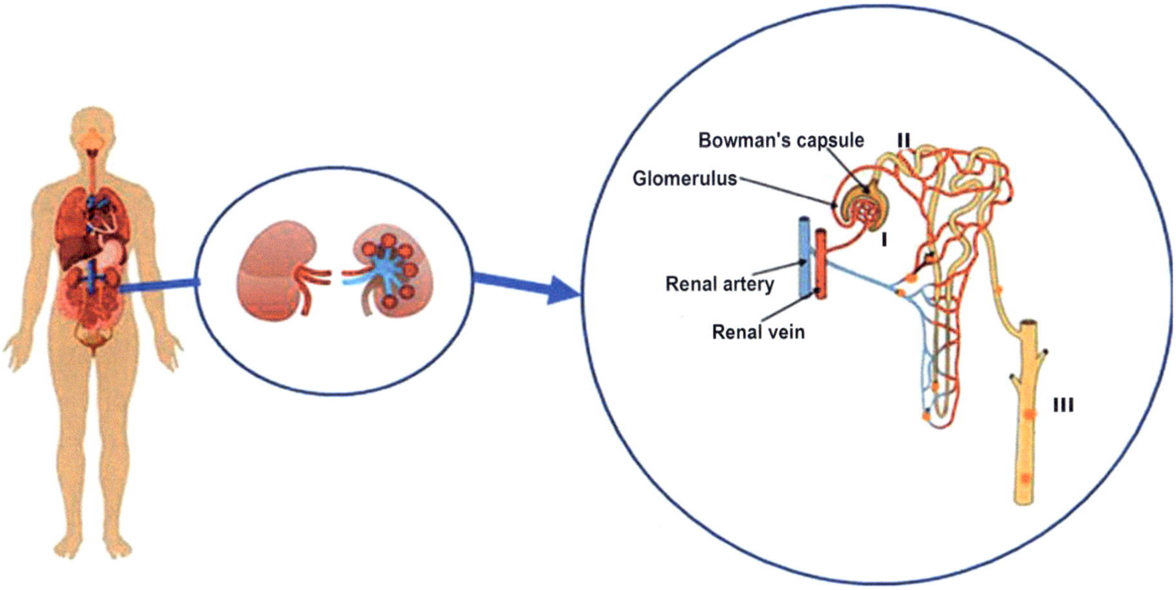

Figure 2.11. Renal excretion the elimination phase of pharmacokinetics.

Source: ResearchGate. (n.d.). *Description of the Renal Excretion of MPs.* https://www.researchgate.net/profile/Luigi-Montano-2/publication/366793821/figure/fig1/AS:11431281110615268@1672662849217/Description-of-the-renal-excretion-of-MPs-I-through-the-bloodstream-MPs-can-flow.jpg.

2.4.2. Biliary Excretion

Pharmacokinetics involves the mechanisms by which the fate of a drug in the body is determined, such as absorption, distribution, metabolism, and elimination. Of these, elimination is particularly important for drug clearance and biliary excretion is a major pathway, particularly for drugs that are metabolized by the liver. The liver not only metabolizes drugs through enzymatic processes like cytochrome P450 isoforms but also actively secretes many drug metabolites into bile, channelling them into the GI tract. This process aids in the elimination of lipophilic compounds that are less suitable for renal clearance. Knowledge of biliary excretion is not only crucial for the prediction of drug elimination kinetics but also for the anticipation of possible DDIs and toxicity since biliary secretion is dependent on specific transporter proteins and enzymatic processes, which can be affected by disease states or co-administered drugs. The effect of disease states on biliary excretion is illustrated in diabetic patients disturbed metabolism of some drugs (Figure 2.12). As an example, investigations of the pharmacokinetics of cyclosporine (CsA) in diabetic kidney transplant patients have demonstrated a substantial decrease in the levels of CsA metabolites in the post-absorptive phase, regardless of equivalent dosing and concomitant ketoconazole administration. This implies diabetes-induced reduction of hepatic cytochrome P450 3A4 activity that is critical for CsA metabolic processing before biliary excretion. Additionally, the decreased metabolite-to-parent drug concentration ratios suggest possible changes in transporter expression or function involved in biliary secretion. These changes can impact drug efficacy and toxicity, demonstrating the necessity of careful TDM in diabetic patients receiving highly biliary excretion-dependent treatment (Akhlaghi et al., 2012). Additional information regarding the mechanism of biliary excretion and its control can be obtained from pharmacokinetic experiments in animal models, for example, Emepronium clearance in dogs. Studies indicate that biliary excretion rates rise proportionally with plasma drug concentration until a maximum rate is reached, which is dependent on bile flow and can then fall as bile flow declines. This saturation kinetics indicates the capacity-limited nature of the biliary transport processes. Also, a considerable portion of the drug dose is removed through intestinal secretion, as evidenced through bile diversion and single intestinal segment perfusion experiments, highlighting the complexity of enterohepatic circulation in drug disposition. These processes are vital to precisely define plasma clearance and dose adjustment, particularly for drugs that have appreciable biliary excretion and metabolism (Hallén et al., 2009).

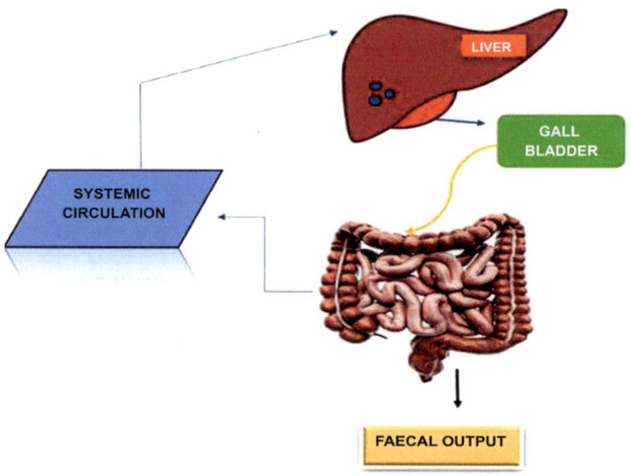

Figure 2.12. Biliary excretion.

Source: https://media.springernature.com/lw685/springer-static/image/chp%3A10.1007%2F978-981-97-4283-7_2/MediaObjects/621006_1_En_2_Fig1_HTML.png.

2.4.3. Factors Influencing Excretion

The capacity of the body to clear drugs is a key determinant of their overall pharmacokinetic profile. Excretion, mainly via the kidneys, liver, and to a lesser degree, the lungs and sweat glands, determines the duration and magnitude of a drug's action. Renal excretion consists of filtration, secretion, and reabsorption mechanisms, all subject to various physiological and pathological influences. For example, aging-related reduction in glomerular filtration rate can dramatically decrease drug clearance, especially for drugs with a narrow therapeutic index. In addition, genetic differences affecting transporter proteins and metabolic enzymes may change rates of excretion, resulting in inter-individual variation in drug elimination. These considerations highlight the importance of dose adjustment in susceptible populations like the elderly and children to prevent toxicity or therapeutic failure. Appreciation of these factors allows clinicians to maximize treatment regimens so that drugs are eliminated at rates that are efficacious yet cause minimal adverse effects. Physiological states and body composition also greatly affect drug excretion kinetics. Changes in fat and muscle mass change the distribution and sequestration of lipophilic and hydrophilic drugs, respectively, indirectly affecting their elimination from the body. For instance, obesity is linked to altered activity of metabolizing enzymes, which can reduce renal and hepatic clearance, requiring dose adjustment. Pregnancy adds another layer of complexity, as physiological changes such as augmented renal blood flow and glomerular filtration increase the elimination of some drugs, and altered metabolism either increases or decreases clearance. Pregnant hormonal changes also affect transporter proteins and enzyme expression with consequences for excretion pathways. These dynamic changes require close therapeutic monitoring to prevent drug toxicity while maintaining drug levels within therapeutic limits, underscoring the need for pharmacokinetic evaluation in unique physiological states (Calderoni et al., 2001). Genetic polymorphism and drug interaction are further layers of complexity that affect drug excretion. Genetic differences in the encoding genes for cytochrome P450 enzymes and efflux transporters like P-glycoprotein are known to significantly alter drug rates of metabolism and elimination, with consequent drug response and toxicity risk variability across patients. Ethnic variations usually translate into these genetic differences, thereby posing difficulties in standardizing dosage regimens for different populations. In addition, the co-administration of drugs that induce or inhibit major transporters and enzymes may change excretion profiles, either by extending drug action or diminishing efficacy. These factors are especially important in the case of drugs which are subject to fine dosing, for example, immunosuppressants or migraine medications, where poor excretion can cause critical clinical consequences (Calderoni et al., 2001; M. S. et al., 2024). An understanding of these factors is necessary to create individualized pharmacokinetic approaches that maximize therapeutic effects while reducing adverse effects.

Test Your Knowledge

1. Which the fate of biliary excretion?
2. How do Renal excretion of pharmacokinetics?

2.5. Pharmacokinetic Models

Learning Outcome

1. One-Compartment Model
2. Multi-Compartment Model
3. Non-Linear Pharmacokinetics

The multivariate nature of drug behavior in the biologic system requires strong models for predicting and quantifying pharmacokinetic characteristics precisely. Pharmacokinetic models (Figure 2.13) act as such models by mathematically representing ADME processes. ADME models can be quite simple, involving compartmental designs, or quite advanced, like PBPK models, that provide space and physiological parameters. Through their ability to represent complex biological interactions in quantifiable terms, pharmacokinetic models enable an appreciation of a drug's temporal profile of concentration in the body. These models are especially useful for anticipating how parameters like age, genetic variability, and disease status can modify drug behavior, and thus direct adjustments in dosage regimen. Application of these models has the potential to connect preclinical discoveries with clinical utility, and thus they are crucial tools for drug development and precision medicine (Abduljalil et al., 2019). Computational advances have greatly improved the ability of pharmacokinetic models to accommodate population heterogeneity and intricate biological interactions. By incorporating *in vitro* data, physiological factors, and physicochemical properties of drugs, modern models model drug kinetics more accurately in varied populations. This incorporation enhances understanding of causes of variability impacting dose-exposure-response relationships, a vital parameter for optimizing efficacy and safety of drugs. An example is how model-informed strategies allow determination of potential herb-drug or drug-drug interactions by using simulations of competitive transport or metabolism. Additionally, application of population pharmacokinetic modeling yields an understanding of differences between individuals to design therapeutics that include provision for such variances. Such advanced modeling approaches are needed to enhance regulatory decision-making and optimize therapeutic results (Bailey et al., 2018). Advances in pharmacokinetic models also cross paths with new biotechnologies, providing fruitful directions for optimizing drug development and therapy strategies.

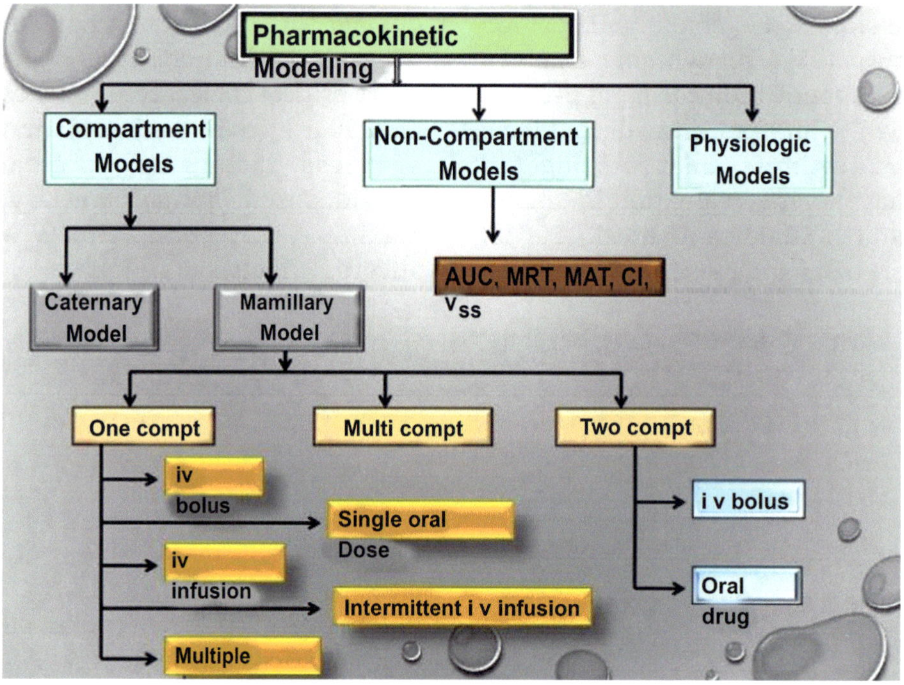

Figure 2.13. Pharmacokinetic models.

Source: Hossain, M. S. (2014). *Pharmacokinetic Models.* https://image.slidesharecdn.com/pharmacokineticmodels-140930004231-phpapp01/95/pharmacokinetic-models-16-638.jpg?cb=1412037860.

New animal models, including those created by CRISPR/Cas9 gene editing, hold the promise of validating pharmacokinetic predictions and investigating the effect of particular genetic alterations on drug transport and metabolism. In addition, non-classical metabolic pathways and hitherto underemphasized enzymes discovered by sophisticated research introduce a level of complexity that contemporary models need to include. These developments challenge old assumptions in pharmacokinetics and demand holistic models that capture actual biological complexities. As such, continuous improvement in pharmacokinetic modeling not only facilitates the creation of improved drugs but also improves clinical practice by allowing more precise, personalized dosing regimens (Abduljalil et al., 2019).

2.5.1. One-Compartment Model

Pharmacokinetic modeling is a basic tool for describing how drugs are absorbed, distributed, metabolized, and eliminated in the body. Of the many models that have been developed, the one-compartment model provides a simple yet effective framework by modeling the body as a single, homogeneous compartment in which the drug concentration is assumed to be uniformly distributed throughout. This model allows for the study of drug kinetics through the emphasis on important parameters like absorption rate, clearance, and volume of distribution. Simple as it is, the one-compartment model is especially useful in situations where drug distribution is fast and does not include complicated tissue binding or multi-phase elimination. For example, to characterize drug kinetics during various stages of severity in COVID-19 in patients who received nadroparin, researchers used a one-compartment model and demonstrated large variations in both rates of absorption and clearance in subgroups of patients (Piwowarczyk et al., 2023). It is frequently necessary when modeling pharmacokinetics in special populations to accommodate physiological and pathological changes in the one-compartment framework by adjusting parameters. The ability of one-compartment models to include covariates including organ function and drug interactions gives it extremely utility in personalized medicine strategies. An example was observed in the research on tacrolimus pharmacokinetics in patients with renal transplantation, where the inclusion of elements like creatinine clearance, hematocrit, and inherent genetic polymorphisms in a one-compartment model worked efficiently. Additionally, it accounted for the drug interaction between tacrolimus and Wuzhi capsule, a Chinese herbal medicine, showing how co-administration influences drug clearance and requires adjustment in doses (Chen et al., 2021). This application speaks to the flexibility of the model in clinical contexts with individualized dosing requirements. Although the one-compartment model simplifies pharmacokinetic analysis under the assumption of uniform drug distribution, it further highlights the necessity of recognizing population variability and clinical implications arising out of model parameters. The application of the model in the selection of dosing adjustments is noted in critically ill patients on anticoagulants or immunosuppressants, in which modified pharmacokinetics necessitate vigilant monitoring to reach therapeutic goals. For instance, the nadroparin study confirmed that dosing regimens in mechanically ventilated or ECMO patients need to be adjusted for changes in the rates of clearance ascertained by the one-compartment analysis (Piwowarczyk et al., 2023). Likewise, renal transplant recipients are benefited from tailored tacrolimus dosing based on population pharmacokinetic models that have provision for the effects of genetics and drug interaction on clearance (Chen et al., 2021). These examples indicate the extent to which the one-compartment model is still a pillar in the effective and effective organization of drug therapy.

2.5.2. Multi-Compartment Model

Sophisticated pharmacokinetic profiles usually cannot be adequately explained by straightforward models that presume the drug distributes evenly throughout the body. Rather, multi-compartment models have been formulated to more accurately depict the kinetics of drug absorption, distribution, metabolism, and elimination (Figure 2.14). These models represent the body as a series of linked compartments, with drugs transferring between a central compartment—usually symbolizing plasma and highly perfused tissues—and one or more peripheral compartments representing tissues with slower drug absorption. Multi-compartment models' flexibility permits scientists to accurately model the complexities of drug concentration over time, including effects like delayed distribution phases or multi-peak absorption patterns. For example, a population pharmacokinetics study of morniflumate and its active metabolite niflumic acid employed a two-compartment multi-absorption model to characterize these drugs, finding important inter-individual variability influenced by physiological determinants like body mass index (Jeong et al., 2023). Another example of the utility of multi-compartment modeling, pharmacokinetic research into isoniazid use in tuberculosis regimens highlights the need for such models in the case of drugs with complex clearance patterns. Non-linear mixed-effects modeling indicated that a two-compartment model with hepatic elimination in closest agreement with isoniazid's behavior, explaining drug metabolism variability associated with genetic factors such as the NAT2 genotype.

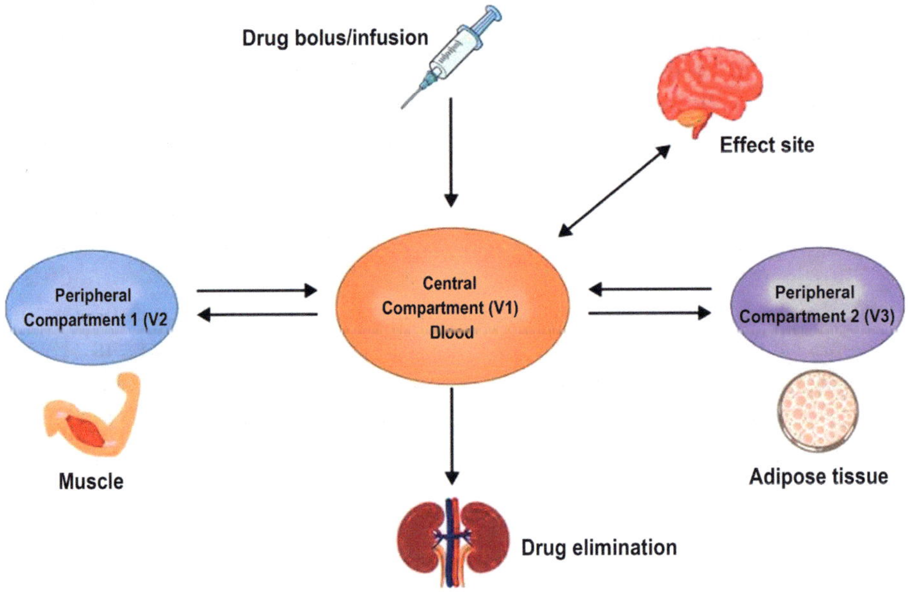

Figure 2.14. Multi-compartment model complex pharmacokinetic profiles.

Source: Cusabio. (2024). *Three-Compartment Model Diagram.*

Moreover, saturable kinetics were noted at higher doses, reflecting higher-order nonlinear pharmacokinetics that are relevant in the understanding of the drug's exposure and risk of toxicity in patients receiving multidrug-resistant tuberculosis (MDR-TB) therapy. This sophistication emphasizes how multi-compartment models not just enhance plasma concentration predictions but also enhance knowledge of DDIs in combination therapies (Gausi et al., 2022). The real-world implications of the use of multi-compartment pharmacokinetic models go beyond theory to influence dose optimization and therapeutic outcomes. By properly modeling drug distribution and elimination, these models help forecast drug levels in various patient subpopulations, including those with diverse body mass indices or co-medication. In the case of morniflumate modeling, it was demonstrated that patients with lower BMI had greater plasma concentrations of the parent drug and its metabolite, leading to greater inhibition of leukotriene B4 synthesis. Conversely, obese patients exhibited reduced drug exposure and efficacy, demonstrating how multi-compartment models can guide personalized medicine approaches by identifying covariates that modulate drug response (Jeong et al., 2023). Such insights are crucial in clinical settings to ensure optimal therapeutic outcomes while minimizing adverse effects.

2.5.3. Non-Linear Pharmacokinetics

Pharmacokinetic events tend to be linear where drug concentration and dose have a predictable association. Clinical evidence in some instances, though, indicates deviation from this as where there are complex biological systems involved or special populations of patients. Non-linear pharmacokinetics occur where drug dose alteration fails to cause corresponding alterations in plasma level or therapeutic response. This can be explained due to factors like saturable metabolism, changed absorption, or changing protein binding, which disturb the linear dynamics that are usually anticipated. Knowledge of these non-linear processes is vital in order to optimize therapeutic regimens, particularly in susceptible groups like pediatric patients, where physiological differences strongly impact drug disposition and efficacy. A dramatic demonstration of non-linear pharmacokinetics is observed during miltefosine therapy of pediatric visceral leishmaniasis, when an increased allometric dose for enhancing therapeutic benefits led to unforeseen lower than proportional drug exposure. This was due to dose-dependent decrease in oral bioavailability, possibly attributable to malabsorption during the early phases of treatment. The drug accumulation stopped prematurely in spite of escalating dosages, showing a non-linear interaction between cumulative dose and GI absorption capacity. However, allometric dosing regimens enhanced early exposure and target achievement compared to traditional dosing, highlighting the value of model-based methods to capture and manage non-linear pharmacokinetics in the clinic (Pali et al., 2020). Likewise, non-linear pharmacokinetics have been reported in vancomycin therapy among pediatric patients with different renal functions. A retrospective population pharmacokinetic analysis emphasized the ways in which physiological development, renal function impairment, and comorbid factors such as cardiothoracic surgery had a pronounced effect on drug clearance and distribution. Modeling methodology within the study allowed for the construction of dosing regimens accounting for age and estimated glomerular filtration rate, mitigating non-linear clearance related to renal function variability. This individualized strategy aided in accomplishing therapeutic goals more accurately along with avoiding nephrotoxicity hazards, demonstrating the urgent necessity of integrating non-linear kinetics into dosing recommendations to enhance clinical results in individuals with complex drug metabolism profiles (Chen et al., 2023).

Test Your Knowledge

1. Which of non-linear pharmacokinetics?
2. What is pharmacokinetic models?

2.6. Clinical Applications of Pharmacokinetics

Learning Outcome

1. Dosing Regimens
2. Therapeutic Drug Monitoring (TDM)
3. Drug Interactions

Optimizing therapeutic drug regimens requires a thorough understanding of pharmacokinetics, particularly when addressing the challenges posed by drugs with poor bioavailability or narrow therapeutic windows. For example, the natural compound rhein, despite its wide pharmacological activities, faces significant clinical limitations due to low water solubility and potential organ toxicity. Pharmacokinetic principles direct modification strategies to enhance clinical outcomes by enabling the development of derivatives with improved absorption profiles and decreased toxicity, as advances in drug formulation and structural optimization have made this possible. These strategies not only reduce adverse effects but also improve the therapeutic efficacy of agents by providing adequate drug exposure at target sites.

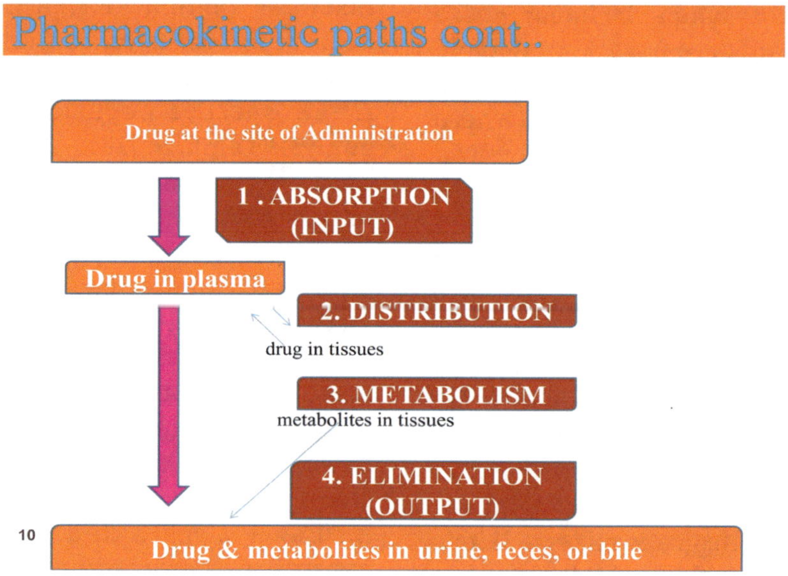

Figure 2.15. Clinical applications of pharmacokinetics.

Source: Ahmedin, M. (2016). *Clinical Pharmacokinetics.*

In addition, combination therapies which take advantage of synergistic benefits highlight the potential of combining pharmacokinetic information to achieve efficacy and safety optimally, culminating in ultimate clinical applications for compounds that hitherto suffered from poor pharmacokinetics (Figure 2.15) (Fu et al., 2024). The merging of pharmacogenetics with pharmacokinetics has seen a dramatic difference in the pharmacological application of drug therapy due to personalized forms of treatment suitable for specific gene profiles. Such intersection enables drug metabolism patient variability to be predicted, thus maximizing therapeutic effect and reducing toxicity through optimized dosing regimens. The shift in paradigm toward precision medicine underlines the requirement for the integration of genetic information into pharmacokinetic models to allow clinicians to better personalize drug selection and dosage.

These approaches are particularly important in the treatment of intricate or chronic conditions where prolonged medication management is needed, in which interpatient variability would potentially have a profound effect on treatment effectiveness. While most of this work is ongoing in human medicine, veterinary pharmacogenomics also holds great promise for individualized therapy in animals, mirroring the general applicability of these principles to clinical specialties (Vaidhya et al., 2023). In the clinical environment, pharmacokinetics is a critical tool for drug development and therapeutic management that provides assurance of maximizing concentration-time profiles for therapeutic intervention. Clinicians are dependent on pharmacokinetic characteristics like rates of absorption, volume of distribution, metabolism, and elimination to individualize treatment for the unique needs of patients, such as special populations such as pediatrics or comorbid conditions influencing drug disposition. TDM utilizes pharmacokinetic information to dynamically alter dosages, avoiding subtherapeutic dosing or toxification. Additionally, comprehension of drug interactions via pharmacokinetic assessments assists in predicting alterations in drug concentration when several agents are simultaneously given, improving safety. Thus, pharmacokinetics is essential not merely in early drug development but across the spectrum of clinical practice, from dosage individualization to prevention of toxicity, thus optimizing outcomes in patients and promoting evidence-based medicine.

2.6.1. Dosing Regimens

Successful drug treatment relies on the intelligent development of dosing regimens based on knowledge of pharmacokinetic principles, including ADME. Each dose must be titrated for timing and amount to produce therapeutic drug concentrations with minimal toxicity. Intranasal preparations such as NRL-1, a new diazepam delivery system for acute seizure emergencies, illustrate how dose-dependent plasma concentrations and rapid absorption can influence dosing schedules. In clinical trials, NRL-1 reached peak plasma concentrations rapidly with dose-proportional increases that correlated with dosage levels, although interindividual variability was observed in peak concentration and area under the curve measurements. These results highlight that dosing regimens should not only be adjusted for dose proportionality but also interindividual variability to provide consistent efficacy during pivotal events like seizure control (Tanimoto et al., 2020). Dosing regimen adjustment is further complicated when accounting for a heterogeneous patient population with differing physiological profiles. More recent pharmacokinetic modeling endeavors have endeavored to integrate and maximize dosing guidelines by examining large datasets within multiple demographic and clinical profiles. An integrated population model established for vancomycin included major covariates including postmenstrual age, weight, and serum creatinine, addressing how clearance and volume of distribution change over the course of a lifetime. These models showed that conventional dosing recommendations usually do not achieve consistent therapeutic exposure, especially in extremes of age and renal function. By optimizing doses to these variables, the authors found better target attainment at lower risks of under- and overdosing, with the authors noting the pivotal importance of customized regimens based on sound pharmacokinetic information (Colin et al., 2019). Combining population pharmacokinetic models and actual-world pharmacodynamic factors promotes the development of dosing regimens that are both safe and effective for mixed patient populations. This trend enables treatment individualization using tools such as TDM and Bayesian prediction, which utilize patient-specific information to adjust dose timing and amount dynamically. The pharmacokinetic variability seen either due to metabolic differences or due to drug formulation variables points toward the fact that one-size-fits-all therapy is not always satisfactory. Rather, dosing regimens need to be flexible, which translates into the dynamic interaction between drug properties and patient physiology. This accuracy in dosing not only maximizes clinical results but also reduces side effects, thereby promoting the quality of personalized medicine in pharmacotherapy (Colin et al., 2019; Tanimoto et al., 2020).

2.6.2. Therapeutic Drug Monitoring (TDM)

Computational modeling and software advances have transformed the clinical use of TDM, improving its accuracy and clinical usefulness (Figure 2.16). In the past, TDM was constrained by less advanced analytical methods and the challenge of individualizing drug dosing based on patient requirements. With access to modeling and simulation software, dosing regimens have been improved to better anticipate drug concentration-time profiles. This conversion enables more tailored therapy, maximizing drug effectiveness with reduced toxicity. Notably, such tools incorporate pharmacokinetic principles to dynamically adjust doses based on patient-specific factors, which conventional methods could not handle satisfactorily.

As a result, TDM has progressed from being a relatively empirical practice to a science-based practice, basically enhancing clinical results in drug therapy management (Karvaly et al., 2024). These advances highlight the increasing overlap between pharmacokinetics and personalized medicine. Drug ADME variability demands the customized intervention that TDM offers. The influence of factors like age, gender, weight, and state of disease profoundly impacts pharmacokinetics and, in turn, the effective antibiotic concentration during treatment. Such intricacy is also augmented by varying routes of administration, i.e., oral versus intravenous administration, which influence drug kinetics and bioavailability. Consequently, real-time monitoring is essential to hold therapeutic concentrations within a narrow therapeutic range to ensure efficacy and restrict resistance or toxicity. New methods, such as deep UV resonance Raman spectroscopy with regression models, are explored for better simulation and prediction of these pharmacokinetic variables. These analytical improvements have promise for augmenting TDM, particularly through enhanced dosing precision for antibiotics such as levofloxacin, thereby illustrating the applied convergence of pharmacokinetic considerations into clinical practice (Domes et al., 2023). The incorporation of sophisticated analytical techniques into TDM reflects a shifting paradigm based on quantitative pharmacokinetics. The potential for applying advanced chemometric analysis, like partial least squares regression, enhances the reliability of monitoring drug levels in different administration forms. Most importantly, the techniques provide more accurate estimation of kinetic parameters, which is important for establishing dosing intervals and quantities among patient populations of heterogeneous characteristics. These innovations illustrate the shift from traditional blood sampling assays to more sophisticated, non-invasive or minimally invasive methods, which improve patient compliance and decrease monitoring turnaround times. As these technologies come of age, they reaffirm the fundamental pharmacokinetic principle that knowledge of drug behavior in the body is critical to maximize therapy. TDM, therefore, increasingly represents an individualized, science-based procedure at the center of optimizing therapeutics in personal patient care (Domes et al., 2023).

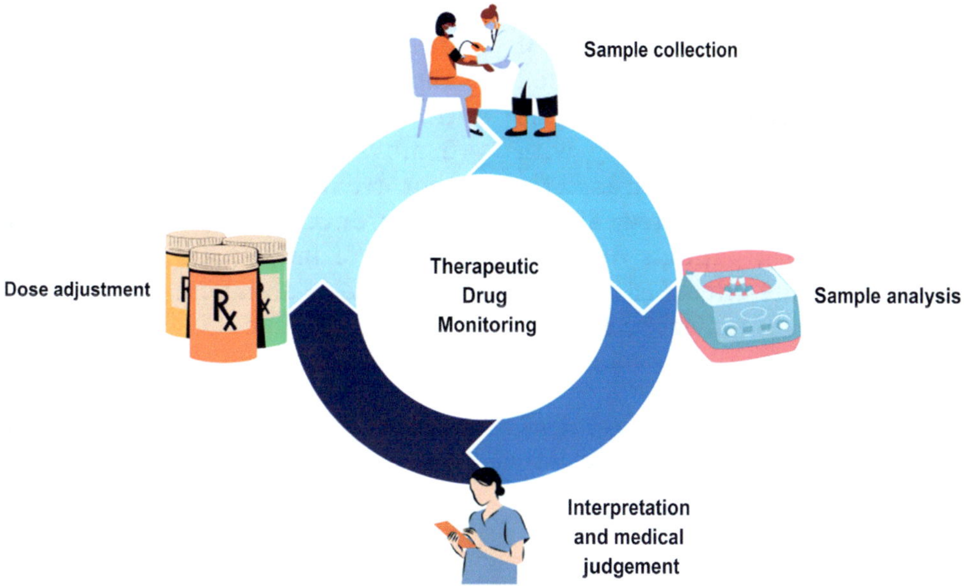

Figure 2.16. Therapeutic drug monitoring (TDM).

Source: Schoretsanitis, G., et al. (2023). Therapeutic drug monitoring in psychiatry: Enhancing treatment safety and efficacy. *Pharmaceuticals, 17*(5), 642.

2.6.3. Drug Interactions

The intricacy of pharmacokinetics is most apparent when one looks at drug interactions, which can drastically modify the ADME of drugs. Such interactions can either increase or decrease the therapeutic response of drugs, at times resulting in detrimental effects or failure of treatment. A good example is antiseizure drugs (ASMs), which are a classic case because of their tight therapeutic windows and common co-administration with other drugs. Pharmacokinetic variability, for example, variation in the activity of enzymes or transporter proteins due to patient-specific factors, also makes it challenging to predict and manage drug interactions. It is thus important to comprehend such interactions for adjusting dosages, as well as for maximizing TDM, which acts as a pragmatic strategy for avoiding unwanted effects and realizing tailored treatments (Landmark et al., 2023). This ground-level knowledge makes the implementation of personalized medicine more safety and efficacy-centered. The changing picture of antiretroviral therapy emphasizes the need to note DDIs in pharmacokinetics. Contemporary research on the two-drug regimen, e.g., dolutegravir plus lamivudine, proves to be non-inferior to classic three-drug regimens, making it necessary to give importance to interaction profiles in reduced treatments. Since HIV patients usually have polypharmacy secondary to age-related comorbid conditions, the risk of DDIs becomes more prominent. Pharmacokinetic profiles of dolutegravir and lamivudine, such as metabolism and protein binding, determine their potential for interaction with other medications. By being able to predict such interactions, clinicians can avoid and counteract adverse interactions and maintain persistent antiretroviral efficacy in the context of concomitant treatments. This strategic blend of pharmacokinetic information is used to drive safer prescribing practices in a high-risk population of complex DDI challenges (Cattaneo et al., 2019). Advances in analytical technology and pharmacogenetics have also advanced our ability to predict and handle drug interactions within pharmacokinetics. The addition of TDM with genetic panels enables individualized assessment of enzyme polymorphisms influencing drug metabolism, especially with drugs of high interaction potential such as ASMs or antiretrovirals. This tailored strategy aids in the identification of at-risk patients for drug clearance alteration or side effects as a result of DDIs, which allows for prophylactic therapy changes. In addition, biochemical markers of drug exposure add depth to the understanding, allowing dynamic monitoring throughout the treatment process. These advances highlight a move towards precision pharmacotherapy that treats drug interactions not as single occurrences but as part of an integrated aspect of individualized patient management, ultimately enhancing clinical outcomes in various therapeutic settings (Cattaneo et al., 2019; Landmark et al., 2023).

Test Your Knowledge

1. The drug interactions of pharmacokinetics?
2. Define of the therapeutic drug monitoring (TDM)?

SUMMARY

The culmination of pharmacokinetic research provides precious information regarding drug behavior in the human body, eventually influencing clinical choices and maximizing the therapeutic effect. During the course of examination of different forms of drugs and metabolism, it becomes clear that knowing about the intricacies of ADME is indispensable for the prediction of drug performance. For example, comparing various delivery forms of a given drug, such as the nano budesonide and Pulmicort Repulse, demonstrates how formulation changes can have critical influences on drug absorption rates and bioavailability while preserving safety profiles, which highlights the promise for enhanced patient compliance and therapeutic results (Beussink et al., 2004). Such reports emphasize the necessity of adapting pharmacokinetic assessment to individual clinical settings in order to obtain more accurate dosing regimens and reduce side effects. In addition, the marriage of sophisticated computational modeling with empirical *in vitro* measurements strengthens the prognostic capacity of pharmacokinetics, making it possible for drug metabolism and clearance to be better understood as a system. Through the use of IVIVE-PBPK methods, scientists are able to close the gap between laboratory results and clinical reality, enabling detailed simulations of drug behavior in adult populations. This combination of empirical evidence and PBPK modeling is a strong methodology for predicting drug kinetics, as seen in the predictive analyses of tramadol clearance and CYP450 enzyme contributions (Allegaert et al., 2014). This simulation not only facilitates drug design but also serves to personalize medicine by considering interindividual variation, thus maximizing therapeutic approaches more precisely. Overall, the science of pharmacokinetics is constantly developing by integrating experimental precision with novel computational techniques, improving our ability to accurately forecast drug disposition and action. Research on individualized drug formulations and metabolic modeling demonstrates how a better understanding of the principles of pharmacokinetics can contribute to more effective, safer therapies designed according to the patient's specific requirements. Such achievements spur further study into the dynamics of physiological and molecular influences governing drug behavior with the ultimate consequence being improved drug design, regulatory assessment, and clinical use. Through the integration of results from heterogeneous methodologies, pharmacokinetics reinforces its position as a pillar of contemporary pharmacology and therapeutic optimization (Allegaert et al., 2014; Beussink et al., 2004).

KEY TERMS FROM THIS CHAPTER

- Clinical Applications of Pharmacokinetics
- Drug distribution
- Physiological
- Routes of Administration
- Metabolism
- Drug concentrations
- Absorption
- Non-Linear Pharmacokinetics
- Pharmacokinetic Models
- Cytochrome P450 enzymes
- Pharmacokinetic evaluation
- Physiological and pathological
- Drug metabolism

CRITICAL THINKING QUESTIONS

1. **Pharmacokinetics is the study of?**
   a. Drug mechanisms of action
   b. How the body processes drugs (Absorption, Distribution, Metabolism, Excretion)
   c. Therapeutic effects of drugs
   d. New drug development
2. **The percentage of a drug that reaches systemic circulation unchanged is called?**
   a. Clearance
   b. Bioavailability
   c. Volume of distribution
   d. Therapeutic index
3. **Which route of administration has the highest bioavailability?**
   a. Oral
   b. Intramuscular
   c. Intravenous
   d. Sublingual
4. **Firstpass metabolism refers to?**
   a. Drug absorption across the liver membranes
   b. Initial drug metabolism by the liver before systemic circulation
   c. Drug elimination by kidneys
   d. Phase II conjugation reactions
5. **A drug highly bound to peripheral tissues would have?**
   a. Low volume of distribution
   b. High volume of distribution
   c. No effect on volume of distribution
   d. High clearance

Short Answer Questions

1. Explain about the Absorption?
2. Which of the Distribution?
3. Explain about Metabolism?
4. What is the Pharmacokinetic Models?
5. What is Clinical Applications of Pharmacokinetics?

Answer to Critical Thinking Questions

1. (b) 2 (b) 3. (c) 4. (b) 5. (b)

REFERENCES

1. Abduljalil, K., Aghazadeh-Habashi, A., Aigrain, L., Aitman, T., Al Za'abi, M., Alegre, O., Alnaqeeb, M., et al. (2019). Current trends in drug metabolism and pharmacokinetics. *Acta Pharmaceutica Sinica B, 9*(6), 1113–1144. https://doi.org/10.1016/j.apsb.2019.10.001.
2. Aebi, C., Shah, A. G., Anderson, B. J., Arlt, W., Barr, G. A., Barthelemy, J., Beiderlinden, M., et al. (2017). Medication complications in extracorporeal membrane oxygenation. *College of Pharmacy Faculty Papers,* 31. https://core.ac.uk/download/129191716.pdf (accessed on 9 May 2025).
3. Ahad, H. A., Barghav, G. C., Challa, M. R., Chinthaginjala, S., et al. (2019). Human organic solute transporters uttered in small intestine, liver, and kidney for homeostasis. *International Journal of Applied Pharmaceutics, 11*(6), 12–17. https://core.ac.uk/download/482243405.pdf (accessed on 9 May 2025).
4. Akhlaghi, F., Dostálek, M., Falck, P., Mendonza, A. E., Amundsen, R., Gohh, R., & Åsberg, A. (2012). The concentration of cyclosporine metabolites is significantly lower in kidney transplant recipients with diabetes mellitus. *Therapeutic Drug Monitoring, 34*, 38–45. https://www.semanticscholar.org/paper/96e38bce7d232db6dce2014229e9e1115ccbe680 (accessed on 9 May 2025).
5. Allegaert, K., Annaert, P., Boussery, K., Colin, P., et al. (2014). Physiology-based IVIVE predictions of tramadol from *in vitro* metabolism data. *Pharmaceutical Research, 32*(1), 260–274. https://core.ac.uk/download/55800839.pdf (accessed on 9 May 2025).
6. Anders, H. (2016). SP0125 renal handling of urate and gout. *Annals of the Rheumatic Diseases, 75*, 30. https://www.semanticscholar.org/paper/a666e947a31c13ab74eff4fd325f885ec12ec7ed (accessed on 9 May 2025).
7. Ates, H. C., Roberts, J., Lipman, J., Cass, A. E. G., Urban, G., & Dincer, C. (2020). On-site therapeutic drug monitoring. *Trends in Biotechnology, 38*, 1262–1277. https://doi.org/10.1016/j.tibtech.2020.03.001.
8. Bailey, A. B., Bon, C., Cox, M., Darwich, A. S., Dorey, J., Duwal, S., Ette, E., et al. (2018). Population variability in animal health: Influence on dose-exposure-response relationships: Part II: Modelling and simulation. https://core.ac.uk/download/159992803.pdf (accessed on 9 May 2025).
9. Beussink, L., Don, B. R., Fitzgerald, K. T., Nancy, K., Greenberg, H. E., & Kraft, W. K. (2004). The pharmacokinetics of nebulized nanocrystal budesonide suspension in healthy volunteers. https://core.ac.uk/download/129190906.pdf (accessed on 9 May 2025).
10. Bois, F. Y., Clewell, H. J., & Jamei, M. (2010). PBPK modelling of inter-individual variability in the pharmacokinetics of environmental chemicals. *Toxicology, 278*(3), 256–267. https://core.ac.uk/download/52669006.pdf (accessed on 9 May 2025).
11. Brunet, M., van Gelder, T., Åsberg, A., Haufroid, V., Hesselink, D., Langman, L., Lemaitre, F., et al. (2019). Therapeutic drug monitoring of tacrolimus-personalized therapy: Second consensus report. *Therapeutic Drug Monitoring, 41*, 261–307. https://www.semanticscholar.org/paper/957dcbb91cc19dd68636abf1d101eec68999ff8c (accessed on 9 May 2025).
12. Calderoni, D., Galli, F., & Guidetti, V. (2001). Up to date on the use of triptans for child and adolescent migraine: "The state of the art." *Journal of Headache and Pain, 2*, S97–S101. https://core.ac.uk/download/54380698.pdf (accessed on 9 May 2025).

13. Cattaneo, D., Capetti, A., & Rizzardini, G. (2019). Drug–drug interactions of a two-drug regimen of dolutegravir and lamivudine for HIV treatment. *Expert Opinion on Drug Metabolism & Toxicology, 15*, 245–252. https://www.semanticscholar.org/paper/11abe0f44cae69b9243beff96e290f78e4e5c626 (accessed on 9 May 2025).

14. Chen, J., Huang, X., Yu, L., Li, J., Yang, R., Li, L., Zhou, J., et al. (2023). Vancomycin population pharmacokinetics analysis in Chinese pediatric patients with varying degrees of renal function and ages: Development of new practical dosing recommendations. *Journal of Antimicrobial Chemotherapy, 78*, 2037–2051. https://www.semanticscholar.org/paper/c9421ee467b2f21ab531c41f1ca92236181acdf5 (accessed on 9 May 2025).

15. Chen, L., Yang, Y., Wang, X., Wang, C., Lin, W. W., Jiao, Z., & Wang, Z. (2021). Wuzhi Capsule dosage affects tacrolimus elimination in adult kidney transplant recipients, as determined by a population pharmacokinetics analysis. *Pharmacogenomics and Personalized Medicine, 14*, 1093–1106. https://www.semanticscholar.org/paper/87c0824b84c718132bef6b648154ea08340528bb (accessed on 9 May 2025).

16. Cho, H. J., Kim, Y. J., Chae, J., Meyer, M. R., Kim, S. K., & Ryu, C. (2023). *In vitro* metabolic characterization of the SARS-CoV-2 papain-like protease inhibitors GRL0617 and HY-17542. *Frontiers in Pharmacology, 14*, 1067408. https://www.semanticscholar.org/paper/e6d9cabf39c31fc8c30143ebfaa3dd86cf5f8ef9 (accessed on 9 May 2025).

17. Colin, P., Allegaert, K., Thomson, A., Touw, D., Dolton, M., de Hoog, M., Roberts, J., et al. (2019). Vancomycin pharmacokinetics throughout life: Results from a pooled population analysis and evaluation of current dosing recommendations. *Clinical Pharmacokinetics, 58*, 767–780. https://www.semanticscholar.org/paper/4a499a07d7bc6d1002601d7bd07e81f10510fb3b (accessed on 9 May 2025).

18. Cun, D., Cvijić, S., Han, M., Ignjatović, M., et al. (2021). *In vitro–in vivo–in silico* approach in the development of inhaled drug products: Nanocrystal-based formulations with budesonide as a model drug. *Asian Journal of Pharmaceutical Sciences, 16*, 350–362. https://core.ac.uk/download/429828824.pdf (accessed on 9 May 2025).

19. Davies, M., Jones, R. D. O., Grime, K., Jansson-Löfmark, R., Fretland, A. J., Winiwarter, S., Morgan, P., et al. (2020). Improving the accuracy of predicted human pharmacokinetics: Lessons learned from the AstraZeneca drug pipeline over two decades. *Trends in Pharmacological Sciences, 41*, 390–408. https://doi.org/10.1016/j.tips.2020.03.004.

20. de Wildt, S. N. (Saskia). (2001). Developmental aspects of midazolam metabolism. https://core.ac.uk/download/18516345.pdf (accessed on 9 May 2025).

21. Domes, C., Popp, J., Hagel, S., Pletz, M. W., & Frosch, T. (2023). Towards therapeutic drug monitoring of antibiotic levels–analyzing the pharmacokinetics of levofloxacin using DUV-resonance Raman spectroscopy. *The Analyst.* https://www.semanticscholar.org/paper/592c8fc9754253e16311b05787de4b96397c77d9 (accessed on 9 May 2025).

22. Fu, Y., Yang, L., Liu, L., Kong, L., Sun, H., Sun, Y., Yin, F., et al. (2024). Rhein: An updated review concerning its biological activity, pharmacokinetics, structure optimization, and future pharmaceutical applications. *Pharmaceuticals, 17*. https://www.semanticscholar.org/paper/0afd5241707c87185d7ccee97d688dd8dbdd7369 (accessed on 9 May 2025).

23. Garrettson, R. B., & Garrettson, L. K. (1974). Practical anticonvulsant pharmacokinetics. *MCV Quarterly, 10*(4), 205–207. https://core.ac.uk/download/51294775.pdf (accessed on 9 May 2025).

24. Gausi, M. K., Chirehwa, E., Ignatius, R., Court, R., Sun, X., Moran, L. E., Hafner, R., et al. (2022). Pharmacokinetics of standard versus high-dose isoniazid for treatment of multidrug-resistant tuberculosis. *The Journal of Antimicrobial Chemotherapy, 77*(9), 2489–2499. https://www.semanticscholar.org/paper/e7763502df0cf2dc6340ab0684f8de09a020a4b5 (accessed on 9 May 2025).

25. Guarin, M., Faelens, R., Giusti, A., de Crozé, N., Léonard, M., Cabooter, D., Annaert, P., et al. (2021). Spatiotemporal imaging and pharmacokinetics of fluorescent compounds in zebrafish eleuthero-embryos after different routes of administration. *Scientific Reports, 11*. https://www.semanticscholar.org/paper/27e271a95d750f2824b0a44b791102f179bd5072 (accessed on 9 May 2025).

26. Habtewold, A., Kassu, A., Tsegaye, A., Habtewold, A., Belanger, A. S., Ward, B. A., Schackman, B. R., et al. (2013). Importance of ethnicity, CYP2B6 and ABCB1 genotype for efavirenz pharmacokinetics and treatment outcomes: A parallel-group prospective cohort study in two sub-Saharan Africa populations. *PLOS ONE, 8*(7), e67946. https://core.ac.uk/download/pdf/18410838.pdf (accessed on 9 May 2025).

27. Hallén, B., Sundwall, A., Elwin, C., & Vessman, J. (2009). Renal, biliary and intestinal clearance of a quaternary ammonium compound, emporium in the dog. *Acta Pharmacological et Toxicological, 44*(1), 43–59. https://www.semanticscholar.org/paper/e07c8bd9d451ce9d36697b30768fc8e633909343 (accessed on 9 May 2025).

28. Horie, T., Oga, E. F., Sekine, S., Shitara, Y., et al. (2015). Pharmacokinetic herb-drug interactions: Insight into mechanisms and consequences. https://core.ac.uk/download/42138675.pdf (accessed on 9 May 2025).

29. Humphreys, S. C., Davis, J. A., Iqbal, S., Kamel, A., Kulmatycki, K., Lao, Y., Liu, X., et al. (2022). Considerations and recommendations for assessment of plasma protein binding and drug–drug interactions for siRNA therapeutics. *Nucleic Acids Research, 50*, 6020–6037. https://doi.org/10.1093/nar/gkac456.

30. Jeong, S. H., Jang, J., & Lee, Y. B. (2023). Modeling population pharmacokinetics of morniflumate in healthy Korean men: Extending pharmacometrics analysis to niflumic acid, its major active metabolite. *Naunyn-Schmiedeberg's Archives of Pharmacology, 397*(2), 843–856. https://www.semanticscholar.org/paper/38c21079e4e0fd15b733c9f1c2fdef7f55a33c22 (accessed on 9 May 2025).

31. Karvaly, G., & Vásárhelyi, B. (2024). Therapeutic drug monitoring and pharmacokinetics-based individualization of drug therapy. *Pharmaceutics, 16*. https://www.semanticscholar.org/paper/e539c9fba1732042dece5a51d040cf11a1049a55 (accessed on 9 May 2025).

32. Kraft, M., Wiedmann, F., Foerster, K., Sauter, M., Paasche, A., Blochberger, P., Yesilgoez, B., et al. (2022). Comparison of the antiarrhythmic potential of doxapram and its metabolite ketodoxaparam. *European Heart Journal, 43*, ehac544.2693. https://www.semanticscholar.org/paper/094e04398e9bd513b3785cbfe976b329d436841d (accessed on 9 May 2025).

33. Kraft, W. K., Lam, E., Lien, Y. T. K., Piraino, et al. (2020). Vancomycin in peritoneal dialysis: Clinical pharmacology considerations in therapy. https://core.ac.uk/download/322850154.pdf (accessed on 9 May 2025).

34. Landmark, C. J., Eyal, S., Burns, M. L., Franco, V., & Johannessen, S. (2023). Pharmacological aspects of antiseizure medications: From basic mechanisms to clinical considerations of

drug interactions and use of therapeutic drug monitoring. *Epileptic Disorders: International Epilepsy Journal with Videotape, 25*(4), 454–471. https://www.semanticscholar.org/paper/d83b97329bf13dbe522342467d7f474b1d0395e9 (accessed on 9 May 2025).

35. Leceta, A., Sologuren, A., Valiente, R., Campo, C., & Labeaga, L. (2017). Bilastine in allergic rhinoconjunctivitis and urticaria: A practical approach to treatment decisions based on queries received by the medical information department. *Drugs in Context, 6*. https://www.semanticscholar.org/paper/1952868436aacb58fd4e5d1915c170ae43616550 (accessed on 9 May 2025).

36. N/A (2022). Drug absorption studies: *In situ*, *in vitro*, and *in silico* models. https://core.ac.uk/download/520262014.pdf (accessed on 9 May 2025).

37. Noh, D., Lee, H., Lee, S., Sun, I. C., & Yoon, H. Y. (2024). Copper-based nanomedicines for cuproptosis-mediated effective cancer treatment. *Biomaterials Research, 28*. https://www.semanticscholar.org/paper/b32e83d52ed95414bcfc06995ee8999c655127d5 (accessed on 9 May 2025).

38. Palić, S., Kip, A., Beijnen, J., Mbui, J., Musa, A., Solomos, A., Wasunna, M., et al. (2020). Characterizing the non-linear pharmacokinetics of miltefosine in pediatric visceral leishmaniasis patients from Eastern Africa. *Journal of Antimicrobial Chemotherapy, 75*, 3260–3268. https://www.semanticscholar.org/paper/f158bbf60bb460bffad7276181dce3552350bf06 (accessed on 9 May 2025).

39. Pang, H., Zhang, X. H., Guo, J. X., Li, Y., Zhao, Y. J., Ibrahim, M. E. H., & Yan, B. C. (2025). Integrating metabolic characterization and pharmacokinetics to uncover the active compounds of *Salvia miltiorrhiza-Ligusticum chuanxiong* for treating cerebral ischemia. *Arabian Journal of Chemistry, 18*, 3212024. https://www.semanticscholar.org/paper/4c91c7ff7098722c5dfe52f7de4ea64ccee32e44 (accessed on 9 May 2025).

40. Piwowarczyk, P., Szczukocka, M., Cios, W., Okuńska, P., Raszewski, G., Borys, M., Wiczling, P., et al. (2023). Population pharmacokinetics and probability of target attainment analysis of nadroparin in different stages of COVID-19. *Clinical Pharmacokinetics, 62*, 835–847. https://www.semanticscholar.org/paper/9eac88578547d82d6bdf3a0bfb806cdea8a95bbb (accessed on 9 May 2025).

41. Raguzin, E. V., Yudin, M., Glushenko, D. D., Vengerovich, N. G., Raguzina, O. G., Pechurina, T. B., Shefer, T. V., et al. (2022). Analysis and evaluation of modern approaches to development of medical drugs using micro- and nanotechnologies. *I.P. Pavlov Russian Medical Biological Herald, 30*(3), 397–410. https://www.semanticscholar.org/paper/9fcd979122a70290a3444e1a083f98cab8b1a1e8 (accessed on 9 May 2025).

42. Salem, A., Jackson, I., Gibbs, A. M., Poirier, Y., Newman, D., Zodda, A., Vujašković, Ž., et al. (2022). Interspecies comparison and radiation effect on pharmacokinetics of BIO 300, a nanosuspension of genistein, after different routes of administration in mice and non-human primates. *Radiation Research, 197*, 447–458. https://www.semanticscholar.org/paper/c086248139b8f598c77ce4ce698e685b9b6811c8 (accessed on 9 May 2025).

43. Sharma, S., Sudhakara, P., Singh, J., Ilyas, R. A., Asyraf, M. R. M., & Razman, M. R. (2021). Critical review of biodegradable and bioactive polymer composites for bone tissue engineering and drug delivery applications. *Polymers, 13*, 2623. https://doi.org/10.3390/polym13162623.

44. Soorya, M. S., Rakshna, M., Pranesh, S., et al. (2024). Understanding the factors influencing

pharmacokinetics of tacrolimus. *International Journal of Research in Medical Sciences, 12*(5), 1769–1775. https://core.ac.uk/download/603896454.pdf (accessed on 9 May 2025).

45. Steffel, J., Verhamme, P., Potpara, T., Albaladejo, P., Antz, M., Desteghe, L., Hæusler, K. G., et al. (2018). The 2018 European Heart Rhythm Association practical guide on the use of non-vitamin K antagonist oral anticoagulants in patients with atrial fibrillation. *European Heart Journal, 39*, 1330–1393. https://doi.org/10.1093/eurheartj/ehy136.

46. Tanimoto, S., Pesco Koplowitz, L., Lowenthal, R., Koplowitz, B., Rabinowicz, A., & Carrazana, E. (2020). Evaluation of pharmacokinetics and dose proportionality of diazepam after intranasal administration of NRL-1 to healthy volunteers. *Clinical Pharmacology in Drug Development, 9*, 719–727. https://www.semanticscholar.org/paper/3821bddb6c50ecebfed621615bc9d10ede0a538a (accessed on 9 May 2025).

47. Vaidhya, A., Ghildiyal, K., Rajawat, D., Nayak, S. S., Parida, S., & Panigrahi, M. (2023). Relevance of pharmacogenetics and pharmacogenomics in veterinary clinical practice: A review. *Animal Genetics, 55*(1), 3–19. https://www.semanticscholar.org/paper/465be9e27c8476fcf4fdafc69b26a8a7022577db (accessed on 9 May 2025).

48. Vitezić, D., & Duraković, Z. (2013). Pharmacodynamics and pharmacokinetics in the elderly. *Periodical Biologorum, 115*(4), 517–520. https://core.ac.uk/download/19545555.pdf (accessed on 9 May 2025).

49. Zou, H., Banerjee, P., Leung, S. S. Y., & Yan, X. (2020). Application of pharmacokinetic-pharmacodynamic modeling in drug delivery: Development and challenges. *Frontiers in Pharmacology, 11*. https://doi.org/10.3389/fphar.2020.00997.

PHARMACODYNAMICS

3

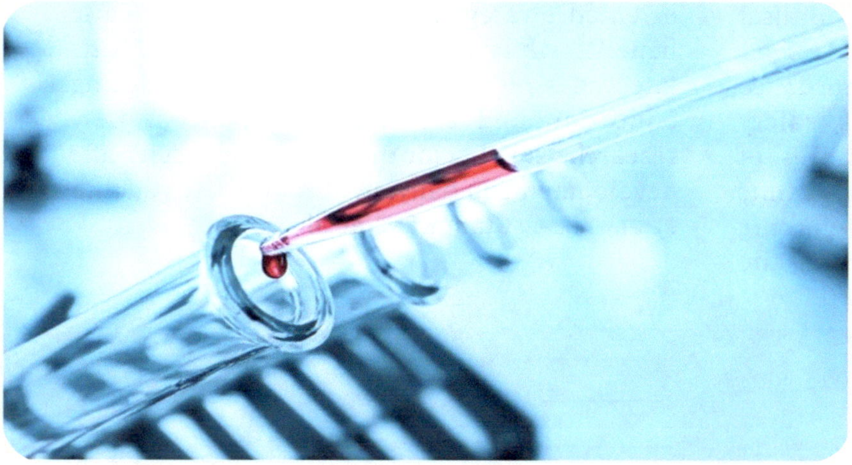

LEARNING OBJECTIVES

After studying this chapter, you will be able to:

1. Explain Mechanisms of Drug Action
2. Identify the Dose-Response Relationships
3. Define Therapeutic Window
4. Explain of Pharmacokinetics Versus Pharmacodynamics
5. Identify the Factors Affecting Drug Response
6. What is Clinical Applications of Pharmacodynamics

Introduction

It is the comprehension of how drugs work within the human body that lies at the heart of enhancing clinical outcomes (Figure 3.1). It is a complex process that encompasses interactions at the cellular and molecular levels, wherein drugs interact with biological targets, resulting in diverse physiological effects. The science of these interactions is referred to as pharmacodynamics, including the mechanisms by which drugs cause therapeutic or toxic effects. It deals with how drug concentration is related to effect, with concern not only for efficacy but also for potency and safety profiles. Understanding these principles allows clinicians to individualize treatment more precisely, maximizing benefit and minimizing risks, an essential area particularly in managing complex diseases such as Major Depressive Disorder where symptom management is a function requiring subtle maneuvers (Cuomo et al., 2024). The theoretical basis of pharmacodynamics is built on a number of axiomatic principles that underpin both research and practice. Of primary importance among these is drug-receptor interaction, in which drugs interact with receptors to trigger a biological effect. The quality of such interactions—agonism, antagonism, and modulation—defines the intensity and direction of the pharmacologic effect. Pharmacodynamics also addresses the dose-response relationship, which shows how the increasing concentrations of drugs affect the magnitude of effects. This information is fundamental to evidence-based medicine, helping practitioners make decisions about therapeutic choices through critical appraisal of clinical evidence and mechanistic insight, so that therapeutic choices have concordance with individual patient requirements, safety factors, and efficacy criteria (Guimarães et al., 2017). Integration of pharmacodynamic principles within clinical decision-making provides healthcare professionals with the instruments for optimisation of therapy. An holistic appreciation encompasses not just the differentiation of mechanisms of action but also the prediction of possible drug interactions and contraindications. It is particularly pertinent in multimodal therapeutic agents, such as psychiatric drugs, where intricate receptor modulation can yield broad-spectrum efficacy and enhanced tolerability. Through the integration of pharmacodynamics with evidence-based practice, clinicians can design patient-oriented strategies that optimize therapeutic benefits while reducing adverse effects. This integration highlights the significance of ongoing education and critical assessment of new research, allowing for the utilization of scientific developments in daily medical practice (Cuomo et al., 2024; Guimarães et al., 2017).

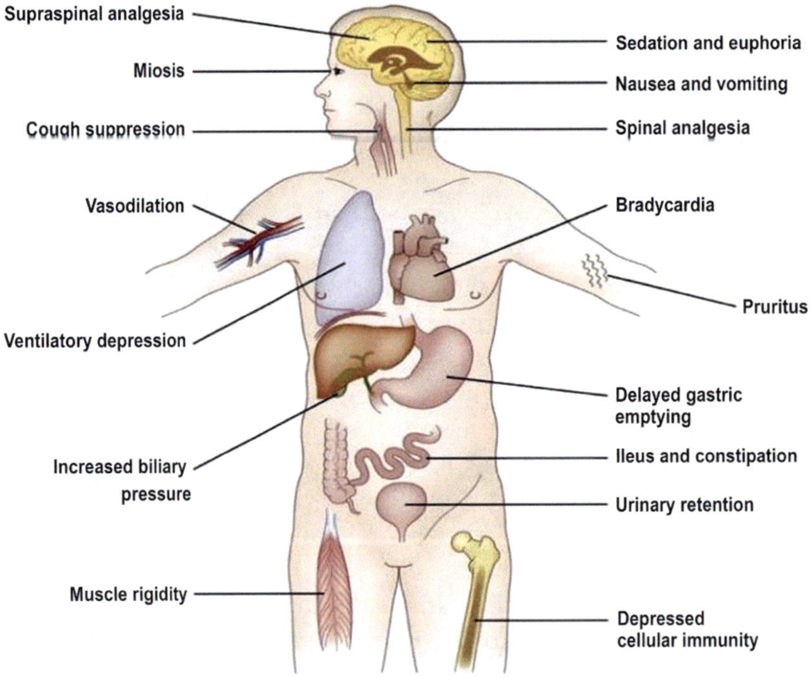

Figure 3.1. Pharmacodynamics effects within the human body.

Source: NYSORA (2022). Ultrasound-Guided Femoral Nerve Block. https://www.nysora.com/wp-content/uploads/2022/06/9.4.jpg.

Definition of Pharmacodynamics

It is only through an understanding of drug interactions with the body that the optimal therapeutic outcome can be achieved. Pharmacodynamics particularly defines the biochemical and physiological responses of drugs on the body and how a substance affects cellular function and body responses. The science describes the concentration-effect relationship of drugs, focusing on receptor binding, signal transduction, and the resulting physiological alterations. Through the study of these interactions at a cellular and molecular level, pharmacodynamics assists in assessing the efficacy and safety of drugs. Therefore, it gives essential information that informs dosage regimens and forecasts therapeutic response, thus allowing clinicians to customize therapies to fit patient needs while avoiding adverse effects. This scientific basis highlights the importance of accurate characterization of drug activity in the general context of medical practice and drug discovery (Visseren et al., 2021). Fundamentally, pharmacodynamics is the binding of a drug molecule to a particular biological target, usually a receptor, enzyme, or ion channel, inducing a cascade of effects that eventually lead to a therapeutic or toxic effect. This affinity for binding and ensuing activation or blockade determines the drug's efficacy and potency and its clinical usefulness. The principle embraces more than receptor interaction alone but also the downstream pathways of signaling and the feedback mechanisms that affect drug response over time. Furthermore, the principles of pharmacodynamics are central to the mitigation of challenges like antimicrobial resistance (AMR), in which knowledge of the mode of action of the drug and the cellular response of the body can inform the creation of new therapeutic drugs with enhanced mechanisms. Such multidisciplinary processes are essential in overcoming the present shortcomings in drug therapy and the improvement of patient care (Miethke et al., 2021). The dynamic relationship studied in pharmacodynamics is distinct yet complementary to pharmacokinetics, which examines the body's effects on the drug. While pharmacokinetics determines drug ADME, pharmacodynamics focuses on the drug's biological impact post-administration. This distinction is essential for clinicians and researchers alike, who must consider both processes to optimize therapeutic strategies effectively. A thorough understanding of pharmacodynamics allows for an understanding of dose-response relationships and therapeutic windows, which can help in the evaluation of drug safety and efficacy. In addition, compliance with changing clinical guidelines provides responsible application of pharmacodynamic knowledge, as it mirrors continuous progress in medical science and regulatory requirements (Visseren et al., 2021).

Importance in Pharmacology

Knowledge of drug interactions at the body level is essential for successful pharmacological treatment (Figure 3.2). Target-mediated drug disposition (TMDD) is a significant aspect that describes the nonlinear pharmacokinetics of drugs that have high-affinity and low-capacity targets. This phenomenon defies classical concepts of dose and systemic exposure relationships, as observed in the case of BI 187004, a selective 11β-hydroxysteroid dehydrogenase-1 inhibitor. The non-intuitive dose-response pattern seen emphasizes the need to build holistic pharmacokinetic models that include TMDD to accurately predict drug behavior. These models not only guide rational dose choice but also optimize the safety and efficacy profiles of novel therapeutics, demonstrating a high-order layer of complexity in pharmacodynamics that has direct implications for clinical outcomes (Yuan et al., 2024). Appreciation of these complexities is essential for the development of personalized medicine approaches. Pharmacodynamics is actually interested in how drugs have their effects through interactions with their biological targets. Conventional approaches tended to relate drug efficacy entirely to systemic drug levels compared with binding affinities. The view ignores, however, other key factors such as drug-target residence time that can significantly determine the magnitude and duration of therapeutic effects regardless of circulating drug concentrations. The residence time model suggests that the drug-target complex lifespan is a better indicator of pharmacodynamic effects than equilibrium affinity in isolation. This realization refocuses interest on the exploration of kinetic parameters that control drug binding and release and hence improves the strategies used to optimize drug construction and therapeutic regimes (Knockenhauer et al., 2023).

The identification of residence time as a determinant highlights the dynamic aspects of drug action above and beyond concentration measures. Advanced pharmacodynamic insight is important for drug development and regulatory processes, where predictions of drug behavior must be accurate. Incorporating ideas such as TMDD and drug-target residence time enables researchers to predict variance between plasma concentrations and clinical effect that would be overlooked by conventional models. This understanding is critical to the creation of drugs with acceptable profiles, reducing adverse effects, and enhancing therapeutic indices. In addition, such pharmacodynamic understanding allows for the detection of biomarkers and surrogate endpoints that are able to accelerate clinical trials. Finally, a deeper understanding of these mechanisms facilitates pharmacologists and clinicians to better personalize treatment approaches that better correspond to patient-specific physiological contexts, thus enhancing more effective and personalized care (Knockenhauer et al., 2023; Yuan et al., 2024).

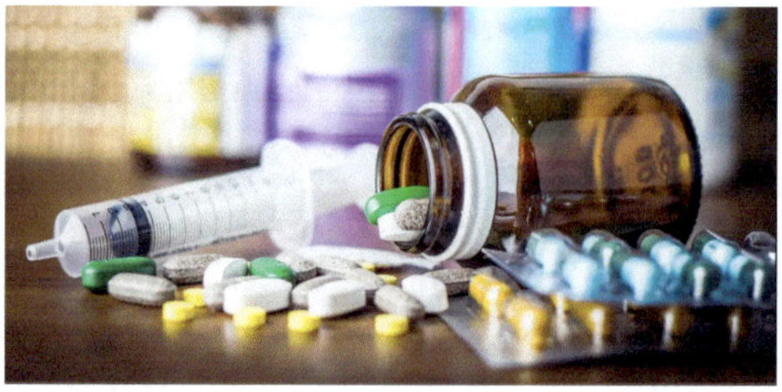

Figure 3.2. Pharmacology.

Source: https://sgtuniversity.ac.in/assets/images/faculty/medicine-health-science/programme/pharmacology.webp.

3.1. Mechanisms of Drug Action

Learning Outcome

1. Receptor Interactions
2. Enzyme Inhibition and Activation
3. Ion Channel Modulation

Identification of the mechanism by which drugs act at the molecular level is vital to an understanding of their therapeutic value and safety profiles. Drugs generally work through interaction with definite cellular targets like receptors, ion channels, enzymes, or transporters and bring about physiological alterations. These interactions trigger a biochemical cascade of events that modify cellular function. Agonists occupy receptors to simulate endogenous molecules, which stimulates signaling cascades, while antagonists prevent receptor activation by blocking cellular response. Moreover, certain drugs behave as enzyme inhibitors, reducing the activity of enzymes essential for the progression of diseases. The drug's selectivity and affinity to their target dramatically affect its efficacy and side-effect profile. These mechanisms are basic to the discipline of pharmacodynamics, since the strength and duration of drug action are a result of the character of these molecular interactions and their consequent biological effects. Pharmacokinetics and drug metabolism also determine to what extent a drug travels to its site of action and maintains its therapeutic activity. Certain drugs need metabolic activation to transform prodrugs into their active state, and other drugs are metabolized into inactive metabolites for excretion. Ticagrelor, a new antiplatelet drug, is one such drug that does not need metabolic activation, unlike other P2Y12 inhibitors but is heavily metabolized by hepatic CYP3A enzymes into its active metabolite AR-C124910XX. This process can be efficiency-constrained according to clinical characteristics including the patient's presence of acute coronary syndromes and concurrent medication of morphine that impacts drug metabolism dynamics. All of these metabolism processes are important for optimizing doses of drugs in populations of patients (Ibanez et al., 2018). Sophisticated pharmacokinetic and pharmacodynamic properties frequently underlie a drug's clinical efficacy and tolerability, particularly in multifactorial conditions such as migraine.

Triptans, selective serotonin 5-HT1B/1D receptor agonists, demonstrate how selective receptor activation can effectively relieve symptoms by modulating neurotransmitter pathways engaged during headache attacks. Eletriptan, a representative of this class, has a sophisticated pharmacokinetic and dynamic profile among other triptans, with metabolism largely mediated by CYP3A4 enzymes. This metabolic process requires careful use when co-administered with inhibitors of CYP3A4 to prevent drug reactions. Herein is an example of the need to know drug-target and metabolic interactions to achieve optimal therapeutic benefits in minimizing risks. This is a demonstration of an inherent delicate balance between drug action mechanisms and patient-related factors in pharmacodynamics (Capi et al., 2016) (Figure 3.3).

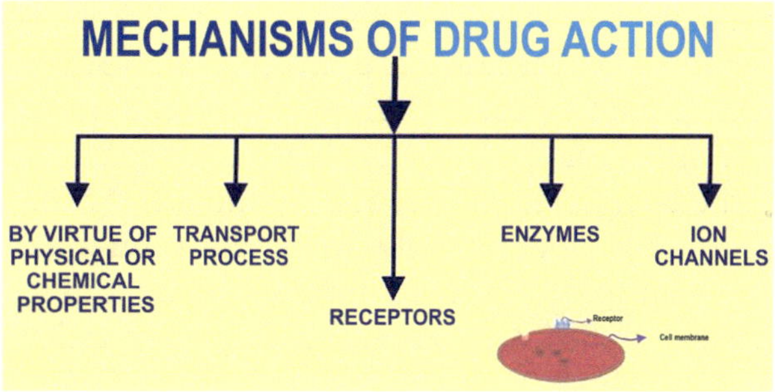

Figure 3.3. Mechanisms of drug action.

Source: https://i.ytimg.com/vi/tBEFtoH5XIc/maxresdefault.jpg.

3.1.1. Receptor Interactions

Knowledge of the dynamic behavior of receptor interactions gives a sophisticated picture of drug efficacy and signaling pathways (Figure 3.4). Receptors, especially G-protein-coupled receptors (GPCRs), have multi-state conformational dynamics that determine their functional states and ensuing cellular response. Receptors are not static; instead, they switch between active-like and inactive-like conformations and can be modulated by ligands like agonists or antagonists. Recent studies employing single-molecule Förster Resonance Energy Transfer (smFRET) technology have shed light on the temporal timescales of these conformational transitions, showing agonist binding causes more rapid dynamics than the receptor's resting state. These results highlight the significance of receptor plasticity in influencing signal transduction and drug action, providing valuable insights into drug design and screening procedures for targeting specific states of a receptor to therapeutic advantage (Maslov et al., 2020). Receptor interaction complexity goes beyond simple ligand binding to include the dynamics between receptor conformations and downstream signaling components. Such dynamics can control not just the quantity but also the specificity of drug responses. For instance, ligands that stabilize a particular receptor conformation can skew signaling pathways, such that specific intracellular cascades are favored over others. This phenomenon, referred to as functional selectivity or biased agonism, is a testament to the complexity of receptor-ligand interactions and their pharmacodynamic consequences. Leveraging these mechanisms, drug design can be made to maximize therapeutic effects with minimal side effects, a departure from traditional receptor theory to an integrated appreciation of receptor function and ligand efficacy modulation.

Although increased understanding of receptor interactions through advances in molecular pharmacology is in place, it is a major challenge to translate such knowledge into clinical use. Success with targeted therapy, especially in cancer, underscores the power of receptor biology in guiding therapeutic approaches. For example, antibody-drug conjugates take advantage of patterns of receptor expression for selective delivery of cytotoxic payloads, enhancing therapy selectivity and efficacy. In addition, immunotherapy research demonstrates that the manipulation of receptor-ligand interactions at immune checkpoints has the potential to bypass resistance mechanisms and thereby improve patient outcomes.

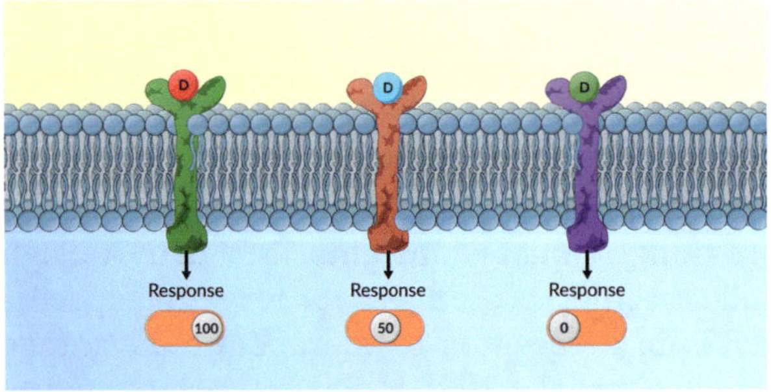

Figure 3.4. Receptor interactions.

Source: JoVE. (n.d.). *Drug-Receptor Interactions.* https://cloudfront.jove.com/files/media/science-education/science-education-thumbs/14379.jpg.

Such clinical paradigms illustrate the translational value of in-depth understanding of receptor interactions, highlighting the significance of incorporating mechanistic studies into drug development to solve unmet medical needs and advance patient care (Ullén, 2019).

3.1.2. Enzyme Inhibition and Activation

The kinetic nature of regulation of enzymes has a large impact on the therapeutic effects of drugs, demonstrating the pivotal function of enzyme inhibition and activation in pharmacodynamics (Figure 3.5). Enzymes are key biological catalysts, and their modulation directly impacts the metabolism of many pharmacological compounds. Inhibition can be achieved through several mechanisms including competitive, non-competitive, or uncompetitive binding, each impacting enzyme activity differently. For instance, competitive inhibitors are structurally similar to the substrate and compete for occupation of the active site, thus decreasing enzymatic rates of conversion. In contrast, enzyme activation is associated with conformational changes that increase substrate binding or catalytic efficiency, which subsequently influences drug efficacy and metabolism. Optimizing drug dosing and reducing unwanted effects is important through knowledge of these mechanisms since enzymes are also involved in the metabolism of endogenous compounds, and when altered, result in physiological imbalance. Pharmacodynamics goes beyond the interaction of receptor and ligand to include the complexity of enzyme modulation, which is a determinant of drug action and efficacy. In drug metabolism, enzymes like cytochrome P450s are central and their inhibition or activation can lead to dramatic changes in drug plasma levels. Such changes can be beneficial by enhancing therapeutic effects or can lead to toxicity, for which caution is needed when planning treatment regimens. In addition, interindividual differences in enzyme activity, subject to genetic, environmental, and pathological influences, complicate pharmacodynamic responses. Recent discoveries have identified non-classical pathways and new enzymes with effects on drug metabolism, stimulating greater insight into enzyme kinetics as part of pharmacology. Such advances highlight the necessity for integrated models that anticipate enzyme-drug interactions and direct safer, more effective pharmacotherapy (Abduljalil et al., 2019).

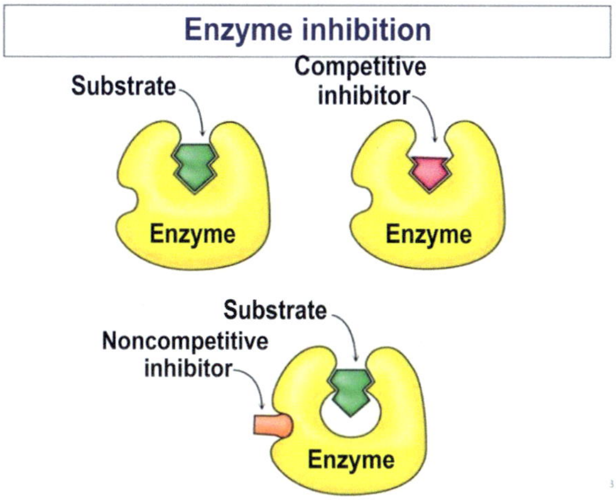

Figure 3.5. Enzyme inhibition and activation.

Source: ImageServe. (n.d.). *Enzyme Inhibition.* https://image3.slideserve.com/5580915/enzyme-inhibition-n.jpg.

Although pharmacokinetic understanding of enzymes has improved, the pharmacodynamic consequences of enzyme modulation of analgesic drug action continue to be an area of research. Genetic factors affecting enzyme activation or inhibition might account in part for the intersubject variation in analgesic effect and pain perception reported among patients. The clinical relevance of such pharmacogenetic factors, especially in enzyme systems controlling drug metabolism and receptor interactions, remains under investigation but is not yet completely understood. Knowledge of enzyme modulation patterns may further advance personalized medicine strategies by individualizing analgesic regimens based on enzymatic profiles, thus maximizing pain relief and minimizing side effects. Yet, inconsistent results and the necessity for additional replication studies highlight that the translation of enzyme-associated pharmacodynamics into everyday clinical practice is still an aim in the future (Branford et al., 2013).

3.1.3. Ion Channel Modulation

The richness of cellular signal cascades emphasizes the vital role ion channels play in ensuring physiological homeostasis, especially in excitable cells like the heart and nervous system. Dynamic modulation of these channels directly affects pharmacodynamic responses, allowing targeted therapeutic intervention (Figure 3.6). Ion channels control the movement of ions through cellular membranes, with a significant impact on cell excitability, signal transduction, and metabolic function. Pharmacologic agents that modify ion channel function either enhance or block ionic currents by interacting with specific channel sites, altering gating kinetics or channel conductance. Modulation can restore altered ionic balances in pathophysiologic conditions, such as myocardial ischemia-reperfusion injury, where calcium ion homeostasis is pivotal. Therapeutic drugs from ancient origins, such as Chinese herbal medicine, have proved to be of potential in affecting mitochondrial ion channels and reducing injury through subtle yet potent modulation of ion fluxes (Tian et al., 2025). This multi-target strategy emphasizes the complex relationship between ion channel dynamics and drug effectiveness within pharmacodynamics. Advances in ion channel modulation include classical pharmacology and emergent bioelectronic paradigms, broadening the therapeutic development toolkit. The developing convergence of organic electrochemical transistor (ECT) technology demonstrates a new approach to interrogating ion channel function and pharmacology. Organic ECTs, which are defined by their bulk electrochemical doping characteristics, offer insight into ionic conductance modulation with high sensitivity and specificity. These devices enable real-time observation of ion flux changes following pharmacological agents, linking molecular interactions to functional readouts. Furthermore, recent research has expanded this idea to two-dimensional materials such as MXenes, further improving detection and modulation capabilities due to their distinct conductive characteristics (Kang et al., 2023). This technology advance not only supports greater mechanistic insight into ion channel function but also promises novel new pathways for drug discovery and precision pharmacology, thus consonant with the objectives of contemporary pharmacodynamics. As part of a larger pharmacodynamics framework, selective ion channel modulation as a strategic initiative, notably in cardiovascular and neurological medicine, presents itself. Stringent control of channel gating and permeability can regulate downstream signaling mechanisms, determining cellular viability, apoptosis, and electrical stability. Modulation of mitochondrial ion channels, for example, regulates ATP generation, reactive oxygen species formation, and calcium handling, all key determinants of ischemic cellular fate. The challenge is to improve drug bioavailability and define precise molecular targets to maximize therapeutic efficacy. Current evidence validates that the convergence of conventional medicinal molecules with novel pharmacokinetic knowledge can amplify the pharmacodynamic properties of ion channel modulators (Tian et al., 2025). Thus, ion channel modulation is a synergistic paradigm in which changing scientific approaches meet proven biological concepts to optimize drug action and ultimately enhance clinical efficacy and safety factors.

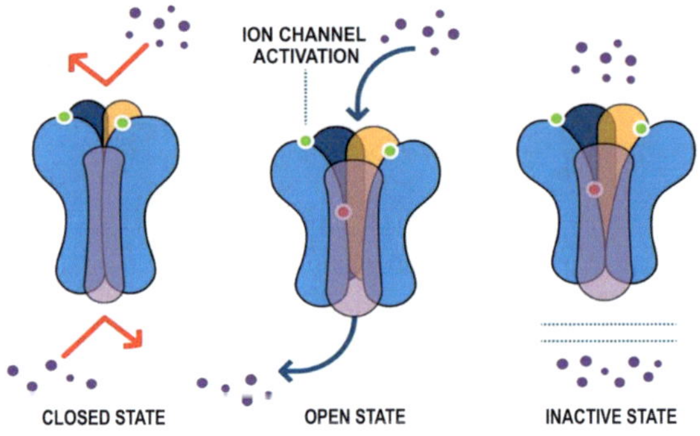

Figure 3.6. Ion channel modulation.

Source: Saniona (2021). *Ion Channels.*

Test Your Knowledge

1. What is mechanisms of drug action?
2. The dynamic behavior of receptor interactions?

3.2. Dose-Response Relationships

Learning Outcome

1. Definition and Significance
2. Types of Dose-Response Curves
3. Factors Influencing Dose-Response

The understanding of how drugs produce their effects in the body is based significantly on the examination of dose-response relationships, an essential principle in pharmacodynamics (Figure 3.7). The relationship demonstrates how drug concentrations of different levels relate to the size of a biological response, with the ability to calculate key parameters of potency and efficacy. These interactions can be quite complicated in cases with drug combinations or interactions, where combined effects do not add up but could reinforce or cancel out each other's action. These combined exposure-response profiles have to be dealt with in sophisticated pharmacodynamic interaction models that facilitate predicting responses and optimizing dosage regimens. The accurate prediction of pharmacodynamic parameters in realistic clinical scenarios is difficult, pointing to the need for pre-knowledge of subject drug responses. When such data are known, they increase the accuracy of dose selection and parameter estimation, leading eventually to better therapeutic outcomes and fewer side effects (Papathanasiou et al., 2018). Investigating dose-response relationships in oncology drug development demonstrates the pivotal contribution of pharmacodynamics to the attainment of therapeutic efficacy with reduced toxicity. New drug candidates, such as liver-specific nucleotide prodrugs, illustrate the value of defining exposure-response relationships through correlations between target-site drug concentrations and biological responses such as DNA damage and tumor inhibition. By this means, dosing requirements that are below those that induce systemic toxicity, for example, in difficult contexts such as hepatocellular carcinoma, can be guaranteed.

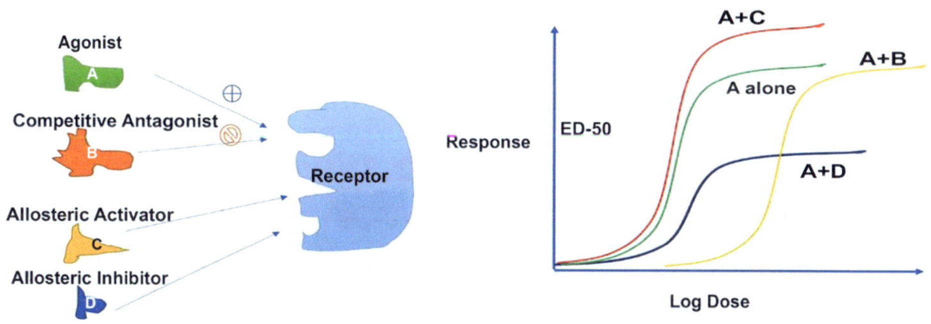

Figure 3.7. Dose-response relationships.

Source: Choudhary, R. (2021). *Drug-Receptor Interaction Dose-Response Curve.*

Information connecting intratumoral drug metabolites to anti-proliferative activities further highlights the therapeutic significance of dose-response experiments, informing dose adjustment and regimen design in an effort to build sustained and effective tumor growth control (Albertella et al., 2017). The real-world application of dose-response relationships goes beyond theoretical model building into concrete clinical and preclinical trial design, calling for optimal study sizes and dosing regimens. Correct description of these relationships aids in understanding the therapeutic window of drugs, weighing the advantages against possible toxicities. In combination therapy scenarios, measurement of pharmacodynamic interactions becomes crucial to determine synergistic or antagonistic effects, which can affect patient management. Although there are inherent difficulties in parameter estimation, combining available monotherapy data with combined drug analysis enhances reliability, showing the dynamic nature of dose-response modeling in pharmacodynamics. This union advances drug development decision-making processes, in the end promoting safer and more efficient pharmacotherapies (Papathanasiou et al., 2018).

3.2.1. Definition and Significance

Grasping the complex correlation between drug concentration and its ensuing effect inside the body is an inherent element of contemporary therapeutics. Pharmacodynamics, in the broadest sense, is the examination of the biochemical and physiologic effects of drugs, as well as the mechanisms of action at the molecular and systemic levels. Pharmacodynamics is essential for describing how drugs interact with cellular receptors, enzymes, and ion channels to bring about therapeutic or toxic responses. By measuring these interactions, pharmacodynamics directs dosage regimens and informs the creation of safer, more effective drugs. Its relevance goes beyond fundamental science, impacting clinical practice and promoting personalized medicine strategies that are specific to individual patient requirements and genetic backgrounds. The clinical relevance of pharmacodynamics is deeply realized in the management of complicated chronic diseases like type 2 diabetes mellitus (T2DM). Considering the variability of patient response to antihyperglycemic drugs, pharmacodynamics explains why the same drugs can have different therapeutic effects in different individuals. Pharmacogenetics provides additional insights by identifying genetic polymorphisms that influence drug efficacy and toxicity, allowing clinicians to tailor pharmacotherapy. This pharmacodynamic integration with genetic information has the capacity to transform treatment paradigms and enable precision medicine approaches that enhance glycemic control with reduced adverse effects in T2DM care (Andreozzi et al., 2019). In addition, pharmacodynamics is central to connecting pharmacokinetics and clinical effectiveness, especially in the treatment of infectious diseases. Therapeutic efficacy is ultimately dependent on the correlation between drug concentration profiles in target tissues and the susceptibility of microorganisms. For instance, research in oxytetracycline against pathogens illustrated the way pharmacodynamic parameters, such as the ratio of area under the concentration-time curve to minimum inhibitory concentration (AUC/MIC), forecast antimicrobial effect. These models guide dosing regimens to maximize eradication of bacteria and minimize development of resistance. Pharmacodynamics hence is crucial in determining effective and rational drug dosage, such that pharmacological action results in their desired clinical impacts (Aliabadi et al., 2018).

3.2.2. Types of Dose-Response Curves

The dose-response curve concept is central to the understanding of drug behavior at different concentrations and its impact on the body. Not all drugs have the same pattern of response; therefore, various forms of dose-response curves (Figure 3.8) assist in explaining the relationship between drug dose and the size of the pharmacological effect. One of the common types is the graded dose-response curve, which is a continuous, proportional rise in effect with an increase in dose until a peak response is achieved. This is particularly helpful in the determination of the efficacy and potency of a drug and in understanding how the effect of a drug varies with concentration. These curves are analyzed to help clinicians identify the best dosage that achieves maximum therapeutic effect with minimum side effects, which is essential when working with drugs with narrow therapeutic windows (Cintron and Putcha, 2025). These patterns form the basis for more sophisticated pharmacodynamic assessments. Aside from the graded dose-response curve, the quantal dose-response curve is of primary importance in pharmacodynamics as it tracks the proportion of a population responding with a certain effect at different doses. In contrast to intensity-measuring graded responses, quantal responses report presence or absence of an effect, for example, therapeutic effect or toxicity, among individuals. This curve plays a crucial role in determining effective dose (ED50), lethal dose (LD50), and toxic dose (TD50) parameters, which determine safety margins and forecast population heterogeneity of drug sensitivity. In addition, the quantal dose-response curve directs the approval of drugs and personalized medicine through highlighting the heterogeneity of people, an aspect that is important for safe management of drugs with a steep dose-response relationship or extensive side effects (Cintron and Putcha, 2025). Therefore, quantal curves supplement graded curves by dealing with population-wide effects instead of individual intensity effects. Besides graded and quantal dose-response curves, biphasic and nonmonotonic dose-response curves elucidate more sophisticated pharmacodynamic phenomena, defying conventional interpretations. Biphasic curves illustrate an initial phase in which a rise in dose increases the effect up to a certain point, after which additional rises decrease the response, typically showing receptor desensitization, toxicity, or regulatory feedback mechanisms. Nonmonotonic curves may have several peaks and troughs, suggesting the action of different receptor subtypes or pathways at different levels of dose. These complex curves reinforce the necessity of simulating multiple dose-response scenarios in order to accurately represent real-world drug behavior. Identification of these curves is crucial in drug development, as they make apparent unanticipated dynamics that are not evident in overly simplistic models, stressing the necessity of robust experimental design and validation to guarantee successful and safe therapeutic interventions.

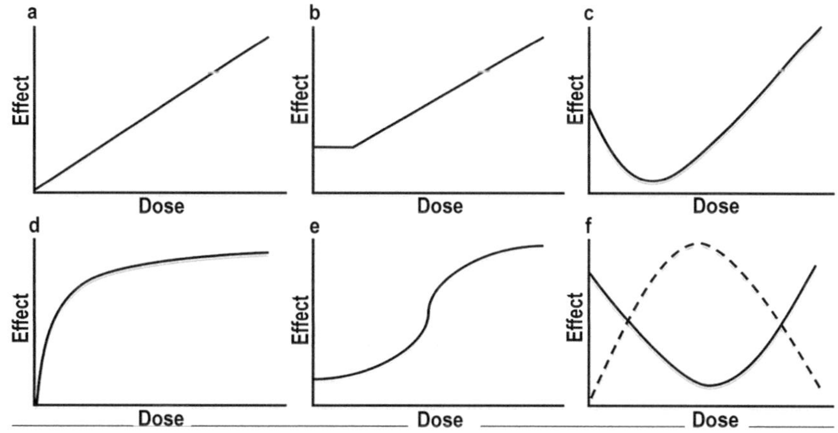

Figure 3.8. Types of dose-response curves.

Source: Ennulat, D. (2016). Illustration of common dose–response curves. In L. Ramaiah, M. J. Hinrichs, & E. V. Skuba (Eds.), *Interpreting and integrating clinical and anatomic pathology results* (p. 1). Wiley.

3.2.3. Factors Influencing Dose-Response

The response of a drug to the biological system on which it acts is not just a function of the dose administered but is complexly regulated by a variety of factors that finally affect the dose-response relationship (Figure 3.9). Of these, patient-specific factors like genetic background and previous history of treatment have key roles. For instance, in antiretroviral therapy, pharmacokinetic variation of drugs such as protease inhibitors and reverse transcriptase inhibitors in plasma can cause large differences in therapeutic responses. This variation results from metabolic, adherence, and resistance differences, which eventually alter the dose-response curve and limit the accuracy of pharmacodynamic predictions. Individualizing dosage regimens in a patient can maximize these effects, but personalization risks loss of efficacy and added side effects, highlighting the nuance of dose-response modulation (Hentig et al., 2012).

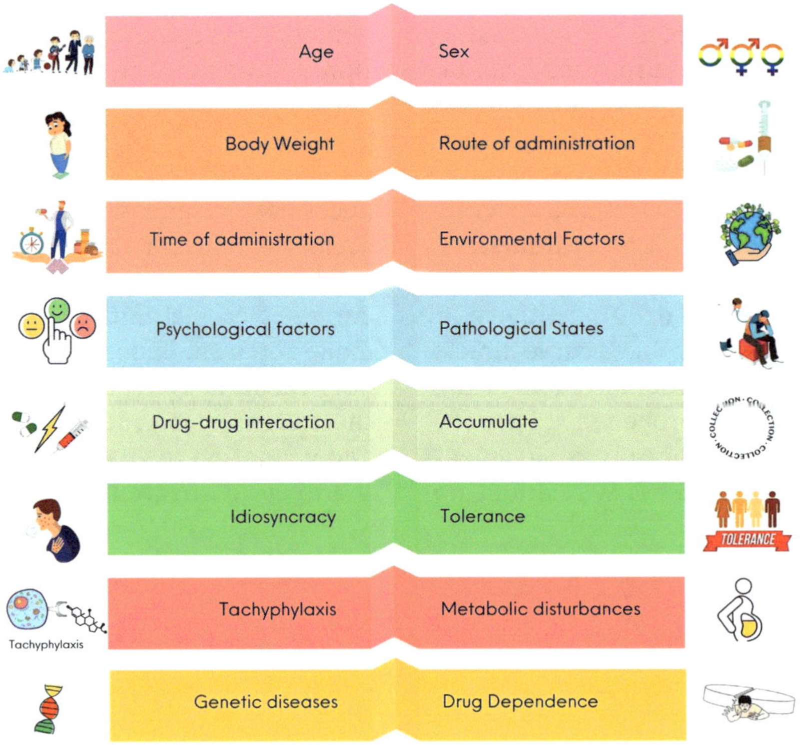

Figure 3.9. Factors influencing dose-response.

Source: LearnAboutPharma (2022). *Posology: Factors Influencing Dose.* https://www.learnaboutpharma.com/wp-content/uploads/2022/09/Posology-_-factors-influencing-Dose.jpg.

Furthermore, biological diversity by nature goes beyond metabolism to involve genetic variation influencing drug targets themselves, changing drug sensitivity and effect. Within the context of analgesic medication, heterogeneity in pain sensitivity and analgesic effect is partially predestined by genetic factors, which affect the pharmacodynamics of such drugs. Whereas metabolic phenomena have been comprehensively investigated via genotype-phenotype correlations, the clinical relevance of inherited drug-receptor interaction variation is not yet well understood. This knowledge deficit hinders the creation of fully personalized analgesic therapy, which captures the complex interplay of variables controlling dose-response relations. The difficulty is in converting these genetic findings into useful therapeutic modifications without losing safety or efficacy (Branford et al., 2013). Physiological, pathological, and environmental conditions complicate the dose-response relationship by modifying drug absorption, distribution, metabolism, and elimination. Age, liver and renal function, and comorbidities modulate bioavailability of drugs and responsiveness of receptors, which consequently affect the magnitude and duration of pharmacologic effects. Additionally, drug interactions may potentiate or diminish drug activity, shifting the dose-response curve either toward increased toxicity or reduced effectiveness. Understanding these multifaceted influences necessitates a comprehensive pharmacodynamic assessment to predict the therapeutic window accurately and minimize adverse reactions. Hence, integrating patient-specific variables into dosing strategies represents an essential step in advancing individualized pharmacotherapy.

Test Your Knowledge

1. Which of Factors Influencing Dose-Response?
2. The Types of Dose-Response Curves?

3.3. Therapeutic Window

Learning Outcome

1. Definition and Importance
2. Determining the Therapeutic Window
3. Implications for Drug Safety

The idea of attaining maximum therapeutic effects in pharmacodynamics goes beyond the mere delivery of a drug; it requires an exact balance between efficacy and safety. This balance is contained within the therapeutic window (Figure 3.10), an essential range of drug concentration where the drug brings about its desired effects without generating severe adverse reactions. Narrow therapeutic windows are particularly problematic, particularly in therapies where tight drug plasma control is necessary to ensure maximum benefit with a minimum of toxicity. Antiretroviral treatments for HIV, for example, exhibit significant inter- and intra-individual variability, making drug level maintenance within this window difficult. Tailored dosing regimens have been suggested to adjust plasma levels to individual factors, thus maximizing therapeutic effect and minimizing side effects. Nonetheless, such individualization threatens to undermine efficacy or promote drug resistance unless well controlled, pointing to the subtlety of preserving the fine balance within the therapeutic window in the clinical setting (Hentig et al., 2012). Individual differences are central to determining the limits and efficacy of the therapeutic window. Genetic variability affects drug metabolism, distribution, and receptor sensitivity, leading to differences in drug response between patients. Pharmacogenetics and pharmacogenomics have become invaluable tools in the discovery of these genetic factors, most prominently polymorphisms in the cytochrome P450 enzymes CYP2D6 and CYP2C19. These enzymes are responsible for metabolizing many drugs, influencing their windows of therapeutic action by changing the plasma drug concentrations required for drug effect without producing toxicity.

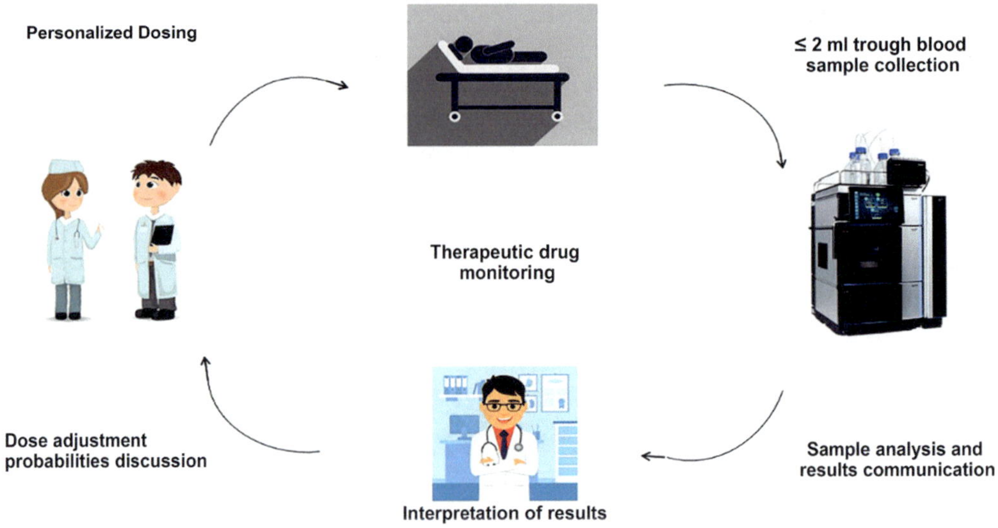

Figure 3.10. Therapeutic window in pharmacodynamics.

Source: Ennulat, D. (2022). *Overview of Therapeutic Drug Monitoring (TDM) Applications in Cytotoxic Anticancer Drug Therapy.*

The incorporation of pharmacogenetic testing into the clinical environment has the potential to further define personalized medicine strategies by enabling medication selection and dosing based on the individual's genetic makeup. Personalized pharmacotherapy can better keep drug concentrations in the therapeutic range by predicting side effects and metabolic variations, thereby maximizing treatment effectiveness (Petek et al., 2009). Even with the progress made in molecular and genetic knowledge, the application of therapeutic window considerations continues to depend on clinical judgment. The process of deciding on a suitable drug, dosing schedule, and tapering plan needs a sophisticated appreciation of pharmacodynamics within the context of individual patient factors. Although pharmacogenetics provides critical information that diminishes doubt about drug metabolism and possible side effects, it is unable to substitute the clinicians function in dynamically adjusting treatment protocols. This interaction between advancing scientific knowledge and clinical acumen highlights the continuing advancement of pharmacodynamics. Finally, keeping drug concentration in the therapeutic window is a keystone of successful therapy, requiring precision and caution to balance efficacy and safety across varied patient populations (Hentig et al., 2012; Petek et al., 2009).

3.3.1. Definition and Importance

Knowing the relationship between drugs and biological systems is the basis for most medical and pharmaceutical therapies. Pharmacodynamics addresses the mechanism of how drugs act on the body, including the drug concentration at the site of action and the produced effect. The discipline explains mechanisms like receptor binding, signal transduction, and modulation of physiological processes. By characterizing these interactions, pharmacodynamics enables the prediction of therapeutic effects and possible adverse effects. This information is important because it guides dosage regimens, maximizing efficacy while minimizing toxicity. Therefore, pharmacodynamics provides a scientific foundation for personalizing treatments to individual patients, complementing personalized medicine strategies that are consistent with ethical and clinical standards in healthcare decision-making (Visseren et al., 2021). The significance of pharmacodynamics goes beyond theoretical comprehension to real-world implementation within clinical practice. It helps clinicians make the right drug choices on the basis of their action mechanisms, potency, and duration of action, thereby enhancing the quality of patient care. Further, pharmaceutical research hinges on pharmacodynamic rules of thumb to create new therapeutics that selectively engage pathologic targets, minimizing off-target effects and enhancing safety profiles. Without the insights of this science, drug development would be directionless, and it could result in ineffective or even dangerous treatments. Thus, pharmacodynamics is an essential bridge between laboratory science and clinical therapeutics, making sure that interventions are scientifically sound as well as clinically applicable (François et al., 2019). Additionally, pharmacodynamics is supported by other pharmacological features like pharmacokinetics to give a complete picture of drug behavior in the body. Whereas pharmacokinetics concerns drug transport via absorption, distribution, metabolism, and excretion (ADME), pharmacodynamics concerns drug action and effect. This combined view facilitates optimal dosing plans, particularly in complicated situations such as polypharmacy or inconsistent patient response. Awareness of the dynamic interaction between drug concentration and effect is also conducive to the prediction of drug interactions and side effects. In this way, pharmacodynamics plays a major role in the development of evidence-based medicine as it allows healthcare providers to personalize treatment successfully, ensuring safer and more effective therapeutic outcomes (François et al., 2019; Visseren et al., 2021).

3.3.2. Determining the Therapeutic Window

Determining the balance between efficacy and toxicity is a foundation in the creation of pharmacological agents, especially in establishing the therapeutic window. This range constitutes the interval between the minimum effective dose and the threshold of side effects, representing a vital sign of a drug's safety profile. Experimental assessment is most often achieved by animal model testing to determine doses that are effective therapeutically without causing adverse effects, allowing researchers to know the margin of safety. The value of these experiments is in the design of dosage regimens to achieve optimal therapeutic benefits with minimal risk, particularly for effective drugs having narrow margins. Having set this window allows future clinical trials to proceed with informed dosing regimens, ultimately bettering patient outcome and minimizing incidence of toxicity by carefully monitoring pharmacodynamics. Advanced formulations and rigorous dosing schedules in preclinical trials are usually utilized to hone the pharmacokinetic and pharmacodynamic profiles critical for establishing the therapeutic window. As an example, the pharmacokinetic assessment of IDD-1040, a new conjugate of lipoic acid with paclitaxel, showed a prolonged circulation half-life and slower metabolism than the parent compound, indicating a potentially wider therapeutic window. These pharmacokinetic parameters, such as volume of distribution and half-life, are key to anticipating drug behavior *in vivo* and directing the optimization of doses. In addition, formulation developments that allow for increased drug content without surfactants indicate enhanced delivery systems that can sustain drug stability and bioavailability, further enhancing a more precise and potentially expanded therapeutic window (Abu-Lafi et al., 2025). These advancements allow for safer dosing regimens and emphasize the multi-dimensional approach needed to precisely identify effective dose ranges. Toxicological studies in multiple rodent models offer precious information for determining secure therapeutic limits since illustrated by evaluation of the peptidomimetic synthetic antimicrobial agent SAMP-1. Markers of dose-dependent lethality and acute toxicity were carefully noted to define its toxic and effective dose limits. These studies resulted in a therapeutic window of intermediate efficacious doses and higher doses that caused distributive shock and death, highlighting the importance of calibrating dose carefully to prevent toxic side effects. Accurate identification of semi-lethal doses provides a quantitative basis for calculation of therapeutic index, an important step in pharmacodynamics that informs clinical dosing strategies. Finally, such toxicological profiling, along with additional cell culture experiments, further enhances insight into the interaction of the drug with biological membranes and helps to safely walk a line between efficacy and toxicity (Lyubushkina et al., 2024).

3.3.3. Implications for Drug Safety

Individual differences in drug response are a major challenge to providing drug safety (Figure 3.11). Genetic variation, notably in drug-metabolizing enzymes like cytochrome P450s, may produce aberrant pharmacodynamic effects.

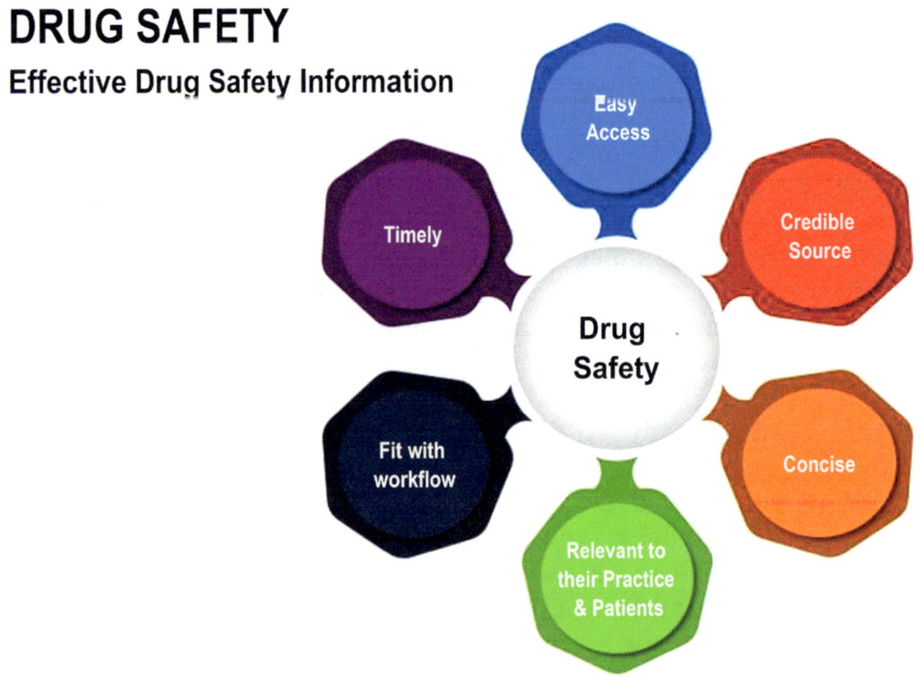

Figure 3.11. Implications for drug safety.

Source: Collidu. (2022). *Drug Safety.* https://www.collidu.com/media/catalog/product/img/2/3/23dc666933552c26eaa987c2fabfbadddc2a485b87f61c2f04b4570fb90a9354/drug-safety-slide3.png.

For instance, enzyme polymorphisms may cause some patients to inactivate drugs too slowly or too rapidly, generating increased toxicity or diminished therapeutic action. This heterogeneity requires meticulous dosing and monitoring to prevent drug side effects, particularly for agents with narrow therapeutic windows. Pharmacometabolomics, a relatively new field of study, provides useful information about these metabolic differences by profiling patients' individual biochemical responses to medications. With these biochemical pathways more fully understood, clinicians can better anticipate patient outcomes and modify treatment regimens to optimize drug efficacy while improving safety overall (Alshamrani et al., 2024). Additionally, population-specific genetic profiles also complicate drug safety landscape. Research on genetic polymorphism in drug metabolizing enzymes in different populations—like Arab populations—evidences major allelic variability impacting drug pharmacodynamics and safety profiles. Differences in enzymes like CYP450, GST, and UGT can vary drug metabolism rates, thus modulating adverse drug reactions (ADRs) or therapeutic failure risk. Identification of these genetic variations allows for the creation of personalized medicine approaches specific to certain ethnic populations. This specificity in designing treatment protocols not only reduces safety concerns but also optimizes drug effectiveness in heterogeneous populations, highlighting the importance of pharmacogenomics in contemporary pharmacodynamics studies (Eitan et al., 2024).

Incorporation of pharmacogenetic and pharmacometabolomic information into clinical practice has revolutionary potential for drug safety. By integrating genetic data with metabolic profiling, clinicians can have an overall picture of an individual's response to drugs and, therefore, make more judicious prescribing decisions. This strategy minimizes the occurrence of ADRs by detecting patients at risk of toxicity or failure of therapy prior to treatment. Therefore, the use of personalized pharmacotherapy through in-depth biochemical and genetic analysis promotes safer drug use and better outcomes for patients. This pharmacodynamic assessment evolution has the potential to close gaps in standard dosing paradigms and progress toward an individualized, proactive model of drug safety management (Alshamrani et al., 2024; Eitan et al., 2024).

Test Your Knowledge

1. How do drug safety response are a major challenge?
2. The Importance relationship between drugs and biological systems?

3.4. Pharmacokinetics Versus Pharmacodynamics

Learning Outcome

1. Definitions and Differences
2. Interplay Between Pharmacokinetics and Pharmacodynamics
3. Clinical Relevance of Both Fields

Understanding the complex interactions between drugs and the human body requires a clear distinction between pharmacokinetics and pharmacodynamics, two fundamental concepts that guide therapeutic strategies (Figure 3.12). Pharmacokinetics involves the ADME of drugs, essentially describing the journey of a drug within the body. In contrast, pharmacodynamics focuses on the drug's biochemical and physiological effects and the mechanisms through which these effects are achieved. This differential emphasis is essential since whereas pharmacokinetics sets the concentration of a drug that arrives at the target site, pharmacodynamics dictates the resulting biological effect. Combining both areas enables clinicians to customize medication regimens for maximized efficacy and reduced toxicity, as in studies where drug concentration-time profiles closely correlate with clinical outcomes in infection therapies (Singh et al., 2024). Also critical is the manner in which pharmacokinetics guides dosage regimens to meet desired pharmacodynamic outcomes, maintaining drug levels within a therapeutic range. As an illustration, time-dependent antibiotics involve sustaining above-the-minimum-inhibitory-concentration concentrations during a proportion of the dosing interval to maximize bacterial killing, a concept gleaned from pharmacokinetic/pharmacodynamic models. This mutual relationship highlights the reason why precise measurement of drug properties like proton dissociation constants can affect both drug absorption and receptor binding affinity, which in turn affects overall drug action (Pálla et al., 2024). Therefore, pharmacodynamics cannot be comprehensively understood without a proper understanding of pharmacokinetics, as the biological effect depends on the concentration and duration of drug exposure at the target site.

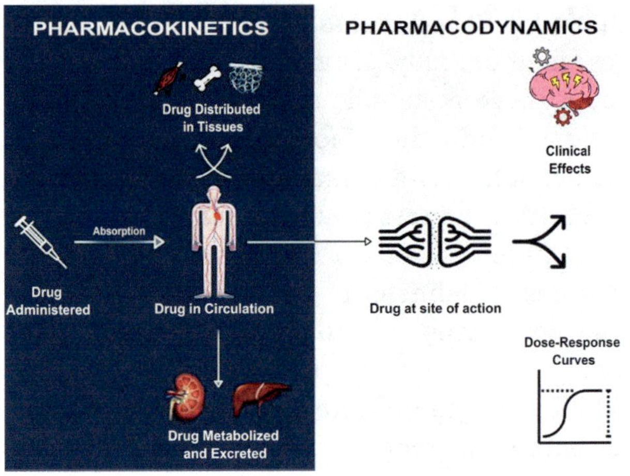

Figure 3.12. Pharmacokinetics Versus pharmacodynamics.

Source: https://i.ytimg.com/vi/jIkQI4cBaBE/maxresdefault.jpg.

The experimental significance of the separation between pharmacokinetics and pharmacodynamics comes alive clinically in drug discovery and clinical practice, where both components need to be optimized simultaneously. For example, recent evidence from antimicrobial drugs illustrates the ways in which pharmacokinetic parameters such as the duration above minimum inhibitory concentration are reflected in pharmacodynamic effect, converting into meaningful enhancement in patient care at the cost of fewer adverse effects (Singh et al., 2024). This interplay increases drug therapy by guiding adjustments in dosing based on patient-specific variables, such as metabolism and disease pathology. Additionally, developments in analytical methods for capturing precise descriptions of molecular behavior, such as with spectroscopic titration protocols, further optimize dosing strategies to capture maximum pharmacodynamic responses (Pálla et al., 2024). Therefore, understanding the complex interplay between pharmacokinetics and pharmacodynamics is still critical towards pushing pharmacotherapy forward.

3.4.1. Definitions and Differences

The interaction of drugs with their biological targets provides the basis for therapeutic effect and possible adverse effects. Pharmacodynamics is essentially concerned with how a drug produces its effect on the body, including mechanisms such as receptor binding, signal transduction, and resultant cellular responses. One of the fundamental differences in pharmacodynamics is the differentiation between affinity and efficacy: affinity is the propensity of a drug to be attracted to its receptor, whereas efficacy is the capacity of the drug-receptor complex to produce a biological response. This distinction is crucial for understanding why two drugs with similar binding capacity can result in enormously different clinical effects. Additional complexity comes in thinking about genetic variability affecting drug responses, particularly evident in analgesics where inherited differences in receptor genes, including the μ-opioid receptor, affect pharmacodynamic responses, underscoring the difficulty in making personalized treatments (Branford et al., 2013). Appreciation of differences in pharmacodynamic mechanisms is important when comparing drug classes, particularly with cardiovascular therapeutics. For instance, antiplatelet drugs work by different mechanisms to inhibit thrombus formation, an essential process in acute myocardial infarction. Aspirin blocks cyclooxygenase, suppressing thromboxane-mediated platelet activation, while newer drugs such as vorapaxar block protease-activated receptors to suppress platelet aggregation through different signaling pathways. These differences not only extend to therapeutic effects but also to safety profiles; vorapaxar, although effective in lowering ischemic events, has an increased risk of bleeding complications. These differences reinforce the need to comprehend particular pharmacodynamic mechanisms to maximize therapy and weigh benefits against risks in clinical decision-making (Farag et al., 2015). In addition, pharmacodynamics is distinguished from pharmacokinetics since the former accounts for drug effects on the body while the latter refers to drug ADME. While pharmacokinetics defines drug concentration at the target tissue, pharmacodynamics describes the resulting physiological or biochemical effect. This distinction explains why two patients with identical drug plasma concentrations may have divergent clinical responses, usually owing to receptor sensitivity, signal transduction efficiency, or downstream regulatory processes. In clinical settings, an understanding of these differences is critical for interpreting drug response variability, informing dose adjustments, and designing novel therapeutic agents. While pharmacokinetic variability has been well characterized, pharmacodynamic mechanisms, particularly genetic determinants of receptor activity, are an essential area for ongoing research to provide personalized medicine (Branford et al., 2013).

3.4.2. Interplay Between Pharmacokinetics and Pharmacodynamics

The safety and effectiveness of any drug treatment depend on the subtle balance between pharmacokinetics—the ADME of drugs—and pharmacodynamics, which characterizes the biochemical and physiological effects caused by the drug on the body (Figure 3.13). Pharmacokinetics controls the drug concentration at its site of action, directly affecting the extent and duration of pharmacodynamic effects. For instance, ticagrelor's metabolic rate, an antiplatelet drug, is regulated by several patient-specific factors like the condition of diabetes or acute coronary syndromes, which change drug metabolism mainly through hepatic enzymes CYP3A. Such metabolism variability impacts the plasma concentration of the parent drug as well as its active metabolite, thus influencing the drug's antiplatelet activity and safety profile (Ibanez et al., 2018). Appreciation of this interaction is essential in the rational optimization of dosing regimens for the enhancement of therapeutic effects and reduction in adverse drug reactions. Pharmacokinetic variability can significantly affect the pharmacodynamic consequences of drug treatment, particularly in multifactorial diseases. Antimalarial drug administration in mass drug administration programs provides an example of how drug pharmacokinetics determine therapeutic efficacy and control of the disease. Long-acting prophylactic drugs offer prolonged protection by sustaining therapeutic drug levels, which enhances the pharmacodynamic effect of long-term malaria parasite suppression. Pharmacodynamic efficacy is compromised, though, if pharmacokinetic parameters like drug absorption or clearance significantly differ between populations or with comorbidities.

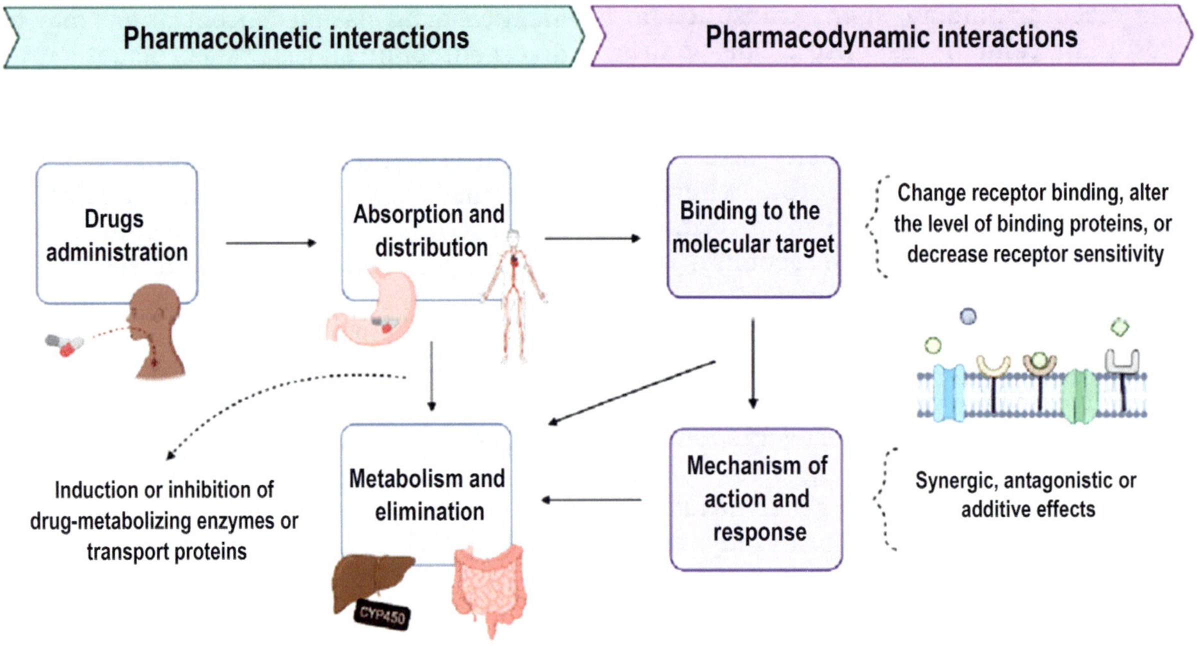

Figure 3.13. Interplay between pharmacokinetics and pharmacodynamics.

Source: Maciel, L. F. (2022). *Pharmacokinetic and Pharmacodynamic Drug Interactions.*

For example, simulations of artemisinin-based combination therapies demonstrate that decreased drug levels resulting from nonadherence or accelerated metabolism lower malaria parasite clearance, emphasizing the necessity of regular drug exposure to meet desirable pharmacodynamic outcomes (Eckhoff et al., 2015). Therefore, the pharmacokinetic profile needs to be taken into account while planning treatment regimens to improve clinical success and public health benefits. The complex interaction between pharmacokinetics and pharmacodynamics is also made more complex by outside influences like drug-drug interactions (DDIs) and individual patient conditions.

For instance, some co-administered drugs like morphine can affect the metabolism of ticagrelor, influencing the rate of conversion to its active metabolite and thereby reducing its pharmacodynamic antiplatelet effect in acute coronary syndromes (Ibanez et al., 2018). Additionally, aspects of lifestyle such as smoking can stimulate hepatic enzymes, stimulating drug metabolism and thus altering the degree of drug action. These interactions highlight the need to incorporate pharmacokinetic information into pharmacodynamic assessments for customized therapies. By critically analyzing these interactions, clinicians will be able to predict therapeutic effects more accurately and adjust treatment regimens accordingly to provide a more accurate balance between efficacy and toxicity.

3.4.3. Clinical Relevance of Both Fields

Pharmacodynamic advances have greatly improved clinical decision-making by giving insight into the complex interplay between drug effect and patient heterogeneity (Figure 3.14). This is particularly critical when population-level differences are considered, which can greatly modify drug efficacy and safety profiles. The use of modeling and simulation tools that incorporate pharmacokinetic information along with species-specific physiological variations enables clinicians to better predict individual and group responses. These methods enable accurate dosing, thus maximizing therapeutic effects and reducing side effects. Practical application of such models is critical in veterinary medicine, where the high diversity of species renders dosing regimes cumbersome. Through investigation of sources of variation using combined pharmacokinetic and *in vitro* data, clinicians may individualize therapy with increased certainty, demonstrating the critical role of pharmacodynamics within human and veterinary medicine to increase the safe and effective application of drugs (Bailey et al., 2018). Clinical significance is reinforced by the influence of patient-related factors like age and sex on pharmacodynamic variation. In disorders such as Attention Deficit/Hyperactivity Disorder (ADHD), where the first line of treatment is with stimulant medications, it is important to recognize these moderating variables to optimize therapeutic management. There is evidence that response to drugs tends to be generally effective in different ages and genders; however, subtleties like decreased effectiveness and enhanced side effects in preschool children reflect the complexity of drug-pharmacodynamic interactions. Although few studies directly evaluate the moderating influences of age and sex on drug response, current data suggest that pharmacodynamics can vary subtly between patient populations. This necessitates more stringent investigation of these factors to optimize dosing parameters and enhance individualized treatment regimens, thus making pharmacodynamic information clinically relevant across diverse populations (Barke et al., 2010). The clinical application of pharmacodynamic principles thus promises much in the realization of personalized medicine. An awareness of the heterogeneity arising from genetic, physiological, and demographic variations enables healthcare professionals to transcend the use of standardized dosing towards a personalized approach that maximizes patient safety and efficacy. This shift in paradigm is dependent on ongoing research into the intricate relationship between drugs and biological systems, underpinned by sound data analytics and predictive modeling. These advances not only fill gaps in the understanding of drug response heterogeneity but also better enable the ability to predict and prevent ADRs. In the end, the convergence of pharmacodynamics and patient-specific factors cement its importance in optimizing therapeutic intervention and improving clinical practice, validating its worth in all areas of medicine and patient populations (Bailey et al., 2018; Barke et al., 2010).

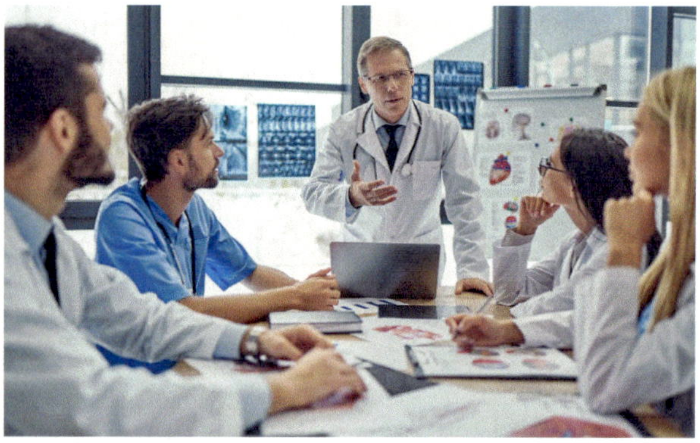

Figure 3.14. Clinical decision-making by relevance of both fields.

Source: Talus. (2020). *Doctors in Clinical Practice.* https://talus.com.au/wp-content/uploads/2020/04/doctors-in-clinical-practice.jpg.

Test Your Knowledge

1. What is clinical relevance of both fields?
2. Define the pharmacokinetics and Pharmacodynamics?

3.5. Factors Affecting Drug Response

Learning Outcome

1. Genetic Variability
2. Age and Gender Differences
3. Environmental Influences

The success of pharmacologic treatment frequently depends on a multifactorial interaction of individual physiological parameters, which may have a marked effect on drug response. Differences in organ function, particularly hepatic and renal function, are critical because these organs are major sites for drug metabolism and excretion. Changes in hepatic enzyme activity may alter the rate of drug metabolism, with possible resultant subtherapeutic effect or toxicity. Likewise, reduced renal clearance influences the elimination of drugs and can lead to accumulation to toxic concentrations. Alterations in the plasma protein composition and binding capacity also influence the free concentration of drugs, affecting their availability at receptor sites. It is important to understand these physiological considerations when evaluating therapeutic regimens, as illustrated in specialized situations like spaceflight, where body fluid distribution, organ perfusion, and metabolic function change, influencing pharmacokinetics and pharmacodynamics. It is by addressing these differences that drug dosing can be optimized to retain effectiveness while reducing adverse effects (Cintron and Putcha, 2025). Another important factor in drug response variability is the route of drug delivery and the individual treatment situation of the patient. For instance, in the treatment of infections in PD patients, drug disposition can be significantly influenced by the dialysis modality and the administration route. Intraperitoneal vancomycin dosing, frequently based on continuous ambulatory PD data, is not necessarily transferable to automated PD patients because of the variation in dwell times and dialysate flow rates. This difference highlights the need for pharmacokinetic studies specific to patient conditions to determine proper dosing. The absence of strong evidence in such cases highlights the dilemma clinicians encounter in reconciling effective antimicrobial action with the potential for toxicity, demonstrating how pharmacodynamic principles need to be combined with patient-specific factors to optimize treatment strategies (Kraft et al., 2020). Genetic heterogeneity and the occurrence of co-morbidities also complicate drug response by modifying receptor sensitivity and downstream signaling pathways. Polymorphisms in drug-metabolizing enzymes, transporters, and target receptors may result in considerable interindividual variations in the efficacy and safety profiles of drugs. Moreover, disease states like liver cirrhosis, congestive heart failure, or infection can interfere with normal physiological function and alter both pharmacokinetic parameters and pharmacodynamic responses. These combined forces require an individualized therapy, where dose modifications and pharmacodynamic monitoring are guided by a detailed knowledge of the patients genetic constitution and medical status. The inclusion of these in clinical practice is essential for attaining the best therapeutic effects with a minimum of ADRs, thus again highlighting the relevance of personalized medicine in pharmacodynamics (Figure 3.15).

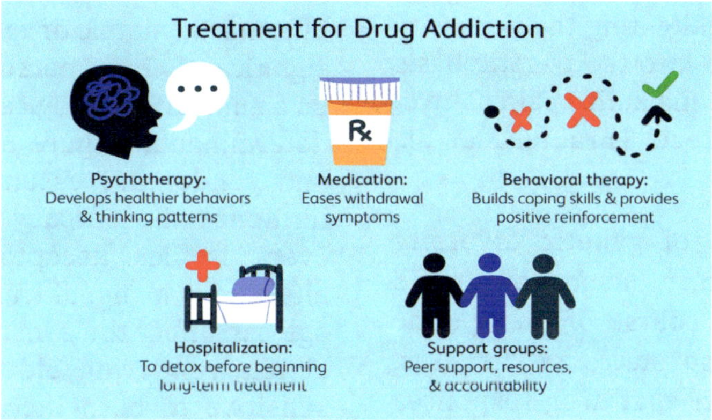

Figure 3.15. Factors affecting drug response; the effectiveness of pharmacological treatment.

Source: Verywell Health. (2023). *The Effects of Drug Addiction.*

3.5.1. Genetic Variability

Elucidation of drug response complexity needs to involve a consideration of the genetic factors behind pharmacodynamics. Pharmacodynamic differences in drug action and toxicity typically arise from genetic variation in drug targets, e.g., receptors, enzymes, and ion channels (Figure 3.16). Instead of concentrating on pharmacokinetic issues like absorption and metabolism, newer studies emphasize polymorphisms involving drug targets themselves. These genetic differences may modify the binding affinity, functional activity, or downstream signaling pathways initiated by drugs, thus modulating therapeutic effects. These findings explain why clinically equivalent doses can result in dramatically dissimilar responses in patients. This increasing interest in genetic variation is essential in the creation of personalized treatment plans, particularly in oncology and orphan diseases, where the interaction between drug-target associations and genetic mutations fundamentally influences efficacy and safety profiles (Altamura et al., 2022). Genetic variability becomes most relevant in clinical practice in the case of analgesic pharmacodynamics. Perception of pain and the effectiveness of analgesic drugs are not consistent between populations, in part because of inherited genetic variation. While pharmacokinetic determinants such as drug metabolism have been well characterized by genotype–phenotype relationships, the genetic regulators of the pharmacodynamic actions of analgesics are less clear. For instance, genetic variation in the μ-opioid receptor gene influences opioid analgesia, but numerous other genes involved in pain modulation and drug response remain to be identified or replicated definitively in studies. This lack of clarity inhibits the achievement of truly personalized analgesic treatment regimens, highlighting the necessity for further investigation into the genetic basis of pharmacodynamics to maximize pain control and reduce adverse effects (Branford et al., 2013).

The incorporation of genetic diversity into pharmacodynamic assessment is gradually changing the course of therapeutic interventions in diverse states of diseases. Current findings indicate that drug responses may be predicted, in addition to assisting in the selection of new drugs that act through variant-specific mechanisms. Clinicians can anticipate the development of resistance or increased sensitivity by realizing the manner in which genetic polymorphism affects drug-receptor interaction. Nonetheless, the challenge persists to convert this information into standard clinical practice, at least partly owing to variable replication of genetic association analyses and the intricate polygenic quality of numerous drug responses. Nevertheless, the development of pharmacogenetics holds potential to increase drug efficacy and safety by providing a more accurate match between an individual's genotype and the pharmacodynamic properties of drugs prescribed (Altamura et al., 2022; Branford et al., 2013).

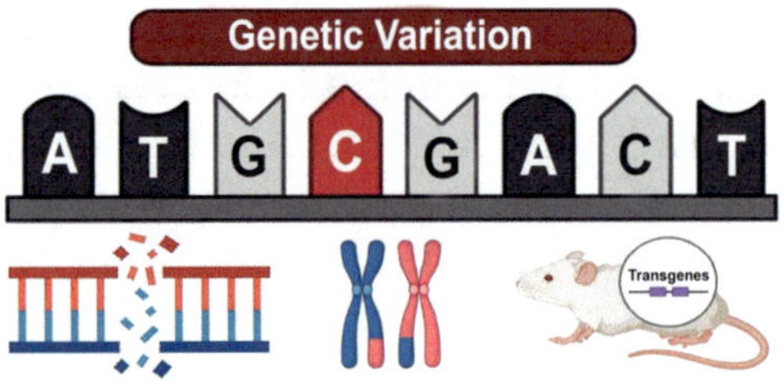

Figure 3.16. Genetic variability.

Source: Microbe Notes. (2022). *Genetic Variation.* https://microbenotes.com/wp-content/uploads/2022/07/Genetic-Variation.jpg.

3.5.2. Age and Gender Differences

Pharmacodynamic drug responses tend to differ significantly from person to person, depending on a number of biological as well as sociocultural determinants (Figure 3.17). Among these, age and gender are essential determinants that influence the efficacy of drugs and adverse event profiles. Receptor density changes and alterations in signal transduction systems with age can affect the sensitivity of tissues to drug action, rendering elderly patients especially sensitive to both increased drug action and toxicity. Simultaneously, gender variations include differences in hormone secretion, enzyme activity, and tissue composition, influencing the interaction between drugs and their sites of action. For example, women in general have a higher receptor binding capacity for psychotropic drugs, leading to improved therapeutic effects at reduced doses compared to men. These differences highlight the requirement of examining age and gender in pharmacodynamic research to achieve optimal dosing regimens and enhance therapeutic outcomes. Additionally, gender-related and aging-related hormonal fluctuations modify pharmacodynamics by controlling the availability of receptors and downstream cascades of signaling. Sex steroids like testosterone and estrogen not only control drug-metabolizing enzyme systems but also affect receptor expression in central nervous system (CNS) and peripheral tissues. The reduction of sex hormones with age, especially in postmenopausal women and andropausal men, can alter immune responses and drug receptor profiles, thus changing both efficacy and susceptibility to side effects. This is further illustrated in the treatment of psychiatric illness, where women, because of hormonal milieu and genetic influences, tend to respond to antipsychotic drugs at lower doses than men, possibly decreasing the risk of dose-related adverse effects. All such individuals highlight the influence of the interplay among gender, age, and inherent genetic profile in the creation of the pharmacodynamic profile (Mary, 2021). Along with biological factors, sociocultural gender roles and lifestyle influences cross paths with age to influence drug response and compliance patterns. Gender-defined behaviors, such as health-seeking activities and adherence to medical regimens, tend to differ between different phases of life and may modulate the therapeutic efficacy. For instance, women's higher health awareness in combination with hormonal fluctuations can influence drug sensitivity and metabolism, whereas men's varied exposure to environmental toxins or workplace hazards can modulate disease progression and response to treatment. More recent studies on sex- and gender-based health disparities, emphasized in pandemic situations like COVID-19, demonstrate how immune responses and therapeutic effects are also influenced by both biological sex and gendered behavior. These observations dictate an integrated strategy in pharmacodynamics that incorporates age and gender as dynamic and interacting variables to tailor precision medicine optimally (Primavera et al., 2020).

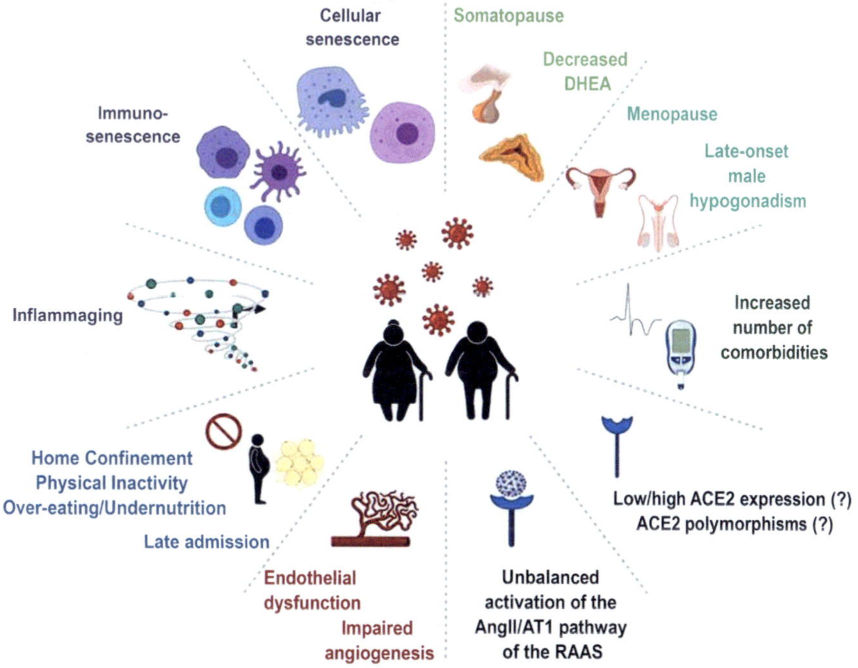

Figure 3.17. Age-related changes in receptor density and signal transduction.

Source: Maciel, L. F., & Marazuela, M. (2022). *Age-Related Endocrine And Immunologic Factors Leading to Severe COVID-19*. In L. F. Maciel, M. Marazuela, & A. Giustina (Eds.), *Aging Versus Youth: Endocrine Aspects of Vulnerability for COVID-19*. Reviews in Endocrine and Metabolic Disorders, 23(2), 1–2.

3.5.3. Environmental Influences

Pharmacodynamic drug responses are not entirely determined by intrinsic genetic influences, but they are also very much shaped by environmental factors that interact with the biochemical systems of the body. Dietary intake, co-administrated drugs, and environmental exposure to toxins are some of the factors that may regulate enzyme activity involved in drug metabolism, consequently modifying the therapeutic effects and side effects of drugs. For example, environmental exposure to inducers or inhibitors of cytochrome P450 enzymes can influence drug metabolism, resulting in differences in drug concentration at the site of action. This interaction presents significant issues in clinical practice, where drug response variability may not be accounted for by genetics alone. Knowledge of these environmental modulators can improve individualized pharmacotherapy by predicting changes in drug efficacy and toxicity under varying external conditions. Besides diet and chemical exposure, lifestyle determinants like smoking, alcohol use, and even stress levels contribute to the environmental profile defining pharmacodynamic effects. Such determinants can stimulate or suppress metabolic enzymes and transport proteins, hence affecting both drug clearance and receptor sensitivity. The intricacies of such interactions are clear when taking the case of drugs such as ketamine, where the metabolism is primarily carried out through polymorphic cytochrome P450 enzymes. Co-administration with other drugs that follow such metabolic pathways adds complexity to such effects through DDIs, which unpredictably increase or decrease drug action. Understanding the dynamic nature of these environmental factors is critical to maximizing dosing regimens and enhancing safety profiles, particularly for drugs with narrow therapeutic windows (Langmia et al., 2022). Furthermore, anesthesiology emphasizes the multifactorial character of environmental factors on drug response, particularly with drugs like propofol. Considerable interindividual variability in the pharmacodynamics of propofol has been noted, resulting not just from genetic polymorphism but also environmental influences on enzyme function and receptor interaction. Environmental factors could encompass co-medication, nutrition, and more general physiological states determined by lifestyle or extrinsic stressors. These factors collectively adjust the metabolism and action of anesthetic drugs, highlighting the difficulty in expecting drug responses on the basis of genetic information alone. The interaction between environment and genetics requires a comprehensive strategy to pharmacodynamic study, as it may enable more accurate anesthetic management and customized therapy planning (Budi et al., 2022).

Test Your Knowledge

1. Define genetic variability in pharmacology?
2. How does age affect drug absorption?

3.6. Clinical Applications of Pharmacodynamics

Learning Outcome

1. Drug Development and Testing
2. Personalized Medicine
3. Case Studies in Pharmacodynamics

Pharmacodynamic advances have largely influenced the method of practice of clinicians through clarification of drug concentration versus pharmacological effect (Figure 3.18). Such scientific knowledge enables one to optimize therapeutic regimens based on the specific needs of the patient, minimizing side effects and optimizing efficacy. For instance, the application of *Holarrhena antidysenterica* in classical Unani medicine illustrates how the understanding of a drug's active ingredients and their interactions at receptor sites guides clinical use. Its flavonoids and alkaloids are responsible for anti-inflammatory and antimicrobial activities, illustrating the relevance of pharmacodynamic principles to the validation and optimization of traditional remedies for contemporary clinical use. Therefore, the incorporation of pharmacodynamic information into treatment protocols is crucial to guaranteeing both the safety and effectiveness of treatments, particularly when translating ancient traditions into modern healthcare systems (Sultana et al., 2025). Theophylline is a good example of pharmacodynamics informing clinical use in respiratory medicine. Its dual action—phosphodiesterase inhibition and adenosine receptor antagonism—accounts for its bronchodilatory and anti-inflammatory activity, which are still useful for the control of asthma and chronic obstructive pulmonary disease (COPD). Furthermore, current research discloses an expanding therapeutic range with immunomodulation and tissue repair, demonstrating the shifting clinical promise guided by pharmacodynamic knowledge. However, the variable pharmacokinetic-sensitive narrow therapeutic index of theophylline emphasizes the need for diligent dosage titration and monitoring to avoid toxicity.

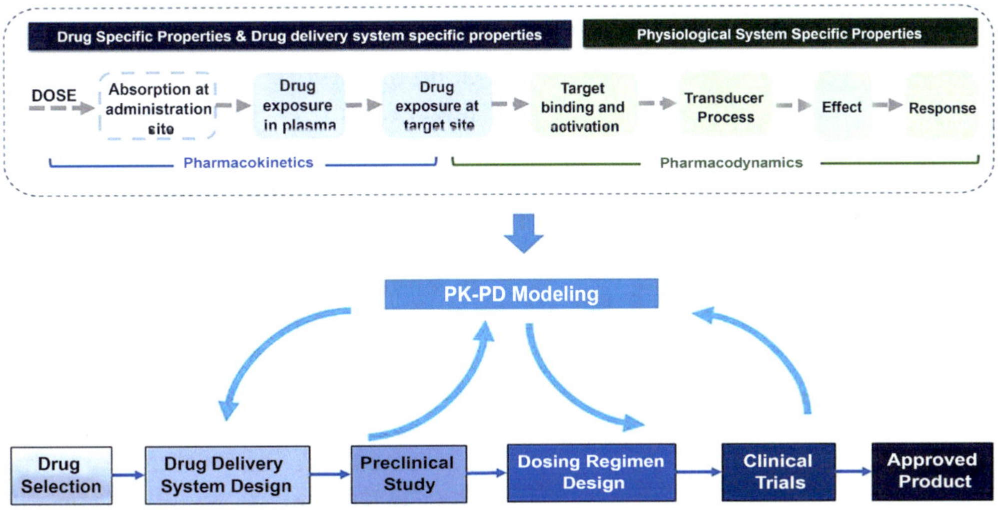

Figure 3.18. Clinical applications of pharmacodynamics.

Source: Frontiers in Pharmacology. (2020). *Screening Protocol for Patients with Suspected COVID-19.*

This thin line between safety and efficacy demonstrates how pharmacodynamic profiling is core in clinical practice to ensure best patient outcomes at the lowest risks (Szar et al., 2025). Pharmacodynamic clinical applications are not limited to respiratory disorders but also cover various therapeutic categories like gastrointestinal (GI) and metabolic conditions. Systematic knowledge of drug-receptor interactions allows identification of dosage regimens that produce desired biological responses with minimal side effects. For example, phytochemicals from indigenous medicines like *Holarrhena antidysenterica* exhibit immunomodulatory as well as hepatoprotective activity and provide novel means of addressing multifactorial disorders like diabetes and inflammatory disease. The juxtaposition of such pharmacodynamic insight with clinical data strengthens personalized medicine practices by allowing practitioners to choose suitable interventions based on patient-related factors. Emerging research on the pharmacodynamics of new and old agents will play a critical role in streamlining therapies and their widening clinical applicability in changing healthcare environments (Sultana et al., 2025; Szar et al., 2025).

3.6.1. Drug Development and Testing

The process of transformation from a theoretical molecule into a licensed therapeutic entity is one that consists of strict testing phases aimed at explaining the drug's response within biological systems. Initial drug development targets deciphering the pharmacokinetics—how the body metabolizes, distributes, absorbs, and excretes the compound—along with pharmacodynamics, which deals with the drug's biochemical and physiological effects. These factors are important not only to establish suitable dosing regimens but also to forecast therapeutic responses and possible adverse effects. Experimental models, such as *in vitro* assays and animal models, yield basic information that informs the progression to human trials. Pharmacodynamic data incorporation at an early stage in development improves candidate selection with favorable efficacy and safety profiles, allowing for highly optimized clinical trial designs where efficacy is balanced with reduced toxicity. These detailed assessments also provide a platform to identify drug interactions and personalize interventions based on mechanistic insight (Flaisher-Grinberg, 2023). Translation into clinical evaluation involves careful human trials to validate the safety, efficacy, and pharmacodynamic qualities observed preclinically. These experiments are phased, having distinct aims: Phase I determines safety and dose in normal volunteers, and the following phases extend to increasingly larger patient groups to determine the therapeutic effect and identify unusual side effects. The pharmacodynamic examination of these trials explains the mechanism of action of the drug and how it affects the target physiological pathways, closing the gap between preclinical promise and clinical use. This phase is critical to establishing therapeutic windows and informing dosing adjustments for optimal efficacy reduction of adverse effects. In addition, the collation and publishing of such information enhance the body of knowledge by the scientific community, facilitating pharmacological agent optimization and development (Lai et al., 2023). Even with strenuous testing processes, inconclusive or negative outcomes of trials pose hurdles to releasing pharmacodynamic observations (Figure 3.19). Resistance of certain scientific journals to publish results without positive outcomes can hide valuable mechanistic data that is crucial to an understanding of drug behavior. Transparency efforts more and more suggest open access to all clinical data regardless of outcome to enable complete knowledge sharing and avoid duplication of efforts in drug development. Public registries and regulatory releases partially fill this void, but peer-reviewed publications are essential for setting data into context within larger scientific paradigms. Improving access to comprehensive and balanced pharmacodynamic profiles via better reporting ensures that drug development is enabled by cumulative knowledge, thereby furthering therapeutic innovation and patient care (Lai et al., 2023).

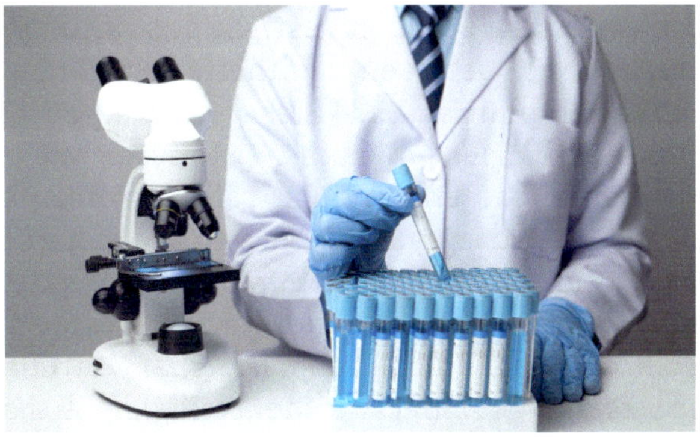

Figure 3.19. Drug development and testing.

Source: Boonchu, P. (2022). *Close-Up View of Scientist Analyzing a Liquid in the Test Tubes in Laboratory*. Vecteezy.

3.6.2. Personalized Medicine

Biomedical research advances have progressively emphasized the importance of personalizing drug treatments to suit patient-specific factors, a key concept of personalized medicine. Personalized medicine has a direct impact on the pharmacodynamics of medications by taking into account specific genetic, environmental, and lifestyle determinants that contribute to drug response heterogeneity. Personalized medicine aims at maximizing therapeutic effectiveness while reducing adverse effects through the selection of appropriately tailored drugs as well as modifying doses. Central to its application is also the merging of genomic information, which may uncover differences in drug target receptors, signaling pathways, and metabolic enzymes, all affecting mechanisms of drug actions. In addition, cutting-edge technology that allows for expedited genetic profiling makes personalized regimens more practical. Governmental agency, academic, and private sector collaborations have played a critical role in driving drug development paradigms that integrate these precision aspects, facilitating streamlined regulatory mechanisms and intellectual property management to bring personalized therapies to market more quickly (N/A, 2010). The increased appreciation for the human gut microbiota's contribution to drug metabolism and response is another key driver of pharmacodynamics in personalized medicine. The complex interplay between the microbial populations and pharmacological agents influences absorption, biotransformation, and excretion mechanisms, finally governing therapeutic effects and toxicity profiles. Changes in the composition of gut microbiota due to diet, prebiotics, and probiotics may introduce considerable interindividual variability in drug disposition. Personalized medicine is therefore required to take these microbial influences into account to provide maximal drug efficacy and safety. Despite this, there are continuing challenges through high inter-individual variability of the microbiomes and limitations in existing analytic models. These issues will need to be overcome through standardized research protocols and high-level bioinformatics focused on defining microbiota-linked drug metabolizing pathways, thus optimizing personalized therapeutic regimens (Satman et al., 2024). In the future, multi-dimensional data sets of genomics, proteomics, and microbiomics hold the promise to revolutionize pharmacodynamics in personalized medicine. Multi-omics research provides an integrated understanding of an individual's drug response through the capture of the rich interplay between genes, proteins, and microbial metabolites that affect drug targets and signaling pathways. This integrated understanding allows for the discovery of new biomarkers of drug efficacy and side effects, opening the door to strongly targeted therapeutic interventions.

In addition, interdisciplinary collaboration involving bioinformatics, pharmacology, and clinical sciences is necessary to translate these molecular findings into effective personalized treatment regimens. Closing existing knowledge gaps in drug–microbiota interactions and creating strong predictive models will greatly improve patient outcomes. Ultimately, the development of personalized medicine (Figure 3.20) through such integrative approaches seeks to revolutionize pharmacodynamics from a one-size-fits-all approach to an exactly tailored science (Satman et al., 2024).

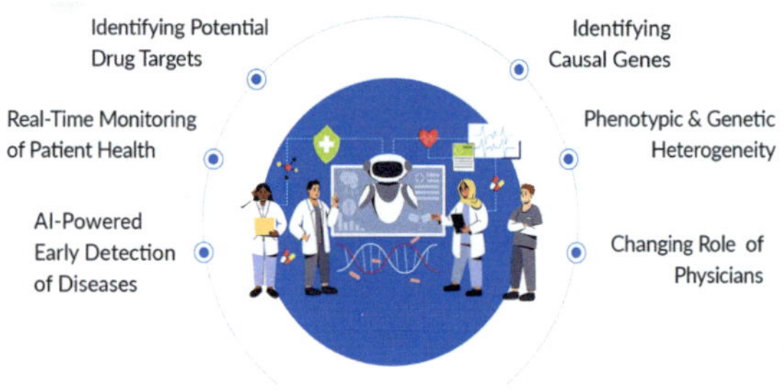

Figure 3.20. Personalized medicine.

Source: https://nextgeninvent.com/wp-content/uploads/2023/10/Artboard-1.jpg.

3.6.3. Case Studies in Pharmacodynamics

Within the complex field of pharmacodynamics, case studies offer incredibly useful information and shed light on the pharmacodynamic correlation between drug concentrations and their toxic and therapeutic actions (Figure 3.21). One important example includes the administration of bedaquiline and clofazimine for the treatment of tuberculosis meningitis. A study integrating evidence from nine studies emphasizes that bedaquiline has better penetration into the CNS and achieves higher concentrations in brain parenchyma than clofazimine. This pharmacodynamic profile is able to account for bedaquiline's improved efficacy against Mycobacterium tuberculosis in cerebrospinal fluid and renders it a potential drug for the treatment of this difficult manifestation of tuberculosis. Limitations remain, including a lack of studies of monotherapy and a requirement for more research to determine optimal dosing regimens. Such case studies highlight the need to consider drug distribution mechanisms and receptor interaction in particular pathological situations, and this is critical for maximizing clinical efficacy (Setyawan et al., 2025). Also important are investigations into the interactions between synthetic drugs and medicinal plants, and these shed light on intricate pharmacodynamic processes which can modify the efficacy and safety profiles of drugs. The widespread concurrent use of herbal preparations with prescription drugs is often done without medical monitoring, resulting in unpredictable drug response changes. Case reports and preclinical evidence highlight that these herb-drug interactions may result in severe therapeutic failures or side effects, depending on the modulation of receptor sites or signaling pathways. This new area of research necessitates extensive pharmacodynamic studies to identify synergistic or antagonistic effects on potential administration of herbal compounds with central or peripheral nervous system medications. As such, these observations support increased pharmacovigilance and educated clinical recommendations aimed at preventing risks, achieving safer and more effective treatment regimens for patients involving the use of herbal products (Bernardo et al., 2024). More critically depicting the relevance of pharmacodynamics in medical practice, case reports frequently demonstrate the subtle heterogeneity between patients in drug responsiveness as a function of genetic, environmental, or pathological influences. That heterogeneity underscores the imperative for personalized strategies, inasmuch as the same drug concentrations can produce different therapeutic or toxic effects in different individuals. For example, pharmacodynamic measurements with antibiotics or neuroactive agents demonstrate varying receptor sensitivities and downstream intracellular signaling efficiencies that can greatly influence therapeutic efficacy. These case studies affirm the utility of combining pharmacodynamic information with pharmacokinetic parameters to optimize dosing recommendations, especially in challenging conditions such as tuberculosis meningitis or neurological disorders. This convergent knowledge encourages the transition to precision medicine, in which personalized pharmacodynamic profiling enhances overall treatment efficacy and safety (Bernardo et al., 2024; Setyawan et al., 2025).

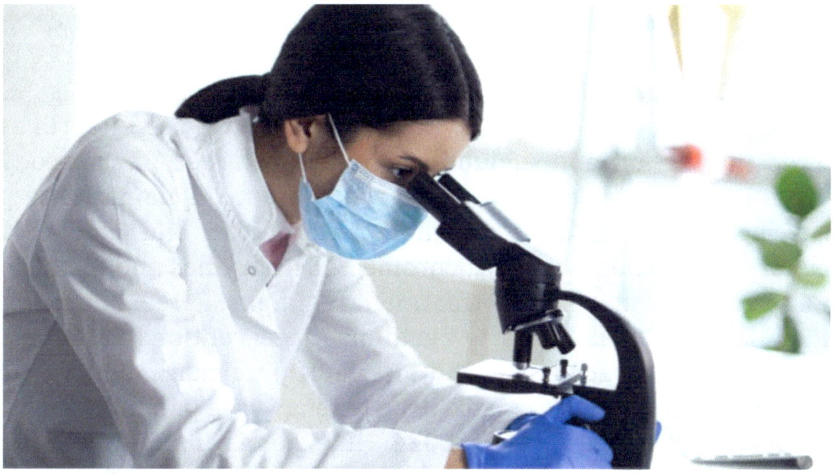

Figure 3.21. Case studies in pharmacodynamics.

Source: https://biotechfarm.co.il/wp-content/uploads/2024/07/Pharmacodynamics-Studies.jpg.

Test Your Knowledge

1. Which pharmacodynamic principle explains this effect?
2. Define preclinical testing in drug development?

SUMMARY

The intricate play of pharmacodynamic mechanisms highlights the importance of a sophisticated approach in the administration of therapeutic agents. Deviations in drug response, as affected by receptor sensitivity, signal transduction processes, and downstream interactions, reinforce pharmacodynamics as a dynamic field that is essential for successful treatment. Beyond mechanistic understanding, it becomes apparent that pharmacodynamic variation is a significant factor influencing clinical endpoints. The incorporation of patient individualization through factors such as genetic polymorphisms and biochemical milieu allows increased ability to anticipate drug action as well as adverse effects. Thus, the future of pharmacotherapy rests on the acceptance of this complexity by integrating personalized strategies focusing on individualized variability of drug response, ultimately enhancing efficacy and safety in the care of patients. Recent progress underlines the significance of incorporating drug interaction and metabolism into the larger pharmacodynamic principle. Antiplatelet therapy is an excellent example of where pharmacodynamics and pharmacokinetics overlap, with DDIs having a significant impact on therapeutic efficacy and safety profiles. Appreciation of these interactions, especially those with cytochrome P450 enzymes and their involvement in drug biotransformation, is critical for maximizing treatment regimens. Personalized approaches, such as genetic testing and TDM, enable clinicians to customize interventions and counteract risks from ADRs and resistance. These approaches portend an age of precision medicine that moves beyond conventional dosing paradigms, seeking to match drug potency with patient-specific variables to meet the optimal clinical outcome (Alshamrani et al., 2024; Huang et al., 2025). In conclusion, the dynamic future of pharmacodynamics calls for a universal understanding of both molecular mechanisms and patient-specific context. The integration of pharmacogenomics and pharmacometabolomic into practice promises a revolutionary transition to individualized pharmacotherapy. These technologies allow the detection of receptor-based and metabolic variations that affect drug action, making precision in drug dosing and selection possible. With the shift toward personalized care models in healthcare, it will be necessary for research and clinical application to work together in order to realize these advances. In the end, such integration is going to be improved in therapeutic effectiveness and safety by minimizing side effects and maximizing patient quality of life through educated, individualized pharmacodynamic treatments (Alshamrani et al., 2024; Huang et al., 2025).

Summary of Key Points

The pharmacodynamic complexities highlight drug concentration and effect relationships, important determinants of therapeutic efficacy as well as safety. To grasp the dynamics behind pharmacodynamics entails comprehending drugs' interactions at the cellular receptors, how their interaction leads to downstream effects, and how potencies and efficacy of the drug determine clinical endpoints. Key concepts such as dose-response relationships and receptor binding affinity provide a framework to predict both desired outcomes and adverse reactions, underscoring the necessity of accurate dosing regimens. Additionally, factors such as receptor sensitivity, the presence of agonists or antagonists, and the concept of drug tolerance further complicate this relationship, requiring comprehensive evaluation during drug development and clinical application. Paraphrasing these key points facilitates better comprehension of how pharmacodynamics inform effective treatment regimens and enhance patient care. Fundamentally, paraphrasing pharmacodynamics points to the ways in which drugs affect biological systems through complex molecular processes. Such processes are not singular but engage within more comprehensive physiological contexts, such as genetic, environmental, and pathological contexts. For instance, variations in receptor expression or mutations may heavily impact drug effectiveness, calling for personalized treatment with medication management. Such a differentiated perspective is equaled in diagnostics, where coordinated information enhances clinical decision-making (Park et al., 2023). Thus, pharmacodynamics cannot be a static entity but a dynamic relationship that guides precision medicine and adaptation therapy, showing the changing world of biomedical sciences. In consolidating the key points of pharmacodynamics, it is essential to recognize their role in optimizing clinical practices and drug development protocols. By systematically summarizing pharmacodynamic principles, healthcare practitioners can prevent inappropriate treatment and enhance patient outcomes, similarly to guidelines established in other healthcare disciplines (Manfredini et al., 2024). This structured approach facilitates consistent therapeutic decision-making and supports ongoing education among healthcare providers. Furthermore, it emphasizes the need to bridge pharmacodynamic insights with useful algorithms that can adjust to different needs of patients. Ultimately, these points form a platform from which to proceed with drug research, clinical use, and policy-making to ensure knowledge is tailored to address diverse medical settings effectively.

KEY TERMS FROM THIS CHAPTER

- Dose-Response Relationships
- Mechanisms of Drug Action
- Drug concentration
- Pharmacodynamics
- Drug absorption
- Polymorphisms
- Drug-receptor interaction
- Safety factors
- Clinical Applications
- Target-mediated drug disposition (TMDD)
- Nonmonotonic
- Dealthcare professionals
- Pharmacogenetic
- Personalized medicine

CRITICAL THINKING QUESTIONS

1. **Pharmacodynamics involves the study of following EXCEPT?**
   a. Biological and therapeutic effects of drugs
   b. Absorption and distribution of drugs
   c. Mechanisms of drug action
   d. Drug interactions
2. **Target proteins which a drug molecule binds include?**
   a. Only receptors
   b. Only ion channels
   c. Only carriers
   d. All of the above
3. **The constant Kd refers to?**
   a. Maximal physiological effect
   b. Maximal receptor binding
   c. Drug concentration to occupy 50% of receptors
   d. Drug concentration that results in halfmaximal physiological response
4. **EC50 mainly reflects a drug's?**
   a. Maximal effect
   b. Potency
   c. Lethality
   d. Ease of elimination
5. **Which are true of competitive inhibition?**
   a. Reversible binding at receptor sites
   b. Dose-response curve shifts to the left
   c. Maximal drug effect cannot be achieved even at high agonist levels
   d. Ease of elimination

Short Answer Questions

1. Which term defines the strength of drug–receptor binding?
2. Explain how Dose-Response Relationships?
3. Pharmacodynamics involves the study of all EXCEPT?s
4. Drug combination where total effect equals the sum of individual effects is called?
5. Which of Clinical Applications of Pharmacodynamics?

Answer to Critical Thinking Questions

1. (b) 2 (d) 3. (c) 4. (b) 5. (a)

REFERENCES

1. Abduljalil, M., Aghazadeh-Habashi, A., Aigrain, L., Aitman, T., Al Za'abi, M., Alegre, L., Alnaqeeb, M., et al. (2019). Current trends in drug metabolism and pharmacokinetics. *Acta Pharmaceutica Sinica B, 9*(6), 1113–1144. https://doi.org/10.1016/j.apsb.2019.10.001.
2. Abu-Lafi, S., Falah, M., Zeidan, M., Rayan, M., & Rayan, A. (2025). Expanding paclitaxel's therapeutic window: Investigating the pharmacokinetic, clinical formulation and mechanistic aspects of paclitaxel-lipoate conjugate. *Oncology Letters*, *29*. https://www.semanticscholar.org/paper/8bb88b39a699dd4f45df88808938a10a2e8ef606 (accessed on 9 May 2025).
3. Albertella, M., Rizoska, B., Kyle, A., Minchinton, A., Linqvist, A., Jurić, S., Sedig, S., et al. (2017). Abstract 5101: Defining exposure-PD and efficacy relationships with the novel liver-targeting nucleotide prodrug MIV-818 for the treatment of liver cancers. *Cancer Research, 77*(1), 5101. https://www.semanticscholar.org/paper/6e29e94790938e0db145717246a3618261d935c2 (accessed on 9 May 2025).
4. Aliabadi, F. S., Aliabadi, M. S., Brentnall, J., Craig, W., Davey, R., de Jong, A., et al. (2018). Pharmacokinetic–pharmacodynamic integration and modelling of oxytetracycline for the calf pathogens *Mannheimia haemolytica* and *Pasteurella multocida*. https://core.ac.uk/download/132194056.pdf (accessed on 9 May 2025).
5. Alshamrani, A., Al-Moashi, H. M. H., Alqunfdi, M. A. M., Alhaqwe, I. A., Alruwaili, A. H., Alenezi, B. H., Almutiry, M. M., et al. (2024). Biochemical mechanisms in drug metabolism: Implications for personalized pharmacotherapy in pharmacy practice. *Egyptian Journal of Chemistry, 67*(13), 1493–1505. https://www.semanticscholar.org/paper/2cf72bf7b8268df46f459a28bfdbd07110e411ef (accessed on 9 May 2025).
6. Altamura, C., Conte, D., Desaphy, J. F., & Carratu, M. R. (2022). Target mutation-driven drug discovery. https://core.ac.uk/download/541260146.pdf (accessed on 9 May 2025).
7. Andreozzi, F., Mannino, G. C., & Sesti, G. (2019). Pharmacogenetics of type 2 diabetes mellitus: The route toward tailored medicine. *Diabetes/Metabolism Research and Reviews, 35*, e3109. https://core.ac.uk/download/231747878.pdf (accessed on 9 May 2025).
8. Bailey, D., Bon, C., Cox, J., Darwich, A., Dorey, R., Duwal, S., Ette, E., et al. (2018). Population variability in animal health: Influence on dose-exposure-response relationships. Part II: Modelling and simulation. https://core.ac.uk/download/159992803.pdf (accessed on 9 May 2025).
9. Barke, E., Coghill, D., & Cornforth, C. (2010). Stimulant drug effects on attention deficit/hyperactivity disorder: A review of the effects of age and sex of patients. https://core.ac.uk/download/55797029.pdf (accessed on 9 May 2025).
10. Bernardo, J., & Valentão, P. (2024). Herb-drug interactions: A short review on central and peripheral nervous system drugs. *Phytotherapy Research, 38*(5), 1903–1931. https://www.semanticscholar.org/paper/c4c3e53c2161bd19cd98e2be79ea2a021b63d341 (accessed on 9 May 2025).
11. Branford, R., Cregg, R., Gubbay, A., & Russo, M. (2013). Pharmacogenetics of analgesic drugs. *British Journal of Pain, 7*(4), 189–208. https://core.ac.uk/download/29416244.pdf (accessed on 9 May 2025).

12. Budić, I., Jevtović-Stoimenov, T., Pavlović, D., Marjanović, V., Djordjević, I., Stević, M., & Simić, D. (2022). Clinical importance of potential genetic determinants affecting propofol pharmacokinetics and pharmacodynamics. *Frontiers in Medicine, 9*. https://doi.org/10.3389/fmed.2022.809393.

13. Capi, M., Curto, M., De Andrés, F., & Gentile, S. (2016). Eletriptan in the management of acute migraine: An update on the evidence for efficacy, safety, and consistent response. *Therapeutic Advances in Neurological Disorders, 9*(5), 414–423. https://core.ac.uk/download/74319151.pdf (accessed on 9 May 2025).

14. Cintron, N. M., & Putcha, L. (2025). Pharmacokinetics and pharmacodynamics in space. https://core.ac.uk/download/pdf/42806060.pdf.

15. Cuomo, A., Barillà, G., Cattolico, M., Pardossi, S., Mariantoni, E., Koukouna, D., Carmellini, P., et al. (2024). Perspectives on the impact of vortioxetine on the treatment armamentarium of major depressive disorder. *Expert Review of Neurotherapeutics, 24*, 465–476. https://www.semanticscholar.org/paper/b5922bfb68aba9e9fd124925c75d7d90e8d4069f (accessed on 9 May 2025).

16. Eckhoff, P., Gerardin, J., & Wenger, E. A. (2015). Mass campaigns with antimalarial drugs: A modelling comparison of artemether-lumefantrine and DHA-piperaquine with and without primaquine as tools for malaria control and elimination. *BMC Infectious Diseases, 15*, 144. http://arxiv.org/abs/1503.09149 (accessed on 9 May 2025).

17. Eitan, L. A., Khair, I., & Alahmad, S. (2024). Drug metabolizing enzymes: An exclusive guide into latest research in pharmaco-genetic dynamics in Arab countries. *Current Drug Metabolism, 25*(7), 465–478. https://www.semanticscholar.org/paper/c14ded482ee415dd099fe5f333c49163ed7e320b (accessed on 9 May 2025).

18. Farag, M., Gorog, D. A., & Patel, H. (2015). Adjunctive therapies to reduce thrombotic events in patients with a history of myocardial infarction: Role of vorapaxar. https://core.ac.uk/download/287581702.pdf (accessed on 9 May 2025).

19. Flaisher-Grinberg, S. (2023). Poppy seed consumption and oral fluid opioids detection: A classroom demonstration of psychopharmacological concepts. *Journal of Undergraduate Neuroscience Education, 22*(1), A37–A44. https://www.semanticscholar.org/paper/82e8eb5241f5469753966cffd288bdb0cd2119b4 (accessed on 9 May 2025).

20. Giovagnoli, A., & Zagoraiou, M. (2025). Simulated clinical trials: Some design issues. https://core.ac.uk/download/pdf/6820410.pdf (accessed on 9 May 2025).

21. Guimarães, H., Pinto, J. L., Pereira, R., & Domingues, C. (2017). From molecule to outcome: Evidence-based medicine and pharmacology applied therapeutic practices in medical learning. https://www.semanticscholar.org/paper/8e20ba561c02a68ee1d6641b6d4d5a7740ca6688 (accessed on 9 May 2025).

22. Huang, X., Song, J., Zhang, X., Wang, M., Ding, Y., Ji, X., Zhou, D., et al. (2025). Understanding drug interactions in antiplatelet therapy for atherosclerotic vascular disease: A systematic review. *CNS Neuroscience & Therapeutics, 31*. https://www.semanticscholar.org/paper/48b4362ad646fbea4dab08d71a11c6d5549098e5 (accessed on 9 May 2025).

23. Ibanez, B., Varenhorst, C., Alexopoulos, D., Aradi, D., Lindholm, D., Zhou, D., Amsterdam, E. A., et al. (2018). Metabolism of ticagrelor in patients with acute coronary syndromes. *Scientific Reports, 8*, 11746. https://core.ac.uk/download/287581672.pdf (accessed on 9 May 2025).

24. Kang, M. A., Shakya, J., Li, J., VahidMohammadi, A., Tian, W., Zeglio, E., Hamedi, M. M., et al. (2023). 2D MXene electrochemical transistors. *Nanoscale*. https://www.semanticscholar.org/paper/5c992f45bf2805f519f02b6d50a87702d9404b63 (accessed on 9 May 2025).
25. Knockenhauer, K., & Copeland, R. (2023). The importance of binding kinetics and drug-target residence time in pharmacology. *British Journal of Pharmacology, 181*(21), 4103–4116. https://www.semanticscholar.org/paper/360a911bf2a96729969a295ae1249a8a33547663 (accessed on 9 May 2025).
26. Kraft, W. K., Lam, E., Lien, Y. T. K., Piraino, P., et al. (2020). Vancomycin in peritoneal dialysis: Clinical pharmacology considerations in therapy. https://core.ac.uk/download/322850154.pdf (accessed on 9 May 2025).
27. Lai, Y., Yanev, S., & Liu, Z. (2023). Editorial: Clinical trials in drug metabolism and transport: 2022. *Frontiers in Pharmacology, 14*. https://www.semanticscholar.org/paper/90707c9575fecf7cbf55c5a39f5cbb665238c9a9 (accessed on 9 May 2025).
28. Langmia, I. M., Just, K. S., Yamoune, S., Müller, J. P., & Stingl, J. C. (2022). Pharmacogenetic and drug interaction aspects on ketamine safety in its use as antidepressant—Implications for precision dosing in a global perspective. *British Journal of Clinical Pharmacology, 88*(11), 5149–5165. https://doi.org/10.1111/bcp.15467.
29. Lyubushkina, E., Bondareva, E., Soldatova, M., & Madonov, P. (2024). Experimental determination of the “therapeutic window” of the synthetic peptidomimetic SAMP-1. *2024 IEEE International Multi-Conference on Engineering, Computer and Information Sciences (SIBIRCON)*. https://www.semanticscholar.org/paper/a6a77584a1f2ed903208ef84e44a8d3eb8a51864 (accessed on 9 May 2025).
30. Mach, F., Baigent, C., Catapano, A. L., Koskinas, K. C., Casula, M., Badimón, L., Chapman, M. J., et al. (2019). 2019 ESC/EAS guidelines for the management of dyslipidaemias: Lipid modification to reduce cardiovascular risk. *European Heart Journal, 41*(1), 111–188. https://doi.org/10.1093/eurheartj/ehz455.
31. Manfredini, D., Häggman-Henrikson, B., Al Jagshi, A., Baad-Hansen, L., Beecroft, E., Bijelic, T., Bracci, A., et al. (2024). Temporomandibular disorders: INfORM/IADR key points for good clinical practice based on standard of care. *Cranio: The Journal of Craniomandibular Practice, 43*(1), 1–5. https://www.semanticscholar.org/paper/6872d48a634f04904ee405af21357149df90a15f (accessed on 9 May 2025).
32. Maslov, I., Volkov, O., Khorn, P. A., Orekhov, P., Gusach, A., Kuzmichev, P., Gerasimov, A., et al. (2020). Sub-millisecond conformational dynamics of the A2A adenosine receptor revealed by single-molecule FRET. *Communications Biology, 6*(1). https://www.semanticscholar.org/paper/c14e294a2bdf380e1282c99713e46edde871824d (accessed on 9 May 2025).
33. Miethke, M., Pieroni, M., Weber, T., Brönstrup, M., Hammann, P., Halby, L., Arimondo, P. B., et al. (2021). Towards the sustainable discovery and development of new antibiotics. *Nature Reviews Chemistry, 5*(11), 726–749. https://doi.org/10.1038/s41570-021-00313-1.
34. N/A. (2010). The new role of academia in drug development. Retrieved from: https://core.ac.uk/download/71353433.pdf (accessed on 9 May 2025).
35. Pálla, T., Mazák, K., Alkhazragee, D. M., Balogh, G. T., Noszál, B., & Mirzahosseini, A. (2024). Comparison of orthogonal determination methods of acid/base constants with meta-analysis. *International Journal of Molecular Sciences, 25*. https://www.semanticscholar.org/paper/d3614453c3790f56dc020a3e1e14210276ca4b52 (accessed on 9 May 2025).

36. Papathanasiou, T., Strathe, A., Hooker, A., Lund, T. M., & Overgaard, R. V. (2018). Feasibility of exposure-response analyses for clinical dose-ranging studies of drug combinations. *The AAPS Journal, 20*. https://www.semanticscholar.org/paper/66d3d9d21879631418f3dc3006bd65b0c60fc7a7 (accessed on 9 May 2025).

37. Park, Y., Vollmuth, P., Foltyn-Dumitru, M., Sahm, F., Ahn, S., Chang, J. H., & Kim, S. H. (2023). The 2021 WHO classification for gliomas and implications on imaging diagnosis: Part 1—Key points of the fifth edition and summary of imaging findings on adult-type diffuse gliomas. *Journal of Magnetic Resonance Imaging, 58*. https://www.semanticscholar.org/paper/2ba3e44bfa288f4df1a088672a9424e9cf9e5f36 (accessed on 9 May 2025).

38. Petek, A., & Filaković, P. (2009). Personalized pharmacotherapy in psychiatry. *Psychiatric Danuban, 21*(3), 341–346. https://core.ac.uk/download/14420495.pdf (accessed on 9 May 2025).

39. Satman, S. L., Mishra, S., Patnaik, S., Behera, H. P., Jani, P. K., Rathore, A., Padhy, R. P., et al. (2024). Exploring the role of gut microbiota in drug efficacy and pharmacological outcomes. Retrieved from: https://core.ac.uk/download/640070317.pdf (accessed on 9 May 2025).

40. Seeman, M. V. (2021). The pharmacodynamics of antipsychotic drugs in women and men. *Frontiers in Psychiatry, 12*. https://doi.org/10.3389/fpsyt.2021.650904.

41. Setyawan, M., Mertaniasih, N., Soedarsono, S., Artama, W., & Matsumoto, S. (2025). Penetration levels and concentration of bedaquiline and clofazimine into the brain parenchyma compared with those in blood plasma: A systematic review and individual case report analysis. *Journal of Public Health and Development, 23*(1), 329–347. https://www.semanticscholar.org/paper/9d56247c1977059c2db4904776a01fd589f35468 (accessed on 9 May 2025).

42. Singh, S., Gumbo, T., Wang, J. Y., Boorgula, G., Burke, A., Huang, H. L., McShane, P. J., et al. (2024). Imipenem pharmacokinetics/pharmacodynamics in preclinical hollow fiber model, dose-finding in virtual patients, and clinical evidence of efficacy for *Mycobacterium abscessus* lung disease. *The Journal of Infectious Diseases,* jiae601. https://www.semanticscholar.org/paper/16c95696b39d2d74f9d7bee0bb2fe77a0a4876b9 (accessed on 9 May 2025).

43. Spagnolo, P. A., Manson, J. E., & Joffe, H. (2020). Sex and gender differences in health: What the COVID-19 pandemic can teach us. *Annals of Internal Medicine, 173*, 385–386. https://doi.org/10.7326/m20-1941.

44. Sultana, R., Rahman, M. N., Yusuf, M. S., & Karim, M. S. (2025). Therapeutic potential of Inderjo Talkh (Holarrhena antidysenterica) in Unani medicine: An in-depth study. *Journal of Drug Delivery and Therapeutics, 15*(4). https://www.semanticscholar.org/paper/3017dbc85443ed5b6e31b658a2e2c550c5e31536 (accessed on 9 May 2025).

45. Szarłowicz, J., Mazur, M., Waz, D., Goliszek, Z., Sobek, K. Ł., Tabin-Barczak, W., Sokołowska, A., et al. (2025). Theophylline revisited: Mechanisms, challenges, and new horizons. *Quality in Sport, 37,* 57009. https://www.semanticscholar.org/paper/f672bc826955c5d746d2fcf1465474bab6c7dce4 (accessed on 9 May 2025).

46. Tian, Y., Hu, X., Zhang, T., Li, B., Fu, Q., & Li, J. (2025). Advances in Chinese herbal medicine in modulating mitochondria to treat myocardial ischemia-reperfusion injury: A narrative review. *Cardiovascular Diagnosis and Therapy, 15*, 207–232. https://www.semanticscholar.org/paper/60333955be679d92e89f41e6fb0d7592e3b5c402 (accessed on 9 May 2025).

47. Ullén, A. (2019). Outside the box of immunotherapy–New hope for patients with advanced urothelial cancer. *Acta Oncological, 58*, 951–952. https://www.semanticscholar.org/paper/b9e90888eba8f2280139278c8594249a79dfc3b8 (accessed on 9 May 2025).

48. Visseren, F. L. J., Mach, F., Smulders, Y. M., Carballo, D., Koskinas, K. C., Bäck, M., Bénétos, A., et al. (2021). 2021 ESC guidelines on cardiovascular disease prevention in clinical practice. *European Heart Journal, 42*(32), 3227–3337. https://doi.org/10.1093/eurheartj/ehab484.

49. von Hentig, N. (2012). Personalizing HIV therapy, mission impossible? *Journal of Antivirals and Antiretrovirals, 5*, 012–020. https://core.ac.uk/download/17028337.pdf (accessed on 9 May 2025).

50. Yuan, X., & An, G. (2024). Characterizing the nonlinear pharmacokinetics and pharmacodynamics of BI 187004, an 11β-hydroxysteroid dehydrogenase type 1 inhibitor, in humans by a target-mediated drug disposition model. *Journal of Clinical Pharmacology, 64*(8), 993–1005. https://www.semanticscholar.org/paper/c5aaadfbdcd7cb97f5b21960530f874c8dbc2d1a (accessed on 9 May 2025).

AUTONOMIC NERVOUS SYSTEM PHARMACOLOGY

4

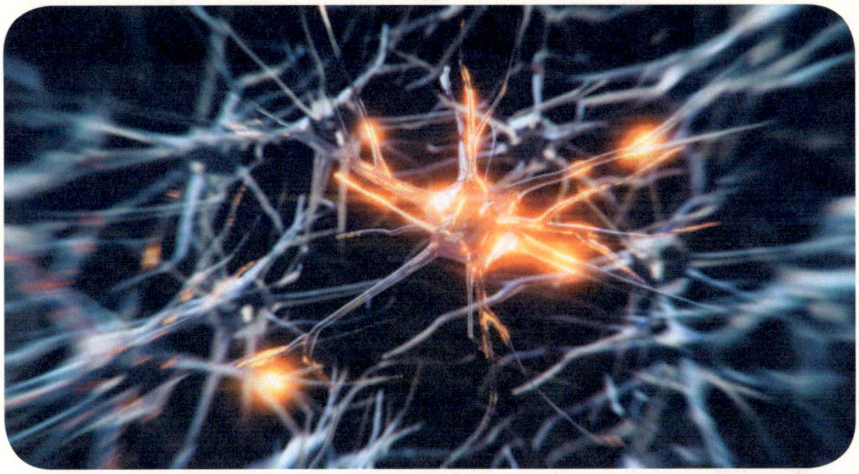

Introduction

The intricate relationship between physiological regulation and the nervous system lies at the heart of understanding autonomic function-focused pharmacological intervention. The autonomic nervous system (ANS) (Figure 4.1), which oversees involuntary body processes like heart rate, digestion, and respiratory rate, functions by way of sympathetic and parasympathetic divisions. Sympathetic and parasympathetic divisions function synergistically to uphold homeostasis and react to environmental stress in a manner usually mediated by neurotransmitters such as acetylcholine and norepinephrine. Pharmacological agents that act on these pathways have a significant impact on cardiovascular, respiratory, and gastrointestinal function and are vital tools in treating hypertension and asthma. Knowledge of the subtle mechanisms that govern these interactions is key to the effective development of therapies that control ANS activity with minimal adverse effects, and strict study of both neural regulation and pharmacological modulation is thus highly relevant (Akkamahadevi et al., 2025). Recent progress

LEARNING OBJECTIVES

After studying this chapter, you will be able to:

1. Define Anatomy of the Autonomic Nervous System (ANS)
2. Understand Neurotransmitters in the Autonomic Nervous System (ANS)
3. Identify the Pharmacological Agents Affecting the Autonomic Nervous System (ANS)
4. Explain Clinical Applications of Autonomic Pharmacology
5. Learn Side Effects and Adverse Reactions
6. Explain about Current Research and Developments

has started to reveal the complex neuroimmune interactions along the autonomic pathways, especially emphasizing the contribution of specific neuronal subsets to immune regulation. Studies employing chemogenetic methods have shown that activation of certain neuronal populations, such as nociceptors that express Trpv1, can modulate immunocyte populations, including regulatory T cells that are critical for immune homeostasis. These observations indicate that pharmacological modulation of the ANS might be more extensive than conventional targets, involving neuroimmune cross-talk in gut physiology and systemic inflammation. Such intricacy requires an advanced pharmacological strategy that considers both neural signaling and immune modulation, shifting the treatment promise of autonomic drugs not only for classical disorders but also for inflammatory and autoimmune diseases (Zhu et al., 2024). The pharmacological profile of the ANS is also complemented by non-pharmacological treatments with a modulating effect upon autonomic tone and consequent enhancement of clinical outcome. Deep breathing maneuvers have been tested for reducing sympathetic outflow with augmentation of parasympathetic output and have been associated with significant drops in the blood pressure of hypertensive patients. This holistic strategy demonstrates the promise of the modulation of autonomic regulation by both pharmacologic and behavioral strategies to maximize cardiovascular health. Such measures highlight the ANS's essential role in managing systemic disease and the requirement for holistic treatment protocols that intervene in neural, immune, and behavioral aspects of autonomic regulation (Akkamahadevi et al., 2025).

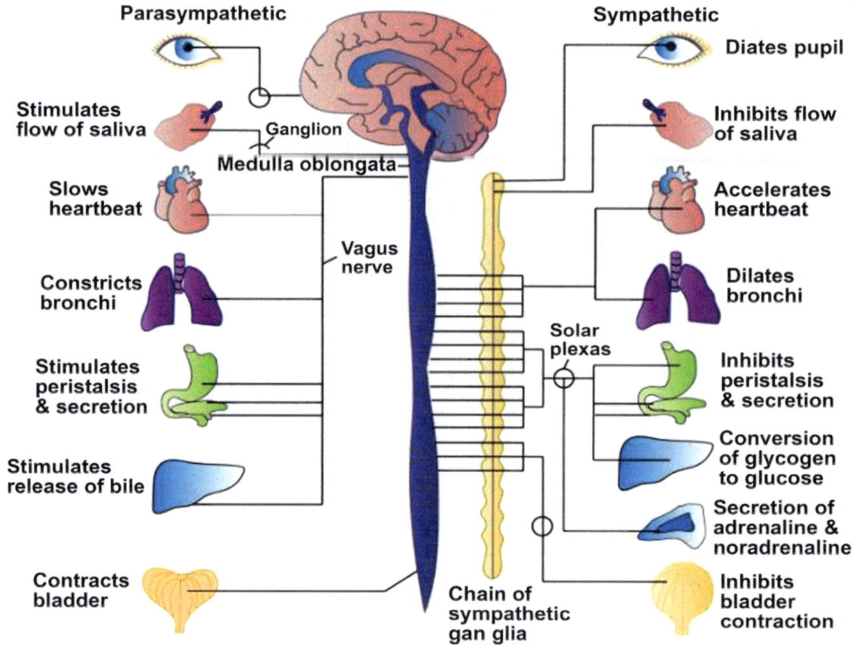

Figure 4.1. Autonomic nervous system (ANS).

Source: Wisconsin Technical College System. (2019). *Autonomic Nervous System*. https://wtcs.pressbooks.pub/app/uploads/sites/10/2019/10/Graphic-1536x1210.png.

Definition of the Autonomic Nervous System

The intricate control of involuntary physiological processes depends on a highly complex network of neural pathways that happen to function largely beyond conscious control. Of all such systems, the autonomic nervous system (ANS) is most important, regulating vital functions like cardiovascular activity, digestion, respiratory rate, and glandular secretion. It operates through a harmonized response constituted by two complementary branches—the sympathetic and parasympathetic nervous systems—which counterbalance excitatory and inhibitory pressures in order to preserve homeostasis. Notably, the ANS interacts with the central nervous system (CNS) to dynamically modulate visceral activities in response to internal and external stimuli. Its regulatory function highlights why knowledge of the ANS is important in pharmacology, since numerous drugs act on these autonomic pathways to treat disorders from hypertension to gastrointestinal (GI) disturbances. The complex neural circuitry of ANS emphasizes the difficulty in creating therapies selectively modulating its activity without the occurrence of unwanted systemic effects. The ANS functions through a two-neuron efferent pathway, coupling the CNS to peripheral target organs through an autonomic ganglia synapse. The preganglionic neuron arises in the CNS and projects to autonomic ganglia, where it synapses with the postganglionic neuron, and the latter innervates effector tissues. This anatomical arrangement presents several drug targets from a pharmacological perspective, such as receptors on post- and preganglionic neurons and mechanisms of neurotransmitter release. The major parasympathetic and sympathetic responses are mediated by acetylcholine and norepinephrine, respectively, with receptor subtypes further increasing the systems pharmacological complexity. Moreover, this dual framework allows fine-tuned control over bodily functions but also presents a challenge in clinical pharmacology, as drugs influencing one branch may inadvertently affect the other, necessitating a nuanced understanding of receptor pharmacodynamics and receptor subtype distribution (Aksu et al., 2019). Basic to the pharmacological control of the ANS is the appreciation for its participation in acute and chronic physiological phenomena, such as pain modulation and maintenance of homeostasis. The interaction between the ANS and pain mechanisms represents its wide-ranging influence, in which sympathetic drive frequently serves to enhance chronic states of pain and thus to make treatment more complicated. This forms part of the justification for the use of multiple methods in the management of autonomic dysfunctions and has led to therapy that includes the use of both pharmacological drugs and neuromodulation methods. In addition, the complex role of the ANS in systemic diseases necessitates that clinicians handle prescribing practice with care for opioid analgesics since these act profoundly on autonomic networks and affect pain modulation and autonomic tone in acute and chronic situations. Detailed assessment of patients and individualized treatment plans are necessary to maximize therapeutic benefits with minimal risks, a philosophy underlying present pharmacological recommendations (Curro, 2017).

Importance of Pharmacology in Autonomic Function

It is important to understand the intricate interaction between pharmacological agents and ANS function for successful therapeutic interventions. The ANS controls essential involuntary functions like cardiovascular, respiratory, and digestive functions; disturbances in its balance can result in serious clinical conditions. Pharmacology has a vital role in modulating these autonomic pathways, especially by acting on neurotransmitter receptors and ion channels that affect sympathetic and parasympathetic activity. For instance, patients with migraine tend to show autonomic dysfunction, as reflected in diminished response to deep breathing and orthostatic tests, which underlines the need for pharmacologic evaluation and management of ANS abnormalities. Drugs like anti-calcitonin gene-related peptide antibodies not only relieve migraine but also potentially alter autonomic function (Figure 4.2), and this underlines an imperative of drug therapy to understand drug effects beyond the control of the fundamental symptom (Antun et al., 2024). The dynamic behavior of the ANS requires cautious management upon administration of pharmacological drugs, particularly during special physiological conditions such as pregnancy. Findings from heart rate variability (HRV) research indicate that autonomic modulation varies greatly across pregnancy, demonstrating complex physiological adaptations. Pharmacological management during this time needs to be mindful of potential changes in autonomic responsiveness since inappropriate treatment might worsen gestational morbidity through interference in the fine balance between sympathetic and parasympathetic outflow. In addition, lifestyle and sociodemographic determinants have a significant impact on HRV, implying that pharmacologic approaches must be integrative and individualized, taking into account both intrinsic autonomic modification and extrinsic factors.

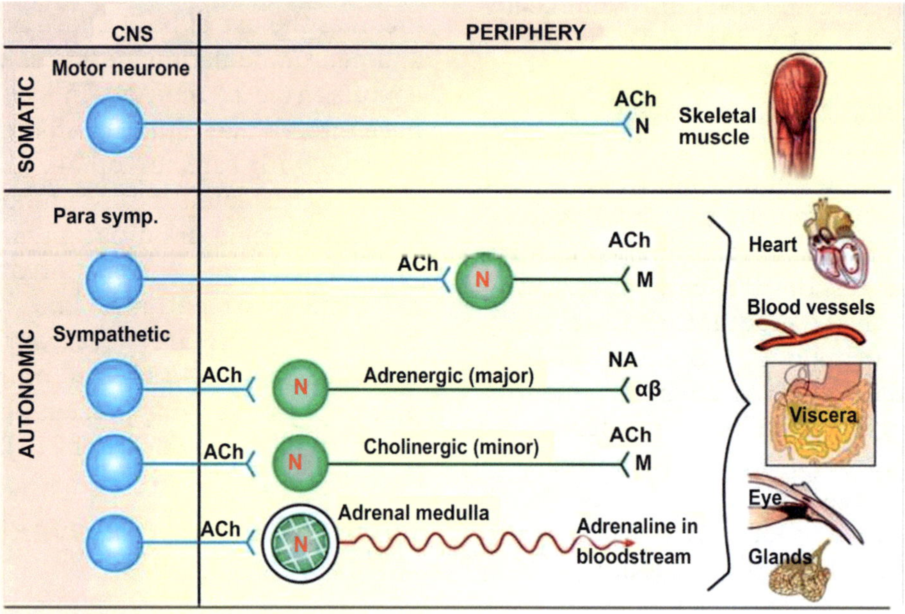

Figure 4.2. Pharmacology in autonomic function.

Source: Pharmacy180. (n.d.). *Pharmacology in Autonomic Function.* https://www.pharmacy180.com/media/imgph01/KuLPziU.jpg.

The insight provided by supervised machine learning models of HRV emphasizes the need for sophisticated pharmacological interventions to preserve autonomic stability during pregnancy and the postpartum period (Sharifi-Heris et al., 2023). Additionally, pharmacological investigation of the ANS is being expanded to include the creation of diagnostic instruments and individually designed therapies that counteract autonomic dysfunctions in a wide range of clinical populations. Determination of precise autonomic impairments, like those associated with migraineurs or with pregnancy-induced cardiovascular stress, directs clinicians in the choice of drugs that correct or improve autonomic balance without sacrificing physiological adaptability. This accuracy of autonomic pharmacology not only enhances therapeutic efficiency but also decreases side effects associated with non-selective autonomic modulation. Synthesis of novel analytical methods and clinical pharmacology is crucial in developing tailored interventions that maximize autonomic health. Therefore, the significance of pharmacology in autonomic function goes beyond symptom control, with a fundamental contribution to disease prevention, patient quality of life, and the optimization of clinical practice guidelines (Antun et al., 2024; Sharifi-Heris et al., 2023).

4.1. Anatomy of the Autonomic Nervous System (ANS)

Learning Outcome

1. Components of the Autonomic Nervous System
2. Sympathetic Versus Parasympathetic Nervous System
3. Role of the Enteric Nervous System (ENS)

Knowledge of the anatomical complexities of the ANS is necessary for an appreciation of the pharmacology of interventions aimed at modulating its activity (Figure 4.3). The ANS has two major divisions: the parasympathetic and sympathetic nervous systems that function in opposition to each other to ensure physiological homeostasis. Both divisions consist of a two-neuron pathway consisting of a preganglionic neuron with its origin in the central nervous system (CNS) and a postganglionic neuron with its termination on effector organs. The spatial anatomy of such neurons also differs, with sympathetic ganglia generally positioned close to the spinal cord and parasympathetic ganglia close to or even inside target organs. This anatomy determines the location and mode of action of drugs, especially with regard to releasing the neurotransmitter and the distribution of receptors. In addition, the identification of purinergic signaling by the early anatomists has broadened the knowledge about neurotransmission in the ANS, demonstrating the function of ATP as a cotransmitter together with traditional agents (Burnstock et al., 2011). These discoveries have significant impacts on the treatment of autonomic disorders. The heterogeneity of neurotransmitter receptors in the ANS reflects the complexity of its anatomical structure and functional regulation. Historically, adrenergic and cholinergic receptors have been the focus of autonomic pharmacology, but research has uncovered a wider range of receptor types such as purinergic receptors for extracellular nucleotides like ATP. The discovery of P1 and P2 purinergic receptor families with a number of subtypes in each family has underlined the subtle regulation of autonomic signaling pathways. These receptors are involved in both rapid synaptic transmission and longer-term trophic actions on neuronal and non-neuronal cells. Their anatomical distribution is different in various autonomic ganglia and effector tissues, mediating responses that influence cardiovascular, gastrointestinal, and genitourinary functions. Identification of the anatomical basis for these receptor distributions is essential for the understanding of pharmacodynamic properties of drugs acting on autonomic functions and for the prediction of their therapeutic and adverse effects (Burnstock et al., 2009). Apart from neurons, the ANS's anatomy includes sophisticated interactions with non-neuronal components like glial cells, which are involved in ensuring neural homeostasis and regulating synaptic activity. Anatomical research has confirmed that interactions between neurons and glial cells in autonomic ganglia are responsible for neurotransmitter metabolism, sensitivity to receptors, and neurovascular coupling. This complex microenvironment is a dynamic biochemical arena that acts as a regulator of autonomic reflexes and responses. Recent breakthroughs underscore the anatomical mapping of modified purinergic transmission in glial cells and pathological conditions such as hypertension and neurodegenerative disorders. Thus, the anatomical knowledge about these cellular constituents and spatial interactions within the autonomic circuitry guides the pharmacological regimens intended to modulate these interactions for therapeutic purposes. Such anatomical integrative information is a basis for the creation of new drugs designed to specific autonomic targets (Burnstock et al., 2009, 2011).

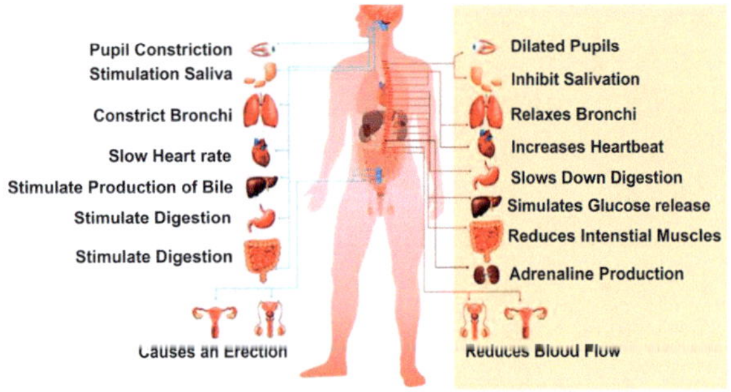

Figure 4.3. Anatomy of the autonomic nervous system (ANS).

Source: GeeksforGeeks. (2019). *Anatomy of the Autonomic Nervous System.* https://media.geeksforgeeks.org/wp-content/uploads/20221202163614/AtomicNervousSystem.jpg.

4.1.1. Components of the Autonomic Nervous System

The human body keeps a fine balance between involuntary physiological activities through an intricate network referred to as the ANS. This system regulates fundamental functions like heart rate, digestion, respiratory rate, and vascular tone by coordinating between its two major branches: the sympathetic and parasympathetic nervous systems. The sympathetic branch basically readies the body for "fight or flight" reactions through elevated heart rate and blood pressure, while the parasympathetic branch encourages "rest and digest" functions, recovering and conserving energy. From a drug pharmacology perspective, it is essential to know about these components as drugs acting at adrenergic receptors manipulate the sympathetic system, while cholinergic agents affect the parasympathetic pathways. In disease conditions like chronic kidney disease (CKD) and cardiovascular disease, a sympathetic predominance over parasympathetic activity has been noted, leading to inflammatory reactions and poor clinical outcomes. Pharmacological intervention to restore this balance can therefore reduce inflammation and enhance prognosis (Zoccali et al., 2025). Besides its systemic regulatory functions, the ANS is also intricately involved in the modulation of immune function in the tumor microenvironment. The sympathetic nervous system, through adrenergic signaling, modulates the growth and mobilization of myeloid-derived suppressor cells (MDSCs), a heterogeneous population of immune cells responsible for promoting cancer development. The parasympathetic action, however, mediated by cholinergic signaling, is involved in the multicellular behavior of these cells. This two-way influence is a paradigm for bidirectional information between immune and neural systems, showing how disturbance of autonomic signals can develop a suppressive immune environment that supports neoplastic growth. Pharmacologic agents that manipulate these neural circuits may thus present exciting avenues for managing cancer growth through modulation of the elements of the ANS that govern MDSC kinetics (Shu et al., 2024). Most influential to successful pharmacologic approaches is a subtle understanding of how the sympathetic and parasympathetic networks interact to modulate inflammation and physiological homeostasis. Beta-blockers, angiotensin-converting enzyme inhibitors (ACEi), and angiotensin II receptor blockers (ARBs) predominantly work by suppressing overactive sympathetic behavior, thus minimizing inflammatory mediators and improving cardiovascular outcomes. On the parasympathetic side, nonpharmacologic treatments such as VNS hold promise in enhancing cholinergic anti-inflammatory mechanisms, leading to reduced systemic inflammation and improved tissue repair. The new appreciation for the fact that autonomic nerve density and signaling significantly influence pathological processes highlights the necessity for pharmacological agents specific to restore autonomic balance. This combined strategy, targeting modulation of both autonomic branches, has great potential for the treatment of a variety of conditions characterized by autonomic dysfunction (Zoccali et al., 2025).

4.1.2. Sympathetic Versus Parasympathetic Nervous System

Grasping the functional dichotomy of the ANS is essential for understanding the pharmacological modulation of body functions. The sympathetic and parasympathetic nervous systems, while anatomically integrated, have different physiological functions. The sympathetic nervous system plays the major role in orchestrating the body's fight or flight reaction under stress, with resultant heightened heart rate, bronchodilation, and mobilization of energy. In contrast, the parasympathetic nervous system allows rest and digestion processes, prioritizing energy conservation and maintenance activities of the body like digestion and salivation. Pharmacologically, agents that act on these systems have to be accurately targeted to either imitate or block neurotransmitters such as norepinephrine and acetylcholine, which control receptor activity. This two-way control is especially relevant to cardiovascular disorders where sympathetic overdrive might require beta-blockade, while parasympathetic stimulation would be therapeutically beneficial (José et al., 2023). Hence, this comprehension of conflicting activities provides pivotal information for the intervention of therapeutic modalities in autonomic disorders. The discrete neurochemical pathways underlying the sympathetic and parasympathetic nervous systems provide a basis for their differing physiological outcomes and drug targets. Sympathetic postganglionic neurons release mainly norepinephrine, which acts on adrenergic receptors that are divided into alpha and beta types, each with specific cellular actions. Parasympathetic postganglionic neurons secrete acetylcholine that acts on muscarinic receptors to produce the effects of slowed heart rate and increased secretions of glands. The specific activation of these receptors enables precise control of autonomic functions in the clinical situation. For instance, parasympathetic agonists may enhance GI motility, whereas sympathetic antagonists may lower hypertension by reducing vasoconstriction. Modern treatments increasingly depend on receptor subtype specificity to limit systemic side effects inherent in autonomic pharmacology. Furthermore, the emerging knowledge of neuropeptides and hormones like glucagon-like peptide-1 uncovers further layers of autonomic control, broadening the pharmacological landscape (Timo et al., 2019). The interplay between sympathetic and parasympathetic nervous system activity exemplifies a delicate physiological balance susceptible to pharmacological intervention for diverse clinical indications. Autonomic dysfunction, whether from pathological excess or deficiency of sympathetic or parasympathetic tone, demands tailored therapeutic strategies. For instance, atrial fibrillation management incorporates modulation of autonomic inputs to restore cardiac rhythm and function, underscoring the importance of autonomic pharmacology guidelines (José et al., 2023). Also, novel agents acting on autonomic pathways demonstrate auspicious neuroprotective and metabolic actions, represented by GLP-1 receptor agonists that modulate cardiovascular and neurodegenerative disease processes through systems integration of autonomic mechanisms (Timo et al., 2019). Such developing comprehension not only enhances therapeutic potential but also requires a sophisticated understanding of autonomic receptor pharmacodynamics. Therefore, the parasympathetic and sympathetic nervous systems continue to be pivotal in furthering pharmacotherapy for systemic and organ-specific diseases (Figure 4.4).

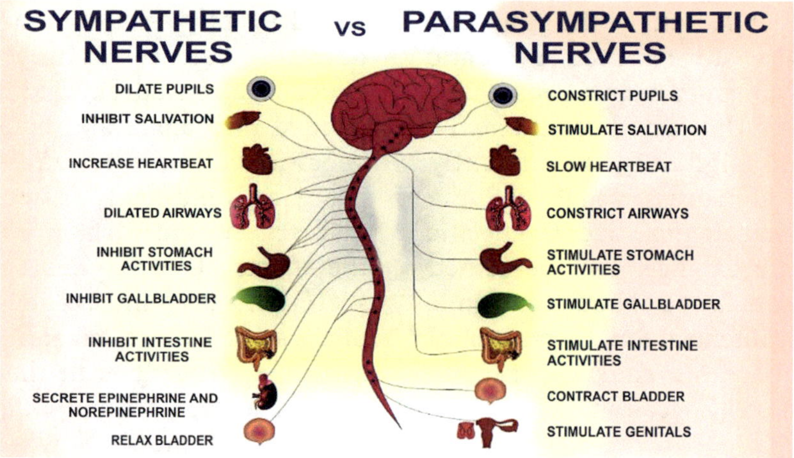

Figure 4.4. Sympathetic versus parasympathetic nervous system.

Source: YouTube. (n.d.). Sympathetic Versus Parasympathetic Nervous System. https://i.ytimg.com/vi/Yo9jZqyZruU/maxresdefault.jpg.

4.1.3. Role of the Enteric Nervous System (ENS)

The intricate interplay between neural, immune, and epithelial elements in the GI tract highlights the importance of intrinsic control mechanisms. Of these, the enteric nervous system (ENS) functions as an independent but integrated system of the ANS, regulating intestinal homeostasis with great intricacy. It is endowed with a vast network of neurons and glial cells, which control motility, secretion, and blood flow, making for the fine-tuned coordination required for digestion and nutrient uptake. Notably, the ENS regulates intestinal barrier function, impacting permeability and immune reactions in order to preserve gut homeostasis. This is mediated via neurotransmitters and neuropeptides that impact epithelial and immune cells, modulating inflammatory mechanisms and gut lining defense. The ENS is therefore a vital interface between luminal environment and host, underpinning the fine balance that underlies GI health and overall wellness (Cuddihey et al., 2022). The role of the ENS is not confined to local control, but it interacts with the CNS through bidirectional pathways of signaling well-known as the gut-brain axis. This comprehensive communication network involves not only neuronal circuits but also immune and endocrine pathways influenced by the gut microbiota. Emerging evidence points to the involvement of microbial metabolites such as short-chain fatty acids (SCFA) in modulating ENS function and neuroimmune interactions, emphasizing the system's adaptability to internal and external stimuli. These insights have profound implications for understanding functional GI disorders and their neuropathophysiology. The ENS is thus a key component that bridges the realms of microbial biology and autonomic regulation to influence neurochemical pathways with implications for both GI and CNS function (Silva et al., 2020). Pharmacologically, targeting the ENS offers novel therapeutic possibilities to modulate numerous digestive diseases. Drugs affecting ENS modulation can affect motility, secretion, and visceral sensitivity, hence treating symptoms of diseases like irritable bowel syndrome (IBS) and inflammatory bowel disease (IBD). The complex interplay between the ENS and endocannabinoid system represents the potential for receptor-specific therapies to modulate gut homeostasis and immune responses effectively. In addition, since the ENS acts somewhat autonomously, pharmacologic manipulation can elicit localized responses with less systemic participation. Ongoing investigation of ENS pharmacodynamics is needed to create targeted ANS therapies that leverage the intrinsic properties of gut neural circuits to restore and preserve GI well-being (Cuddihey et al., 2022).

Test Your Knowledge

1. What is the enteric nervous system (ENS)?
2. What is the role of the enteric nervous system as part of the ANS?

4.2. Neurotransmitters in the Autonomic Nervous System (ANS)

Learning Outcome

1. Acetylcholine and Its Functions
2. Norepinephrine and Its Role in Sympathetic Activation
3. Other Neurotransmitters Involved

Appreciation of the complexity of neurotransmitter dynamics in the ANS is key to understanding its pharmacological manipulation (Figure 4.5). Neurotransmitters serve as vital chemical messengers, mediating communication between the sympathetic and parasympathetic branches and peripheral target organs. Of these, acetylcholine and norepinephrine have predominant roles, mediating opposing physiological effects that preserve homeostasis. The complexity of receptor subtypes and their tissue distribution makes drug targeting more difficult, requiring a subtle understanding of neurotransmitter action. In addition, the role of modulatory peptides and endogenous opioids adds further layers of regulation, as opioid receptors found throughout autonomic pathways modulate neurotransmitter release and affect autonomic functions like cardiovascular control and stress responses (Walwyn et al., 2022). Therefore, the interaction among classical neurotransmitters and neuropeptides constitutes a multifunctional network that plays a critical role in determining autonomic pharmacological approaches. Cellular signaling pathways involved in neurotransmitter discharge and receptor triggering within the ANS uncover new mechanisms pivotal to the therapeutic approach. Intracellular messengers like Ca^{2+} and cAMP have been shown to synergistically interact in controlling exocytosis of neurotransmitters in autonomic neurons. This Ca^{2+}/cAMP interaction regulates neurotransmitter release by affecting calcium channel function and intracellular stores of calcium, thereby influencing synaptic transmission efficacy. Pharmacological agents that inhibit or enhance this intracellular interaction have the potential to increase or decrease autonomic signaling, providing new therapeutic options for controlling disorders characterized by sympathetic hyperactivity or parasympathetic dysregulation. Interestingly, calcium channel blockers—widely prescribed antihypertensives—have paradoxical actions by enhancing neurotransmitter release through this Ca^{2+}/cAMP cross talk, which underscores the complexity of autonomic neurotransmitter regulation and the requirement for accurate drug modulation (Bergantin et al., 2017). Such findings emphasize the role of intracellular signaling pathways in ANS pharmacology. Beyond traditional neurotransmitters, the endogenous opioid system illustrates the multidimensional modulation of autonomic neurotransmission. Opioid peptides like enkephalins, beta-endorphins, and dynorphins act on mu, delta, and kappa opioid receptors found pre- and post-synaptically in autonomic pathways. These G protein-coupled receptors suppress neuronal excitability and release of neurotransmitters via mechanisms such as inhibition of adenyl cyclase and ion channel modulation and thereby modulate autonomic output. The differential expression and capacity of opioid receptors to heteromerize raise the level of complexity of their regulatory function, and they modulate autonomic functions such as pain sensation, stress reaction, and cardiovascular regulation (Walwyn et al., 2022). Modulation of opioid receptors in the ANS is promising for creating therapeutics that selectively act on autonomic neurotransmitter discharge, offering elegant treatments for diseases like hypertension, addiction, and stress disorders.

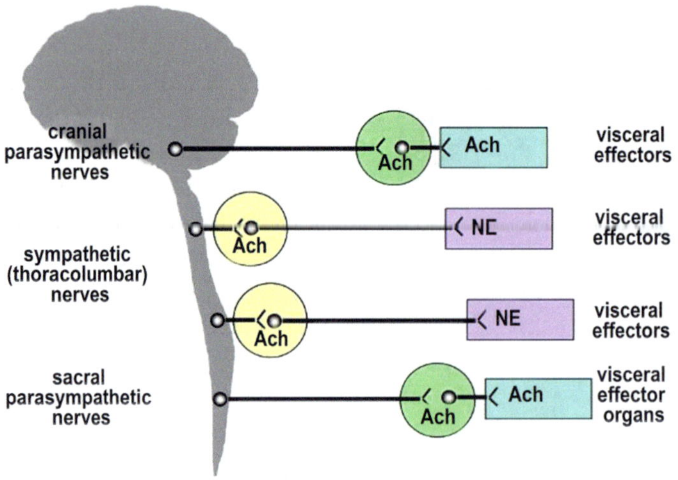

Figure 4.5. Neurotransmitters in the autonomic nervous system (ANS).

Source: Slideserve. (n.d.). *Neurotransmitters in the Autonomic Nervous System.* https://image3.slideserve.com/6110536/neurotransmitters-of-the-ans1-l.jpg.

4.2.1. Acetylcholine and Its Functions

The complex mechanisms involved in autonomic regulation underscore the crucial role played by neurotransmitters in ensuring physiological homeostasis. Of these, acetylcholine is the key neurotransmitter of the parasympathetic nervous system, its actions being mediated through binding to muscarinic and nicotinic receptors (Figure 4.6). Such interaction at postsynaptic locations initiates various physiological responses including modulation of heart rate, glandular secretion, and smooth muscle contraction in visceral organs. Interestingly, the effect of acetylcholine goes beyond traditional neurotransmission to encompass regulatory roles in peripheral tissues, as seen in its modulation of ovarian function via parasympathetic mechanisms. This cholinergic regulation is involved in the fine-tuning of steroid hormone release and follicular growth, which are critical for reproductive well-being. This neural-endocrine interaction highlights acetylcholine's wider influence on systemic function, especially in disorders with autonomic dysbalance such as polycystic ovary syndrome (PCOS) (Yu et al., 2024). Apart from its traditional function of neurotransmission, acetylcholine has important immunomodulatory roles via the cholinergic anti-inflammatory pathway. This includes acetylcholine's binding to α7 nicotinic acetylcholine receptors on immune cells, downregulating pro-inflammatory cytokine release and facilitating immune homeostasis. This pathway disruption can be a cause of pathological conditions due to immune dysfunction. For example, prenatal exposure to environmental xenobiotics such as Deca brominated diphenyl ether (BDE-209) has been known to disrupt parasympathetic signaling with consequences on modified acetylcholine interactions at the receptors on immune cells. Such interference impacts immune defense through the modulation of crucial signaling cascades, for example, JAK2/STAT3 signaling pathway, thereby resulting in offspring with immunotoxic effects. This finding supports acetylcholine's dual nature as both a neurotransmitter and an immunoregulatory molecule in ANS pharmacology (Mao et al., 2024). Pharmacological interference with autonomic disorders relies on understanding acetylcholine's diverse functions. Agents augmenting or blocking cholinergic transmission corrects aberrant parasympathetic activity, which affects cardiovascular function, GI motility, and immune function. For instance, therapeutic modulation of acetylcholine receptors has been promising in the restoration of sympathetic-parasympathetic imbalances seen in disease states such as PCOS, where enhanced sympathetic and reduced parasympathetic outputs underlie pathophysiology. Another pharmacological approach lies in the prevention of environmental toxin-induced impairments in cholinergic pathways to restore immune competence. Accordingly, ongoing studies on the pharmacodynamics of acetylcholine and its receptors will improve the discovery of more targeted autonomic treatments that can target both neural and immunological disorders (Mao et al., 2024; Yu et al., 2024).

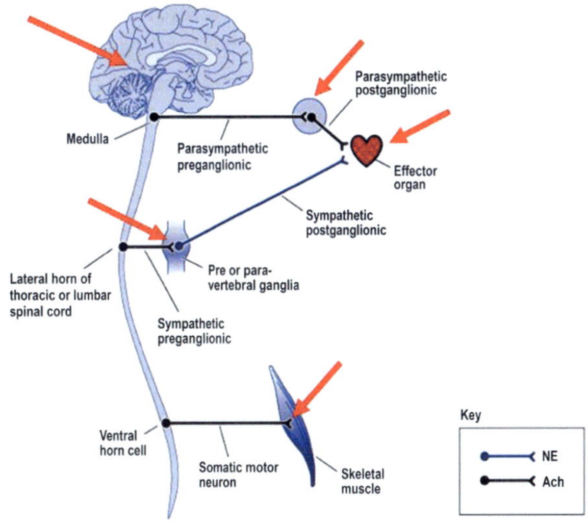

Figure 4.6. Acetylcholine and its functions.

Source: The Pepproject. (2022). *Acetylcholine and Its Functions.*

4.2.2. Norepinephrine and Its Role in Sympathetic Activation

The ANS coordinates quick physiological responses essential for survival, particularly under stress or threat. At the heart of this quick response is the sympathetic nervous system, which mobilizes body resources through a rise in heart rate, expansion of airways, and diversion of blood to vital muscles. This integration is highly reliant on the release of norepinephrine from sympathetic nerve terminals. Norepinephrine is both a neurotransmitter and a hormone, binding to adrenergic receptors on target cells to trigger biochemical cascades that allow the fight-or-flight response. Its mechanisms of synthesis, release, and reuptake guarantee rapid onset and timely termination of sympathetic stimulation. Such control mechanisms enable the organism to achieve homeostasis while responding to external stimuli effectively. In addition, norepinephrine's effects upon the system are not limited to direct sympathetic stimulation, acting upon metabolic and cardiovascular functions to position it as a key player within autonomic regulation (John et al., 2019). In peripheral tissues, the action of norepinephrine is emphasized through its activation of adrenergic receptors that are G-protein coupled receptors categorized into α and β types. Norepinephrine activates these receptors when sympathetic nerves are activated, regulating various physiological processes. For instance, in cardiac tissue, stimulation of β1-adrenergic receptors increases contractility and heart rate, thus increasing cardiac output. In vascular smooth muscle, stimulation of α1-adrenergic receptors results in vasoconstriction, raising systemic vascular resistance and blood pressure. Norepinephrine also regulates energy metabolism by stimulating lipolysis in adipose tissue, releasing free fatty acids as alternative substrates for energy during stress. This complex receptor interaction broadens the range of norepinephrine's actions, coordinating the nervous system's messages with peripheral organ reactions necessary for adaptive physiological modifications (Castillo et al., 2019). Modulation of norepinephrine signaling offers important pharmacological opportunities to manage diverse autonomic and cardiovascular disorders. Norepinephrine-mimetic drugs, including sympathomimetics, may increase sympathetic tone in instances of hypotension or cardiac arrest. In contrast, adrenergic antagonists, α and β blockers, block the binding of norepinephrine and downstream responses, invaluable in treating hypertension, arrhythmias, and anxiety disorders. Current studies highlight the understanding of receptor subtype selectivity to maximize therapeutic effects and minimize unwanted side effects. Furthermore, pathological abnormalities in norepinephrine pathways, for example, inappropriate release or deficient reuptake, are the basis for disease conditions such as heart failure and chronic stress disorders. Intervening on these disruptions presents highly promising lines for intervention in the autonomic pharmacological context, illustrating norepinephrine's place at the center of both physiological and therapeutic investigation (Figure 4.7).

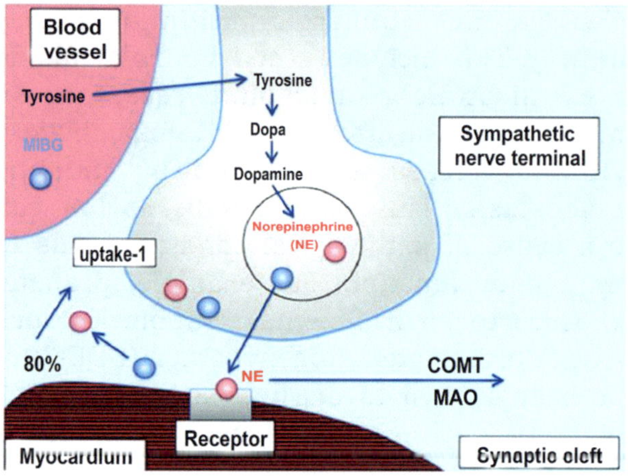

Figure 4.7. Norepinephrine and its role in sympathetic activation.

Source: de Brito, A. X., et al. (2021). Norepinephrine and MIBG metabolic pathways in the sympathetic cardiac nerve terminal. In *Autonomic Innervation Evaluation in Cardiac Disease. ResearchGate.*

4.2.3. Other Neurotransmitters Involved

Outside the traditional catecholamines and acetylcholine, numerous other neurotransmitters have a profound influence on the ANS's activity, extending the pharmacologic horizon. Serotonin, for instance, has a complex role in controlling cardiovascular and autonomic responses. Antidepressant medication acting on serotonin reuptake exhibits varied actions on blood pressure and autonomic balance.

Selective serotonin reuptake inhibitors (SSRIs) are found to have little effect, showing a safer profile for cardiovascular patients. On the other hand, medications affecting both serotonin and norepinephrine levels, like serotonin-norepinephrine reuptake inhibitors, may increase sympathetic nervous system activity, leading to hypertension at times. In addition, dopamine and histamine systems overlap with autonomic pathways, mediating vascular tone and heart rate modulation. The intricacy of these interactions underscores the need for a sophisticated appreciation of how pharmacological modulation of these neurotransmitters can be beneficial or complicated for autonomic regulation, especially in comorbid patients with cardiovascular or psychiatric disorders (Calvi et al., 2021). Besides classical neurotransmitters, new evidence points to the role of other biochemical mediators and natural products in autonomic regulation. Essential oils, for example, have exhibited anxiolytic, antidepressant, and sedative activities due to their action on multiple neurotransmitter systems such as the GABAergic, serotonergic, and dopaminergic systems. Animal models revealed that these compounds are able to modulate physiological parameters that are closely linked with autonomic function, such as heart rate and blood pressure, suggesting a direct effect on autonomic output.

Nonetheless, clinical verification is inevitable to completely disclose their mechanisms and possible therapeutic applications. It can reveal new perspectives regarding adjunct treatments of conditions with autonomic dysregulation by knowing how natural products act upon several neurotransmitter systems (Lorena, 2020). The interaction of varied neurotransmitters and their receptors also highlights the complexity and plasticity of autonomic control. Neurotransmitter drugs manipulating norepinephrine, dopamine, serotonin, and others like histamine or melatonin receptors modulate the autonomic tone in the face of fluctuating physiological as well as pathologic states. Such is illustrated by the irregular blood pressure response to various antidepressants that exert their effects across multiple transmitter mechanisms. For example, certain agents will enhance the sympathetic outflow to cause hypertension, whereas other agents induce orthostatic hypotension from varied receptor engagements.

This complex pharmacodynamic matrix requires prudent therapeutic attention, particularly to the risks of drug interaction, side effects, and cardiovascular risk specific to the patient. Thus, broadening investigation to these other neurotransmitters increases the potential for therapeutic intervention while drawing attention to mechanistic nuance in ANS pharmacology (Figure 4.8) (Calvi et al., 2021).

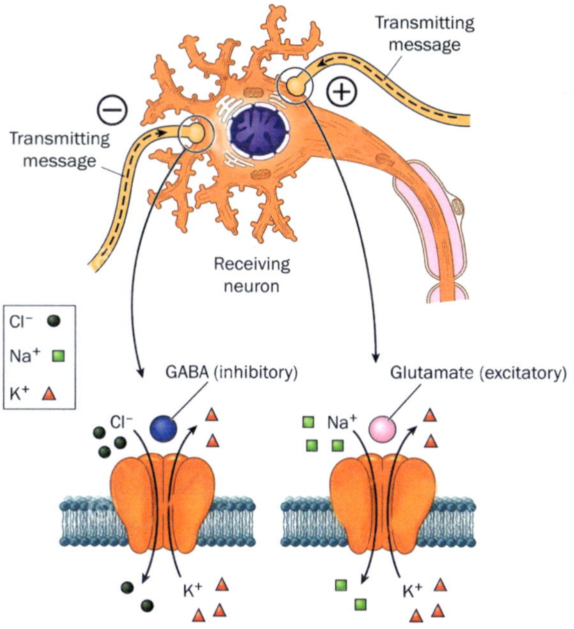

Figure 4.8. Other neurotransmitters involved.

Source: Dreamstime. (n.d.). *Neurotransmitters Involved in Epilepsy.* https://thumbs.dreamstime.com/z/neurotransmitters-involved-epilepsy-12522920.jpg.

Test Your Knowledge

1. How does norepinephrine affect heart rate and blood pressure?
2. How does dopamine act as a neurotransmitter in the ANS?

4.3. Pharmacological Agents Affecting the Autonomic Nervous System (ANS)

Learning Outcome

1. Cholinergic Drugs and Their Mechanisms
2. Adrenergic Drugs and Their Applications
3. Other Classes of Autonomic Pharmacological Agents

The complex ANS network controls involuntary physiologic processes, from cardiovascular control to GI motility. The pharmacologic modulation of the ANS utilizes agents acting on the sympathetic and parasympathetic divisions, which commonly have opposite actions on organ systems. drenergic agonists and antagonists, for example, selectively stimulate or block receptors that respond to norepinephrine and epinephrine, controlling vascular tone and cardiac output. In contrast, cholinergic drugs act on acetylcholine pathways, altering neurotransmission in parasympathetic synapses. The therapeutic uses of these medications involve varied clinical settings such as hypertension, arrhythmias, and asthma. Receptor subtypes and their pharmacodynamics are critical to understand since selective activation or blockade can reduce side effects with increased efficacy. The sophistication of autonomic pharmacology is emphasized by the foundational research achievements characterizing neurotransmission mechanisms and purinergic transmission, which have deepened our understanding of receptor diversity and functional consequences (Burnstock et al., 2011). Growing evidence indicates that the interaction of the ANS with peripheral systems goes beyond traditional neurotransmission and includes immune and GI realms modulated by drugs. Diseases like Parkinson's disease illustrate the clinical relevance of this network, in which autonomic dysfunction precedes motor symptoms. Modulation of the gut-brain axis by microbiota and immune signaling pathways has implications for autonomic control as well as neurodegeneration. Pharmacologic interventions in dysbiosis-related inflammation or the stabilization of intestinal barrier function can secondarily regulate ANS activity. Toll-like receptors (TLRs) are pivotal to innate immunity and are new targets that modulate neuroimmune communication. Therefore, medications that alter the microbiota-gut-brain axis are a new field in autonomic pharmacology, modulating systemic and neuronal inflammation to correct autonomic and ENS dysfunctions (Caputi et al., 2018). The selectivity and specificity of pharmacological compounds acting on the ANS are essential to maximize therapeutic effects while avoiding off-target activities. Progress in receptor subtype identification has created drugs with improved receptor affinity profiles, including beta-1 selective blockers for cardiac disease or muscarinic antagonists for respiratory disease. Moreover, the identification of purinergic receptors has provided new possibilities for novel therapies aimed at ATP-mediated signaling within autonomic pathways, expanding the range of available neuropharmacological interventions (Burnstock et al., 2011). The therapeutic value of these drugs is further augmented by the knowledge of their mechanisms at molecular and systemic levels, enabling personalized medicine strategies. In-depth understanding of autonomic pharmacology not only enhances existing clinical practice but also stimulates innovation in the treatment of diseases with autonomic dysregulation, providing better quality of life for patients with complex neurophysiological disorders.

4.3.1. Cholinergic Drugs and Their Mechanisms

Knowledge of the subtlety of the interaction in the ANS illustrates the mode of action of cholinergic drugs to achieve their therapeutic impact through the stimulation of certain receptors to alter parasympathetic activity. The drugs act mainly on muscarinic and nicotinic acetylcholine receptors, which are found in widespread tissues such as smooth muscles, cardiac muscles, and glands. Muscarinic agonists, for instance, simulate the effect of acetylcholine to produce increased secretions, reduced heart rate, and enhanced GI motility. In contrast, muscarinic antagonists inhibit such receptors, lowering parasympathetic tone and are therapeutically beneficial in conditions such as bradycardia or overactive bladder. Nicotinic receptor modulators, though targeted less frequently in therapeutics, act on autonomic ganglia and neuromuscular junctions and affect both sympathetic and parasympathetic systems. The subtype specificity of cholinergic drugs is the foundation for their multiple clinical uses and side effect profiles, which emphasizes the role of receptor pharmacodynamics in the design of autonomic agents (Fromer et al., 2014). The pivotal role of the cholinergic system in modulating both cognitive and autonomic processes emphasizes the complexity of its pharmacological mechanisms. The limbic system, specifically the hippocampus, integrates cholinergic input to modulate memory and behavioral output, interacting with autonomic outputs through hypothalamic mechanisms. Drugs like scopolamine are muscarinic antagonists in this system, reducing cholinergic output and eliciting clinically significant effects such as mitigation of motion sickness and cognitive impairment. This shows how cholinergic drugs (Figure 4.9) can affect both peripheral autonomic targets and CNS pathways. In addition, cholinergic modulation crosses with the other neurotransmitter systems, including dopamine and norepinephrine, to give the subtle regulation of autonomic and cognitive activities (Kohl and Odell, 2025). Such modulation highlights the importance of accuracy when developing drugs that modulate cholinergic neurotransmission without central or peripheral side effects. Pharmacological manipulation of cholinergic transmission requires a knowledge of enzyme regulation and the availability of synaptic acetylcholine, which are essential determinants of drug action. Acetylcholinesterase inhibitors extend the synaptic action of acetylcholine by inhibiting its degradation, thus potentiating parasympathetic response. These inhibitors have been used from the treatment of myasthenia gravis to the prevention of neurodegenerative loss seen in Alzheimer's disease (AD), where cholinergic loss is responsible for cognitive defect. But such increased cholinergic tone can also trigger unwanted effects like bronchoconstriction or bradycardia, reflecting the therapeutic dilemma of achieving safety alongside efficacy. Progress in selective cholinergic drug design continues to improve these agents' selectivity, aiming for subtype-selective receptor agonists or inhibitors to maximize clinical efficacy while limiting systemic cholinergic side effects (Fromer et al., 2014). This delicate balance is crucial in ANS pharmacology, where targeted modulation of cholinergic mechanisms has major therapeutic potential.

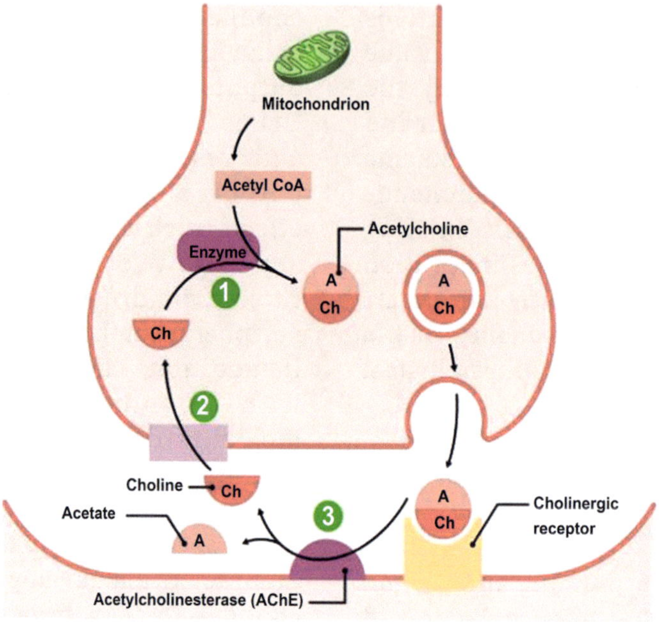

Figure 4.9. Cholinergic drugs and their mechanisms.

Source: Lecturio. (n.d.). *Cholinergic Drugs and Their Mechanisms.* https://cdn.lecturio.com/assets/Acetylcholine-Secretion-and-Reabsorption.png.

4.3.2. Adrenergic Drugs and Their Applications

The delicate equilibrium that is preserved by the ANS is highly dependent on adrenergic receptor modulation and, therefore, adrenergic drugs are critical in therapeutic strategies (Figure 4.10). Adrenergic drugs act by mimicking or blocking the action of endogenous catecholamines, i.e., norepinephrine and epinephrine, on α and β adrenergic receptors found in many organ systems. Their varied mode of action allows for selective targeting of physiological effect, e.g., vasoconstriction, bronchodilation, and enhanced cardiac output. For this reason, these agents prove to be exceedingly valuable in controlling cardiovascular disease, respiratory disease, and even some anaphylactic crises. Investigation into the pharmacodynamics of these substances identifies a complicated interplay between receptor subtypes and drug specificity and serves to emphasize the relevance of receptor selectivity in reducing unwanted effects while maximizing therapeutic benefit. With changing clinical guidelines, healthcare professionals are required to constantly upgrade their knowledge so that adrenergic pharmacotherapies can be used optimally within patient-focused care paradigms (Kirchhof et al., 2016). Clinical utility of adrenergic agents penetrates deeply into emergency medicine, where hemodynamic stabilization is often needed quickly. Agents like epinephrine are used as first-line therapy in anaphylaxis and cardiopulmonary arrest because of their strong α and β adrenergic receptor activity, which brings about vasoconstriction and increased myocardial contractility. Moreover, β2-selective agents like albuterol have transformed the treatment of asthma by causing relaxation of airway smooth muscle and increased airflow obstruction. Still, systemic side effects from these drugs, such as tachycardia and hypertension, pose problems with clinical use in requiring cautious dose titration and monitoring. Pharmacokinetics of these drugs, such as their duration of action and metabolic fate, also impact their clinical choices. Therefore, an in-depth understanding of adrenergic receptor pharmacology provides the correct choice and administration of these drugs in diverse clinical settings, striking the right balance between efficacy and safety issues (Kirchhof et al., 2016). In addition to this, adrenergic antagonists or beta-blockers and alpha-blockers have proved to play a vital part in the chronic control of disease states. Beta-blockers, through competitively inhibiting β-adrenergic receptors, reduce heart rate and myocardial oxygen consumption, rendering them essential in managing hypertension, angina, and arrhythmias.

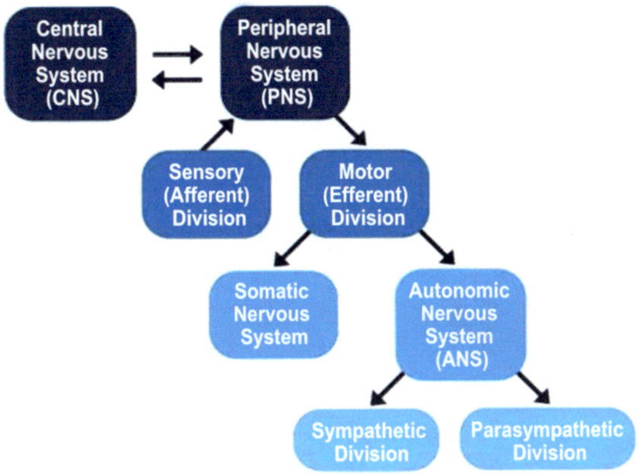

Figure 4.10. Adrenergic drugs and their applications.

Source: Elsevier. (n.d.). *Adrenergic Drugs and Their Applications*. https://ars.els-cdn.com/content/image/3-s2.0-B978032395901800016X-f15-01-9780323959018.jpg.

Likewise, alpha-blockers reduce peripheral vascular resistance by avoiding vasoconstriction, which is useful in benign prostatic hyperplasia and some forms of hypertension. Choice of these drugs is frequently influenced by receptor selectivity profiles and patient comorbidities, emphasizing the requirement for individualized therapeutic strategies. These agents illustrate how adrenergic medications move beyond acute uses to shape chronic disease management, highlighting their adaptability in the pharmacology of ANS. Practice according to up-to-date clinical guidelines and best evidence is essential to optimize patient outcomes while avoiding possible drug interactions and contraindications (Kirchhof et al., 2016).

4.3.3. Other Classes of Autonomic Pharmacological Agents

In addition to the familiar adrenergic and cholinergic drugs, the ANS pharmacology also involves a range of additional classes with important clinical actions (Figure 4.11). These involve ganglionic blockers, which disrupt transmission at autonomic ganglia and influence both sympathetic and parasympathetic outflow. These agents are no longer commonly employed because of their wide, non-selective blockade and severe side effects but are important to consider because they reveal so much about the integrated activity of autonomic pathways. Moreover, neuromodulators with action on particular neurotransmitter release or reuptake processes, e.g., monoamine oxidase inhibitors and reuptake blockers, affect autonomic tone indirectly and play key roles in treating depression and neurodegenerative disease. Such multifaceted pharmacotherapies depict the intricate interaction between autonomic outflow and systemic physiological control, the necessity of therapeutic specificity and the creation of agents with more selectively profiled action. Another significant category consists of drugs that act on the ENS, a separate branch of the ANS that governs GI function. Drugs that target this system play a critical role in the treatment of a variety of GI disorders, from motility disturbances to acid secretion disturbances. For example, advances in gastroenterology pharmacology have utilized fiberoptic endoscopy to enhance mucosal biology, enabling more effective therapeutic interventions that act on autonomic gut modulators. New pharmacologic agents, such as prokinetics and secretagogues, exert their effects through the modulation of autonomic receptors in the GI tract to normalize function or relieve symptoms. These therapies highlight the subtle role of autonomic pharmacology over wide systemic actions, illustrating its importance in organ-specific situations and the potential for improving patient outcomes in specialized practice (Camilleri et al., 1999). In addition, the ANS's interaction with higher brain systems provides another multifaceted dimension for pharmacological control. Various drugs exert their autonomic actions via mechanisms that include the limbic system, hippocampus, and hypothalamus, thus modulating hormonal as well as neurochemical responses. For instance, drugs like scopolamine and amphetamine are well known to counteract motion sickness through action on cholinergic transmission in the septohippocampal pathway, which then modulates autonomic outputs. Such effects transcend mere peripheral receptor modulation to involve intrinsic neurochemical processes responsible for coordinating endocrine and behavioral responses to stress and environmental challenge. Such an understanding is fundamental to the formulation of therapeutic strategies that not only correct autonomic dysfunction but also address the cognitive and emotional aspects of autonomic regulation (Kohl and Odell, 2025).

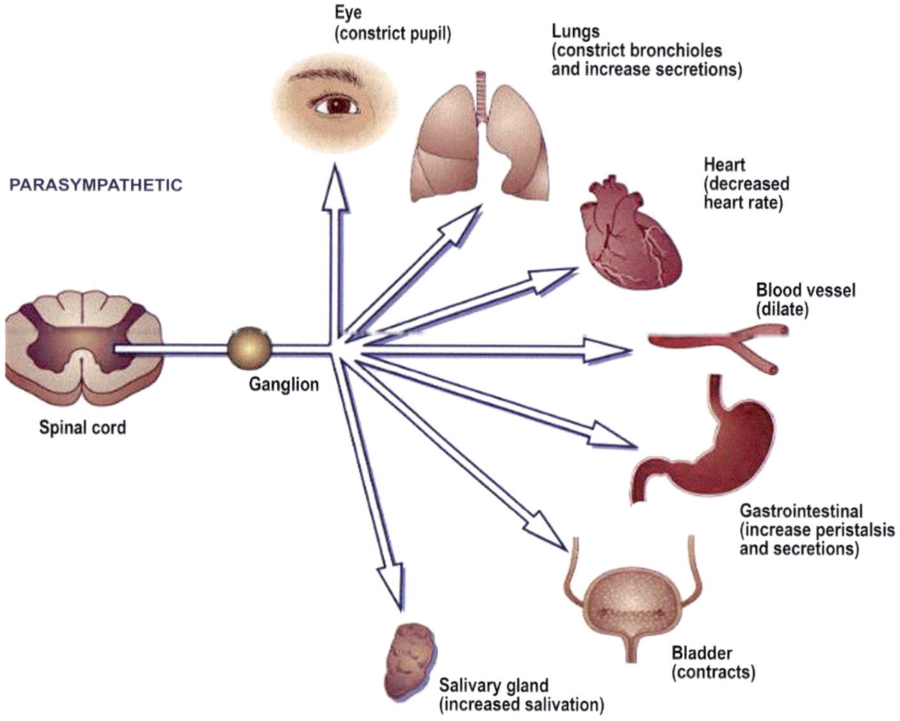

Figure 4.11. Autonomic nervous system (ANS) pharmacology and cholinergic.

Source: https://basicmedicalkey.com/wp-content/uploads/2017/04/image02323.jpeg.

Test Your Knowledge

1. What are adrenergic drugs?
2. What are autonomic pharmacological agents?

4.4. Clinical Applications of Autonomic Pharmacology

Learning Outcome

1. Treatment of Hypertension
2. Management of Asthma
3. Use in Gastrointestinal (GI) Disorders

The therapeutic implication of autonomic pharmacology resides in its power to regulate the parasympathetic and sympathetic nervous system and thereby to correct a myriad of clinical states. Adrenergic and cholinergic receptors can be specifically modified with drugs to control selectively cardiovascular, respiratory, and GI functions for treating conditions such as hypertension, asthma, and chronic obstructive lung disease (COPD). Sympathomimetic agents, such as, cause bronchodilation due to the activation of beta-2 adrenergic receptors, yielding symptomatic relief during acute exacerbation of asthma, whereas cholinergic antagonists decrease secretions and spasms of smooth muscle in respiratory illnesses. Careful autonomic agent selection based on receptor specificity and systemic actions optimizes patient responses and prevents untoward reactions. This strategy is the epitome of the clinical significance of autonomic pharmacodynamics and pharmacokinetics in designing personalized treatment strategies that maximize efficacy and safety, illustrating the critical role of autonomic agents in modern medical practice (Ahmed et al., 2023). In psychiatric and stress-related disorders, autonomic pharmacology provides avenues to counteract the physiological expressions of anxiety and depression through modulation of autonomic tone. Sympathetic dominance, which is commonly seen in these disorders, interferes with homeostasis and amplifies symptoms, making interventions that restore equilibrium necessary. Although pharmacologic interventions addressed to neurotransmitter mechanisms can reduce symptoms, recent data show the significant impact of non-pharmacologic interventions on autonomic regulation. Interventions like meditation and regulated breathing influence parasympathetic activity, thus suppressing sympathetic overdrive and balancing cardiovascular and respiratory responses. This integrated view argues that the merger of pharmacologic agents with behavioral therapies may add therapeutic potency to such interventions and address more adequately the systemic and emotional aspects of these disorders. Further, inquiry into autonomic pharmacology as an approach underscores the need for multidisciplinary care in neuropsychiatry (Barnes et al., 2015). Autonomic pharmacology plays a vital role in the treatment of conditions that are dominated by dysregulation of autonomic control in cardiovascular medicine. Beta-blockers and alpha-adrenergic antagonists are used on a regular basis to slow heart rate and vascular resistance, thereby managing hypertension and avoiding such complications as heart failure and arrhythmias. These drugs take advantage of targeted receptor sites to dampen inappropriate sympathetic nervous system activity that contributes to pathophysiology. Parasympathetic modulators also can treat bradyarrhythmia's and enhance cardiac function by augmenting vagal tone. The accuracy provided by autonomic pharmacology enables doctors to individualize interventions that correct autonomic dysequilria, decrease morbidity, and enhance quality of life. The clinical application does not just reflect a thorough appreciation of receptor pharmacology but is also an expression of the bridge of translation among physiological insight and therapeutic development (Ahmed et al., 2023).

4.4.1. Treatment of Hypertension

Regulation of blood pressure is an intricate play of neural and hormonal messages, and the ANS has an integral role. The pathogenesis of hypertension is usually caused by dysregulation in this system, requiring treatment that involves correcting autonomic imbalances (Figure 4.12). Pharmacologic agents aimed at the sympathetic nervous system, like beta-adrenergic blockers, reduce sympathetic outflow and lower cardiac output, hence reducing blood pressure. In addition, alpha-adrenergic blockers lower peripheral vascular resistance through enhancement of vasodilation. These drugs are excellent examples of the efficacy of modulation of autonomic pathways in the management of hypertension. Nonpharmacological interventions, such as lifestyle changes that minimize sympathetic activation—stress management and aerobic exercise—augment pharmacotherapy. Thus, treatment regimens incorporating both pharmacological and nonpharmacological interventions can better restore autonomic balance and maximize hypertensive control outcomes. Where traditional pharmacologic therapies are ineffective or contraindicated, emerging therapies aimed at autonomic dysfunction are promising. Pulmonary arterial hypertension (PAH) is an example of the wider importance of autonomic participation in vascular disease, and heightened sympathetic nervous system activation worsening disease progression. Therapies including renal denervation and pulmonary artery denervation seek to interrupt pathological sympathetic nerve activity (SNA), thus lowering vascular resistance and enhancing cardiac function (Mylène et al., 2017). Although these strategies are mainly investigated in PAH, they demonstrate a translational application for resistant systemic hypertension treatment by regulating autonomic tone. Elucidation and harnessing these neurogenic mechanisms would revolutionize therapeutic strategies, particularly in refractory hypertension, by directly addressing the autonomic mechanisms responsible for the maintenance of elevated arterial pressure. Further, the incorporation of ANS pharmacology spans the treatment of blood pressure regulation to incorporate comorbid autonomic dysfunctions frequently encountered with chronic diseases. For instance, in neurodegenerative illnesses such as Parkinson's disease, impairment of the autonomic system is responsible for orthostatic hypotension and other circulatory dysfunctions, making it difficult to treat hypertension (Jose-Palma et al., 2018). Personalized drug therapy to mitigate certain autonomic deficits enhances the quality of life of patients and decreases cardiovascular risk. This requires careful agent selection that optimizes the reduction of blood pressure efficacy with maintenance or restoration of the autonomic functions. Therefore, in addition to routine antihypertensive treatment, physicians need to take into account the larger autonomic picture, knowing that integrated treatment of autonomic dysregulation is essential to maximize hypertension treatment and patient outcome.

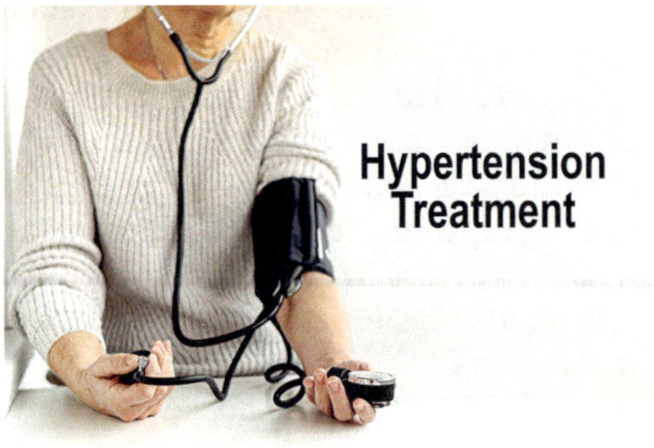

Figure 4.12. Treatment of hypertension.

Source: Dr. Benny Jose. (2021). *Treatment of Hypertension.*

4.4.2. Management of Asthma

Optimal control of asthma requires a complex comprehension of the ANSs function in airway regulation. Bronchoconstriction is mediated by the parasympathetic nervous system, mostly through vagal innervation, by the release of acetylcholine on muscarinic receptors in the airway smooth muscle. On the other hand, sympathetic stimulation causes bronchodilation through β2-adrenergic receptors. Pharmacological agents that act upon these mechanisms form the foundation of asthma treatment. β2-agonists, being bronchodilators, cause relaxation of airway smooth muscle through the stimulation of adenylate cyclase, increasing cyclic AMP concentration. This pharmacodynamic concept is the basis for both short-acting drugs in acute relief and long-acting drugs in maintenance. In addition, anticholinergic drugs inhibit muscarinic receptors and thus parasympathetic-induced bronchoconstriction. The subtle regulation of these autonomic mechanisms allows for specific therapeutic approaches, prioritizing bronchodilation and anti-inflammatory control to achieve maximum asthma control. Adjuvant treatments continue to support autonomic-targeted pharmacological interventions by treating inflammatory and metabolic aspects interwoven with asthma pathophysiology. Corticosteroids, which do not modulate autonomic receptors directly, suppress airway inflammation, thereby reducing hyperresponsiveness frequently elevated by neural reflex arcs. Other recent findings relating to the influence of free fatty acid receptors (FFARs) explain the potential indirect effects of autonomic influences in asthma through immune and metabolic control. FFARs, which are sensitive to a range of fatty acid ligands, regulate inflammatory mediators and may be new targets for therapeutic interventions that balance metabolic and immune pathways that affect airway function (Kimura et al., 2019). Incorporating such strategies expands the pharmacological repertoire beyond traditional autonomic agents, promoting a more holistic asthma management paradigm. Clinical guidelines repeatedly emphasize the importance of individualized treatment plans based on patient response and evidence-based protocols. Although the European Society of Cardiology guidelines are most concerned with cardiovascular implications, their approach to the proper evaluation of risk, patient-specific variables, and compliance with progressive therapeutic guidelines applies well to asthma care (Figure 4.13). Standardized guidelines have to be balanced against clinical acumen, particularly where autonomic pharmacology interacts with comorbid disease and polypharmacy (Josép Brugada et al., 2019). Such an integrated approach guarantees that asthma treatment not only entails autonomic modulation that is specifically targeted but also broader patient health considerations, safety, and new evidence in order to maximize therapy results.

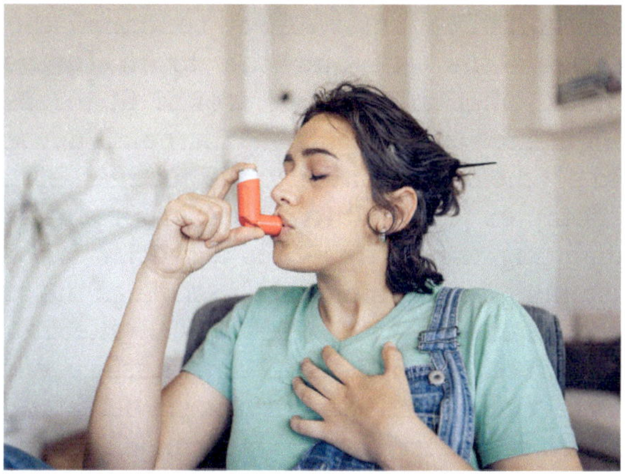

Figure 4.13. Management of asthma.

Source: Hill Regional Hospital. (n.d.). *Effective Strategies for Asthma Management: Expert Insights*. https://www.hillregionalhospital.com/assets/img/blogs/effective-strategies-for-asthma-management-expert-insights.jpg.

4.4.3. Use in Gastrointestinal (GI) Disorders

The complex interaction between the ANS and GI function has been widely explored in recent pharmacological literature, especially within disorders involving abnormal gut-brain communication. This interaction is particularly important to understand since the ANS controls essential processes like motility, secretion, and GI blood flow, all of which play significant roles in maintaining homeostasis. New technologies, including wearable sensors, have further informed this knowledge by providing real-time measurements of autonomic parameters beyond the confines of laboratory testing. Such sensors enable the evaluation of physiological indicators such as respiratory sinus arrhythmia and vagal efficiency, which act as surrogates for parasympathetic tone and general autonomic balance. In GI diseases such as cyclic vomiting syndrome, where psychosocial stressors exacerbate ANS dysregulation, these advances present hope for personalized therapeutic interventions to treat autonomic dysfunction (Kolacz, 2024). The two-way communication between the gut and the brain further renders pharmacologic control of GI disease complicated by bringing in microbial, neural, and psychological variables. The gut microbiota, a complex community of microorganisms inhabiting the GI tract, has a crucial role in sustaining neural and GI health through the gut microbiome-brain axis. Dysbiosis, or alteration in microbial composition, can interfere with this regulatory pathway, resulting in heightened blood-brain barrier (BBB) permeability and resultant GI and neurological diseases. ANS modulates these effects by acting directly on gut motility, secretion, and permeability, which in turn dictates the microbial environment. Such dynamic interaction emphasizes the role of pharmacological agents that modulate autonomic pathways in restoring microbial balance and alleviating GI symptoms, and the necessity for integrative approaches encompassing both neuropharmacology and microbiome-targeted therapies (Janet et al., 2023). Pharmacologic modulation of the ANS in GI disease requires a balanced understanding of both central and peripheral processes impacting gut function. Drugs modifying sympathetic and parasympathetic mechanisms are capable of strongly affecting gut motility and secretion, bringing about symptomatic benefit in IBS and functional dyspepsia. But heterogeneity of such diseases and mediation of psychological stressors via autonomic dysregulation continue to pose challenges towards the best of therapeutic modalities. In addition, incorporation of wearable sensor technology into clinical use provides even more layers of customized evaluation, allowing clinicians to observe autonomic function non-stop and modify treatments according to individual autonomic patterns. These developments show potential to enhance diagnostic precision and the effectiveness of pharmacologic treatments for reestablishing autonomic equilibrium in GI diseases (Kolacz, 2024) (Figure 4.14).

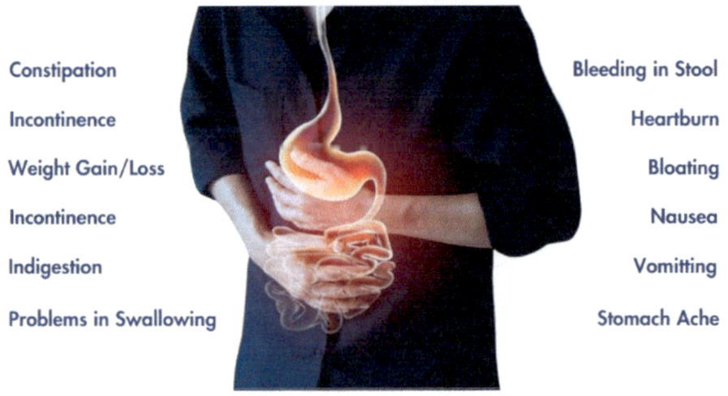

Figure 4.14. Use in gastrointestinal disorders.

Source: Dr. Abhishek Jain Gastroenterology (2025). *Gastrointestinal Diseases: Symptoms and Treatments.*

Test Your Knowledge

1. What are the main functions of the gastrointestinal (GI) tract?
2. What are asthma management?

4.5. Side Effects and Adverse Reactions

Learning Outcome

1. Common Side Effects of Cholinergic Agents
2. Adverse Effects of Adrenergic Drugs
3. Considerations for Special Populations

The pharmacology of ANS is made more complex by the development of side effects and adverse reactions (Figure 4.15), which tend to result from the wide distribution of autonomic receptors across the body. These unwanted effects tend to occur when drugs bind to non-target tissues, resulting in off-target effects that may compromise patient compliance or require alterations in dosage. For example, monoclonal antibodies against GD2 in neuroblastoma therapy illustrate how pharmacological therapies influencing autonomic pathways can trigger consequential unfavorable events. The acute side effects such as pain and sympathetic skin response changes observed demonstrate the fine line between benefit and autonomic disruption, emphasizing the necessity of receptor location and action in drug development and delivery (Mora et al., 2024). These discoveries necessitate the creation of sophisticated delivery protocols to be both non-toxic and retain efficacy, demonstrating the subtle intricacies in ANS pharmacology. Adaptive mechanisms to overcome autonomic-associated side effects prove the dynamics of changing pharmacological intervention. The use of novel protocols, including the Step-Up infusion system for anti-GD2 monoclonal antibody infusion, takes advantage of tachyphylaxis to regulate the response of the ANS.

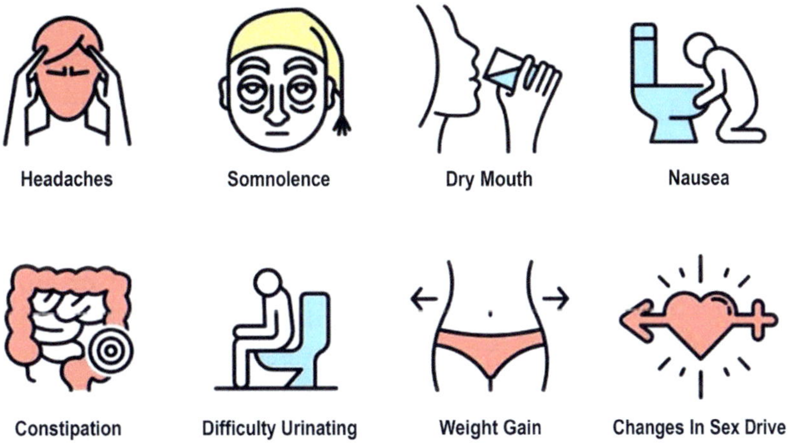

Figure 4.15. Side effects and adverse reactions.

Source: Addiction Resource (2023). *Amitriptyline Side Effects.*

Through judicious control of drug exposure and timing, this strategy takes advantage of the transient desensitization of autonomic pathways to minimize untoward side effects without sacrificing therapeutic benefits (Mora et al., 2024). This strategy is an example of how mechanistic understanding of autonomic pharmacodynamics not only explains the mechanism of side effects but also provides insight into useful solutions, leading to safer and more effective clinical use. These innovations highlight the importance of combining pharmacological information with patient-specific considerations for addressing side effects associated with autonomic drug targets. In investigating autonomic pharmacology, it is important to appreciate the constraints presented by drug toxicity and intolerance, especially for therapies involving intricate signaling pathways like in B-cell malignancies. The recent introduction of targeted drugs such as Bruton's tyrosine kinase inhibitors provides hopeful options with fewer side effects compared to traditional chemotherapies.

These drugs also have no absence of side effects, reflecting the ongoing problem of adverse reactions in the autonomic system and body physiology. It is crucial to comprehend these drug-induced autonomic derangements to maximize patient benefit, personalize interventions to reduce hazards, and enhance tolerance. The continuous fine-tuning of therapeutic interventions through judicious observation of side effects is a standing tribute to the complex interplay between pharmacologic specificity and ANS integrity.

4.5.1. Common Side Effects of Cholinergic Agents

The pharmacological manipulation of the ANS, especially by cholinergic agents, must be done with caution given their very potent effect on parasympathetic action. These drugs simulate the effect of acetylcholine, exerting action mainly through muscarinic and nicotinic receptors, which are ubiquitous in the body. Although therapeutic uses of cholinergic agents—like in glaucoma, myasthenia gravis, and AD—have been rewarding, their general therapeutic effects tend to produce a variety of side effects. Since cholinergic activation increases parasympathetic tone, it has the potential to induce signs and symptoms of hypersalivation, enhanced GI motility, and bradycardia. Such side effects are the result of muscarinic receptor overactivation and demonstrate the difficulty in obtaining target specificity without disrupting homeostatic physiological regulation within other autonomic regions (Zoccali et al., 2025). Uncovering the deeper effects of adverse reactions to cholinergic agents reveals their effects on various organ systems, tending to cause clinical management challenges. GI upset in the form of nausea, vomiting, abdominal cramping, and diarrhea is common and results from increased smooth muscle contractility and secretions. Stimulation of muscarinic receptors in the respiratory system may also trigger bronchoconstriction and augmented bronchial secretions, with risks particularly in patients with underlying respiratory conditions.

Cardiovascular side effects, including bradycardia and hypotension, arise from vagal stimulation that slows atrioventricular conduction and decreases heart rate. Knowledge of these widespread effects promotes safer prescribing habits by projecting complications and adjusting dosing to reduce patient discomfort while maximizing therapeutic benefit (Zoccali et al., 2025). The wider significance of cholinergic side effects goes beyond immediate symptomatic distress to impact the continued evolution of autonomic pharmacotherapies. Drug design innovations are intended to overcome these systemic side effects by maximizing receptor subtype specificity or utilizing new delivery modalities. As an example, with atrial fibrillation treatment where autonomic input is highly active, affecting unique pathways without initiating global parasympathetic activation continues as a therapeutic aim. New technologies like gene therapy and tissue engineering provide potential new alternatives to conventional cholinergic drugs by better targeting autonomic function. Finally, successful control of cholinergic side effects is part of the key to furthering ANS pharmacology as well as enhancing patient compliance to therapies involving these drugs (Figure 4.16).

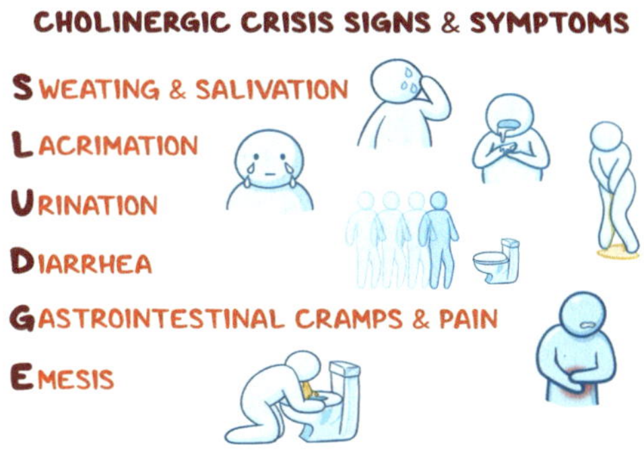

Figure 4.16. Common side effects of cholinergic agents.

Source: Addiction Resource. (2023). Amitriptyline Side Effects. https://d16qt3wv6xm098.cloudfront.net/YRq1qzV_SIyJY_RQ3FGpqqH-SpOFKAt8/_.png.

4.5.2. Adverse Effects of Adrenergic Drugs

Adrenergic medications, which are commonly used for their capacity to adjust sympathetic nervous system activity, have powerful physiological effects that may also cause serious side effects (Figure 4.17). These drug molecules target alpha and beta adrenergic receptors, affecting cardiovascular, respiratory, and metabolic function. Although their therapeutic advantages in hypertension, heart failure, and asthma, overstimulation or blockade of the adrenergic receptors can interfere with homeostatic equilibrium and produce side effects such as tachycardia, arrhythmias, and hypertension. In addition, adrenergic agents could further exacerbate pro-inflammatory conditions by manipulating sympathetic nervous system control, especially in susceptible patients with chronic conditions. The interaction between adrenergic receptor stimulation and immune modulation highlights the sophistication of these side effects, since excessive sympathetic drive is responsible for increased inflammation and tissue injury, a process most evident in CKD and cardiovascular disease (Zoccali et al., 2025). Therefore, awareness of these risks is paramount to maximizing clinical management and avoiding harm. Aside from their cardiovascular effects, adrenergic drugs also affect neurological functions, leading to a range of negative consequences. Beta-blockers, for example, can pass the BBB to produce CNS side effects including fatigue, depression, and insomnia. These neurological effects are indicative of the foundational role of adrenergic signaling in controlling mood and cognitive processes in the brain. Additionally, adrenergic antagonists may disrupt ANS balance by blocking normal sympathetic tone, potentially inducing orthostatic hypotension, dizziness, or syncope, which may lower the patient's compliance with prescribed regimens. Variability in receptor subtype specificity among adrenergic drugs contributes to differences in side effect profiles, making therapeutic choice more problematic. In light of this complexity, clinical caution is indicated to control adverse neuropsychological consequences while preserving the desired cardiovascular effects inherent in adrenergic pharmacotherapy (Zoccali et al., 2025).

Outside of human health, the environmental impact of adrenergic drugs has become a serious issue owing to their persistence and biological activity in aquatic environments. Studies have found that drugs like propranolol and moxisylyte, which are representative beta- and alpha-adrenergic antagonists respectively, cause harmful effects on the development of aquatic animals, especially fish larvae. While such drugs might have little impact on survival or on gross morphological abnormalities at levels of environmental exposure, there is subtle but vital disruption in cardiovascular and nervous system functions in such species as zebrafish. These alterations occur from varying mechanisms of action, as reflected in changes in gene transcription and enzymatic functions, suggesting that adrenergic drugs interfere with physiological control beyond their intended site. These results underscore the more general relevance of adrenergic pharmacology, including emphasis on prudent stewardship in the environment as well as clinical use to prevent unproductive ecological damage.

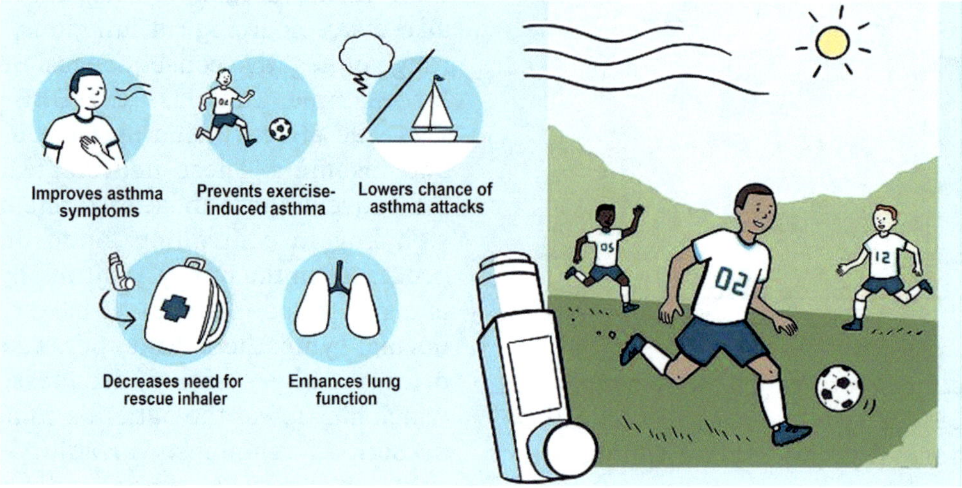

Figure 4.17. Adverse effects of adrenergic drugs.

Source: Verywell Health. (n.d.). *Beta-2 Agonists*. https://www.verywellhealth.com/thmb/6X4FSw4STxrePtk1KB3O1twgF-w=/1500x0/filters:no_upscale():max_bytes(150000):strip_icc()/beta-2-agonists-200960_FINAL-31a308ef0f324533a98ed5bd12ecae26.jpg.

4.5.3. Considerations for Special Populations

Special population variability in drug response requires specific pharmacologic strategies for ANS agents (Figure 4.18). Pediatric patients, for instance, have different pharmacokinetic and pharmacodynamic profiles from adults, reflecting developmental variations in enzyme function, receptor sensitivity, and autonomic control. This variability is manifest when treating disorders like performance anxiety, in which sympathetic nervous system activation can create dramatic physiological effects as well as psychological symptoms. Attentive regard for age-related factors is critical in order to prevent adverse consequences and maximize therapeutic effectiveness. In child athletes with performance anxiety, intervention should minimize side effects from agents such as propranolol or benzodiazepines that directly affect the ANS, against the benefits of symptom reduction. Cognitive behavioral therapy is still key, but pharmacologic adjuncts must be used with caution based on developmental pharmacology considerations (Katherine et al., 2025). Therefore, knowledge of these developmental subtleties is paramount for anesthesiologists, cardiologists, and psychiatrists who prescribe ANS-active medications to children. Pharmacological treatment in older subjects demonstrates further complexity secondary to age-related autonomic decline and polypharmacy. Elderly individuals frequently display reduced baroreflex sensitivity and changed receptor responsivity, which can increase sensitivity to both adrenergic and cholinergic drugs. Additionally, prevalence of comorbidities and regular use of drugs metabolized via similar liver pathways enhance risks of drug-drug interactions (DDIs) and adverse reactions. These concerns underscore the value of individualized dosing schedules and careful monitoring during autonomic pharmacotherapy in order to avert orthostatic hypotension, bradyarrhythmia's, or worsening underlying conditions. Utilizing model-based meta-analysis for the design optimization of clinical trials and treatment approaches has demonstrated potential in customizing interventions among such special groups through quantitative estimation of drug response and interindividual variation. Current methodologies, though, need further development for increased application in geriatric cohorts (Yang et al., 2024). Hence, careful modification of autonomic agents continues to be a bedrock of effective and safe pharmacologic management in geriatrics. Pregnant and breastfeeding women are another key special population requiring focused autonomic pharmacology principles. Physiological changes in pregnancy, including expanded blood volume, changed renal clearance, and changed autonomic tone, have a significant impact on drug disposition and response. These alterations make it difficult to use medication that affects the ANS, particularly beta-blockers or anticholinergic medications, which have the potential to affect fetal growth and neonatal outcomes.

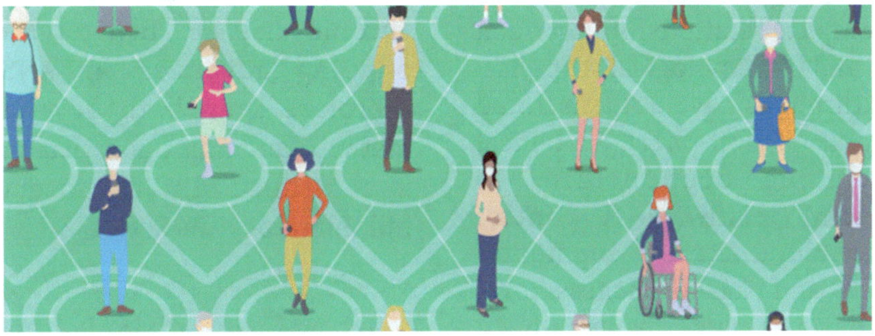

Figure 4.18. Considerations for special populations.

Source: Centers for Disease Control and Prevention (CDC). (n.d.). *Special Populations and COVID-19.*

Additionally, placental transfer and possible teratogenic potential of ANS drugs require careful benefit-risk evaluation to maintain maternal well-being at the expense of fetal safety. Multidisciplinary evaluation is necessary, bringing together obstetric, pharmacological, and neonatological knowledge to formulate safe management strategies. In addition, acknowledgment of sparse data from ANS-targeted clinical trials during pregnancy highlights the importance of sophisticated meta-analytical methods for extrapolating conclusions and informing evidence-based practice among this vulnerable population (Yang et al., 2024). Consequently, ANS-targeted pharmacotherapy in pregnancy requires accuracy, prudence, and ongoing assessment of newly emerging data.

Test Your Knowledge

1. Which of considerations for special populations?
2. How do cholinergic agents affect heart rate?

4.6. Current Research and Developments

Learning Outcome

1. Advances in Autonomic Pharmacology
2. Novel Therapeutic Targets
3. Future Directions in Research

New research into ANS pharmacology further emphasizes the complex relationship between neural modulation and immunological response. More recent breakthroughs have demonstrated the therapeutic value of non-pharmacological approaches, including acupuncture, in modulating autonomic pathways to control immune function. Acupuncture's segmental effect on sympathetic and vagal branches shows promising therapeutic impacts, especially in reducing systemic inflammation from diseases like sepsis. These discoveries emphasize the subtle role of autonomic control in inflammatory regulation and point towards a paradigm shift towards bioelectronic medicine that selectively activates individual autonomic circuits. By addressing parameters like acupoint specificity and stimulation frequency, future studies intend to further refine these interventions for clinical applications. An appreciation of the sympathetic nervous system's immunomodulatory function via such methods might lead to new treatments for a range of inflammatory diseases beyond current pharmacological options (Zhang et al., 2024). Concurrently, human investigations of autonomic-immune cross-talk offer key insights into the manner in which dysfunction within autonomic branches intensifies chronic inflammation. Studies among HIV-infected individuals demonstrate that compromised parasympathetic vagal function has a high correlation with raised pro-inflammatory cytokines such as IL-6, highlighting the link between autonomic control and immunity. Additionally, autonomic neuropathy involving reduced sympathetic function correlates with specific immune profiles typified by elevated CD8+ T-cell levels and increased type 1 cytokine presence.

These observations indicate that autonomic control deficits not only intensify systemic inflammation but also play a role in disease severity and comorbidity burden. This study highlights the value of therapeutics aimed at autonomic function recovery as a strategy to counteract inflammation-driven pathology in chronic disease (Bridget et al., 2024). Such ongoing advances in ANS pharmacology therefore span both novel neurostimulation methods and immunological profiling, indicating a multidisciplinary intervention against inflammatory diseases.

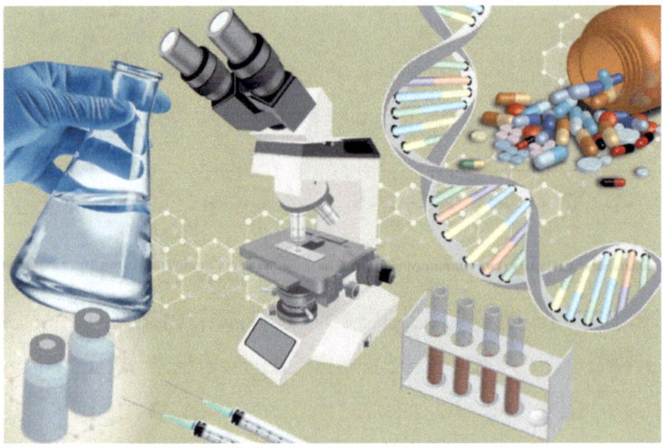

Figure 4.19. Current research and developments.

Source: https://www.cbo.gov/sites/default/files/2021-04/57025-home-cover.png.

The convergence of bioelectronic medicine, with lessons learned from autonomic neuropathy research, guides a future in which therapies will potentially integrate targeted neural modulation with immune-targeted pharmacology. This cross-disciplinary breakthrough holds the potential for more effective and tailored interventions, enhancing outcomes by restoring autonomic balance and modulating immune responses simultaneously. Sustained research into autonomic-immune crosstalk, mechanistic and clinical, must serve to translate these findings to the common practice of therapy, to develop new pharmacological compounds and bioelectronic devices targeting inflammation via the autonomic axis (Figure 4.19).

4.6.1. Advances in Autonomic Pharmacology

Substantial progress in elucidating the intricacies of the ANS has driven dramatic advances in drug development. Contemporary research has increasingly emphasized selectivity in receptor targeting to regulate autonomic functions with improved potency and fewer side effects. Advances in agent specificity enable more specific control of sympathetic and parasympathetic pathways, essential in managing cardiovascular, GI, and respiratory disease. Advances in the design of new drug formulations have also improved bioavailability and therapeutic efficacy. Further, an understanding of the interaction between central and peripheral structures of the ANS has made it possible to formulate drugs that can penetrate the BBB and affect autonomic control centers. These advances collectively demonstrate how a sophisticated understanding of autonomic pharmacology is transforming clinical practice and augmenting therapeutic options in this area. New evidence on the ENS has dramatically shaped progress in autonomic pharmacology, especially in relation to GI function. The complexity of the ENS, labeled as the "brain-in-the-gut," highlights its autonomy and regulatory role, governing smooth muscle function and mucosal secretions through a connective web of neurons and glial cells (Zizzo et al., 2011). Understanding the functional and chemical similarity of this system with the CNS has provided avenues for pharmacological agents directly targeting enteric neurons. Such precision is crucial in treating disorders such as IBS, gastroparesis, and other dysmotility's. These developments highlight the significance of the ENS in the overall autonomic system and demonstrate how contemporary pharmacology is progressing toward responding to the complexity of GI autonomic regulation with improved accuracy and efficacy (Zizzo et al., 2011). Advances in technology have further accelerated development in autonomic pharmacology through the introduction of advanced drug delivery systems that enhance therapeutic targeting while limiting systemic exposure. Nanotechnology, for example, has allowed the creation of carriers that release autonomic agents under controlled conditions at desired locations, improving drug efficacy while decreasing adverse effects. Also, developments in molecular biology have enabled the characterization of new receptor subtypes and signal transduction pathways, which represent potential sites of drug action. These have made it possible to design more selective agents able to modulate autonomic responses with greater discrimination. The coming together of genetic and proteomic information has also helped in personalized strategies in autonomic pharmacology, enabling treatment to be optimized according to individual autonomic profiles, thereby enhancing clinical efficacy and expanding the horizon of therapy.

4.6.2. Novel Therapeutic Targets

The convergence of peripheral signals with CNS processes has increasingly highlighted the therapeutic potential of ANS targeting in new ways. Recent developments have highlighted the importance of interoception—the brains processing of internal bodily stimuli—in mental health, and proposed that disorders like anxiety and depression may result from disruptions in interoceptive pathways. New treatments target the modulation of these pathways in order to restore equilibrium, with both pharmacological therapy and psychological treatment designed to improve perception and interpretation of body signals. For instance, antidepressants have demonstrated ability to modulate interoceptive processes, and certain psychotherapies involve controlled respiratory exercises to rebalance autonomic activity. This overlap of central and peripheral targets presents a promising route for therapeutic innovation, where not only are neural mechanisms addressed but also bodily feedback loops responsible for emotional processing and general mental well-being reconfigured (Camilla et al., 2022). Cardiovascular disease (CVD) is just one such frontier where targeting the ANS via new modalities has been highly promising. The intricacy of vagal nerve anatomy and its governing role over cardiac physiology has inspired the evolution of VNS as a therapeutic device. While early clinical uses of VNS in CVD patients provided variable results, continued research targets improved neuromodulation methodologies. Refinements in neural interface technology and closed-loop stimulation protocols are designed to amplify specificity and efficacy of VNS, further optimizing its influence upon autonomic balance. These strategies highlight a move toward precision neuromodulation, where selective activation of autonomic pathways may reverse cardiovascular homeostasis more precisely than conventional pharmacotherapy alone. This new pathway also emphasizes the possibility of using bioelectronic medicine as a part of normal care for long-term cardiovascular conditions (Ottaviani et al., 2022). Treating both mental illness and cardiovascular disease through modulation of the ANS illustrates a general principle: new therapeutic targets tend to lie at the interface between central and peripheral systems. Understanding the dynamic interplay between brain, body, and immune function opens the door to interdisciplinary approaches that combine pharmacology, neuromodulation, and behavioral therapy. For example, blocking afferent vagal pathways not only impacts cardiac function but also modulates inflammation and mood disorders, demonstrating the therapeutic flexibility of autonomic targets. To maximize the potential of these opportunities, future studies must clarify mechanisms that control interoceptive signaling and establish more precise methods to selectively alter autonomic circuits. These efforts will allow for treatments to be developed that are specifically designed for individual physiological profiles, marking a new frontier in ANS pharmacology beyond symptom suppression to reach systemic homeostasis (Camilla et al., 2022; Ottaviani et al., 2022).

4.6.3. Future Directions in Research

Neuromodulation innovations hold promising directions for the development of ANS pharmacology. Cardioneuroablation, an ablation technique that specifically targets parasympathetic ganglia in the heart, is an example of this innovation in that it provides an emerging therapeutic approach to treatment-refractory conditions like vasovagal syncope. Although existing modalities of treatment for such autonomic dysfunctions prove moderately successful, further streamlining of mapping techniques and ablation endpoints could significantly improve clinical outcomes. This strategy not only enhances insight into autonomic pathways but also links interventional cardiology with drug therapies. Future studies need to clarify the procedural heterogeneity and long-term efficacy of cardioneuroablation in order to confirm its place in clinical use (Figure 4.20). Furthermore, the combination of electrophysiological knowledge with pharmacodynamics may provide new combinatorial approaches, justifying the necessity for multidisciplinary research in this new area (Shen et al., 2023). In parallel, the intersection of pharmacology and new technologies promises great promise for ANS investigation. Autonomic computing principles borrowed from the Internet of Things designs provide a theoretical framework for building smart, learning therapeutic systems responsive to dynamic changes in physiology. These systems have the potential to transform drug delivery by allowing real-time monitoring and autonomous adjustment of pharmacological therapies according to subject-specific autonomic responses. The resource limitation and complexity typical of autonomic networks are similar to issues seen in heterogeneous IoT networks, suggesting a rich sharing of methodologies between the two areas. Future research should involve the integration of self-governing algorithms and feedback loops into drug delivery devices to maximize therapeutic accuracy and reduce side effects (Ashraf et al., 2023). Additionally, advancing biomarker identification and molecular stratification will be key to personalizing autonomic pharmacotherapy. Since the ANS controls a myriad of physiologic processes, its pharmacological manipulation requires highly selective targeting to prevent off-target activity. Advances in genomics, proteomics, and metabolomics will allow the discovery of new biomarkers that predict drug sensitivity and toxicity, setting the stage for precision medicine strategies.

Subsequent investigation must focus on determining the molecular underpinnings of autonomic dysregulation in order to guide the design of selective receptor modulators and signal transduction modifiers. Moreover, incorporating these molecular findings into noninvasive neuromodulation methods and intelligent drug delivery systems could have a profound impact on therapeutic efficacy and patient quality of life. These modalities combined present an integrated vision in ANS pharmacology research.

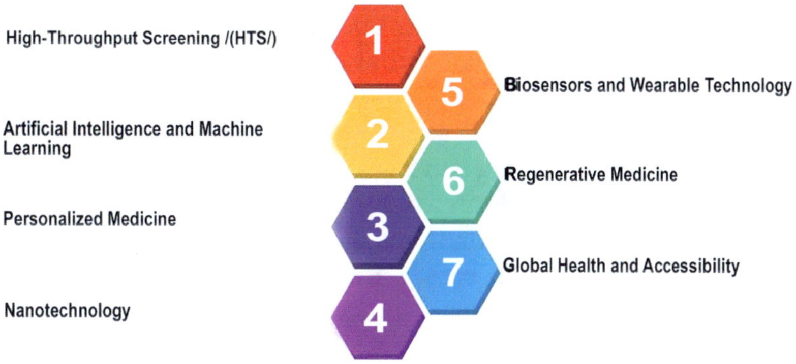

Figure 4.20. Future directions in research.

Source: FasterCapital. (2025). *Clinical Laboratory Pharmacology: Laboratory Techniques for Drug Analysis—Future Directions in Laboratory Pharmacology.*

Test Your Knowledge

1. How could artificial intelligence (AI) assist in ANS-related research?
2. How to advances in autonomic pharmacology?

SUMMARY

The delicate interaction among the ANS and drug regimens highlights the multifaceted nature of treatments for disorders affecting autonomic regulation. Studies addressing cardiovascular aspects of autonomic control, particularly during challenging environments of spaceflight, show the significance of precise therapeutic strategies to help reduce risks of conditions such as orthostatic intolerance. These observations underscore the importance of both non-pharmacological and pharmacological interventions in the upkeep of autonomic balance that benefit specialized environments as well as shedding light on the treatment of autonomic-linked cardiovascular disease here on Earth. This holistic comprehension can influence clinical practice, which stresses the need to adapt treatments taking into account the dynamic nature of autonomic responses to environmental and physiological stressors (Jordan et al., 2022). In addition, the new understanding of the microbiota-gut-brain axis has broadened the pharmacological background concerning ANS modulation. Appreciation that the autonomic network is not just limited to traditional neural circuits but also encompasses microbial influences makes the scope for new therapeutic targets more profound. The two-way communication between the vagus nerve and microbial metabolites implies a multifaceted regulatory mechanism impacting neuropsychiatric and neurodegenerative diseases. This new paradigm promotes the incorporation of microbiota-directed interventions in conjunction with conventional pharmacologic modalities to enhance autonomic function and global homeostasis, furthering patient care through enhanced understanding of autonomic pharmacology (John et al., 2019). Overall, the integration of current research emphasizes the need to address ANS pharmacology with multi-dimensional approaches. Breakthroughs in appreciating autonomic adaptations within singular habitats and the microbiota-gut-brain axis open the door for novel therapeutics involving the integration of both systemic and microbial factors. Further investigation into these areas holds the promise of greater pharmacological effectiveness and safety, ultimately leading to better clinical outcomes. The intersection of these disciplines provides an integrated platform, such that interventions in the future will respond to the variability and complexity associated with autonomic control and pharmacological manipulation thereof (John et al., 2019; Jordan et al., 2022).

Summary of Key Points

The ANS is involved in the regulation of homeostasis by its parasympathetic and sympathetic branches, which have opposite effects on different organs. Pharmacological modulation of these branches is the key to the management of a variety of clinical conditions, such as hypertension, asthma, and cardiac arrhythmias. The subtle control of SNA reflects considerable heterogeneity between vasculature of peripheral and core locations, with more exaggerated responsiveness in peripheral locations to stimuli like cold stress. Methods such as photoplethysmography (PPG) and spectral analysis of heart rate variability yield quantitative estimates of this differential autonomic control. These techniques unveil the strong central autoregulation that maintains core circulation during stress, which is in contrast to the increased peripheral sympathetic responses, a discovery that is central for directed pharmacotherapy of selective vascular beds (Ainslie et al., 2019). Such physiological understanding highlights site-specific autonomic modulation as central to advancing more accurate therapeutic interventions. In addition, autonomic pharmacology unlocks the complex interaction between the nervous system and wider physiological processes outside of cardiovascular control. Emerging research points to the way that the ANS interacts with psychosocial variables and homeostatic processes, affecting systemic measures like stress responses, metabolism, and immune response. For example, autonomic changes triggered by stress not only enable short-term adaptive reactions but also affect brain energy allocation, which can influence behaviors that are pertinent to energy intake and expenditure. These interactions highlight that autonomic regulation is extended to behavioral and emotional realms, where pharmacological treatments may modulate not only peripheral sites but also central processes associated with attachment and emotional regulation. Appreciation of these bio-behavioral interfaces increases the therapeutic value of autonomic drugs in the treatment of disorders with both physiological and psychological aspects (Ainsworth et al., 2014). This integrative approach expands the clinical reach of ANS pharmacology. Overall, the most important points in ANS pharmacology are the differential control of sympathetic and parasympathetic action across organ systems, the quantitative determination of sympathetic nerve function, and the broadened perspective regarding autonomic regulation of health and behavior. The interplay between central and peripheral control mechanisms for the autonomic nervous system requires careful pharmacologic targeting to maximize therapeutic effects while minimizing side effects. Sensitivity to the variability in autonomic function determined by physiological, environmental, and psychosocial influences further improves treatment strategies. Developments in monitoring technologies and conceptual frameworks for integrating autonomic physiology and behavioral health allow a holistic view crucial for the future generation of pharmacological interventions. These factors individually emphasize the polyvalent character of autonomic pharmacology and its core role in contemporary clinical practice (Ainslie et al., 2019; Ainsworth et al., 2014).

KEY TERMS FROM THIS CHAPTER

- Autonomic Nervous System (ANS)
- Norepinephrine
- Microenvironment
- Autonomic Pharmacology
- Modulating hormonal
- Autonomic dysfunction
- Cholinergic Drugs
- Parasympathetic Nervous System
- Neuromodulation
- Pharmacological Agents
- Gastrointestinal (GI)
- Central nervous system (CNS)

CRITICAL THINKING QUESTIONS

1. **Which of the following organs is innervated only by parasympathetic nerves?**
   a. Sweat glands
   b. Ciliary muscle
   c. Iris muscles
   d. Splenic capsule
2. **The termination of acetylcholine action at synapses is primarily via:**
   a. Reuptake by presynaptic neurons
   b. Metabolism by monoamine oxidase
   c. Breakdown by acetylcholinesterase
   d. Enzymatic destruction by COMT
3. **Neostigmine enhances cholinergic transmission by:**
   a. Blocking nicotinic receptors
   b. Inhibiting acetylcholinesterase
   c. Stimulating βadrenergic receptors
   d. Enhancing dopamine release
4. **Which classic triad describes cholinergic crisis from organophosphate poisoning?**
   a. SLUDGE and miosis (Salivation, Lacrimation, Urination, Diarrhea, GI distress, Emesis)
   b. Tachycardia, dry skin, hypertension
   c. Hyperthermia, seizures, mydriasis
   d. Bradycardia, bronchospasm, hypotension
5. **A nonselective beta-blocker that may cause bronchoconstriction in asthma is:**
   a. Albuterol
   b. Atropine
   C. Propranolol
   d. Epinephrine

Short Answer Questions

1. Which of Anatomy of the Autonomic Nervous System (ANS)
2. How do Neurotransmitters in the Autonomic Nervous System (ANS)
3. Why do Pharmacological Agents Affecting the Autonomic Nervous System (ANS)
4. Mechanisms & Clinical Use of Adrenergic Agents
5. What do you Side Effects and Adverse Reactions
6. What are Current Research and Developments

Answer to Critical Thinking Questions

1. (b) 2 (c) 3. (b) 4. (a) 5. (c)

REFERENCES

1. Ainslie, A., Anderson, P., Appelhans, B., Billman, G., Budidha, K., Budidha, R., Budidha, N., et al. (2019). Photoplethysmography for quantitative assessment of sympathetic nerve activity (SNA) during cold stress. *Frontiers in Physiology*, *9*, 1863. Retrieved from: https://core.ac.uk/download/169434493.pdf (accessed on 9 May 2025).
2. Ainsworth, B., Avitsur, R., Baumeister, H., Beedie, C., Biomarker Definitions Working Group, Bolger, E., Bowlby, J., et al. (2014). The attachment system and physiology in adulthood: Normative processes, individual differences, and implications for health. *Journal of Personality*, *82*(6), 515–527. https://doi.org/10.1111/jopy.12052.
3. Aksu, C., & Gürkan, Y. (2019). ESRA19-0475 chronic pain neuromodulation for the anesthesiologist not in practice, but why not in the future. *Regional Anesthesia & Pain Medicine*, *44*, A62–A63. https://www.semanticscholar.org/paper/8774ef9cee1b50192dea8185d533b5468f31419a (accessed on 9 May 2025).
4. Ashraf, Q., Tahir, M., Habaebi, M., & Isoaho, J. (2023). Toward autonomic internet of things: Recent advances, evaluation criteria, and future research directions. *IEEE Internet of Things Journal, 10*, 14725–14748. https://www.semanticscholar.org/paper/28eadc8265fcedbfe42fb4efaf94456a137faab2 (accessed on 9 May 2025).
5. Barnes, V. A., Crawford, M. W., Harden, K., Ravinder, P., et al. (2015). Self-regulation of breathing as a primary treatment for anxiety. Retrieved from: https://core.ac.uk/download/131210063.pdf (accessed on 9 May 2025).
6. Beenen, K. T., Vosters, J. A., & Patel, D. R. (2025). Sport-related performance anxiety in young athletes: A clinical practice review. *Translational Pediatrics, 14*, 127–138. https://www.semanticscholar.org/paper/bf32cfa4e140ea6c4fa70ef73def438fb2de1521 (accessed on 9 May 2025).
7. Bergantin, L., & Caricati-Neto, A. (2017). Advances for the pharmacotherapy of depression: Presenting the rising star—Ca^{2+}/cAMP signaling interaction. *Frontiers in Pharmacology, 3*. https://www.semanticscholar.org/paper/3ebb23eea6481f8bc76209302dffe5f881dd7f9d (accessed on 9 May 2025).
8. Bergeri, A. S., & Daruwala, S. S. (2025). Effectiveness of abdominal deep breathing exercises in managing blood pressure among hypertensive patients. *Cures*, *17*. https://www.semanticscholar.org/paper/50e6b1ba80127b895fe4e133a095f97ed212c8e0 (accessed on 9 May 2025).
9. Brugada, J., Katritsis, D. G., Arbelo, E., Arribas, F., Bax, J. J., Blomström-Lundqvist, C., Calkins, H., et al. (2019). 2019 ESC Guidelines for the management of patients with supraventricular tachycardia. *European Heart Journal, 41*, 655–720. https://doi.org/10.1093/eurheartj/ehz467.
10. Burnstock, G. (2009). Purinergic signaling: Past, present and future. *Brazilian Journal of Medical and Biological Research*, *42*, 3–8. Retrieved from: https://core.ac.uk/download/1670991.pdf (accessed on 9 May 2025).
11. Burnstock, G. (2011). Purinergic signaling in the gastrointestinal tract. *World Journal of Gastrointestinal Pathophysiology*, *2*(2), 31–34. Retrieved from: https://core.ac.uk/download/1676059.pdf (accessed on 9 May 2025).

12. Calvi, A., Fischetti, I., Verzicco, I., Belvederi Murri, M., Zanetidou, S., Volpi, R., Coghi, P., et al. (2021). Antidepressant drugs effects on blood pressure. *Frontiers in Cardiovascular Medicine, 8*. https://doi.org/10.3389/fcvm.2021.704281.

13. Camilleri, M. (1999). Functional bowel disease: A challenging frontier in gastroenterology. *Maltese Medical Journal, 11*(1, 2), 4. Retrieved from: https://core.ac.uk/download/46601769.pdf (accessed on 9 May 2025).

14. Caputi, V., & Giron, M. C. (2018). Microbiome-gut-brain axis and toll-like receptors in Parkinson's disease. *International Journal of Molecular Sciences, 19*(1689). Retrieved from: https://core.ac.uk/download/168404181.pdf (accessed on 9 May 2025).

15. Castillo-Armengol, J., Fajas, L., & López-Mejía, I. C. (2019). Inter-organ communication: A gatekeeper for metabolic health. *EMBO Reports, 20*. https://doi.org/10.15252/embr.201947903.

16. Cryan, J. F., O'Riordan, K. J., Cowan, C. S. M., Sandhu, K. V., Bastiaanssen, T. F. S., Boehme, M., Codagnone, M. G., et al. (2019). The microbiota-gut-brain axis. *Physiological Reviews, 99*, 1877–2013. https://doi.org/10.1152/physrev.00018.2018.

17. Cuddihey, H., MacNaughton, W. K., & Sharkey, K. A. (2022). Role of the endocannabinoid system in the regulation of intestinal homeostasis. *Cellular and Molecular Gastroenterology and Hepatology, 14*, 947–963. https://doi.org/10.1016/j.jcmgh.2022.05.015.

18. Curro, F. (2017). Opioids for the treatment of pain: The risk of treating a multivariate symptom. *The Journal of Clinical Pharmacology, 57*. https://www.semanticscholar.org/paper/0473b0f0e47a551e8c6d624bb9ade2a6b36a1c26 (accessed on 9 May 2025).

19. Fromer, L., Kaplan, A., Price, D., Román-Rodríguez, et al. (2014). Is there a rationale and role for long-acting anticholinergic bronchodilators in asthma? Retrieved from: https://core.ac.uk/download/25497566.pdf (accessed on 9 May 2025).

20. Gamal, S. M., Hussein, M. I. H., Salih, T. S. M., Waseem, et al. (2023). Pharmacology of the autonomic nervous system. Retrieved from: https://core.ac.uk/download/588401322.pdf (accessed on 9 May 2025).

21. Joglar, J. A., Chung, M. K., Armbruster, A. L., Benjamin, E. J., Chyou, J. Y., Cronin, E. M., Deswal, A., et al. (2023). 2023 ACC/AHA/ACCP/HRS guideline for the diagnosis and management of atrial fibrillation: A report of the American College of Cardiology/American Heart Association Joint Committee on Clinical Practice Guidelines. *Circulation, 149*. https://doi.org/10.1161/cir.0000000000001193.

22. Jordan, J., Limper, U., & Tank, J. (2022). Cardiovascular autonomic nervous system responses and orthostatic intolerance in astronauts and their relevance in daily medicine. *Neurological Sciences, 43*, 3039–3051. https://doi.org/10.1007/s10072-022-05963-7.

23. Kimura, I., Ichimura, A., Ohue-Kitano, R., & Igarashi, M. (2019). Free fatty acid receptors in health and disease. *Physiological Reviews, 100*, 171–210. https://doi.org/10.1152/physrev.00041.2018.

24. Kirchhof, P., Benussi, S., Kotecha, D., Ahlsson, A., Atar, D., Casadei, B., Castellá, M., et al. (2016). 2016 ESC Guidelines for the management of atrial fibrillation developed in collaboration with EACTS. *European Heart Journal, 37*, 2893–2962. https://doi.org/10.1093/eurheartj/ehw210.

25. Kirchhof, P., Benussi, S., Kotecha, D., Ahlsson, A., Atar, D., Casadei, B., Castellá, M., et al. (2016). 2016 ESC Guidelines for the management of atrial fibrillation developed in collaboration with EACTS. *EP Europace, 18*, 1609–1678. https://doi.org/10.1093/europace/euw295.

26. Kohl, R. L., & Odell, S. (2025). Neurophysiological responses to stressful motion and anti-motion sickness drugs as mediated by the limbic system. https://core.ac.uk/download/pdf/42853678.pdf (accessed on 9 May 2025).

27. Kolacz, J. (2024). Autonomic assessment at the intersection of psychosocial and gastrointestinal health. *Neurogastroenterology and Motility*. Retrieved from: https://www.semanticscholar.org/paper/2d73c3b0df829225be39590c2e01ba4a7e76bc98 (accessed on 9 May 2025).

28. Lizarraga-Valderrama, L. R. (2020). Effects of essential oils on central nervous system: Focus on mental health. *Phytotherapy Research, 35*, 657–679. https://doi.org/10.1002/ptr.6854.

29. Lv, J., Sun, F., Li, Z., Qin, Y., Sheng, R., & Sun, L. (2024). Comparative study of the effects of drugs targeting adrenergic receptors on the early life stages of zebrafish. *Toxics, 12*. https://www.semanticscholar.org/paper/efe1829b3313957e38fe125105d02493b712d65c (accessed on 9 May 2025).

30. Mao, G., Tang, J., Xu, M., Okeke, E., Dong, F., Chen, Y., Gao, J., et al. (2024). Role of autonomic nervous system in BDE-209 maternal exposure induced immunotoxicity in female offspring. *Environmental Toxicology*. Retrieved from: https://www.semanticscholar.org/paper/75f750e9a1960151cb2820c9fccba68e82e20f72 (accessed on 9 May 2025).

31. Mora, J., Climent, A., Roldan, M., Flores, M. C., Varo, A., Perez-Jaume, S., Jou, C., et al. (2024). Desensitizing the autonomic nervous system to mitigate anti-GD2 monoclonal antibody side effects. *Frontiers in Oncology, 14*. https://www.semanticscholar.org/paper/81c44d6d8a1b7de8666226a632173c053944bb73 (accessed on 9 May 2025).

32. Mueller, B. R., Mehta, M., Campbell, M., Neupane, N., Cedillo, G., Lee, G., Coyle, K., et al. (2024). The autonomic nervous system (ANS)-immune network in people living with HIV. *Research Square*. https://www.semanticscholar.org/paper/73e87083528ffaf1df59db7d942c68e30392ea1b (accessed on 9 May 2025).

33. Müller, T. D., Finan, B., Bloom, S. R., D'Alessio, D. A., Drucker, D. J., Flatt, P. R., Fritsche, A., et al. (2019). Glucagon-like peptide 1 (GLP-1). *Molecular Metabolism, 30*, 72–130. https://doi.org/10.1016/j.molmet.2019.09.010.

34. Nord, C. L., & Garfinkel, S. N. (2022). Interoceptive pathways to understand and treat mental health conditions. *Trends in Cognitive Sciences, 26*, 499–513. https://doi.org/10.1016/j.tics.2022.03.004.

35. Ottaviani, M. M., Vallone, F., Micera, S., & Recchia, F. A. (2022). Closed-loop vague nerve stimulation for the treatment of cardiovascular diseases: State of the art and future directions. *Frontiers in Cardiovascular Medicine, 9*. https://doi.org/10.3389/fcvm.2022.866957.

36. Palma, J. A., & Kaufmann, H. (2018). Treatment of autonomic dysfunction in Parkinson disease and other synucleinopathies. *Movement Disorders, 33*, 372–390. https://doi.org/10.1002/mds.27344.

37. Pavelic, A. R., Zebenholzer, K., & Wöber, C. (2024). Reconceptualizing autonomic function testing in migraine: A systematic review and meta-analysis. *The Journal of Headache and Pain, 25*. https://www.semanticscholar.org/paper/64496e5960aedbf0bdfd33223aa51a1f42d8d986 (accessed on 9 May 2025).

38. Sasso, J. M., Ammar, R., Tenchov, R., Lemmel, S., Kelber, O., Grieswelle, M., Zhou, Q., et al. (2023). Gut microbiome–brain alliance: A landscape view into mental and gastrointestinal

health and disorders. *ACS Chemical Neuroscience, 14*, 1717–1763. https://www.semanticscholar.org/paper/f1bf6755b6475c0a9aeba054a64f46a92ab4ad77 (accessed on 9 May 2025).

39. Sharifi-Heris, Z., Yang, Z., Rahmani, A. M., Fortier, M. A., Sharifiheris, H., & Bender, M. (2023). Phenotyping the autonomic nervous system in pregnancy using remote sensors: Potential for complication prediction. *Frontiers in Physiology, 14*. https://www.semanticscholar.org/paper/4a05281f624a3cbb9fcb6983829ccdc2a6c5ab93 (accessed on 9 May 2025).

40. Shen, W., Ko Ko, N. K., Kowlgi, G. N., Juan, A., Pachón, J., & Pachon-M, E. (2023). Selective modulation of the cardiac autonomic nervous system: A new therapeutic strategy for cardioinhibitory vasovagal syncope. *Medical Research Archives*. https://www.semanticscholar.org/paper/9720d85d51499aaba85acb33d6aaf1fef32aed39 (accessed on 9 May 2025).

41. Shu, L., Ding, Y. D., Zhang, J. Y., He, R. S., Xiao, L., Pan, B. X., & Deng, H. (2024). Interactions between MDSCs and the autonomic nervous system: Opportunities and challenges in cancer neuroscience. *Cancer Immunology Research*. https://www.semanticscholar.org/paper/4f96767f3ae35c59bc0af21b1e57e2681c5c7c05 (accessed on 9 May 2025).

42. Silva, Y. P., Bernardi, A., & Frozza, R. L. (2020). The role of short-chain fatty acids from gut microbiota in gut-brain communication. *Frontiers in Endocrinology, 11*. https://doi.org/10.3389/fendo.2020.00025.

43. Vaillancourt, M., Chia, P., Sarji, S., Nguyen, J., Hoftman, N., Ruffenach, G., Eghbali, M., et al. (2017). Autonomic nervous system involvement in pulmonary arterial hypertension. *Respiratory Research, 18*. https://doi.org/10.1186/s12931-017-0679-6.

44. Walwyn, W., & Valenza, M. (2022). Editorial: Kappa opioid receptors revealed: Disentangling the pharmacology to open up new therapeutic strategies. *Frontiers in Pharmacology, 13*. https://www.semanticscholar.org/paper/3d9a7ec2be62c853eb9004ec00bb0279aeb01a53 (accessed on 9 May 2025).

45. Wong, C. K., & Tse, H. (2020). New methodological approaches to atrial fibrillation drug discovery. *Expert Opinion on Drug Discovery, 16*, 319–329. https://www.semanticscholar.org/paper/1032280e5785b4be0d3816d772669ca4af8d1eaa (accessed on 9 May 2025).

46. Xing, Y., Zhao, K., Zhang, Y., & Wang, Y. (2024). BTK inhibition in primary central nervous system lymphoma: Mechanisms, clinical efficacy, and future perspectives. *Frontiers in Oncology, 14*. https://www.semanticscholar.org/paper/2bb2a1d7e02f6eedc649af553c1fe371d9260d6f (accessed on 9 May 2025).

47. Yang, Z., He, H., Wang, R., Liu, D., Li, G., & Sun, F. (2024). Application and quality of model-based meta-analysis in pharmaceutical research: A systematic cross-sectional analysis and practical considerations. *Clinical Pharmacology and Therapeutics*. https://www.semanticscholar.org/paper/5ebd3bd76f2be7443bbf73cfc04f493e4bbfc4cd (accessed on 9 May 2025).

48. Yu, Y., Chen, T., Zheng, Z., Jia, F., Liao, Y., Ren, Y., Liu, X., et al. (2024). The role of the autonomic nervous system in polycystic ovary syndrome. *Frontiers in Endocrinology, 14*. https://www.semanticscholar.org/paper/42c3ba40b4dbea1af47812c77341dc2541c89841 (accessed on 9 May 2025).

49. Zhang, Z., Zhang, D., Lin, Q., & Cui, X. (2024). Therapeutically fine-tuning autonomic nervous system to treat sepsis: A new perspective on the immunomodulatory effects of acupuncture. *Journal of Inflammation Research, 17*, 4373–4387. https://www.semanticscholar.org/paper/9f0d6153157e4f95ca5cc6874649b8e15b8fe73d (accessed on 9 May 2025).

50. Zhu, Y., Meerschaert, K. A., Galván-Peña, S., Bin, N. R., Yang, D., Basu, H., Kawamoto, R., et al. (2024). A chemogenetic screen reveals that Trpv1-expressing neurons control regulatory T cells in the gut. *Science, 385*. https://www.semanticscholar.org/paper/8cc3e68d4dce42d24766cb1f7f30192a194ad616 (accessed on 9 May 2025).

51. Zizzo, G., Mastropaolo, M., & Serio, R. (2011). The enteric nervous system: New developments and emerging concepts. Retrieved from: https://core.ac.uk/download/46602300.pdf.

52. Zoccali, C., Mallamaci, F., Kanbay, M., Tuttle, K. R., Kotanko, P., De Caterina, R., Grassi, G., et al. (2025). The autonomic nervous system and inflammation in chronic kidney disease. *Nephrology, Dialysis, Transplantation: Official Publication of the European Dialysis and Transplant Association–European Renal Association*. Retrieved from: https://www.semanticscholar.org/paper/c7fcd3879e3f1aec860981eaff25f18e476ac253 (accessed on 9 May 2025).

DRUGS AFFECTING THE CARDIOVASCULAR SYSTEM

5

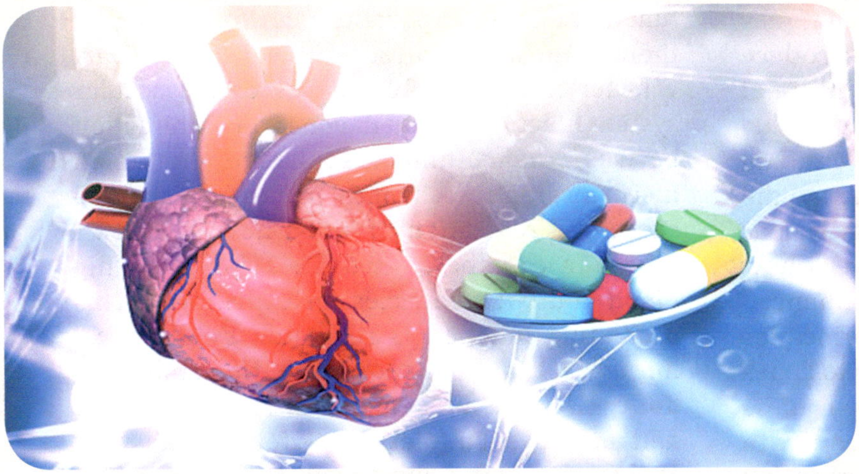

LEARNING OBJECTIVES

After studying this chapter, you will be able to:

1. Explain Types of Cardiovascular Drugs
2. Define Mechanisms of Action
3. Define Therapeutic Uses
4. Identify the Side Effects and Risks
5. Discuss the Drug Interactions
6. Explain the Current Research and Developments

Introduction

The cardiovascular system (Figure 5.1) is a highly organized network designed to provide hemodynamic stability and oxygen and nutrient delivery to the body. Dysfunctions of this system, including hypertension and heart failure, account for most global morbidity and mortality. Therefore, pharmacologic interventions have become critical in the management of cardiovascular disease (CVD) by modulating different physiological pathways to restore normal function or slow progression. Understanding how these drugs function is important in order to maximize therapeutic effects and reduce side effects. Advances in drug discovery, especially those directed towards enzyme inhibitors or new drug delivery systems, have had a significant impact on treatment modalities, giving clinicians a wider arsenal to treat cardiovascular diseases (Kapse et al., 2024; Li et al., 2024). At the center of most cardiovascular diseases lies hypertension, a multicausal disease defined by chronically elevated blood pressure. An interesting biochemical contributor to hypertension is the angiotensin-converting enzyme (ACE), which catalyzes the conversion of angiotensin I to the powerful vasoconstrictor angiotensin II. Vasoconstriction and sodium retention are favored by this enzymatic activity, compounding high blood pressure and enhancing cardiovascular risk. The discovery and application of ACE inhibitors have revolutionized hypertension treatment by effectively inhibiting this pathway, leading to decreased vascular resistance and improved patient outcomes. Investigations into the enzyme and its inhibitors have further enriched drug design approaches, applying techniques such as molecular docking in order to produce more effective therapeutics with minimal side effects (Li et al., 2024). Emerging drug delivery systems further augment conventional pharmacological therapies by enhancing the efficacy and bioavailability of cardiovascular medications. Of these, phytosomes are a new type of formulation that facilitates enhanced absorption of plant-based bioactive principles that have cardioprotective activities. Phytosomes enhance solubility and therapeutic effectiveness through complexation of phytoconstituents with phospholipids and, therefore, present promising adjuncts or alternatives to cardiovascular therapy. These systems illustrate better safety profiles and have the potential to lower the dosage and toxicity of traditional drugs. Since CVDs need to be managed long-term, such innovative drug delivery not only enhances clinical effectiveness but also patient compliance and quality of life (Kapse et al., 2024).

Definition of Cardiovascular System

Human physiology complexity is diverse in terms of numerous interrelated systems that perform homeostasis and survival. Of these, cardiovascular system is a key network tasked with delivering oxygen, nutrients, and signaling molecules throughout the body. The system is comprised of the heart, which is a muscular pump, and a large network of blood vessels such as arteries, veins, and capillaries. The hearts rhythmic contractions generate the force necessary to propel blood through these vessels, maintaining circulation to all tissues. Additionally, the cardiovascular system plays a role in waste removal and immunological defense by transporting immune cells and metabolic by-products. Understanding the cardiovascular system's structure and function is fundamental when discussing pharmacological interventions, as drugs affecting this system influence heart rate, vascular tone, and blood composition. This delicate equilibrium is vital to physiological function and an important focus for numerous therapeutic agents directed toward CVDs (Bart van der Hee et al., 2021). The cardiovascular system functions through concerted interaction between heart and vasculature, in which mechanical and biochemical processes guarantee successful regulation of blood flow. The heart has four chambers: two atria for receiving blood and two ventricles for expelling it. This oscillating function is regulated by electrical impulses that emanate from the sinoatrial node to provide synchronized contraction and effective circulation. Arteries transport oxygenated blood away from the heart, while veins transport deoxygenated blood back to be reoxygenated in the lungs. Capillaries, the most diminutive of blood vessels, allow for nutrient and gas exchange at the tissue level. Notably, the dynamic responsiveness of the cardiovascular system is regulated by endogenous mechanisms including hormones and the autonomic nervous system (ANS), both of which are the targets for drugs that act on the cardiovascular system. These drugs can exert their action through the modulation of receptor pathways, regulating vascular resistance or cardiac output to restore pathological conditions like hypertension or heart failure (Bikbov et al., 2020). Beyond its primary function in circulation, the cardiovascular system also interacts closely with other physiological systems, influencing overall organismal health. For instance, impaired kidney function has been shown to exacerbate CVD risk due to fluid and electrolyte imbalances, further complicating treatment approaches.

This cross-talk underscores why cardiovascular medications frequently must be viewed in the context of overall systemic health, especially in the presence of chronic diseases such as diabetes that affect cardiovascular risk factors. Moreover, metabolites like short-chain fatty acids (SCFAs) affect cardiovascular control by signaling through certain receptors found on vascular and immune cells, illustrating the pleiotropic nature of regulatory mechanisms. Clinical pharmacology directed towards the cardiovascular system must thus be geared towards this complexity, maximizing therapeutic effects with minimal side effects caused by systemic interactions (Bart van der Hee et al., 2021).

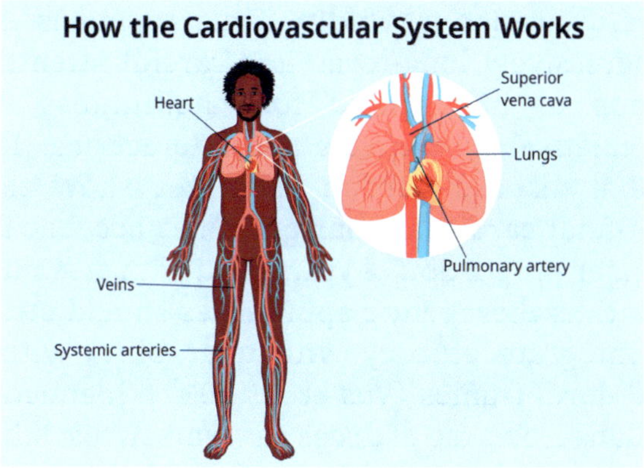

Figure 5.1. Cardiovascular system.

Source: Verywell Health. (n.d.). *How the Cardiovascular System Works.* https://www.verywellhealth.com/thmb/rdWbM4pFhsfDPy7DfSkPmoD_LCE=/1500x0/filters:no_upscale():max_bytes(150000):strip_icc()/HowtheCardiovascularSystemWorks-notext-final-6c82a8b033834fd59c2a3f3b089a581c.png.

Overview of Drugs Affecting the Cardiovascular System

Advancements in molecular biology have already vastly increased the comprehension of how mitochondrial function affects cardiovascular health, and new therapeutic targets for vascular disease have been identified. At the molecular level, one protein that stands out as relevant is uncoupling protein 2 (UCP2), found within the inner mitochondrial membrane. UCP2 has a crucial role to help prevent oxidative stress by decreasing mitochondrial membrane potential and dispersing metabolic energy. Experiments have also indicated that deficiency of the UCP2 gene aggravates atherosclerosis development and reduces lifespan in animal models, and downregulation makes individuals more susceptible to renal and cerebrovascular injury in hypertensive states. On the other hand, overexpression or pharmacologic induction of UCP2 expression by agents like fenofibrate and natural products such as curcumin has been reported to have protective action against endothelial dysfunction and target organ damage in hypertension. These results place UCP2 not only as a crucial mediator in cardiovascular pathophysiology but also as a potential target for new interventions that will prevent vascular complications in obesity, diabetes, and hypertension (Forte et al., 2017). The management of hypertension continues to be a cornerstone in preventing the burden of cardiovascular morbidity and mortality, but controlling the condition is challenging in its multifaceted nature. Recent clinical research among veteran populations has revealed that adherence to antihypertensive medication regimens is a significant independent predictor of systolic blood pressure control. These findings underscore that beyond the pharmacodynamic properties of antihypertensive drugs, patient-related factors such as compliance critically influence therapeutic outcomes. Since the management of hypertension is complicated, upcoming studies must clarify patient-specific determinants of drug compliance, using uniform hypertension definitions based on endorsed guidelines such as JNC-7. Elucidation of these dimensions can promote intervention design maximally empowering drug effectiveness by facilitating prolonged blood pressure control and, in turn, minimizing the risks of stroke, heart attack, and CKD that attend uncontrolled hypertension (Liu et al., 2013). A broad overview of cardiovascular drugs demonstrates a complex pharmacological profile with multiple mechanisms of action against diverse pathophysiological processes to improve heart and vascular diseases. Cardiovascular drug classes like beta-blockers, ACE inhibitors, calcium channel blockers, and diuretics together treat abnormal hemodynamic values by controlling heart rate, vascular resistance, and blood volume. Lipid-lowering drugs and antiplatelet drugs also play a role in preventing atherosclerotic plaque development and thrombotic complications. New data further support the therapeutic promise of modulating the mitochondrial protein UCP2, since adjunctive measures can complement conventional therapies to prevent oxidative stress and endothelial dysfunction. The combination of pharmacological treatments with a sophisticated understanding of patient compliance, co-morbidities, and molecular targets presents a systems-based strategy for CVD management that enhances clinical outcomes and quality of life for patients afflicted with these ubiquitous diseases.

Importance of Understanding Drug Effects on Cardiovascular Health

The complex interaction between pharmacologic agents and cardiovascular physiology requires a thorough comprehension of the drug effect to maximize patient benefits and reduce untoward effects. Cardiovascular drugs represent a diverse array that includes antihypertensives, anticoagulants, and lipid-lowering drugs, each having a different mechanism that affects hemodynamics, myocardial performance, and vascular integrity. A knowledge of these effects enables clinicians to customize therapeutic regimens according to the patient's profile, including comorbid illnesses and underlying cardiac disease. Further, knowledge of the drugs' pharmacodynamics and pharmacokinetics provides assurance for minimizing possible hazards like arrhythmias, hypotension, or thromboembolic events. This individualized strategy is at the forefront of efficient cardiovascular risk treatment, as highlighted in guidelines designed to harmonize evidence-based treatment with clinical acumen for patient-driven care (François et al., 2019). Such extensive information about drug effects is therefore crucial in enhancing therapeutic effectiveness while preserving cardiovascular well-being. In addition to short-term pharmacological effects, understanding the long-term cardiovascular drug effects is important for counteracting chronic disease evolution and enhancing quality of life. With a growing population of an aging global population and increasing incidence of cardiovascular morbidity, drug regimens are progressively long-term, and careful attention needs to be applied to watchfulness for cumulative drug effects and interactions. The global disease burden estimates show that non-fatal cardiovascular outcomes account for a major proportion of years lived with disability, and thus therapeutic approaches should strive to integrate efficacy with tolerability within long-term frames (Vos et al., 2017). Ineffective or dangerous use of drugs can worsen disability, emphasizing the importance of clinicians' grasp of cardiovascular pharmacotherapy. Matching drug selection with changing CVD pathophysiology allows clinicians to more effectively avert progression and complications, emphasizing the value of ongoing education and research in this fluid field. In addition, applying drug effect knowledge into the context of changing clinical guidelines and regulatory policies is crucial for ensuring high-quality care. The intricacy of cardiovascular pharmacotherapy requires following new recommendations while at the same time enabling tailored decision-making that considers patient-specific attributes and ethical obligations (François et al., 2019). Evidence-based guidelines are valuable tools to help guide therapeutic decisions, but they are never a substitute for the subtle decision-making involved with varied clinical cases. Practitioners need to be aware of inconsistencies or confusions between sources, check regulations regarding drugs, and look towards new evidence so as to make patient safety and efficacy optimal. This double reliance on policy and clinical judgment emphasizes how essential a complete understanding of drug effects is in encouraging cardiovascular well-being and guaranteeing prudent medication stewardship within contemporary healthcare systems.

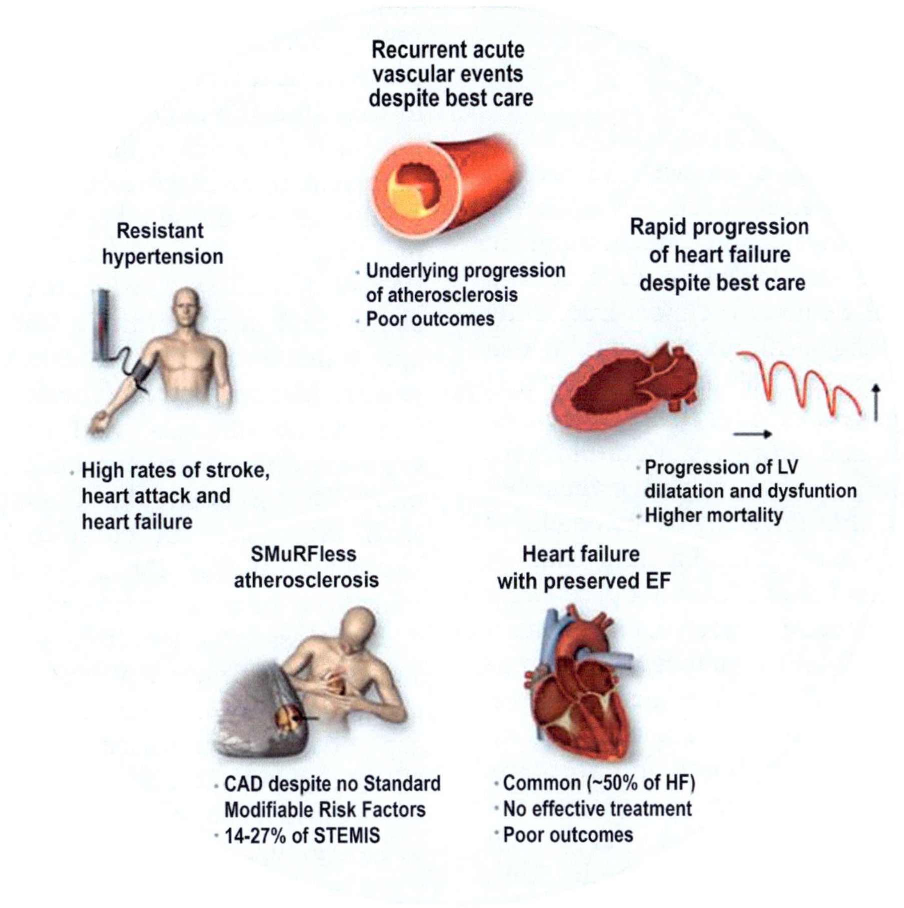

Figure 5.2. Drug effects on cardiovascular health.

Source: American Heart Association. (n.d.). *Illustration of Cardiovascular Disease Pathways. Circulation.* https://www.ahajournals.org/cms/10.1161/CIR.0000000000000981/asset/95d0d67c-5d63-4e79-94c4-9990de354485/assets/graphic/cir.0000000000000981.fig01.jpg.

5.1. Types of Cardiovascular Drugs

Learning Outcome

1. Antihypertensives
2. Anticoagulants
3. Lipid-Lowering Agents

The treatment of cardiovascular disease (CVD) depends largely on a wide variety of pharmacological agents, each acting on a particular pathophysiologic mechanism in order to restore and maintain cardiac and vascular function. Some of the most frequently prescribed are the antihypertensives, which are divided into a number of subclasses that include beta-blockers, calcium channel blockers, ACE inhibitors, and diuretics. Beta-blockers act by decreasing heart rate and myocardial contractility and thus lowering oxygen demand and managing hypertension. Calcium channel blockers produce vasodilatation by relaxing vascular smooth muscle to decrease peripheral resistance. ACE inhibitors suppress the renin-angiotensin system to block vasoconstriction. Diuretics allow excretion of excess sodium and water, decreasing blood volume and pressure. These drugs alone or together make up the backbone of treatment for hypertension and heart failure and permit modulation of cardiovascular load and ventricular performance to enhance outcome in patients. Besides antihypertensives, antiplatelet and anticoagulant drugs are pivotal in the prevention and management of thromboembolic events, which often complicate cardiovascular disease. Antiplatelet medications like aspirin and P2Y12 inhibitors prevent platelet aggregation, thus limiting the development of arterial clots that are involved in myocardial infarction and stroke. Anticoagulants such as warfarin and direct oral anticoagulants (DOACs) work by interfering with the coagulation cascade, reducing the risk of venous thromboembolism and stroke in atrial fibrillation. Clinical application of these drugs calls for precise balancing of efficacy and risk of bleeding, which necessitates thorough patient assessment. The emergence of personalized medicine and enhanced *in vitro* models for cardiovascular drug testing, such as the utilization of patient-derived iPSCs, holds the promise of more targeted therapeutic intervention and safer drug profiles in this area (Chandy et al., 2020). In addition, lipid-lowering drugs like statins and fibrates represent another critical class of cardiovascular drugs that are designed to alter the root causes of atherosclerotic disease. Statins suppress HMG-CoA reductase, respectively lowering LDL cholesterol and exhibiting anti-inflammatory properties at the vascular endothelium, which retards plaque growth. Fibrates chiefly reduce triglyceride and raise HDL cholesterol levels. With continued cardiovascular morbidity and mortality, in particular among populations with high rates of complex comorbidities like severe mental illness, incorporating such therapies into comprehensive care models becomes essential. Monitoring of cardiovascular side effects of some psychotropic drugs and promotion of collaborative care models fill the gap between cardiovascular and mental health, enhancing both compliance with and outcomes of cardiovascular drug therapies (Braga et al., 2018) (Figure 5.3).

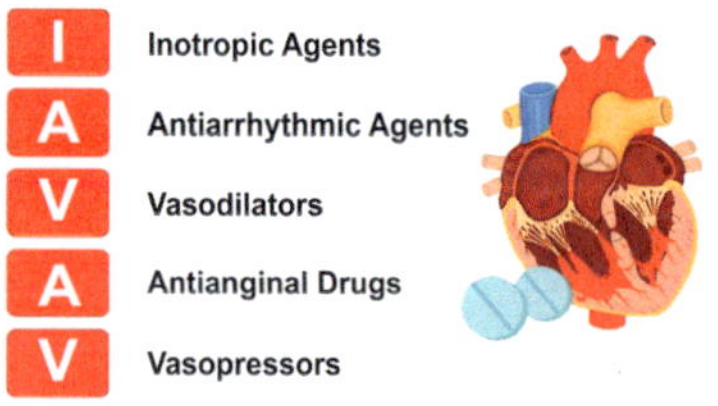

Figure 5.3. Types of cardiovascular drugs.

Source: Respiratory Therapy Zone. (2022). *Types of Cardiovascular Drugs.* https://www.respiratorytherapyzone.com/wp-content/uploads/2022/06/Types-of-Cardiovascular-Drugs-Illustration.png.

5.1.1. Antihypertensives

The management of cardiovascular disease habitually requires management of high blood pressure, itself a leading global cause of morbidity. Clinical practice relies upon antihypertensive drugs (Figure 5.4) as an anchor for treating hypertension, that if untreated exposes patients to subsequent complications including stroke, myocardial infarction, and congestive heart failure. The pharmacologic arsenal is varied and includes agents exerting their effects by means of vasodilation, lowering cardiac output, and altering fluid balance. Agents that are not only critical in primary hypertension but also in pregnancy-related complications, in which hypertensive disorders have severe implications on both maternal and fetal health, are equally important. Modern protocols highlight the importance of early detection and individually optimized treatment plans to maximize benefit and avoid complications, representing an emerging paradigm in cardiovascular pathophysiology within diverse patient populations (Freeman et al., 2013). In addition to their fundamental cardiovascular actions, some antihypertensive drugs have nuanced interactions with neuropsychiatric illness, demonstrating the intersection of cardiovascular and mental well-being. There is emerging evidence that certain categories of antihypertensives can impact mood disorders, both worsening and possibly improving symptoms. For example, ACE inhibitors and angiotensin receptor blockers (ARBs) have been linked with reduced admission rates for mood disorders, suggesting a protective effect. Beta-blockers and calcium channel antagonists, on the other hand, increase the risk of mood disturbances and thus require cautious selection in vulnerable individuals. These observations highlight the need for taking into account comorbidities and patient-specific attributes while prescribing antihypertensive treatment in order to maximize both cardiovascular and mental health (Boal et al., 2016). Clinical use of antihypertensive treatment goes beyond mere blood pressure lowering, with the need for a sophisticated understanding of individual patient attributes and concomitant conditions. During pregnancy, for instance, hypertensive disorders are increasing in tandem with maternal age and coexisting comorbidities, necessitating rapid and accurate intervention to avoid poor perinatal outcomes. The modalities of treatment need to weigh the effectiveness against safety, taking into consideration fetal exposure and long-term cardiovascular risk to the mother. This heightened complexity serves to underscore continued research and guideline maturation that incorporates new epidemiological findings and advances in screening. In this way, healthcare professionals are able to more effectively counteract the immediate dangers of hypertension and its consequences while also dealing with the wider implications for maternal and child cardiovascular health (Freeman et al., 2013).

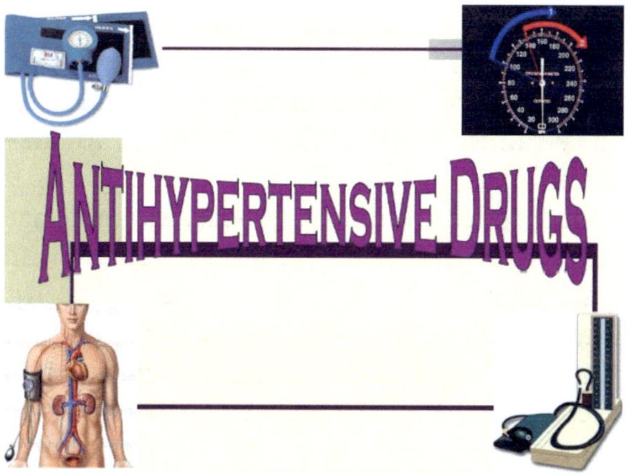

Figure 5.4. Antihypertensive drugs serve.

Source: Slideserve (n.d.). Antihypertensive Drugs Serve. https://image2.slideserve.com/4024782/slide1-l.jpg.

5.1.2. Anticoagulants

The issue of stroke prevention, especially ischemic stroke, is a fundamental issue in cardiovascular medicine because of the high morbidity and mortality of this condition. Of all the causes of stroke, atrial fibrillation is one of the major risk factors, largely because it facilitates the generation of thrombi within the atria that can embolize to cerebral arteries. Anticoagulants have therefore become central drugs in clinical guidelines directed at minimizing stroke risk in patients with atrial fibrillation (Figure 5.5). The efficacy of these medications is not only dependent on their biochemical actions but also on patient compliance, which is usually undermined by poor knowledge of the disease and treatment significance. Educational interventions targeting enhanced patient comprehension have shown statistically significant knowledge score improvements, directly related to enhanced adherence and lowered stroke incidence. Therefore, the function of anticoagulants goes beyond pharmacodynamics and involves patient education as an integral part of stroke risk management in cardiovascular practice (Jeyasingh et al., 2022). Vitamin K is a key component in coagulation-related physiological processes, representing an indispensable nexus between nutrition and anticoagulation therapy. The vitamin occurs in two main forms—phylloquinone (vitamin K1) and a group of menaquinones (vitamin K2)—each characterized by unique bioavailability, tissue distribution, and physiological activity. These vitamers control clotting factor synthesis, and thus they are both a natural target and a potential confound in anticoagulant therapy, especially with vitamin K antagonists like warfarin. New evidence underscores the wider health relevance of vitamin K beyond hemostasis, including certain protective actions on CVD, which is an issue for patients receiving anticoagulant therapy. Elucidation of personal vitamin K status and its nutritional supplementation may provide means for maximizing therapeutic response with reduced side effects, thus closing the divide between pharmacologic intervention and dietary intervention in cardiovascular well-being (Araujo et al., 2020). Clinical use of anticoagulants involves an intricate weighing of efficacy for prevention of thrombosis against the potential for bleeding complications, for which rationale it is necessary to monitor carefully and tailor therapy to the patient. Newer anticoagulants, such as DOACs, have revolutionized cardiovascular therapy by offering alternatives to historic vitamin K antagonists with better pharmacokinetics and less restrictive diets. This change is indicative of a continuing attempt to optimize patient quality of life through fewer hospitalizations and adverse effects of therapy nonadherence. All these advances notwithstanding, optimal anticoagulation still involves the removal of patient education, nutrition, and comorbid barriers. Ongoing investigations and quality improvement efforts directed toward improving knowledge regarding anticoagulation have proved to have tangible effects in clinical outcomes, which emphasizes the value of the multidisciplinary management of CVDs with drug therapy (Araujo et al., 2020; Jeyasingh et al., 2022).

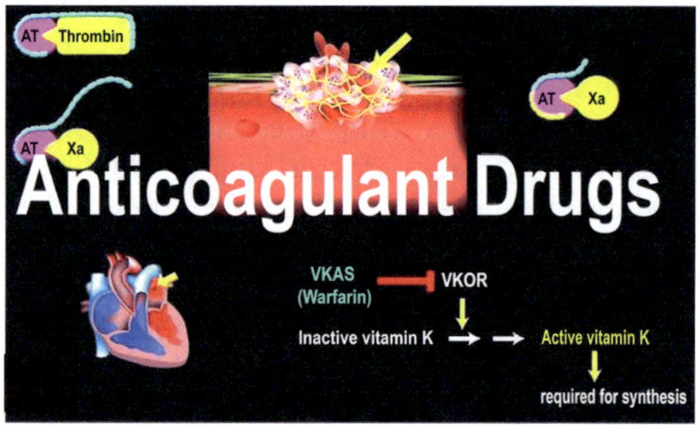

Figure 5.5. Anticoagulants drugs.

Source: YouTube. (n.d.). *Anticoagulants drugs.* https://i.ytimg.com/vi/3GN5L2ugfvk/sddefault.jpg.

5.1.3. Lipid-Lowering Agents

Successful cardiovascular risk control is heavily reliant on the manipulation of lipid concentration, especially that of low-density lipoprotein cholesterol (LDL-C), which has a key role to play in atherosclerosis pathogenesis. Statins have drastically changed lipid lowering because of the strong LDL-C lowering and resultant cardiovascular event reduction, but clearly, their constraints are obvious. Some patients tolerate statins, while others neither achieve lipid endpoints with statin monotherapy alone nor tolerate maximum tolerated statin doses, indicating the need for adjunctive lipid management strategies. One such strategy is the use of ezetimibe, which blocks intestinal cholesterol absorption by binding to the Niemann-Pick C1-like 1 protein. The combination of ezetimibe with statins has shown incremental LDL-C reductions, offering a second option for high-risk patients in need of more stringent lipid control. Continued assessment of the safety and efficacy of ezetimibe continues to define its place in cardiovascular pharmacotherapy, highlighting its value in various clinical settings where monotherapy is inadequate (Dayspring et al., 2012). The process of managing lipid risk is more challenging in the presence of comorbid conditions like chronic kidney disease (CKD) or kidney transplantation. These patients have very high cardiovascular risk profiles, which are propelled by a clustering of factors such as dyslipidemia, hypertension, and the side effects of immunosuppressive drugs. With the significance of CVD as a cause of morbidity and mortality in this group, lipid-lowering drugs become an integral part of total care. Pharmacologic management, such as the use of statins and other lipid-altering drugs, needs to be individualized for consideration of changes in drug metabolism and possible interaction with immunosuppressants. Optimization of the lipid profile in kidney transplant recipients not only plays a role in the reduction of cardiovascular risk but also in graft survival, highlighting the complex interrelationship between lipid management and transplant success (Jardine et al., 2014). In addition to statins and cholesterol absorption inhibitors, the therapeutic armamentarium of lipid-lowering agents continues to grow with the advent of new therapies directed at various aspects of lipid metabolism. Agents like PCSK9 inhibitors have emerged as effective alternatives that can induce impressive LDL-C decreases in patients resistant or intolerant to standard treatment. These monoclonal antibodies facilitate LDL receptor recycling, with increased clearance of circulating LDL particles. Such breakthroughs represent strides towards personalized cardiovascular management, allowing clinicians to intervene on the diverse lipid profiles and risk factors faced. However, the choice of lipid-lowering drugs needs to take into account efficacy, safety, patient compliance, and cost-effectiveness to maximize cardiovascular benefits. Future research and clinical trials will continue to define the roles and permutations of these treatments in reducing CVD burden (Dayspring et al., 2012).

Test Your Knowledge

1. What is low-density lipoprotein cholesterol?
2. Define antihypertensive drugs?

5.2. Mechanisms of Action

Learning Outcome

1. How Antihypertensives Lower Blood Pressure?
2. Mechanisms of Anticoagulants in Preventing Clot Formation
3. Role of Lipid-Lowering Agents in Cholesterol Management

To comprehend the complex mechanisms through which drugs affect the cardiovascular system is to appreciate the interplay between pharmacological targets and physiological pathways (Figure 5.6). Most cardiovascular drugs act by modifying the renin-angiotensin-aldosterone system (RAAS), an important regulator of blood pressure and fluid balance. Agents like ACE inhibitors and ARBs break this system, thus inhibiting vasoconstriction and sodium retention and eventually lowering blood pressure and cardiac workload. Furthermore, these drugs have an important function in the management of vascular complications of comorbid conditions like diabetes, where endothelial dysfunction and inflammation worsen cardiovascular risk. Through their action on oxidative stress and inflammatory pathways, these therapeutic interventions not only enhance hemodynamics but also assist in preventing the exacerbation of vascular injury in coexistence with metabolic disease (Guzik et al., 2018). In addition to traditional antihypertensive drugs, some drugs target specifically cardiac contractility and rhythm by modulating adrenergic receptors and ion channels. Beta-adrenergic blockers decrease sympathetic stimulation, which results in decreased heart rate and myocardial oxygen demand, helpful in ischemic heart disease and arrhythmias. Calcium channel blockers, by contrast, block calcium influx in vascular smooth muscle and cardiac cells, resulting in vasodilation and decreased myocardial contractility. These mechanisms all together decrease the workload on the heart and help in enhanced cardiac efficiency. Yet the heterogeneity of the mechanisms suggests the need for tailored therapeutic choice according to pathophysiology in individual patients in order to maximize outcomes while reducing side effects. With emergent therapeutic dilemmas, like cancer-related cardiovascular complications, analysis of drug action mechanisms includes awareness of cardiotoxicity from anticancer drugs. More recently developed chemotherapeutic agents, specifically those antagonizing vascular endothelial growth factor signaling pathways, are capable of inducing hypertension, thrombosis, and myocardial damage through endothelial dysfunction and increased oxidative stress. These disease states illustrate the fine balance that must be achieved when treating complicated patients at risk for both oncologic and cardiovascular morbidity. Cooperative care plans that combine cardiovascular pharmacology and oncologic therapy offer a platform to counteract untoward cardiovascular effects with maintained anticancer activity (Cameron et al., 2015). This dynamic environment necessitates continuous studies on mechanisms of action to devise treatment with maximum efficiency and minimum collateral cardiovascular impact.

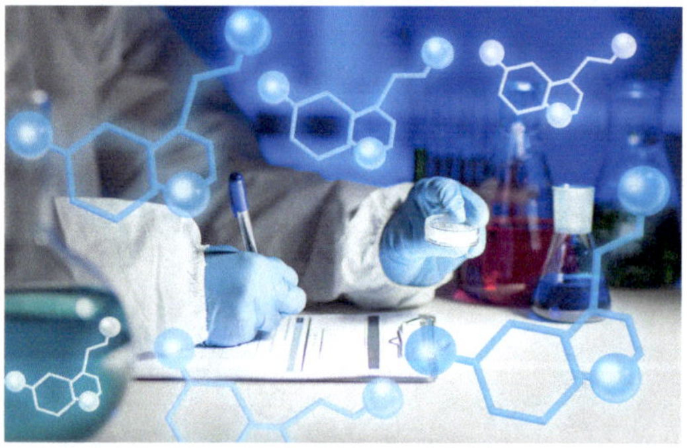

Figure 5.6. Mechanisms of action by which drugs influence.

PTCB Test Prep. (2020). *Top mechanisms of action.*

Source: https://ptcbtestprep.com/wp-content/uploads/2020/05/top-mechanisms-of-action.jpg.

5.2.1. How Antihypertensives Lower Blood Pressure?

Effective control of cardiovascular well-being depends on knowing how antihypertensive medications decrease blood pressure (Figure 5.7). They act via different mechanisms that ultimately decrease vascular resistance and cardiac load. For example, diuretics stimulate the excretion of sodium and water, hence reducing blood volume and decreasing arterial pressure. Other drugs, including beta-blockers, blunt the effect of the sympathetic nervous system by decreasing heart rate and myocardial contractility, which decreases cardiac output. Also, ACE inhibitors block the RAAS, restricting vasoconstriction and sodium retention. Through the inhibition of various physiological processes, antihypertensives as a group lower arterial pressure, enhancing overall cardiovascular function and lowering the risk of end-organ damage. This multi-dimensional strategy highlights the value of these medications in preventing and controlling hypertension-induced complications. In addition to blood pressure reduction, a number of antihypertensive agents provide other protective mechanisms for the cardiovascular system. Calcium channel blockers, for instance, not only reduce vascular tone by blocking the influx of calcium into smooth muscle cells but potentially have neuroprotective effects that are useful in cerebrovascular disease. This is important with the rising dementia burden that will place a strain on medical resources worldwide. Clinical evidence indicates improved antihypertensive therapy diminishes cerebrovascular disease and amyloid deposition caused by hypoxia—a pathological feature of Alzheimer's disease (AD)—suggesting a preventative action on cognitive impairment in addition to cardiovascular effects (Demuro et al., 2012). Therefore, antihypertensive mechanisms go beyond basic hemodynamic modification to more intricate interactions with neurovascular cascades, with wider therapeutic potentials. Clinical evidence also supports the effectiveness of tight blood pressure control with antihypertensive treatment. Comparative research shows that keeping blood pressure below 130 mmHg considerably reduces the occurrence of stroke compared to conventional control levels between 130 and 139 mmHg (Abraham et al., 2020). Although this more stringent control did not definitively lower rates of myocardial infarction, decreased stroke risk underscores the value of intensive blood pressure control for cerebrovascular protection. These data also mirror the pivotal role of antihypertensives in preventing vascular events, solidifying treatment recommendations that promote lower target pressures in targeted populations. Yet, the heterogeneity of individual response and the requirement to weigh benefits against possible side effects emphasize the demand for individualized therapeutic approaches in cardiovascular pharmacotherapy.

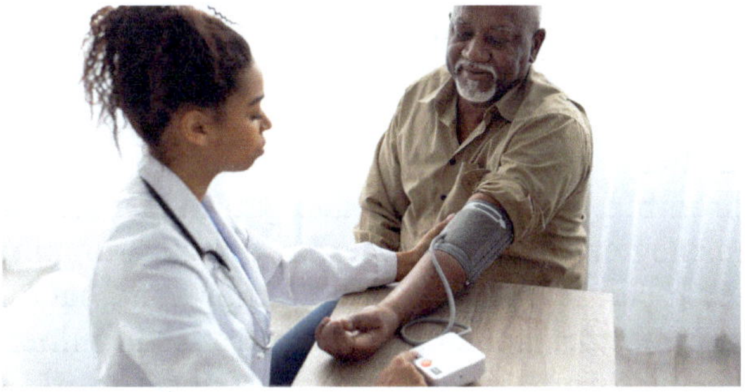

Figure 5.7. Antihypertensives lower blood pressure.

Source: Hospital Pharmacy Europe. (2023). *Low-Dose Combination Antihypertensives Effective First-Line Treatment.*

5.2.2. Mechanisms of Anticoagulants in Preventing Clot Formation

Grasping the biochemical mechanisms of thrombus formation is crucial to an understanding of the mechanism of anticoagulants in cardiovascular treatment. Hemostasis, or blood clotting, is a complicated cascade of cellular and molecular elements, mostly platelets and coagulation factors, that interact with each other to produce fibrin mesh stabilizing the thrombus. Anticoagulants act at one or more stages of this cascade, acting against specific proteins or enzymes essential to the propagation of clot. For instance, vitamin K antagonists such as warfarin inhibit the synthesis of vitamin K-dependent clotting factors II, VII, IX, and X by blocking vitamin K epoxide reductase. This reduces the availability of functional clotting proteins required for fibrin generation, thus impairing clot stability and growth. Through alteration of these molecular targets, anticoagulants interfere with the balance between procoagulant and anticoagulant forces, potentially reducing the risk of pathologic clot formation in conditions like atrial fibrillation or venous thromboembolism, as per existing clinical recommendations (José et al., 2023). DOACs have become crucial agents with unique mechanisms over conventional therapies. These medications exert their effects through selective inhibition of either thrombin (factor IIa) or factor Xa, both key players in the common pathway of the coagulation cascade. Direct thrombin inhibitors like dabigatran inhibit the fibrinogen to fibrin conversion, directly stopping fibrin clot formation. On the other hand, factor Xa inhibitors apixaban and rivaroxaban inhibit the prothrombin to thrombin activation, thus reducing thrombin availability and activity. This targeted interference not only decreases clot formation efficiency but also possesses benefits in terms of pharmacodynamics and safety profiles, such as fewer dietary limitations and monitoring. The functional specificity of DOACs maximizes their clinical application in conditions that demand anticoagulation, which further solidifies their position in contemporary cardiovascular pharmacotherapy (José et al., 2023). While anticoagulants are effective in the prevention of thrombotic complications, their administration must be done with careful patient selection and monitoring because of the inherent risk of bleeding complications. The balance between inhibiting the formation of a clot and preserving hemostasis is tenuous, as aggressive anticoagulation can cause hemorrhagic events, while inadequate dosing will not prevent thrombosis. Clinical factors involve patient age, gender, comorbid conditions like chronic myeloid leukemia, and having cardiac devices, which affect drug metabolism and response. Moreover, combining anticoagulant therapy with diagnostic techniques such as cardiac magnetic resonance enhances treatment and risk stratification outcomes. Appreciation of these subtleties highlights the value of personalized therapeutic strategies using the mechanistic benefits of anticoagulants in the overall management of CVD.

5.2.3. Role of Lipid-Lowering Agents in Cholesterol Management

Cholesterol management is key to lowering cardiovascular risk, and this requires the use of pharmacologic agents that can modulate lipid profiles. Lifestyle modification remains central, but most patients need to be treated with lipid-lowering agents to reach target cholesterol values, specifically LDL-C (Figure 5.8). Statins have become the keystone in cholesterol management because of their strong inhibition of HMG-CoA reductase, lowering endogenous cholesterol production. Yet, not every patient tolerates statins or achieves optimal LDL-C levels on these medications alone. In such instances, supplementary therapies such as ezetimibe are useful adjuncts by reducing intestinal cholesterol absorption via the Nieman Pick C1 like 1 protein, causing additional LDL-C lowering. Ezetimibe is known to be effective and safe, an important alternative in integrated cholesterol treatment regimens to reduce cardiovascular event risk (Dayspring et al., 2012). Statins' advantages lie beyond cholesterol lowering, and it is because of this that they play a key role in preventing CVD. Statins pleiotropic actions on vascular endothelium have been brought into focus by studies, such as enhanced endothelial function, inflammation reduction, and atherosclerotic plaque stabilization, and these combined could decrease ischemic events. In particular, statins have proved to be effective in reducing the occurrence of stroke and cerebral ischemia, especially in hypercholesterolemic patients and those with previous cerebrovascular disease. These pleiotropic effects indicate that the benefits of statins cannot be entirely explained by their lipid-lowering ability but also by vasculoprotective mechanisms. Although there is a degree of doubt regarding the relative contribution of these effects, clinical wisdom favors statins as cornerstone drugs in the prevention of coronary as well as cerebrovascular complications (Al Sulaiman et al., 2017). Lipid-lowering agent developments further expand therapy options for controlling cholesterol, complementing statin monotherapy limitations. Synergistic combinations of agents like bile acid sequestrants, fibrates, and emerging therapy options like PCSK9 inhibitors offer customized strategies for patients with different dyslipidemia profiles and tolerances to therapy. Each drug has a different mechanism of action, e.g., increasing cholesterol clearance or altering lipoprotein metabolism, thereby expanding therapeutic effects. As knowledge of cholesterol's role in cardiovascular disease increases, maximizing lipid-lowering interventions continues to be key to decreasing morbidity and mortality. Physicians need to balance patient-specific risk factors, drug interactions, and side effect profiles to achieve maximal benefit, reflecting the dynamic and individualized process of cholesterol management in cardiovascular pharmacotherapy.

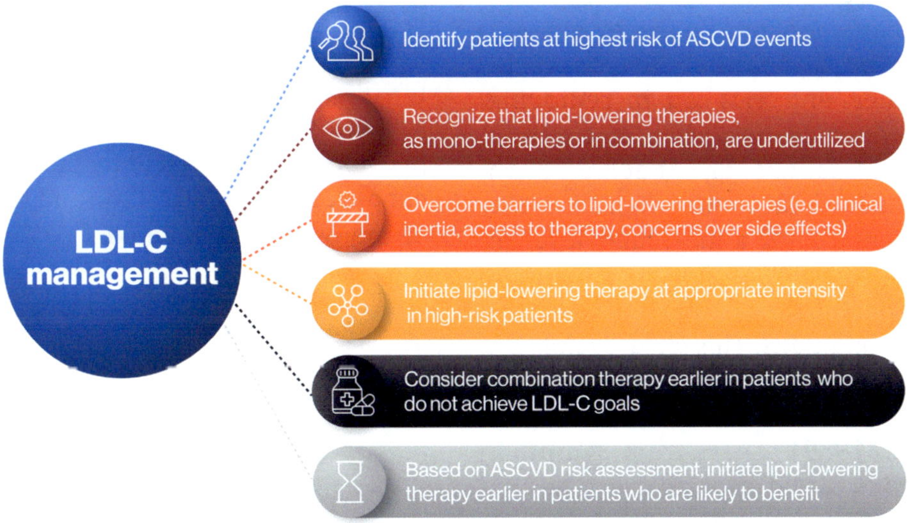

Figure 5.8. Role of lipid-lowering agents in cholesterol management.

Source: American Heart Association. (n.d.). *Role of Lipid-Lowering Agents in Cholesterol Management.* https://www.ahajournals.org/cms/asset/3645b260-60e3-437b-a732-e5b9c49edadb/jah38493-fig-0001.png.

Test Your Knowledge

1. How do diuretics lower blood pressure?
2. What are lipid-lowering agents?

5.3. Therapeutic Uses

Learning Outcome

1. Management of Hypertension
2. Prevention of Stroke and Heart Attack
3. Treatment of Dyslipidemia

The treatment of CVDs may frequently require pharmacologic interventions that address specific physiological mechanisms to reinstate and preserve cardiac function. The therapeutic applications of cardiovascular drugs cover a wide variety of conditions including hypertension, heart failure, arrhythmias, and angina pectoris (Figure 5.9). For example, beta-adrenergic blockers are used mostly to decrease myocardial oxygen demand through reduction of heart rate and contractility and thus to treat symptoms of angina and to enhance survival following myocardial infarction. In the same manner, diuretics aid in removing excess fluid, which is essential in treating congestive heart failure and edema. Such highly customized treatments highlight the role of comprehension at a molecular level in drug action, which allows clinicians to tailor therapy based on the severity of disease and patient-specific conditions. This ensures not just symptom control but also improvement in long-term prognosis for cardiovascular pathologies (Hastings et al., 1959). Apart from symptom control, numerous cardiovascular drugs have a central role to play in the prevention of disease progression and adverse cardiovascular events. ACE inhibitors and ARBs are generally employed to counteract the impact of the RAAS, which plays a significant role in causing hypertension and cardiac remodeling. These drugs have been shown to be effective in reducing blood pressure, decreasing afterload, and preventing structural injury to the heart and vasculature. Antiplatelet medications and anticoagulants are also important in preventing thrombotic illnesses like stroke and myocardial infarction by blocking platelet aggregation or pathways of coagulation. These preventive measures illustrate the therapeutic value of cardiovascular medication beyond relieving acute symptoms, with a focus on long-term health benefit and mortality decline (Hastings et al., 1959).

The incorporation of drug treatment in cardiac treatment also entails the management of comorbidities that increase cardiac risk and complicate drug treatment protocols. Medications that influence the cardiovascular system, thus, need to be chosen with regard to their effects on cognitive and neurological well-being, particularly among elderly groups. Polypharmacy and patient compliance issues, together with the risk of adverse interactions, are still compelling considerations for therapeutic success. Emerging innovations in drug development are increasingly focusing on targeted treatments with better safety profiles and tailored dosing regimens. Such a comprehensive treatment strategy not only prevents cardiovascular pathology but also enhances the quality of life and functional status of the patient as a whole.

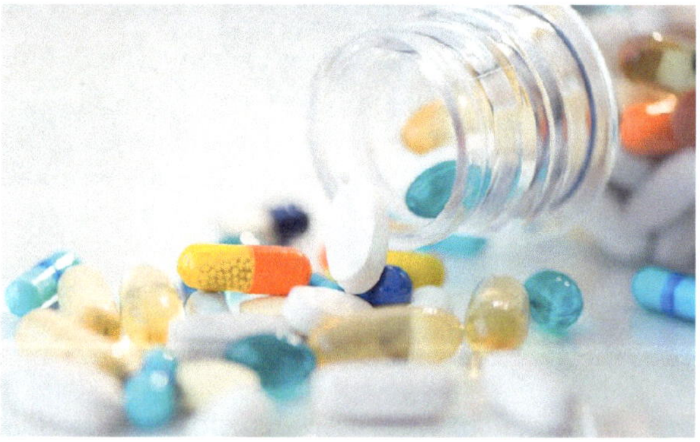

Figure 5.9. Therapeutic uses of cardiovascular drugs.

Source: Atlanta Medicare. (2019). *Therapeutic Drugs.* https://www.atlantamedicare.co.th/wp-content/uploads/2019/05/Therapeutic-Drugs-01.jpg.

5.3.1. Management of Hypertension

Optimal control of hypertension needs to be a multimodal process that goes beyond mere blood pressure control to deal with related cardiovascular risk (Figure 5.10). Contemporary practice guidelines stress the importance of thorough risk stratification, such as for target organ damage like left ventricular hypertrophy, which may affect therapy. Ambulatory blood pressure monitoring thus becomes a useful tool in this regard, revealing such patterns as increased pulse pressure in younger patients with hypertension and possibly indicating sympathetic nervous system activation. It is knowledge of these physiological subtleties that guides the choice of proper pharmacological agents, not just to reduce blood pressure but also to prevent unfavorable cardiovascular remodeling. Treatment plans, therefore, need to be tailored, considering age, the occurrence of comorbidities, and cardiovascular risk factors in order to maximize outcomes as well as decrease morbidity related to hypertension (Mattioli et al., 2024). Pharmacotherapy is the foundation of treating hypertension and consists of a wide variety of drug classes acting on the cardiovascular system. Initial drugs—such as ARBs, calcium channel blockers, and diuretics—are selected for their effectiveness, safety profile, and tolerability. Recent clinical studies have highlighted the additional advantages of some medications, emphasizing their ability to enhance cognitive function and decrease sympathetic hyperactivity, which could potentially lead to better long-term outcomes. Additionally, developing evidence into adjunct therapies, including vitamin D supplementation, has started to uncover significant interactions with cardiovascular disease through modulation of vascular function and inflammatory mechanisms. Such observations indicate that individualized treatment based on biochemical markers and comorbidities might augment the therapeutic effect of traditional antihypertensive therapies (Mattioli et al., 2024). Financial factors play an important role in the management strategies for hypertension considering the high direct and indirect cost burden of the chronic disease. Medication covers most of the direct costs, and hence there is a strong need for cost-effective prescribing without affecting clinical outcomes. Evidence is in favor of early and persistent blood pressure control lowering the cost of cardiovascular complications and related hospitalizations. Novel pharmacoeconomic models propose that maximizing treatment compliance and taking advantage of agents with multiple benefits—e.g., cognitive protection—may result in significant savings for healthcare systems while enhancing patient quality of life. Therefore, future studies need to strike a balance between clinical outcomes and economic viability, with longer-term cost-benefit assessments to inform policy and clinical practice in hypertension management (Himmelmann et al., 2002).

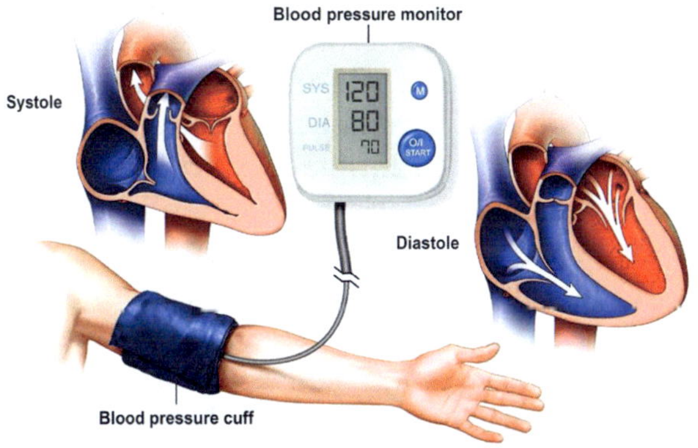

Figure 5.10. Management of hypertension.

Source: Mayo Clinic. (2023). *Blood Pressure Measurement.* https://www.mayoclinic.org/content/dam/media/en/images/2023/02/10/blood-pressure-measurement.jpg.

5.3.2. Prevention of Stroke and Heart Attack

The intricacy in avoiding stroke and heart attack is mostly rooted in the multi-factorial pathophysiology of CVDs, which requires a multilateral pharmacological strategy (Figure 5.11). Drugs acting on modifiable risk factors like hypertension, hyperlipidemia, and diabetes form the basis for lowering the incidence of these events. Antihypertensive agents, for instance, reduce blood pressure, hence the amount of work exerted on arterial walls and the risk of rupture or blockage of vessels. In the same manner, statins have a vital role to play in the reduction of cholesterol, inhibiting the development of atherosclerotic plaques that lead to ischemic events. Individualized drug treatment based on the patient's risk factors prevents the measures from being ineffective and detrimental. These are elaborate choices that necessitate the clinician to balance guideline advice with the patient's unique conditions and preferences to ensure maximum outcomes (Cosentino et al., 2019). This individualized medicine strategy is a pillar in the current prevention of cardiovascular tragedies. In addition to control of blood pressure and cholesterol, antithrombotic therapy plays a crucial role in preventing stroke and myocardial infarction by blocking platelet aggregation and thrombus formation. Aspirin, an extensively used antiplatelet drug, decreases clot formation, especially in established CVD or high-risk patients. Newer medications, like P2Y12 inhibitors, have alternatives or additions in selected individuals to further increase prevention. Bleeding hazards associated with these medications, however, need to be carefully weighed against the advantages, requiring cautious clinical evaluation and observation. Moreover, glycemic control in diabetic individuals lowers vascular comorbidities responsible for causing stroke and myocardial infarction; hypoglycemic agents are therefore indirectly preventive. Recommendations highlight the importance of comprehensive approaches involving lifestyle, pharmacologic therapy, and periodic monitoring in lowering cardiovascular events (Paul et al., 2017). This multidisciplinary management illustrates contemporary preventive cardiology. The final aim of drug treatment of stroke and heart attack prevention is to recognize and counteract the pathophysiologic processes underlying before clinical events take place. This requires continuous research and evidence-based revision to guidelines such that drug regimens keep pace with new evidence of efficacy and safety. Joint efforts of cardiology societies and public health agencies have yielded strict clinical practice guidelines that guide drug choice, dose, and risk stratification algorithms. Clinicians have to remain skilled at applying the guidelines but not lose clinical judgment on a case-by-case basis. In addition, patient compliance with drugs prescribed is still a key determinant of outcome in prevention, which indicates that education and communication are essential. By this holistic practice, cardiovascular drug use has the potential to minimize morbidity and mortality due to stroke and heart attack (Cosentino et al., 2019; Paul et al., 2017).

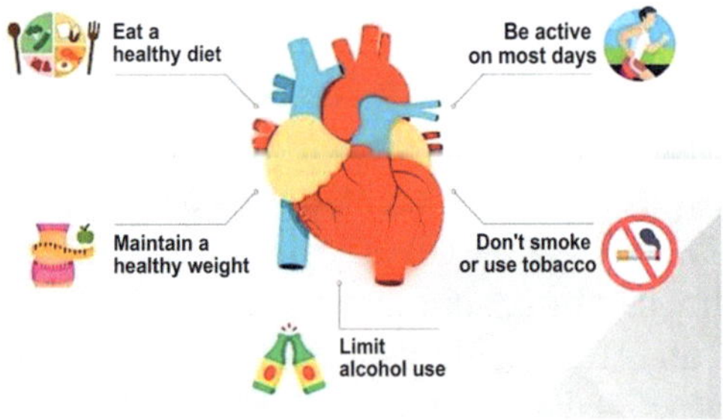

Figure 5.11. Prevention of stroke and heart attack.

Source: CK Birla Hospitals. (n.d.). *Prevention of Stroke and Heart Attack.* https://ckbh.ckbirlahospitals.com/storage/rbh/uploadedfiles/gallery/article/rbh-health-habits.webp.

5.3.3. Treatment of Dyslipidemia

Effective control of cardiovascular health must take priority over the complex issues raised by dyslipidemia, a disease state due to abnormal lipid composition that highly predisposes to atherosclerosis and subsequent cardiac events. Management strategies are mainly centered on pharmacological interventions for the normalization of lipid levels as a means to decrease the morbidity and mortality of CVD. Statins are the mainstay of therapy, with their action being to inhibit HMG-CoA reductase, resulting in reduced cholesterol production and an increase in LDL receptors. Their extensive use is justified by ample evidence for LDL cholesterol and cardiovascular event reductions. Nonetheless, treatment regimens need to be carefully weighed, particularly in comorbid populations with serious mental illness where metabolic side effects of psychotropic medications complicate lipid control (Braga et al., 2018). This highlights the requirement for personalized approaches in balance with efficacy and safety in vulnerable groups. In addition to statins, adjunctive therapies such as fibrates, niacin, and PCSK9 inhibitors are important in the management of targeted lipid abnormalities. These drugs act on triglycerides, high-density lipoprotein (HDL), and LDL cholesterol by various mechanisms, offering alternatives to patients who do not reach lipid targets with statins alone or have contraindications. Fibrates, for instance, bind to peroxisome proliferator-activated receptors to stimulate triglyceride degradation, while niacin inhibits hepatic production of VLDL. The introduction of PCSK9 inhibitors presents a new mechanism by increasing the recycling of LDL receptors to remove LDL cholesterol more efficiently. Combining these treatments necessitates the constant monitoring of metabolic parameters and the modification of treatment regimens accordingly, particularly in patients taking antipsychotic drugs known to worsen lipid disorders and metabolic syndrome (Moreno et al., 2016). This vigilance optimizes the reduction of cardiovascular risk while avoiding adverse effects. In the overall context of cardiovascular pharmacotherapy, dyslipidemia treatment needs to be placed within a comprehensive framework that also treats lifestyle change and comorbid conditions. Patients with concomitant mental illness, for example, tend to have increased cardiovascular risk in part due to the metabolic effects of psychotropic medications and inadequate preventive services (Braga et al., 2018). This requires models of care that combine primary and psychiatric health services to enable systematic screening and active management of lipid disorders. Health provider education interventions have been reported to enhance follow-through with guidelines for lipid screening, especially for patients on second-generation antipsychotics (Moreno et al., 2016). Finally, the therapeutic success in dyslipidemia as part of CVD depends on multidisciplinary collaboration, patient counseling, and individualized pharmacological regimens taking into account the intricate cross-play among drugs influencing numerous physiological systems (Figure 5.12).

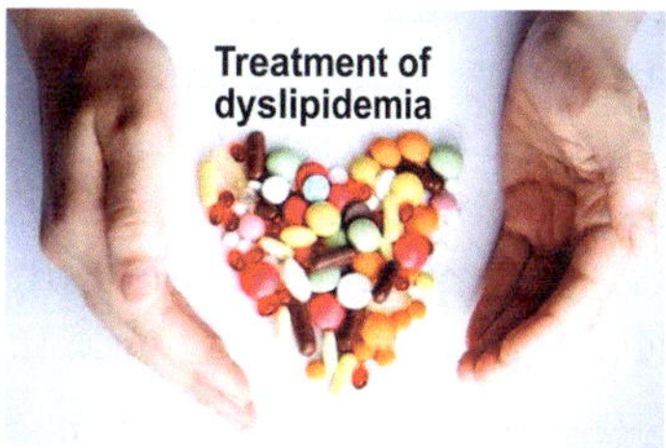

Figure 5.12. Treatment of dyslipidemia.

Source: SlideShare (2015). *Treatment of Dyslipidemia.* https://image.slidesharecdn.com/treatmentofdyslipidemia-150531125104-lva1-app6892/95/treatment-of-dyslipidemia-1-638.jpg?cb=1433076985.

Test Your Knowledge

1. Define hypertension?
2. How do statins help in treating dyslipidemia?

5.4. Side Effects and Risks

Learning Outcome

1. Common Side Effects of Antihypertensives
2. Risks Associated with Anticoagulant Therapy
3. Potential Adverse Effects of Lipid-Lowering Medications

The drug administration aimed at the cardiovascular system requires utmost care owing to the intricate physiological interaction they control. Although these drugs are critical in regulating conditions like hypertension, arrhythmia, and heart failure, their adverse effects sometimes pose considerable threats to patient safety and compliance with treatment (Figure 5.13). For instance, beta-blockers, which are frequently used to treat hypertension and heart rhythm abnormalities, can produce fatigue, dizziness, or worsen bronchospastic states. Analogously, diuretics, as effective as they are in decreasing blood volume and pressure, are usually responsible for causing electrolyte disturbances, the dangers of which include arrhythmias or muscle weakness. Knowledge of these possible adverse effects is important for clinicians to optimally weigh therapeutic gain against potential harm, pointing to the importance of personalized risk assessment and ongoing monitoring during treatment (Visseren et al., 2021). Adverse reactions to cardiovascular drugs can on occasion complicate established comorbidities, requiring interdisciplinary strategies in the management of patients. Statins, used extensively for lipid reduction and cardiovascular risk, have been associated with myopathy and, in extreme instances, rhabdomyolysis, which can drastically affect muscle integrity. Apart from side effects concerning muscle, some antihypertensive drugs such as ACE inhibitors can cause angioedema or severe cough, restricting tolerability. These risks reflect the necessity of continuous pharmacovigilance and patient education, enabling early detection and prevention of side effects. The outcome of untreated adverse reactions not only decreases the efficacy of drugs but also imposes healthcare burdens from hospitalization or treatment withdrawal (François et al., 2019). Additionally, patient heterogeneity in response to cardiovascular medications makes risk-benefit assessments even more challenging, underscoring the importance of individualized therapeutic approaches. Genetic factors, physiological changes with age, and pre-existing organ dysfunction can impact drug metabolism and sensitivity, thereby contributing to heterogeneous side effect profiles. For instance, older adults are particularly susceptible to orthostatic hypotension from vasodilators, increasing fall risk, while patients with renal impairment require cautious dosing to avoid toxicity.

These complexities highlight that guidelines must be integrated with clinical discretion, ensuring that treatments are tailored with attention to potential side effects, interactions, and individual patient contexts. Finally, it is the responsibility of healthcare providers to remain updated regarding changing evidence and regulatory guidance to maximize cardiovascular drug safety (François et al., 2019; Visseren et al., 2021).

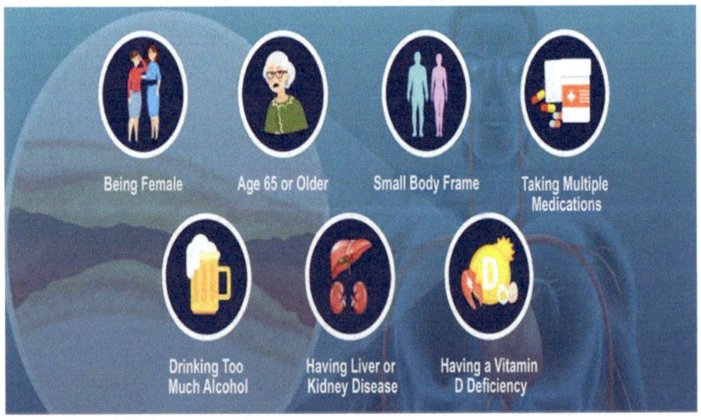

Figure 5.13. Side effects and risks.

Source: Jockers, D. (2021). Statin Drug Side Effects. https://drjockers.com/wp-content/uploads/2021/06/Statin-Drug-Side-Effects.jpg.

5.4.1. Common Side Effects of Antihypertensives

Treating CVDs frequently requires the administration of antihypertensive drugs, which play a critical role in lowering morbidity and mortality. Unfortunately, their therapeutic effectiveness is usually associated with a variety of side effects that may impact compliance in patients. Such adverse reactions depend on the drug group, but dizziness, fatigue, and gastrointestinal (GI) upset are among the most frequent reactions. The development of these side effects can present challenges in the clinical setting since they can require dosage changes or even a shift to other medications. Familiarity with the pharmacodynamics and patient-specific dynamics is important in avoiding these side effects and providing optimum treatment. Hence, healthcare providers need to be watchful for any new developing side effects and weigh benefits against risks while prescribing antihypertensive drugs. Of the antihypertensive drug categories, beta-blockers and diuretics are especially known for their unique side effect profiles. Beta-blockers, although good for decreasing cardiac workload, often produce bradycardia, lethargy, and cold limbs, which can result in discontinuation in susceptible patients. Diuretics, another cornerstone of hypertension management, commonly lead to electrolyte disturbances like hypokalemia and hyponatremia, together with excessive urination and dehydration. These presentations require close monitoring of renal function and electrolyte levels during treatment. Additionally, side effects such as angioedema and cough are most frequently related to ACE inhibitors, and thus proper patient education and early detection of side effects are crucial to avoid severe consequences. Pharmacovigilance is still a vital aspect of risk management for antihypertensive therapy, given the potential to compromise patient safety and healthcare resources through adverse drug reactions (ADRs). Research has demonstrated that most side effects are mild, yet a significant proportion can be severe enough to necessitate intervention or hospitalization. These effects illustrate the complexity of caring for cardiovascular medications, where polypharmacy raises the risk of drug interactions and cumulative adverse effects. Clinical protocols thus place emphasis on the necessity of extensive monitoring to identify early toxicity or intolerance signs. Focusing on patient compliance and reporting, along with clinician recognition, is critical in reducing the impact of side effects, hence maximizing overall cardiovascular pharmacotherapy effectiveness (Adhikari et al., 2009; Freeman et al., 2013).

5.4.2. Risks Associated with Anticoagulant Therapy

Anticoagulant treatment is a foundation of treatment of numerous cardiovascular illnesses, most especially those involving the thromboembolic phenomena. Nonetheless, because of its therapeutical merits, this therapeutic group possesses intrinsic hazards that deserve clinical vigilance (Figure 5.14). Hemorrhage is the most dangerous and common complication that ranges from isolated episodes of blood loss to dangerous hemorrhage including intracranial or GI bleeding. The fine balance between inhibiting clotting and triggering inappropriate bleeding is patient-specific and varies with patient age, renal status, and concurrent medications. In addition, patient compliance with dosing regimens and frequent monitoring, especially with vitamin K antagonists such as warfarin, are important factors in lessening these risks. The dynamic pathophysiology of CVDs, added to by factors like hypertension and metabolic derangements intrinsic to the renin-angiotensin system, also increases the complexity of anticoagulation management (Ahmad et al., 2023). In addition to bleeding complications, some anticoagulants are also accompanied by other challenges with drug interactions and cardiovascular adverse effects. The introduction of DOACs has enhanced therapeutic convenience but not without issues of interaction with other cardiovascular medications, with the resultant possible variation in efficacy and safety profiles. Infections such as COVID-19 complicate this, as their inflammatory effects on cardiovascular pathways and the common necessity for polypharmacy in infected patients create difficulties. SARS-CoV-2 acts upon the angiotensin-converting enzyme 2 (ACE2) receptor, affecting vascular function and potentially heightening susceptibility to thrombotic events and myocardial injury. This interaction requires increased alertness when anticoagulant-treated patients become infected with COVID-19, as they are doubled at risk for arrhythmias, heart failure, and thromboembolism, complicating anticoagulant dosing and monitoring even further (Philip et al., 2023).

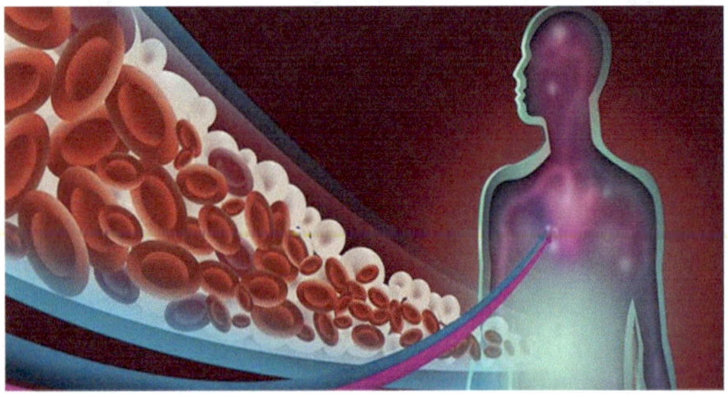

Figure 5.14. Risks associated with anticoagulant therapy.

Source: Sanident. (n.d.). *Terapia Anticoagulante.* https://www.sanident.com/wp-content/uploads/2019/09/terapia-anticoagulante.jpg.

Anticoagulant therapy can also lend itself to long-term complications that compromise cardiovascular stability. The long-term management of CVD patients includes the alleviation of risks like hypertension, diabetes, and atherosclerosis—diseases that anticoagulants can affect indirectly by their action on vascular endothelium and hemostatic processes. Anticoagulation, for example, can worsen microvascular bleeding or negate compensatory reactions in individuals with inadequate blood pressure control, which is often controlled by mechanisms targeted by cardiovascular medications like ARBs and ACE inhibitors (Ahmad et al., 2023). In addition, the interaction between anticoagulants and chronic comorbidities demands clever clinical approaches to avert harmful consequences, underlining the need for individualized treatment and ongoing risk-benefit evaluation in cardiovascular drug therapy.

5.4.3. Potential Adverse Effects of Lipid-Lowering Medications

The extensive application of lipid-lowering drugs, most notably statins, has transformed the control of cardiovascular risk, but it is important to appreciate their possible side effects (Figure 5.15). Statins, which are generally well tolerated, may at times result in muscle symptoms from a simple myalgia through to the more severe, though extremely rare, rhabdomyolysis. Another fear is elevation of hepatic enzymes, although such elevations are frequently asymptomatic and transient. Patients can also have GI disturbances or new-onset diabetes mellitus, which are allegedly related to statin-induced alterations in glucose metabolism. Comorbid conditions and genetic variables may affect the heterogeneity of adverse effects, emphasizing individualized treatment. Once concerns are raised, however, the benefit-risk ratio strongly supports the use of statins for CVD prevention, particularly in view of their ability to prevent major adverse cardiovascular events. Clinical awareness and patient counseling continue to be important to maximizing therapy and effectively controlling side effects. Outside of statins, other lipid-lowering drug classes have unique safety profiles deserving cautious attention. Fibrates, commonly used to lower triglycerides, are associated with GI distress, elevated liver enzymes, and, infrequently, myopathy, especially when used in combination with statins. Niacin, despite elevating HDL cholesterol, commonly produces flushing, pruritus, and possibly hepatotoxicity, which limits its tolerability. The discovery of newer agents, including PCSK9 inhibitors, has provided additional treatment options with reduced metabolic side effects but with possible injection site reactions and high expense. The choice of therapy should take these side effects into account, together with efficacy and patient-specific factors, to adjust cardiovascular risk reduction appropriately (Mary et al., 2023). In addition, lipid-lowering drugs can have effects beyond immediate side effects, affecting patient health in intricate ways. There is also emerging evidence to suggest that statins might impact non-hepatic systems such as cognitive status and the susceptibility to developing fatty liver disease, which raises some concerns regarding longer-term safety within specific groups of patients. Patients with existing liver disease need vigilant monitoring to differentiate drug-induced from progression of the underlying disease as suggested in managing patients with hepatic and metabolic comorbidities (Mary et al., 2023). The multifactorial etiology of adverse effects highlights the importance of continued research and post-marketing monitoring to further clarify and neutralize the risks of lipid-lowering therapy while preserving cardiovascular benefits.

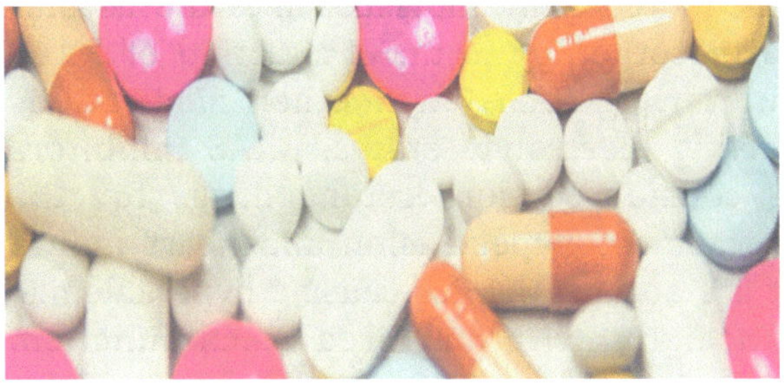

Figure 5.15. Potential adverse effects of lipid-lowering medications.

Source: eCare. (n.d.). Lipid Lowering Medications: Uses of Statins. https://1.bp.blogspot.com/-0z98yg4C92A/YHKAxbdWpmI/AAAAAAAAEkQ/JpLB7hTSGNcO5AGXaTEj05Bn Nwpawu8PACLcBGAsYHQ/w1200-h630-p-k-no-nu/lipid_lowering_ medications_uses_ statin_ ecare%255B1%255D.png.

Test Your Knowledge

1. What is the most common side effect of diuretics?
2. Which lipid-lowering drug is least likely to cause systemic side effects?

5.5. Drug Interactions

Learning Outcome

1. Interactions Between Antihypertensives and Other Medications
2. Impact of Anticoagulants on Surgical Procedures
3. Effects of Lipid-Lowering Agents on Liver Function

The treatment of CVDs commonly requires polypharmacy, which increases the risk of drug interactions that can make treatment more complex (Figure 5.16). Most cardiovascular drugs have shared metabolic pathways, specifically cytochrome P450 enzymes, that may result in changes in the plasma levels of co-administered drugs. For example, co-administration of some antiarrhythmics and statins may enhance the risk of side effects such as myopathy caused by impaired metabolism. In addition, medications such as beta-blockers and calcium channel blockers may interact at the pharmacodynamic level to cause inordinate bradycardia or hypotension. These kinds of interactions require proper dose adjustments and constant monitoring to achieve maximal therapeutic benefit with minimal adverse consequences. Awareness of these mechanisms is essential to provide patients with maximally beneficial and safe cardiovascular treatment. One of the more significant issues in cardiovascular pharmacotherapy is the interaction of RAAS inhibitors (RAASi) with other medications affecting electrolyte status. RAAS inhibitors are considered cornerstone drugs for the treatment of hypertension and heart failure but are at high risk for causing hyperkalemia, particularly with impaired renal function. The recent introduction of novel potassium-binding medications like patiromer and sodium zirconium cyclosilicate has been a great addition to avoid this risk. These drugs safely reduce serum potassium concentrations, enabling the maintenance of RAAS inhibitors that enhance cardiovascular outcomes. However, the risk of drug-drug interactions (DDIs) with these potassium binders is an area to be explored in order to comprehensively understand their long-term safety profiles and pharmacological interactions in intricate cardiovascular regimens (Agewall et al., 2019; Rosano et al., 2017). Drug interactions in the cardiovascular area go beyond pharmacokinetic and pharmacodynamic interactions to involve the modification of drug absorption. Antacids, for instance, and bile acid sequestrants can decrease the bioavailability of cardiovascular agents by formation of complexes or pH changes of the GI tract. The action can decrease the curative effect of drugs like digoxin or statins, requiring proper scheduling of drug administration. Moreover, concomitant effects among oral anticoagulants and other cardiac drugs can modify clotting times and have hazardous consequences of bleeding or thrombosis when not carefully controlled. These complex interactions highlight the need for an integrative approach to prescribing and monitoring cardiovascular therapy that ensures clinicians prevent and counteract potential side effects and concomitantly preserve therapeutic objectives.

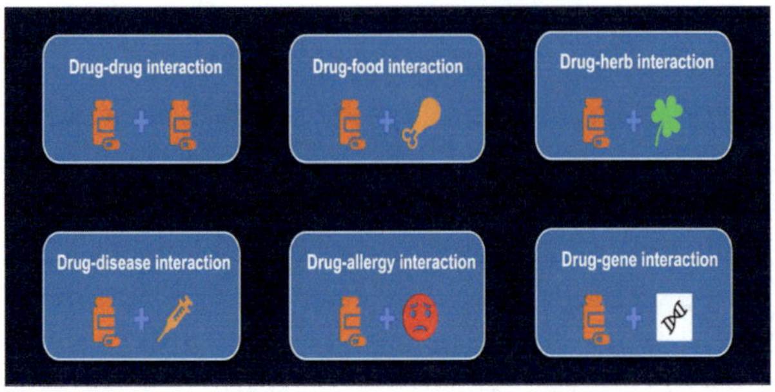

Figure 5.16. Drug interactions.

Source: Altexsoft. (2021*). Drug Interactions.* https://content.altexsoft.com/media/2021/01/word-image-25.png.

5.5.1. Interactions Between Antihypertensives and Other Medications

Hypertension management in older adults poses special challenges because of polypharmacy and the higher probability of comorbidities. Antihypertensive prescribing to older patients is often a matter of careful weighing of possible drug interactions (Figure 5.17), which can undermine therapeutic effectiveness or enhance adverse effects. For instance, the co-administration of diuretics like furosemide with other cardiovascular drugs might increase the risk of electrolyte disturbances culminating in arrhythmias or reduced efficacy of the drugs. It has been established through studies that monotherapy is still common among elderly patients despite the guideline recommendations for combined therapy, in part due to reluctance to initiate complicated regimens likely to induce adverse interaction. Furthermore, the increased prevalence of potentially inappropriate medications prescribed to very old patients highlights the necessity for more stringent medication review processes to reduce harmful interactions in this at-risk population (Akıcı et al., 2023). Such caution is important since inappropriate combinations can compromise blood pressure control and overall cardiovascular risk reduction. In addition to the physiological intricacies of aging, the impact of patient health literacy on the management of medications cannot be overemphasized, especially in the case of antihypertensive drug-drug interactions. Clear communication and education enable patients to learn about their regimen better, identify adverse effects, and comply with treatment regimens. For end-of-life patients, optimizing medication therapy entails counterbalancing therapeutic benefit against quality-of-life factors, and in this context, polypharmacy may be particularly pernicious by causing inimical drug interactions that worsen morbidity. Interventions aimed at promoting health literacy in older adults can assist them in taking an active role in medication management, with results enabling individualized adjustments minimizing inimical interactions between antihypertensives and other prescribed medications. As a result, this patient-oriented strategy not only enhances curative outcomes but also preserves autonomy and dignity in the treatment of complex medication regimens (Leschisin et al., 2018). The pharmacodynamic and pharmacokinetic interactions between other drugs and antihypertensives require detailed clinical evaluation, particularly in light of the varied mechanism of action of these drugs. Beta-blockers, which are typically used in the treatment of hypertension, can interact with nonsteroidal anti-inflammatory drugs (NSAIDs) and diminish antihypertensive activity by blunting vasodilatory actions. Likewise, calcium channel blockers have the potential to affect the metabolism of statins and some antiarrhythmics, raising the risk of toxicity. Diuretics, which are useful for blood pressure management, need to be monitored cautiously when used with lithium or corticosteroids because of the changed renal clearance and electrolyte imbalance. A grasp of such complex DDIs is necessary for clinicians to maximize cardiovascular therapy, minimize harmful outcomes, and provide assurance that combinations of antihypertensives and other drugs continue to be safe and effective in various patient populations.

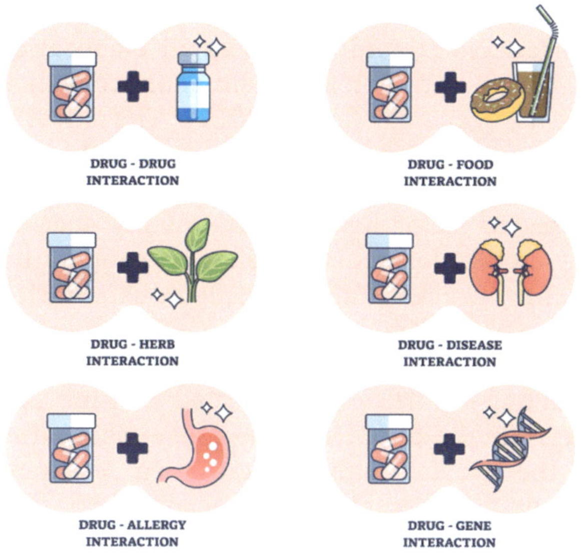

Figure 5.17. Interactions between antihypertensives and other medications.

Source: Docs Education. *(n.d.). BL_EX_2.* https://www.docseducation.com/sites/default/files/inline-images/bl_ex_2.jpg.

5.5.2. Impact of Anticoagulants on Surgical Procedures

The care of patients for surgery who are on anticoagulation therapy requires careful balancing between avoiding risk for thrombosis and managing hemorrhagic complications. The pharmacodynamics of anticoagulants, which interfere with the coagulation cascade to inhibit clotting, necessarily enhance bleeding tendency during invasive medical procedures (Figure 5.18). Surgeons and anesthesiologists need to cautiously consider each patient's characteristics, such as the indication for anticoagulation, half-life of drug, and urgency of surgery, to decide if therapy is interrupted or bridged. Premature or inadmissible discontinuation can result in thromboembolic events, while continuation increases the risk of intraoperative and postoperative bleeding. It relies intensively upon evidence-based recommendation to maximize the results through risk stratification for bleeding vs thrombotic consequences, and illustrates an elaboration on perioperative management of anticoagulant agents (Vahanian et al., 2021). The adverse outcomes caused by using anticoagulants with surgery range from a simple increment in blood losses to major hemostatic adversity such as hematomas formation, extended postoperative healing process, and surgical re-exploration for haemorrhagic control. Anticoagulant choice further complicates perioperative planning—warfarin's protracted half-life and unpredictable patient response compared to the shorter-acting DOACs, each requiring unique perioperative management. The advent of reversal agents has revolutionized clinical practice, allowing for rapid neutralization in instances of excessive bleeding or emergent surgical requirements. These maneuvers, however, demand compliance with established guidelines and patient-specific evaluations, since unrestrained use may trigger thrombotic events or be insufficient for hemostasis when required (Cosentino et al., 2019). Moreover, the perioperative management model should include interdisciplinary consultation and patient-specific risk assessment to prevent adverse outcomes related to anticoagulants. Laboratory tests prior to surgery, such as coagulation studies and renal function, direct timing of discontinuation and reinitiation of therapy. Elective procedures usually allow for planned discontinuation with or without bridging anticoagulation, whereas emergent procedures require immediate assessment and use of reversal agents or blood components. Care after surgery is also important as early resumption of anticoagulation leads to bleeding, and delayed resumption results in enhanced thrombotic risk. Therefore, maximization of surgical results in anticoagulated patients requires stringent use of clinical guidelines in addition to individualized therapeutic choices reflective of changing evidence and patient profiles (Cosentino et al., 2019; Vahanian et al., 2021).

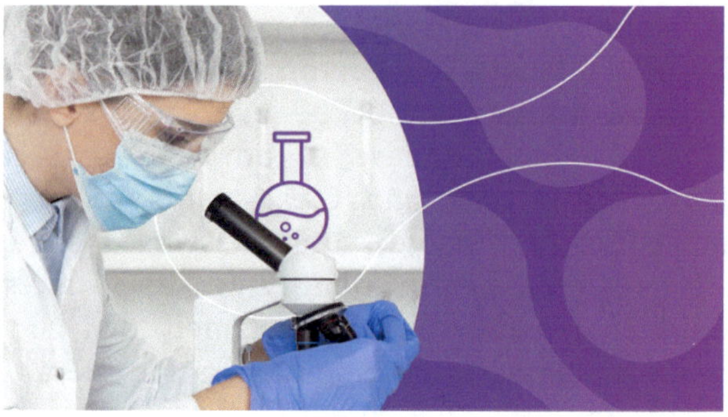

Figure 5.18. Anticoagulants on surgical procedures.

Source: BRF Ingredients. (n.d.). *How Heparin Aids Anticoagulant Treatments And Its Applications In Medicine.* https://www.brfingredients.com/assets/images/posts/saiba-como-a-heparina-auxilia-os-tratamentos-anticoagulantes-e-suas-aplicacoes-na-medicina/image.webp.

5.5.3. Effects of Lipid-Lowering Agents on Liver Function

The liver is at the center of lipid metabolism and hence a prime target for lipid-lowering drugs, which are central to the treatment of CVDs. Statins, the most commonly prescribed lipid-lowering drugs, exert their effect by inhibiting the enzyme HMG-CoA reductase and thereby inhibiting cholesterol production in hepatocytes. Although potent in lowering LDL cholesterol and in preventing cardiovascular events, these drugs may also cause hepatocellular stress. Mild increases in transaminase levels are fairly frequent on statin therapy, an indication of liver cell adaptation or injury. Clinically important liver damage is unusual. The pathogenesis of these hepatic effects is multifactorial and includes disruption of cholesterol biosynthesis, mitochondrial stress, and inflammatory reactions. Monitoring liver enzymes during treatment is thus necessary, though discontinuation is rarely necessary unless transaminase levels increase to greater than three times the upper limit of normal. The equilibrium between cardioprotective effects and possible hepatic harm characterizes clinical decision-making in the administration of lipid-lowering drugs (Al Sulaiman et al., 2017). Aside from statins, other lipid-lowering drugs like fibrates and niacin have unique hepatic effects based on their mechanisms of action. Fibrates stimulate peroxisome proliferator-activated receptors (PPARs), increasing lipid breakdown but occasionally inducing cholestatic liver damage, as well as liver transaminase elevations. Niacin, which lowers lipoprotein(a) and raises HDL, is linked to occasional hepatotoxicity in the form of steatohepatitis or fulminant liver failure in a minority of instances. These hepatic side effects require judicious patient selection and routine liver function tests, particularly in patients with preexisting liver disease. The hepatic effects of such agents highlight the intricate interaction between lipid metabolism modulation and liver function, especially when treating patients with concomitant metabolic conditions like hypertension and diabetes that augment cardiovascular risk (Guzik et al., 2018). The combined treatment of CVD with lipid-lowering drugs must take into account liver-related safety profiles to maximize patient benefits. Although statins pleiotropic activity significantly contributes to stroke prevention and vascular protection, their effect on liver enzymes requires clinician awareness to recognize early hepatic impairment. New research indicates that certain lipid-lowering drugs also possess a beneficial effect on endothelial function and systemic inflammation, which may counterbalance the negative hepatic impact in the long run. Furthermore, advancing therapeutic approaches are exploring agents with more targeted hepatic action to minimize liver injury risks while maintaining lipid control. Consequently, understanding the liver-specific consequences of lipid-lowering drugs remains crucial in the context of cardiovascular pharmacotherapy, ensuring maximized efficacy with minimized complications (Al Sulaiman et al., 2017; Guzik et al., 2018).

Test Your Knowledge

1. Why must anticoagulants often be stopped before surgery?
2. Which class of lipid-lowering agents may cause elevated liver enzymes?

5.6. Current Research and Developments

Learning Outcome

1. Innovations in Antihypertensive Drugs
2. Advances in Anticoagulant Therapies
3. Emerging Lipid-Lowering Treatments

The recent developments in deciphering the interaction between neurotransmitters and cardiovascular function have created new therapeutic possibilities, especially concerning the vascular modulation role of serotonin (5-HT). Serotonin, classically investigated in the central nervous system (CNS), is presently known to play a role in vascular tone, cardiac performance, and overall circulation. Recent research investigates how imbalance between levels of 5-HT and receptor stimulation contributes to comorbid cardiovascular disease often noted with obstructive sleep apnea (OSA). With the fact that OSA worsens cardiovascular risk by intermittent hypoxia and sympathetic activation, approaches targeting serotonergic pathways offer a promising method to counteract harmful cardiovascular consequences. Pharmacologic drugs affecting 5-HT receptors show promise in enhancing respiratory as well as cardiovascular indices, indicating wider applications than sleep disease alone. Such consolidation of neurotransmitter control and cardiovascular pharmacotherapy is a testament to ongoing progress toward more targeted, multi-dimensional treatment strategies in cardiovascular disease (Witkowska et al., 2024). Concurrent with neurotransmitter-directed interventions, hormone-based treatments are being noted for their subtle impacts on cardiovascular risk factors among targeted populations. Menopausal hormone therapy (MHT), when properly given to middle-aged women, has been effective in lowering the occurrence of cardiovascular events like hypertension and angina pectoris. Extensive clinical assessments document that MHT is beneficial for cardiovascular outcome without the major impact on lipid profiles or glucose metabolism, which continue to be important variables in cardiovascular risk determination. Yet, MHT also affects hematologic parameters linked to thrombosis risk, such as platelet count and fibrinogen, highlighting the significance of individualized risk-benefit assessment prior to therapy initiation. Such outcomes reflect the intricate trade-off between the means whereby hormonal modulation provides cardiovascular protection but requires careful monitoring for prothrombotic predilection (Zahorodnia et al., 2024). Current research into cardiovascular pharmacotherapy remains focused on personalized medicine, combining molecular information with patient-specific variables. The overlap of neurotransmitter modulation and hormone therapy reflects the drift toward synergy between mechanistic insight and clinical expediency. Future research seeks to elucidate how these treatments interact with genetic susceptibility and comorbid states, tailoring their functions in CVD prevention and management. Further, investigation of new receptor targets and downstream signaling pathways will continue to augment the arsenal of drugs capable of modulating cardiovascular function with maximum efficacy and minimal risk. These advancements are crucial as the burden of CVD changes with aging populations and modifying epidemiological trends, requiring responsive and individualized therapeutic interventions. This continuous evolution is a manifestation of an age of changing innovation based on translational research and clinical relevance (Figure 5.19).

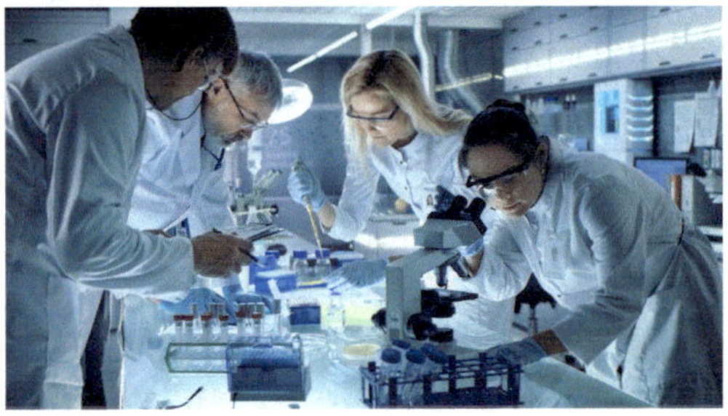

Figure 5.19. Current research and developments.

Source: Future Healthcare Today. (2021). *Current Research And Developments.* https://futurehealthcaretoday.com/wp-content/uploads/2021/01/shutterstock_691541095-scaled.jpg.

5.6.1. Innovations in Antihypertensive Drugs

The ongoing development of treatment approaches in cardiovascular medicine mirrors the multifaceted nature of treating hypertension and the requirement to optimize efficacy with fewer side effects. Recent advances in antihypertensive therapy have targeted novel mechanisms outside conventional targets, such as new agents that affect RAAS with increased specificity and lower side effects (Figure 5.20). Other advances involve drug combinations with lower doses to provide additive blood pressure reduction with decreased toxicity. These smart medicines are designed to enhance compliance through pill burden reduction and reduction of side effects. Additionally, some innovations seek to bring into play genetic and biomarker-based therapies with individualized patient profiles, a move toward personalized care for hypertension. In spite of such advances, long-term outcome and real-world deployment in various populations pose challenges, highlighting the necessity for continued research and assessment of the impact of new drugs on cardiovascular mortality and morbidity (Dent et al., 2011). Aside from efficacy, the safety profile of new antihypertensive drugs is an essential consideration in their development and clinical application. Current systematic reviews bring into focus potential harms of specific classes of drugs, including photosensitizing actions with diuretics and calcium channel blockers, potentially increasing susceptibility to skin cancer. While the quality of evidence is diverse, these observations emphasize the need to examine non-cardiovascular safety endpoints concurrently with blood pressure lowering. This has been met by innovations that have come to develop drugs with reduced off-target actions and enhanced receptor specificity. In addition, continuous pharmacovigilance and meta-analyses further enhance the comprehension of dose-response relationships and identification of patient subgroups at risk, informing safer prescribing. Ultimately, weighing therapeutic benefits against possible adverse effects continues to be a central theme in antihypertensive drug development and cardiovascular pharmacology (Cohen et al., 2024). Supplementing pharmacological advances, technology integration has promoted the emergence of precision therapeutics and enhanced hypertension management tools. Computerized health programs currently enable compliance monitoring and continuous blood pressure monitoring, allowing patient activation and tailored treatment adjustment. Pharmacogenomics advances are increasingly identifying gene variants that affect drug response, potentially leading to tailoring antihypertensive therapy according to genetic characteristics. This new paradigm promises to decrease trial-and-error use of medications and maximize therapeutic results. In parallel, population-level data analysis can identify high-risk "hotspots" so that targeted public health interventions to prevent hypertension and its complications can be implemented more effectively. Although such innovations need vigorous validation and ethics considerations, incorporation into clinical practice represents a paradigm shift in the delivery of cardiovascular care that makes antihypertensive drug use more effective and safer (Dent et al., 2011).

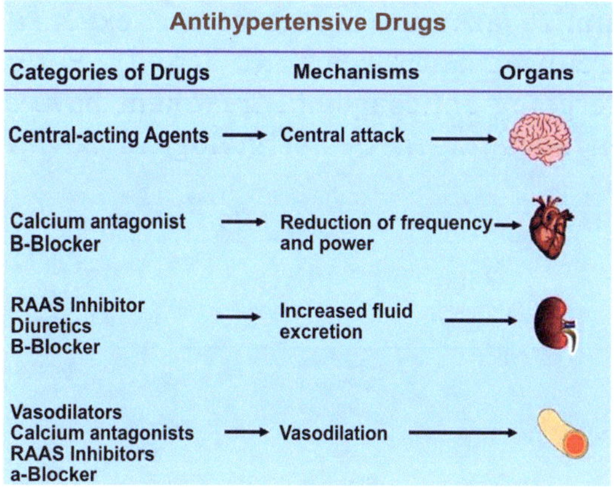

Figure 5.20. Innovations in antihypertensive drugs.

Source: WeCare Golp. (2022). *Antihypertensive Drugs.* https://wecaregolp.com/wp-content/uploads/2022/12/Antihypertensive-Drugs.jpg.

5.6.2. Advances in Anticoagulant Therapies

Current advances in cardiovascular medicine have radically altered the treatment of thromboembolic disorders to the point where anticoagulant therapies have been refined for greater efficacy and safety. In the past, vitamin K antagonists such as warfarin were the primary agents used in anticoagulation; however, their unpredictable pharmacodynamics and food interactions usually made therapeutic management difficult. DOACs have changed this paradigm with their provision of reliable pharmacokinetics and reduced interactions, thereby simplifying patient compliance and monitoring issues. These advances not only enhance stroke prevention for atrial fibrillation but also treat venous thromboembolism more accurately. Notably, these advances in treatment have created more of a personalized treatment landscape, recognizing heterogeneity in patient response and comorbidities. This progress is accompanied by emerging knowledge of cardiovascular risk factors and incorporation of new biomarkers, in total providing personalized anticoagulant regimens that minimize adverse events at the expense of no reduced antithrombotic activity. Patients undergoing anticoagulant treatment have also been advantaged by technological advances transcending pharmacology, particularly in assistance with patients' maintenance of good overall health, including oral health. Anticoagulant patients tend to have bleeding complications, and these can be worsened by inadequate oral hygiene, sometimes causing misinterpretation of drug side effects. Recent research highlights the importance of adjunctive treatments, including the application of dental irrigators, which create a pulsatile water jet to dislodge plaque and food particles better than simple brushing. Clinical examinations show that adding these devices to daily oral hygiene practices significantly reduces gum bleeding and inflammatory markers in periodontal tissues for patients on both traditional and new anticoagulants.

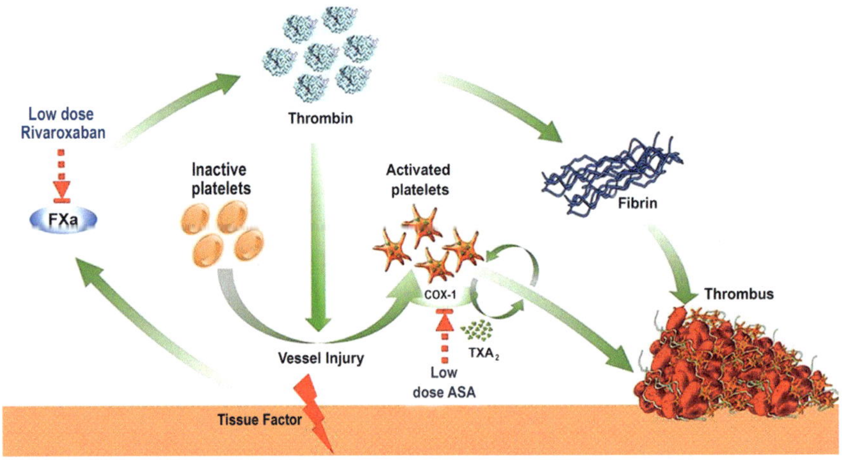

Figure 5.21. Advances in anticoagulant therapies.

Source: American Heart Association. (2019). *Advances in Antithrombotic Therapy.* https://www.ahajournals.org/cms/10.1161/ATVBAHA.118.310960/asset/c50f8541-6dd8-440c-8757-21332f211c20/assets/graphic/7ga1.jpg.

In turn, promoting oral health not only reduces bleeding hazards but also breaks a cycle of viciousness where periodontal inflammation aggravates cardiovascular diseases, showing the complex nature of anticoagulant therapy management (Kaygorodov et al., 2024). Concurrently with therapeutic advances, the more general interdetermination of cardiovascular health factors and drug response has come into focus, notably the changing role of vitamin D. New evidence points toward vitamin D affecting vascular function, inflammatory processes, and metabolic homeostasis, determinants central to CVD development. While vitamin D's direct anticoagulant activity continues to be explored, its regulation of risk profiles is a strong ancillary approach to conventional anticoagulant therapy. Individualized supplementation based on baseline vitamin D status and specific cardiovascular risk factors could improve the overall effectiveness of pharmacological interventions, lowering mortality from cardiovascular events. This complementary approach reflects a paradigm shift toward comprehensive management in which drug treatment is supported by correcting modifiable deficiencies and comorbidities to promote better long-term outcomes for patients undergoing anticoagulation (Mattioli et al., 2024).

5.6.3. Emerging Lipid-Lowering Treatments

Recent advances in pharmacotherapy in the cardiovascular field confirm the growing importance of treatments aimed at lipid disturbances beyond conventional statin therapy. Despite the foundation of statin utilization to reduce LDL-C, many patients are not achieving maximal levels of lipids or demonstrate intolerance to these drugs. This clinical problem has motivated researchers to look for alternative agents to complement or substitute statin therapy. For instance, cholesterol absorption inhibitors such as ezetimibe have emerged as significant adjunctive treatments. By selective inhibition of proteins involved in intestinal cholesterol absorption, these agents reduce LDL-C with an acceptable safety profile. This development underscores the sophisticated understanding of lipid metabolism and the requirement for a complete approach in reducing cardiovascular risk, particularly in patients who require more aggressive or additive lipid-lowering treatment (Dayspring et al., 2012). In addition to cholesterol absorption inhibitors, other studies have indicated the potential for modulating pro-inflammatory pathways that play a role in atherosclerosis, one of the key determinants of CVD. Fundamental science research increasingly supports the hypothesis that immune-inflammatory processes play a central causal role in the development and instability of plaques. Therefore, novel therapies to inhibit vascular inflammation promise to be an exciting new frontier in lipid management. However, translating such findings into clinical practice remains challenging, as conclusive evidence regarding the safety and efficacy of immune modulation to lower cardiovascular events remains lacking. Nevertheless, such emerging strategies indicate growing therapeutic targets, from lipid modulation itself to simultaneous regulation of both lipids and vascular inflammation, promising more personalized and best cardiovascular therapy (Abbas et al., 2017). Another promising area of lipid therapy is embodied by gene-silencing and monoclonal antibody therapy that has proved to be quite effective in reducing LDL-C and other atherogenic lipids. Drugs such as PCSK9 inhibitors increase the clearance of LDL-C from the circulation and have been proved to cause profound LDL reduction even in statin-resistant individuals. In addition, therapies for lipoprotein(a), another well-established CVD risk factor, also are being clinically tested. These novel therapies not only possess significant lipid-lowering effects but also offer possibilities for statin-intolerant subjects or those requiring more intense therapy. Their clinical implementation may revolutionize dyslipidemia treatment, complementing existing therapies and contributing to improved cardiovascular outcomes in high-risk individuals. Thus, the future for lipid-lowering drugs holds a lot and foresees the future of precision medicine for cardiovascular disease.

Test Your Knowledge

1. What role between neurotransmitters in current drug development?
2. What is emerging lipid-lowering treatments?

SUMMARY

The complex dynamic between pharmacologic interventions and cardiovascular well-being calls for a fine appreciation of both therapeutic effects and possible harms. Though drugs acting on the cardiovascular system may benefit patient recovery considerably, ADRs are still a cause for great concern in clinical practice. The effects may be mild or even lethal, making monitoring compulsory and the choice of drug combination deliberate to avoid harm. An example of the complexity involved in antimicrobials and CNS agents is the implication of ADRs in their usage. Accordingly, prevention of morbidity and mortality in cardiovascular therapy relies significantly on stringent ADR monitoring programs integrated into daily medical practice environments (Adhikari et al., 2009). Investigating newer generations of cardiovascular drugs, including Dipeptidyl peptidase-4 (DPP-4) inhibitors, uncovers their dualistic effect on cardiac function. Studies on drugs such as Sitagliptin and Vildagliptin show profound chronotropic and inotropic effects, with suppressant effects on heart rate and contrasting inotropic effects. These subtle effects underscore the need to individualize treatment regimens and dose considerations to maximize therapeutic benefits while reducing adverse cardiovascular events. Although their potential myocardial metabolic advantages, variable results from cardiovascular outcome trials create ongoing need for experimental and clinical assessment to completely define their safety profiles and roles in patient-specific scenarios (Bhatti et al., 2019). In the end, the dynamic nature of cardiovascular pharmacotherapy supports a balanced strategy combining clinical watchfulness, targeted medicine, and adequate awareness of drug-specific cardiovascular impacts. This strategy ensures that therapeutic practices not only treat the root cause of cardiovascular pathology but also reduce unforeseen systemic complications. Systematic research and monitoring systems are critical to further enhance drug safety, maximize efficacy, and minimize adverse outcomes in the clinical environment. With ongoing advances in the medical field, a patient-centric approach will remain essential to taking full advantage of cardiovascular drugs without exposing patients to risks associated with their use (Adhikari et al., 2009; Bhatti et al., 2019).

Summary of Key Points

Recognizing the many-sided effect of drugs on the cardiovascular system is only possible with an understanding of both their curative effects and their mechanisms. Among these medications, risk-reducing interventions for atherosclerotic cardiovascular disease (ASCVD) have proved to hold tremendous significance. For example, coronary artery calcium (CAC) scoring is a key diagnostic that informs preventive therapy. Its utilization, though, is dependent upon the knowledge and self-assurance of healthcare professionals, which can greatly be enhanced by educational interventions focusing on specific needs. Such interventions not only increase proper risk evaluation but also resolve important issues such as racial imbalances in cardiovascular treatment. Research proves considerable improvements in physician self-confidence and awareness following these education programs, which result in fairer and better clinical practices, highlighting the important role of ongoing education in maximizing cardiovascular drug therapy and outcomes (Daga et al., 2024). In the treatment of cardiovascular complications secondary to systemic diseases like type 2 diabetes, pharmacotherapy plays a crucial role, especially in younger individuals where precocious onset influences disease evolution. Emerging drug clinical trials examining drugs like dapagliflozin underscore its ability to provide improved glycemic control, and hence decrease cardiovascular burden from hyperglycemia. On the other hand, other drugs like saxagliptin, although safe, do not have the same efficacy in this population, thereby determining the therapeutic options landscape. Notably, both drugs have acceptable safety profiles without appreciably raising adverse cardiovascular events such as hypoglycemia, and this reiterates the importance of drug precision to prevent cardiovascular risk in at-risk patients (Shehadeh, 2024). Altogether, the merger of diagnostic improvements and drug treatments for CVD displays an encompassing method to handle CVD. The priority given to refining knowledge on aids such as CAC scoring works together with the increasing range of pharmacological agents focused on combating cardiovascular risk indicators and consequences. With filling of education gaps and personalized medication according to clinical trials data, the health system has the capacity to enhance outcomes of care in the patient and reduce differences. This two-way approach supports the dynamic character of cardiovascular therapy, where ongoing learning and innovation are essential to meeting the challenges of CVDs through evidence-based drug use and preventive measures (Daga et al., 2024; Shehadeh, 2024).

KEY TERMS FROM THIS CHAPTER

Drug Interactions
Lower Blood Pressure
Cardiovascular system
Mechanisms
Antihypertensive treatment
Cholesterol management
gastrointestinal (GI)
Developments
Cardiovascular disease (CVD)
Calcium channel blockers
Bioavailability
Pharmacotherapy
Monitoring
Cardiovascular Drugs

CRITICAL THINKING QUESTIONS

1. **Which of the following is a cardioselective β-blocker?**
   a. Propranolol
   b. Metoprolol
   c. Carvedilol
   d. Labetalol
2. **Which class of diuretics is most effective for treating acute pulmonary edema?**
   a. Thiazide diuretics
   b. Potassium-sparing diuretics
   c. Loop diuretics
   d. Osmotic diuretics
3. **Digoxin toxicity is increased in the presence of which electrolyte imbalance?**
   a. Hyperkalemia
   b. Hypocalcemia
   c. Hypokalemia
   d. Hypermagnesemia
4. **Statins exert their lipid-lowering effect primarily by inhibiting?**
   a. Cholesterol absorption
   b. HMG-CoA reductase
   c. Bile acid synthesis
   d. Lipoprotein lipase
5. **Which antihypertensive drug can cause a dry cough as a side effect?**
   a. Losartan
   b. Amlodipine
   c. Enalapril
   d. Metoprolol

Short Answer Questions

1. Which of Types of Cardiovascular Drugs?
2. Explain the mechanism of action, therapeutic uses, and adverse effects of ACE inhibitors in cardiovascular diseases?
3. Explain about the Therapeutic Uses?
4. Classify antiarrhythmic drugs based on the Vaughan-Williams classification and describe their mechanisms, indications, and potential side effects?
5. What is Drug Interactions?
6. Here is an overview of current research and developments drugs affecting the cardiovascular system?
7. Current Research and Developments?

Answer to Critical Thinking Questions

1. (b) 2 (c) 3. (c) 4. (b) 5. (c)

REFERENCES

1. Abbas, M., Agca, R., Ait-Oufella, H., Albert, M. A., Alexander, J. K., et al. (2017). Targeting inflammation to reduce cardiovascular disease risk: A realistic clinical prospect? *British Journal of Pharmacology, 174*, 3898–3913. https://core.ac.uk/download/80697766.pdf (accessed on 9 May 2025).
2. Abela, S., Innes, A., & Scerri, C. (2010). Pharmacotherapeutic aspects of dementia care in Malta. *Malta Medical Journal, 22*(3), 6–12. https://core.ac.uk/download/46602264.pdf (accessed on 9 May 2025).
3. Abraham, B. E., Almasri, N., Alyas, F., Budzynska, K., et al. (2020). Tight versus standard blood pressure control on the incidence of myocardial infarction and stroke: An observational retrospective cohort study in the general ambulatory setting. *BMC Family Practice, 21*, 91. https://core.ac.uk/download/327711582.pdf (accessed on 9 May 2025).
4. Adhikari, P., Padmaja, U., & Pereira, P. (2009). A prospective analysis of adverse drug reactions in a South Indian hospital. *Journal of Health and Allied Sciences, 8*(3), 1–6.
5. Agewall, S., Rosano, G. M. C., & Spoletini, I. (2019). Pharmacology of new treatments for hyperkalaemia: Patiromer and sodium zirconium cyclosilicate. *European Heart Journal Supplements, 21*(Suppl A), A28–A33. https://core.ac.uk/download/228160208.pdf (accessed on 9 May 2025).
6. Ahmad, H., Khan, H., Haque, S., Ahmad, S., Srivastava, N., & Khan, A. (2023). Angiotensin-converting enzyme and hypertension: A systemic analysis of various ACE inhibitors, their side effects, and bioactive peptides as a putative therapy for hypertension. *Journal of the Renin-Angiotensin-Aldosterone System, 2023*. https://www.semanticscholar.org/paper/0a223b5045b768c6386797e6e063da2ec0dae1f3 (accessed on 9 May 2025).
7. Akıcı, A., Ataç, Ö., Aydın, V., Kaşkal, M., et al. (2023). Comparison of primary care prescriptions for old and very old hypertensive patients. *Turkish Journal of Medical Sciences, 53*, 572–585. https://core.ac.uk/download/568287256.pdf (accessed on 9 May 2025).
8. AlSulaiman, W. (2017). Assessing the effect of statins in lowering the risk of stroke and preventing cerebral ischemia in patients with hypercholesterolemia. *Boston University*. https://open.bu.edu/bitstream/2144/23752/5/AlSulaiman_bu_0017N_12798.pdf (accessed on 9 May 2025).
9. Araujo, N. C. P., Marreiros, C., Simes, D., & Viegas, C. (2020). Vitamin K as a diet supplement with impact in human health: Current evidence in age-related diseases. *Nutrients, 12*(138), 1–24. https://core.ac.uk/download/288958659.pdf (accessed on 9 May 2025).
10. Bhatti, A. S. A., Shehzad, A. W., Shabbir, A., & Bhatti, M. A. (2019). Non incretin effects of DPP-4 inhibitors: Comparative study. *Journal of Shalamar Medical and Dental College (formerly Medical Journal of Sakina Begum Institute), 1*(1), 8–12. https://core.ac.uk/download/603616199.pdf (accessed on 9 May 2025).
11. Bikbov, B., Purcell, C., Levey, A. S., Smith, M., Abdoli, A., Abebe, M., Adebayo, O., et al. (2020). Global, regional, and national burden of chronic kidney disease, 1990–2017: A systematic analysis for the Global Burden of Disease Study 2017. *The Lancet, 395*, 709–733. https://doi.org/10.1016/S0140-6736(20)30045-3.

12. Boal, A. H., Dominiczak, A. F., McCallum, L., & Muir, L. (2016). Monotherapy with major antihypertensive drug classes and risk of hospital admissions for mood disorders. *Antihypertensive Drugs and Mood Disorders*. https://core.ac.uk/download/46559113.pdf (accessed on 9 May 2025).

13. Braga, O. G. (2018). Antipsychotic drug use: Managing cardiometabolic and cost effects. *Healthy Policy and Management Student Publications*, 6. https://core.ac.uk/download/212899184.pdf (accessed on 9 May 2025).

14. Cameron, A. C., Lang, N. N., & Touyz, R. M. (2015). Vascular complications of cancer chemotherapy. *Core*. https://core.ac.uk/download/42370677.pdf (accessed on 9 May 2025).

15. Chandy, M., Paik, D. T., & Wu, J. C. (2020). Patient and disease-specific induced pluripotent stem cells for discovery of personalized cardiovascular drugs and therapeutics. *Core*. https://core.ac.uk/download/323062894.pdf (accessed on 9 May 2025).

16. Cohen, O. G., Giordano, S. H., Hinkston, C. L., & Langan, S. M. (2024). Antihypertensive medications and risk of melanoma and keratinocyte carcinomas: A systematic review and meta-analysis. *Core*. https://core.ac.uk/download/619412707.pdf (accessed on 9 May 2025).

17. Cosentino, F., Grant, P. J., Aboyans, V., Bailey, C. J., Ceriello, A., Delgado, V., Federici, M., et al. (2019). 2019 ESC Guidelines on diabetes, pre-diabetes, and cardiovascular diseases developed in collaboration with the EASD. *European Heart Journal, 41*, 255–323. https://doi.org/10.1093/eurheartj/ehz486.

18. Daga, P., Devanand, D., Umer, M., Sagheer, U., Menon, T., Singh, G., & Kalra, D. (2024). Abstract 4136462: Provider understanding of coronary artery calcium scoring (CAC) testing in atherosclerotic cardiovascular disease risk stratification and racial disparities study (CAC-CARD) to reduce healthcare disparities. *Circulation*. https://www.semanticscholar.org/paper/b9991c2d3491c214089d77dab2de690d01f6a6a0c.

19. Dayspring, T. D., Phan, B. A. P., & Toth, P. P. (2012). Ezetimibe therapy: Mechanism of action and clinical update. *Core*. https://core.ac.uk/download/323069011.pdf.

20. Demuro, A., Popa-Wagner, A., Semplicini, A., Korczyn, A. D., Korenkov, A. I., Dufouil, C., et al. (2012). Antihypertensives for combating dementia? A perspective on candidate molecular mechanisms and population-based prevention. *Core*. https://core.ac.uk/download/pdf/8717924.pdf.

21. Dent, T., Greenhalgh, T., Mathur, R., & Meads, C. (2011). Risk models and scores for type 2 diabetes: Systematic review. *Core*. https://core.ac.uk/download/20271037.pdf (accessed on 9 May 2025).

22. Forte, M., Migliarino, S., Perelli, M., Pierelli, C., et al. (2017). Uncoupling protein 2: A key player and a potential therapeutic target in vascular diseases. *Core*. https://core.ac.uk/download/153367400.pdf.

23. Freeman, D., Huda, S., Jarvie, E., McKenna, et al. (2013). How to assess and manage hypertension during and after pregnancy. https://core.ac.uk/download/19888252.pdf (accessed on 9 May 2025).

24. Guzik, T. J., Petrie, J. R., & Touyz, R. M. (2018). Diabetes, hypertension, and cardiovascular disease: Clinical insights and vascular mechanisms. https://core.ac.uk/download/153444565.pdf (accessed on 9 May 2025).

25. Hastings, E. P. (1959). The inotropic effects of quinidine and procaine amide: An experimental study. https://open.bu.edu/bitstream/2144/26810/1/Hastings_Elliot_P_1959_web.pdf (accessed on 9 May 2025).

26. Himmelmann, A., Hansson, L., & Hedner, T. (2002). The price you pay for hypertension management: Incorporation of economic factors into clinical decision making. *Blood Pressure, 11*(4, 5). https://www.semanticscholar.org/paper/ee914b5c256b15e7e912e50dd920cc3fe0268b75 (accessed on 9 May 2025).

27. Jardine, A. G., Mark, P. B., & Stoumpos, S. (2014). Cardiovascular morbidity and mortality after kidney transplantation. https://core.ac.uk/download/42353945.pdf (accessed on 9 May 2025).

28. Jeyasingh, R. C. (2022). Improving knowledge of the importance of adhering to anticoagulation therapy among patients with atrial fibrillation to reduce stroke risk: A quality improvement project. https://core.ac.uk/download/548485959.pdf (accessed on 9 May 2025).

29. Joglar, J. A., Chung, M. K., Armbruster, A. L., Benjamin, E. J., Chyou, J. Y., Cronin, E. M., Deswal, A., et al. (2023). 2023 ACC/AHA/ACCP/HRS guideline for the diagnosis and management of atrial fibrillation: A report of the American College of Cardiology/American Heart Association Joint Committee on Clinical Practice Guidelines. *Circulation*, *149*. https://doi.org/10.1161/cir.0000000000001193.

30. Kapse, M. V., & Mulla, J. A. S. (2024). Unlocking the potential of phytotomies: A review of formulation techniques, evaluation methods, and emerging applications. *Acta Materia Medica*. https://www.semanticscholar.org/paper/f9da36e73421380e7c1764cee2ed937186103c7f (accessed on 9 May 2025).

31. Kaygorodov, V., Nurieva, N., & Tezikov, D. (2024). Influence of irrigator on the severity of inflammatory processes in periodontal tissue in patients under anticoagulant therapy. *Actual Problems in Dentistry*. https://www.semanticscholar.org/paper/7ea1d3693892dbaf7701fba67b26cdd5ec70a1a6 (accessed on 9 May 2025).

32. Leschisin, H. (2018). End of life care medication health literacy pertaining to aging adult populations. https://core.ac.uk/download/287187974.pdf (accessed on 9 May 2025).

33. Li, S., & Zhu, M. (2024). Functional structure of angiotensin-converting enzyme (ACE) and its targeted drugs. *Theoretical and Natural Science*. https://www.semanticscholar.org/paper/0c0dca16e1eb0365b5972ce1d328a3284ecb86c9 (accessed on 9 May 2025).

34. Liu, J. H. (2013). Exploring factors impacting veterans' hypertension control. https://core.ac.uk/download/154560538.pdf (accessed on 9 May 2025).

35. Lyon, A. R., López-Fernández, T., Couch, L. S., Asteggiano, R., Aznar, M. C., Bergler-Klein, J., Boriani, G., et al. (2022). 2022 ESC Guidelines on cardio-oncology developed in collaboration with the European Hematology Association (EHA), the European Society for Therapeutic Radiology and Oncology (ESTRO) and the International Cardio-Oncology Society (IC-OS). *European Heart Journal, 43*, 4229–4361. https://doi.org/10.1093/eurheartj/ehac244.

36. Mach, F., Baigent, C., Catapano, A. L., Koskinas, K. C., Casula, M., Badimón, L., Chapman, M. J., et al. (2019). 2019 ESC/EAS Guidelines for the management of dyslipidemias: Lipid modification to reduce cardiovascular risk. *European Heart Journal, 41*, 111–188. https://doi.org/10.1093/eurheartj/ehz455.

37. Mattioli, A., Coppi, F., Severino, P., Penna, C., Pagliaro, P., Dei Cas, A., Bucciarelli, V., et al. (2024). A personalized approach to vitamin D supplementation in cardiovascular health beyond the bone: An expert consensus by the Italian National Institute for Cardiovascular Research. *Nutrients, 17*. https://www.semanticscholar.org/paper/e9fb70deec717f580346335abdcd54fb8e55fe73 (accessed on 9 May 2025).

38. Moreno, A. (2016). Metabolic syndrome screening in seriously mentally ill patients: A quality improvement project. https://core.ac.uk/download/286607497.pdf (accessed on 9 May 2025).

39. Philip, B., Mukherjee, P., Khare, Y., Ramesh, P., Zaidi, S., Sabry, H., & Harky, A. (2023). COVID-19 and its long-term impact on the cardiovascular system. *Expert Review of Cardiovascular Therapy, 21*, 211–218. https://www.semanticscholar.org/paper/e051341c9d7e72e51f3f94d5c490f17bae94ac24 (accessed on 9 May 2025).

40. Rinella, M. E., Neuschwander-Tetri, B. A., Siddiqui, M. S., Abdelmalek, M. F., Caldwell, S. H., Barb, D., Kleiner, D. E., et al. (2023). AASLD practice guidance on the clinical assessment and management of nonalcoholic fatty liver disease. *Hepatology*, *77*, 1797–1835. https://doi.org/10.1097/hep.0000000000000323.

41. Rosano, G. M. C., Spoletini, I., & Agewall, S. (2017). Pharmacology of new treatments for hyperkaliemia: Patiromer and sodium zirconium cyclosilicate. https://core.ac.uk/download/pdf/228160208.pdf (accessed on 9 May 2025).

42. Shehadeh, N. (2024). Dapagliflozin or saxagliptin in pediatric type 2 diabetes: A plain language summary. *Current Medical Research and Opinion*. https://www.semanticscholar.org/paper/c590c0b83e11ed9375c27cf9c7d0c8cb69e82e76 (accessed on 9 May 2025).

43. Vahanian, A., Beyersdorf, F., Praz, F., Milojevic, M., Baldus, S., Bauersachs, J., Capodanno, D., et al. (2021). 2021 ESC/EACTS Guidelines for the management of valvular heart disease. *European Heart Journal, 43*, 561–632. https://doi.org/10.1093/eurheartj/ehab395.

44. van der Hee, B., & Wells, J. M. (2021). Microbial regulation of host physiology by short-chain fatty acids. *Trends in Microbiology, 29*, 700–712. https://doi.org/10.1016/j.tim.2021.02.001.

45. Visseren, F. L. J., Mach, F., Smulders, Y. M., Carballo, D., Koskinas, K. C., Bäck, M., Bénétos, A., et al. (2021). 2021 ESC guidelines on cardiovascular disease prevention in clinical practice. *European Heart Journal*, *42*, 3227–3337. https://doi.org/10.1093/eurheartj/ehab484.

46. Vos, T., Abajobir, A. A., Abate, K. H., Abbafati, C., Abbas, K., Abd-Allah, F., Abdulkader, R. S., et al. (2017). Global, regional, and national incidence, prevalence, and years lived with disability for 328 diseases and injuries for 195 countries, 1990–2016: A systematic analysis for the Global Burden of Disease Study 2016. *The Lancet*, *390*, 1211–1259. https://doi.org/10.1016/s0140-6736(17)32154-2.

47. Whelton, P. K., Carey, R. M., Aronow, W. S., Casey, D. E., Collins, K. J., Dennison Himmelfarb, C., DePalma, S. M., et al. (2017). 2017 ACC/AHA/AAPA/ABC/ACPM/AGS/APhA/ASH/ASPC/NMA/PCNA guideline for the prevention, detection, evaluation, and management of high blood pressure in adults: A report of the American College of Cardiology/American Heart Association Task Force on Clinical Practice Guidelines. *Hypertension*, *71*. https://doi.org/10.1161/hyp.0000000000000065.

DRUGS AFFECTING THE RESPIRATORY SYSTEM

6

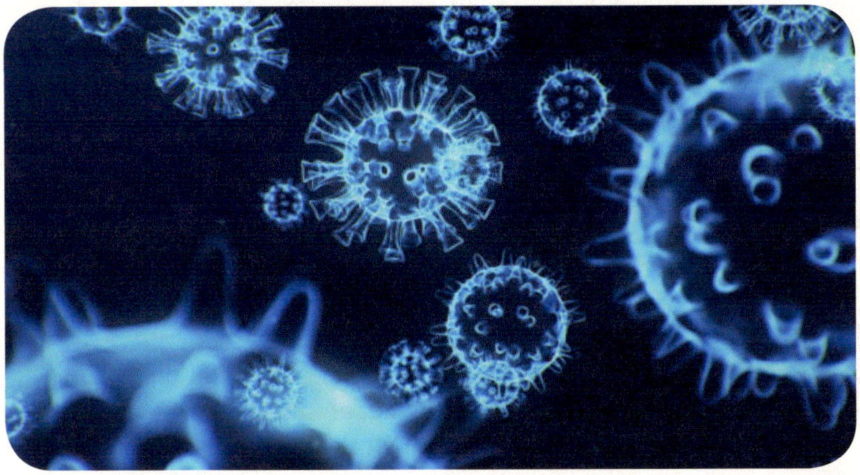

LEARNING OBJECTIVES

After studying this chapter, you will be able to:

1. Understand Types of Drugs Affecting the Respiratory System
2. Explain the Mechanisms of Action
3. Describe Common Respiratory Conditions Treated with Drugs
4. Discuss the Side Effects of Respiratory Drugs
5. Explore Impact of Drug Abuse on the Respiratory System
6. Define Current Research and Developments

Introduction

The complex interaction between pharmacology and respiratory physiology has been of great interest because of the global prevalence of respiratory diseases. The respiratory system is affected significantly by a range of drugs on processes such as airway resistance, gas exchange, and pulmonary circulation. Knowledge of these effects is vital for maximizing therapeutic interventions in conditions such as asthma, chronic obstructive pulmonary disease (COPD), and respiratory infections. In addition, the occurrence of diseases like COVID-19 has increased the necessity to investigate how drugs interact with respiratory pathology, especially in view of systemic implications and comorbidities. This complex interconnection calls for an extensive study of drugs that influence respiratory processes, positively as well as negatively, to improve patient outcomes and reduce complications. The complexity of respiratory pharmacotherapy is further accentuated by the systemic effects that most drugs with respiratory effects can induce. For example, drugs initially designed for use in neurological or cardiovascular applications may indirectly affect respiratory parameters by acting via CNS mechanisms or cardiac-respiratory relationships. Such crossover underscores the need for multidisciplinary study in assessing drug efficacy and safety, particularly in susceptible groups of patients such as those suffering from both pulmonary and systemic diseases. The risk of respiratory impairment through centrally acting drugs and their effect on phenomena such as hypoxia and arrhythmias shows significant balance needed by clinicians during treatment. As such, research on respiratory effects of drugs goes beyond localized pulmonary issues and incorporates wider physiological factors (Visrodia et al., 2021). Current studies on drugs targeting the respiratory system have also adopted sophisticated techniques like bioinformatics and systems biology to determine molecular targets and drug candidates. These techniques allow the understanding of common genetic and biochemical pathways involved in respiratory diseases and accompanying systemic disorders.

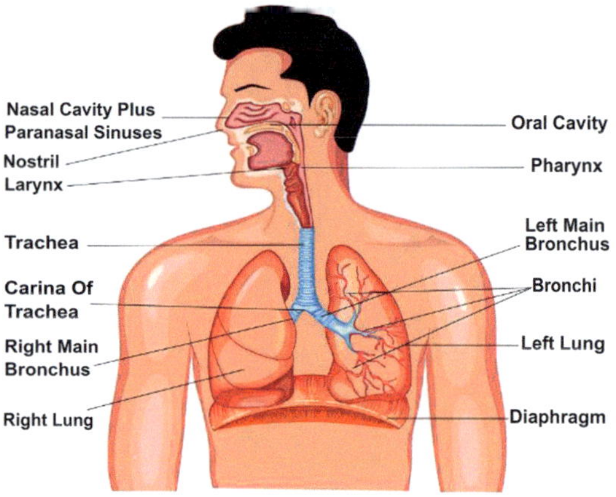

Figure 6.1. Drugs affecting the respiratory system.

Source: American Addiction Centers (2018). *The Potential Repercussion of Substance Abuse on the Respiratory System.* https://admin.americanaddictioncenters.org/wp-content/uploads/2018/10/the-potential-repercussion-of-substance-abuse-on-the-respiratory-system.jpg.

For instance, studies investigating the interface between viral respiratory illnesses and chronic conditions have unveiled pivotal gene expressions and possible pharmacological drugs that can curb disease complications or progression. Such a dynamic knowledge base provides promising directions for individualized interventions, inculcating the ever-changing character of respiratory pharmacology as it evolves to address new health issues and incorporates new scientific methods (Zhou et al., 2024).

Definition of the Respiratory System

The human body depends significantly on a sophisticated system of organs to sustain essential functions, one of which is ensuring that oxygen is transported effectively to tissues and carbon dioxide is removed. This essential function is carried out by the respiratory system (Figure 6.2), a sophisticated collection of structures that consists of the nasal passages, trachea, bronchi, lungs, and alveoli. All the components function together to facilitate gas exchange, a process critical for cellular metabolism and homeostasis. In addition to its mechanical role of transporting air, the respiratory system is also involved in defense against infection through filtering out airborne pathogens and particles. Knowing the anatomy and physiology of the system is crucial, particularly as several drugs aim at these components to treat or manage respiratory illnesses. Consequently, examining the basis of the respiratory system's definition provides the background for distinguishing the manner in which pharmacological substances engage with and influence respiratory function (Christopher et al., 2022). In addition to the anatomical definition, the respiratory system might be envisioned as a dynamic boundary between the extrinsic environment and the circulatory system, having the function of sustaining the respiratory rhythm of the body and maintaining oxygen homeostasis. This system's effectiveness relies upon the coordinated interaction between muscular and neural components governing ventilation, so that suitable air volume is introduced into and removed from the lungs. Further, the role of the respiratory system includes the regulation of blood pH through the management of carbon dioxide levels so as to impact systemic acid-base balance. Perturbations caused by infection, inflammation, or blockage have the capacity to drastically impact respiratory effectiveness, where pharmaceutical intervention becomes obligatory. Similarly, drugs targeting the respiratory system are intended not only to modulate airway patency but also to regulate inflammatory processes and microbial dangers, an idea of special significance in light of bacterial resistance and coagulopathy during infectious illnesses such as COVID-19 (Christopher et al., 2022).

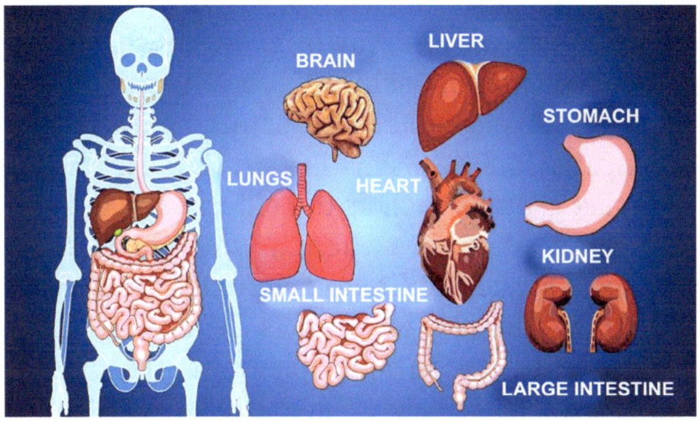

Figure 6.2. The human body respiratory system.

Source: https://i.ytimg.com/vi/R5f9pmgXhIY/maxresdefault.jpg.

An awareness of the integrated functions of the respiratory system makes it possible to have a more sophisticated understanding of how drugs can modulate its elements, especially in disease states. Pharmacologic agents vary from bronchodilators and anti-inflammatory medications to anticoagulants, all aimed at treating particular dysfunctions in this system. Anticoagulant therapy with heparin has been effective, for instance, in decreasing mortality from pulmonary micro-thrombi and coagulopathy, processes that worsen respiratory insufficiency and impair gas exchange. This demonstrates the overlap between respiratory pathophysiology and systemic illnesses in which drugs exert pleiotropic effects beyond their major target organs. Therefore, the definition of the respiratory system is not just a scholarly exercise but a critical milestone in appreciating the extent and mode of action of drugs on respiratory health and disease processes.

Overview of Drugs Affecting the Respiratory System

The gas exchange and respiratory system responsible for oxygen supply are susceptible to multiple diseases that make pharmacological therapy necessary. Pharmaceuticals for the respiratory system include an array of broad classes aimed at treating conditions from asthma and chronic obstructive pulmonary disease (COPD) to infection and allergic reaction. Bronchodilators including beta-agonists and anticholinergics act on relaxing airway smooth muscle so as to ease airflow and also symptoms such as wheezing and dyspnea. Corticosteroids inhibit airway inflammation and are key to the management of chronic inflammatory respiratory diseases. Furthermore, mucolytics promote the clearance of mucus, enabling easier respiration in patients with hypersecretion of sputum. A knowledge of these basic drug classes forms a foundation for understanding their contribution to maintaining respiratory well-being and the problem of optimizing therapeutic benefit. Respiratory infections form a prominent zone where pharmacotherapy is most decisive, due to their widespread and possible severity. Antibiotics still form the drugs of choice in bacterial respiratory infections, though used should be under careful scrutiny so as to counteract antimicrobial resistance (AMR), an issue complicating treatment efficacy. Responsible antibiotic stewardship policies are essential and will need collaborative approaches across the global health sector if they are to be efficacious. Multisectoral strategies, such as infection surveillance and infection prevention, add value to such policies, particularly in multifaceted economic environments where resource distribution diverges significantly. Such factors underscore the importance of integrated strategies to achieve effective infection management and reduce the development of resistant organisms, while guaranteeing that antibiotic treatments remain effective in respiratory therapy (Aarestrup et al., 2015). Outside of traditional pharmaceutical drugs, adjunctive therapy is increasingly known to have the ability to shape respiratory drug use, especially in infection prevention. Probiotic supplementation has been a potential way to lower acute respiratory tract infection incidence and severity, which could thus minimize the demand for antibiotic therapy. Systematic review of randomized controlled trials of infants and children suggests that probiotics are effective in reducing antibiotic prescribing rates, which indicates their function in augmenting host immune defense against prevalent infections. Though promising as an adjunct to conventional drugs, more research is necessary to confirm their efficacy across larger populations and determine the framework for their incorporation into the management of respiratory disease (Connors et al., 2019).

Importance of Understanding Drug Effects on Respiratory Health

The intricacy of the respiratory system requires a multifaceted knowledge of how drugs interact with its processes to prevent unforeseen complications (Figure 6.3). Drugs for respiratory diseases, including bronchodilators and corticosteroids, can significantly affect airway mechanics and immune reactions. Without thorough knowledge of these drug actions, there is a likelihood of worsening existing pulmonary diseases or causing unwanted side effects. Additionally, certain systemic medications, which are not originally intended for respiratory therapy, might unknowingly compromise lung function or initiate harmful inflammatory sequences. Careful awareness on the part of healthcare professionals and patients regarding these interactions promotes safer treatment strategies and allows for early recognition of side effects. This awareness is essential for maximizing therapeutic benefit while reducing harm, assuring respiratory health remains maintained throughout pharmacological therapy (Amaducci et al., 2018). Additionally, understanding the multifarious mechanisms of drug influence on respiratory health promotes personalized therapy and improved outcomes in patients. Respiratory illnesses tend to come with differing pathophysiological designs, which call for customized pharmacotherapy that treats the unique demand without damaging lung structure. Knowledge of drug-induced respiratory manifestations, such as drug-induced bronchospasm or pulmonary fibrosis, helps clinicians choose safer alternatives and watchful strategies. This is especially crucial in high-risk groups, such as the elderly and chronic respiratory disease patients, who might show increased susceptibility to drug-induced adverse effects. Educating physicians regarding these complexities encourages prudent prescribing habits and increases awareness in identifying early warning signs of respiratory insufficiency, ultimately enhancing disease control and patient safety (Amaducci et al., 2018). Furthermore, the general public health implications of drug influences on respiratory well-being highlight the necessity of informed drug administration and regulation. Overuse or abuse of respiratory drugs can contribute to drug resistance, reduced therapeutic efficacy, and greater morbidity. Public health efforts need to place strong emphasis on the pivotal role of education on proper drug use, side effects, and compliance with prescribed regimens. In addition, continued research and pharmacovigilance efforts are required to recognize and manage risks from newly emerging or repurposed drugs influencing respiratory function. Researchers, clinicians, and policymakers need to work together to streamline treatment regimens and make sure pharmaceutical advances are integrated safely into respiratory management.

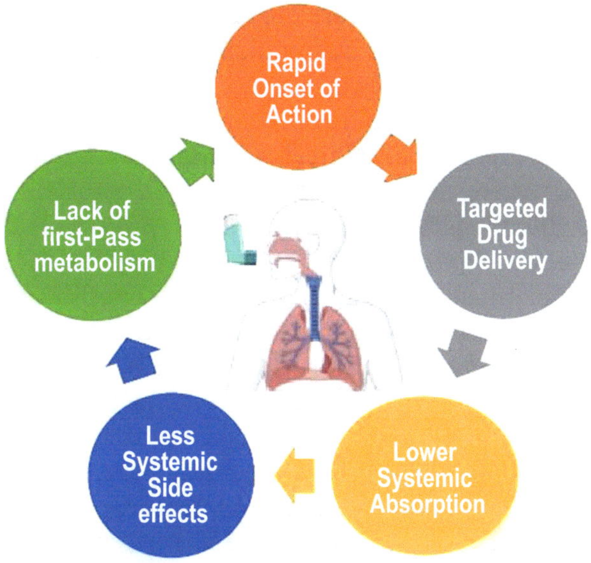

Figure 6.3. Drug effects on respiratory health.

Source: Springer Nature. (2022). *Drug Effects on Respiratory Health.* https://media.springernature.com/lw1200/springer-static/image/art%3A10.1007%2Fs13346-022-01251-1/MediaObjects/13346_2022_1251_Fig1_HTML.png.

6.1. Types of Drugs Affecting the Respiratory System

Learning Outcome

1. Bronchodilators
2. Corticosteroids
3. Antihistamines

The human respiratory system is prone to numerous conditions that necessitate pharmacological treatments, and this has resulted in the creation of several drug classes designed for respiratory health (Figure 6.4). Bronchodilators are one of these classes that work by calming muscles around the airways, thus allowing enhanced airflow in diseases such as asthma and chronic obstructive pulmonary disease (COPD). These medications are mostly classified as beta-agonists and anticholinergics, which work through alternative receptor pathways to reverse bronchoconstriction. Corticosteroids are also routinely used to suppress airway inflammation, a key element in the control of asthma. Their anti-inflammatory action minimizes the immune response causing airway inflammation and mucous accumulation. All of these drugs show a rational strategy in enhancing respiratory function by targeting separate pathophysiologic mechanisms in the respiratory tract. Another remarkable group of drugs influencing respiratory wellness is mucolytics and expectorants, which act on the elimination of mucus from the airways. Mucolytics act by depolymerizing the chemical composition of mucus, decreasing its viscosity so that it may be expelled more readily by coughing. Expectorants make this process easier by stimulating the creation of thinner mucus, which allows for better clearance and greater airway patency. Such medications are especially crucial in treating chronic bronchitis and other respiratory illnesses with excessive mucus production. In addition, some antibiotics and antivirals are added to respiratory treatment regimens when infection complicates underlying respiratory disease. The function of drug therapies goes beyond controlling symptoms to modulating underlying microbial communities and inflammatory mechanisms that may contribute to respiratory disease (Hou et al., 2022). Clinical decision-making in the pharmacotherapy of respiratory disorders, however, in the presence of these drugs, needs to be guided by guidelines focusing on individual treatment strategies. The European Society of Cardiology guidelines, for example, focus on healthcare providers taking into account the entire range of patient-specific variables and the most up-to-date scientific knowledge in deciding to prescribe respiratory medication. This entails thoughtful assessment of comorbid conditions, possible drug interactions, and understanding of changing respiratory pathophysiology. These guidelines emphasize the professional obligation to modify treatments flexibly and communicate closely with patients to obtain the best results while ensuring that therapeutic methods are aligned with both current protocols and unique health requirements (Visseren et al., 2021). The incorporation of such evidence-informed guidelines is critical for the development of patient care in respiratory medicine.

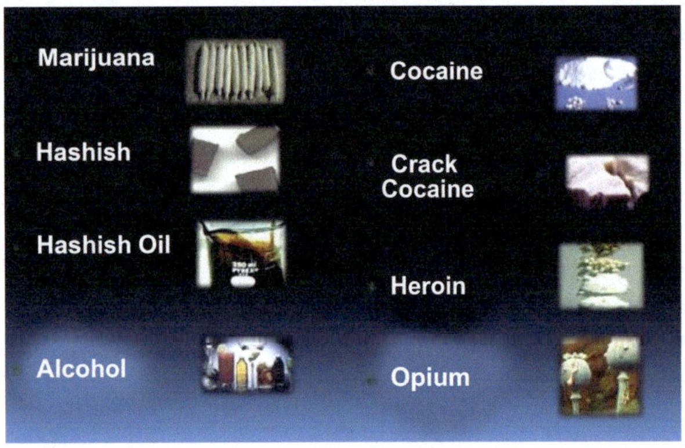

Figure 6.4. Types of drugs affecting the respiratory system.

Source: Shiva Kumar, T. (2014). *Drugs Abuse 3.* SlideShare.

6.1.1. Bronchodilators

The treatment of respiratory illnesses commonly requires therapeutic drugs that can directly affect airway dynamics to control symptoms and enhance pulmonary function. Among such drugs, bronchodilators play an important function by causing relaxation of the smooth muscle covering the bronchi and the bronchioles, thus decreasing airway resistance. This drug action is especially important in diseases like asthma and COPD, where bronchoconstriction hinders the effective flow of air. Bronchodilators include various classes, such as beta-2 adrenergic agonists, anticholinergics, and methylxanthines, all of which have different mechanisms and onset of action. Their capacity to enhance ventilation and alleviate symptoms such as wheezing and shortness of breath not only increases patient comfort but also lowers the rate of exacerbations that can result in hospitalization. Considering the high morbidity of respiratory diseases, the optimization of bronchodilator therapy continues to be the core of clinical respiratory medicine, and continued research measures subtleties of their safety and efficacy. The interaction of infectious pathogens with respiratory function underlines the relevance of bronchodilators as part of the overall therapeutic strategy for treating respiratory disease. For example, respiratory syncytial virus (RSV) is identified as a significant etiology of acute respiratory illness in older persons, frequently precipitating exacerbations of chronic respiratory disease. In these situations, the administration of bronchodilators can be helpful in reversing airway obstruction due to inflammation and mucus plugging. Clinical surveillance research indicates that RSV-caused acute respiratory infection (ARI) has similar severity and outcome to influenza-caused ARI, such as high hospital admission and mortality rates (Symes et al., 2025). Accordingly, the use of bronchodilators in acute care, in addition to antivirals and support, can assist with airway patency, reduce symptoms, and ideally shorten hospital duration among high-risk groups. This emphasizes the critical contribution of bronchodilators not just to chronic care but also to acute respiratory infections. Progress in anesthesia and critical care further broadens the therapeutic environment in which bronchodilators impact respiratory outcomes. Interestingly, volatile anesthetic agents like sevoflurane have inherent bronchodilatory effects, which help improve lung function during acute respiratory distress syndrome (ARDS). Recent clinical trials like SESAR explore inhaled sedation's ability to increase oxygenation and reduce lung inflammation in contrast to conventional intravenous sedation (Blondonnet et al., 2022). This would indicate that bronchodilation could be an advantageous adjunct in treating severely impaired lungs, improving ventilation and minimizing damage due to mechanical ventilation. Investigational as these may be, such findings offer the possibility of more extensive use of bronchodilatory mechanisms beyond the management of respiratory issues on an outpatient basis into critical care interventions. Comprehension of these dynamics supports the idea that bronchodilators (Figure 6.5) are a critical element of the pharmacologic armamentarium directed toward enhancing respiratory system function in a wide range of clinical situations.

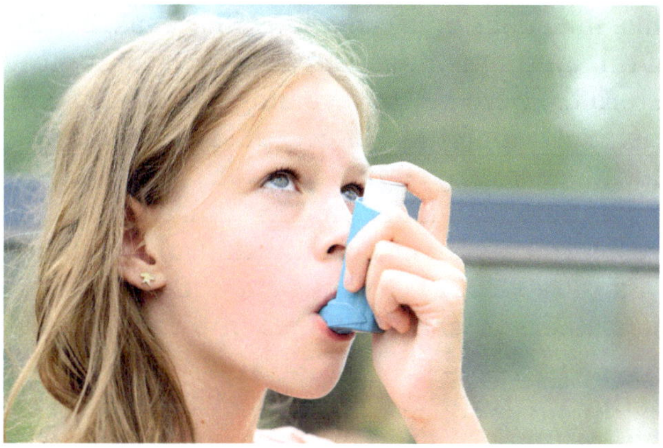

Figure 6.5. Bronchodilators.

Source: NHS24. (2023). *Bronchodilator.* https://appnhs24wp41a8c38064.blob.core.windows.net/blobappnhs24wp41a8c38064/wp-content/uploads/2023/03/bronchodilator.jpg.

6.1.2. Corticosteroids

The treatment of chronic respiratory diseases, including asthma and COPD, frequently requires a multidimensional pharmacological intervention. Of the drugs used, corticosteroids are important in the reduction of airway inflammation and enhancement of lung function. These medications, usually delivered through inhalation, are intended to inhibit the immune response that underlies airway hyperreactivity and mucus secretion. By acting on inflammatory pathways, corticosteroids not only reduce acute symptoms but also the rate of exacerbations. In reality, corticosteroids are often added to long-acting β(2)-agonists, and this combination therapy produces a dual strategy for providing both symptomatic and long-term control. Nevertheless, the specific role of corticosteroids in contrast to β(2)-agonists within these combination regimens continues to be an issue in need of further clinical clarification (Agarwal et al., 2011). Concerns regarding safety have been raised about the use of corticosteroids, particularly when combined with long-acting β(2)-agonists like salmeterol. Epidemiological evidence in the past had indicated a link between β(2)-agonists and higher asthma mortality, leading to a cautious review of their safety profile when combined with corticosteroids. Systematic meta-analyses of randomized controlled trials have also identified no statistically significant increase in fatal or severe adverse events in the combination of corticosteroids and salmeterol compared to corticosteroids only. These observations suggest that the anti-inflammatory activity of corticosteroids may counteract putative risks with β(2)-agonists, though the evidence is currently somewhat limited due to the number of severe adverse events reported being relatively small. The ratio between favourable symptom control and the unpredictability of infrequent but severe side effects has to inform clinical choice in long-term respiratory treatment (Altman et al., 2009). Although their undisputed effectiveness is well known, corticosteroids are not problem-free. They are associated with chronic local side effects, such as oral candidiasis and dysphonia, and with systemic absorption inducing adrenal suppression and metabolic disturbances. Accordingly, therapeutic guidelines stress employing the least effective dose to achieve control over airway inflammation with minimal toxicity. Patient compliance and inhaler technique are crucial factors of therapeutic efficacy, since incorrect delivery can ruin drug delivery and raise the likelihood of undesirable effects. In addition, research continues to further develop corticosteroid formulations and delivery technologies toward maximizing efficacy and safety. Whereas corticosteroids (Figure 6.6) are still a mainstay in the treatment of respiratory disease, their inclusion in holistic plans of care needs to be balanced against both therapeutic advantage and caution regarding possible harms (Agarwal et al., 2011; Altman et al., 2009).

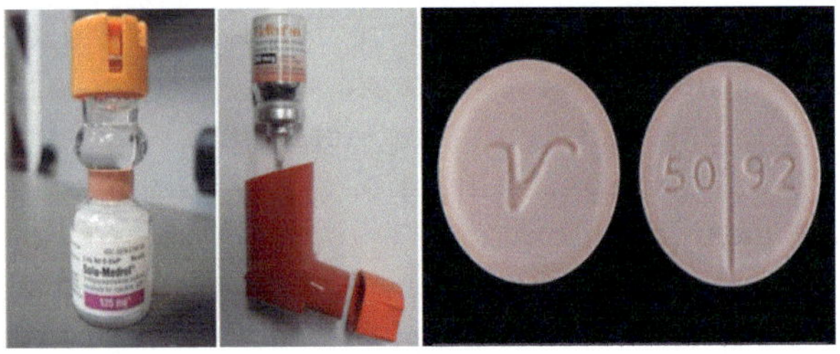

Figure 6.6. Corticosteroids.

Source: https://external-content.duckduckgo.com/iu/?u=https%3A%2F%2Ftse3.mm.bing.net%2Fth%3Fid%3DOIP.4gZGLxzp_OTxGc4ho60u0gHaCc%26pid%3DApi&f=1&ipt=708a388602f5a95b44da97c11b862c9b48f15845aaf950493cb761bb5442ffe7.

6.1.3. Antihistamines

The control of respiratory illnesses is typically a multidisciplinary process involving the management of allergic response as well as inflammatory reactions. Drugs like antihistamines are important in this regard because they act by blocking histamine receptors and hence alleviating symptoms such as nasal congestion, sneezing, and rhinorrhea. Antihistamines were initially used mainly for their sedative properties; however, their use has come to include ancillary actions in respiratory therapy. In pediatric dentistry, for instance, antihistamines are not only appreciated for their low sedative qualities but also for their antiemetic and antisialagogue action that are useful to the patient during minimal to moderate sedation procedures (Regina et al., 2023). This points towards the dynamic pharmacological profile of antihistamines that goes beyond mere allergy relief to the provision of supportive care to patients during respiratory-related medical treatments. The efficacy of antihistamines in respiratory treatment is further highlighted by their versatility in treating symptoms related to immune system stimulation. A fascinating clinical phenomenon includes the application of antihistamines for the prevention of injection site reactions (ISR) that are a side effect of some biologic therapies. In two reported cases, patients administered the PCSK9 inhibitor alirocumab experienced transient ISRs with erythema and itching after immune challenges like infections or vaccinations (Bär et al., 2022). Oral antihistamines, in addition to topical steroids, were key to reversing these reactions, demonstrating their effectiveness in managing localized allergic-type reactions that can be potentiated by underlying inflammation of the respiratory system or activation of immunity (Bär et al., 2022). This program highlights the usefulness of antihistamines in bringing relief against secondary complications which can influence respiratory patient care. Although antihistamines are beneficial with regard to therapeutic outcomes, it is necessary to balance their utility against possible adverse reactions, particularly if they are being used concomitantly with other central nervous system (CNS) depressants. For example, interaction between antihistamines and opioid analgesics may heighten the risk of respiratory depression, emphasizing cautious dosing and monitoring in practice (Regina et al., 2023). Knowledge of pharmacokinetic characteristics like onset, duration, and metabolism is important for optimizing antihistamine application in respiratory treatment protocols. These factors are aimed at maximizing patient safety and optimizing the effectiveness of antihistamines (Figure 6.7) in controlling respiratory manifestations and associated allergic disorders. Research and clinical surveillance, therefore, continue to be crucial to effectively position antihistamines within the entire range of drugs that influence the respiratory apparatus.

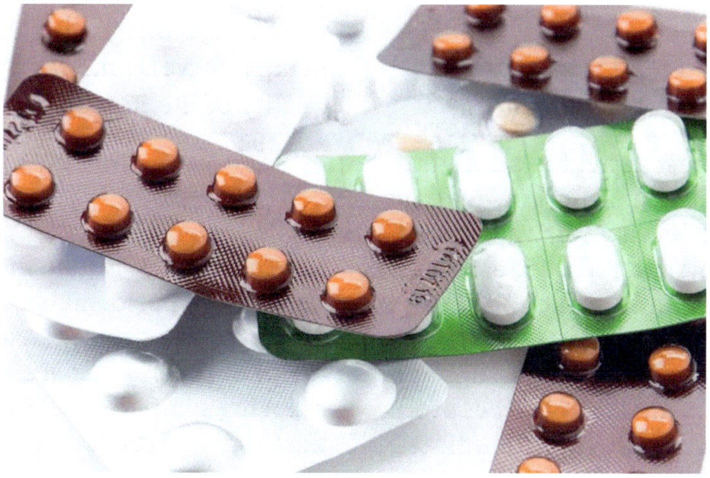

Figure 6.7. Medications such as antihistamines.

Source: Health Jade. (2019). *Antihistamine.* https://healthjade.net/wp-content/uploads/2019/04/antihistamine.jpg.

Test Your Knowledge

1. What are antihistamines action?
2. What are corticosteroids and where are they produced in the body?

6.2. Mechanisms of Action

Learning Outcome

1. How Bronchodilators Work?
2. The Role of Corticosteroids in Inflammation Reduction
3. Antihistamines and Their Effect on Mucus Production

The diversity of viral respiratory infections requires a broad spectrum of pharmacologic therapies, several of which depend on unique mechanisms of action that attack different steps of viral replication. Antiviral agents commonly work by inhibiting enzymes essential to the viral life cycle, including proteases and polymerases, which block the virus from producing vital proteins or copying its genome. In addition, certain agents inhibit viral entry into host cells, breaking the early steps of infection. This multi-pronged strategy is crucial since there is a lack of approved antivirals against lower respiratory tract infections, a major global health issue. Attempts have been made to increase efforts in repurposing drugs and synthesizing new compounds that target viral functions, increasing treatment effectiveness against pathogens such as SARS-CoV-2. Such targeted interventions exemplify how understanding viral biology underpins the design of respiratory therapeutics aimed at mitigating morbidity and mortality due to viral infections (Jim et al., 2021). Bronchodilators represent another critical drug class influencing respiratory mechanics through their interactions with adrenergic receptors and smooth muscle relaxation pathways. Beta-2 adrenergic agonists, for example, activate adenylate cyclase via G-protein coupling, increasing intracellular cyclic AMP levels in airway smooth muscle cells. This molecular cascade results in muscle relaxation and bronchodilation, thus enhancing airflow in disease states like asthma and COPD. Anticholinergic drugs, on the other hand, block muscarinic receptors to decrease parasympathetically mediated bronchoconstriction. These dual mechanisms highlight the balanced interaction between autonomic control and drug therapy in respiratory medicine. Comprehension of these pathways allows for individualized treatment regimens to maximize respiratory function and patient outcome, emphasizing the importance of receptor-selective drug action in preventing airway obstruction.

In pulmonary arterial hypertension (PAH), the mode of action for targeted respiratory drugs involves vascular modulation and enhanced tissue oxygenation beyond bronchodilation. Agents like endothelin receptor antagonists and phosphodiesterase-5 inhibitors work by relaxing pulmonary vasculature, lowering pulmonary arterial pressure, and enhancing cardiac output. These hemodynamic gains are vital to the relief of exertional dyspnea and prevention of right heart failure progression. Recent understanding also highlights the importance of combined pharmacological and rehabilitative approaches, wherein drug-induced augmentation of cardiopulmonary physiology increases patients' ability to participate in supervised exercise programs, further augmenting therapeutic gains. The systemic actions of these drugs, positive modulation of skeletal muscle function and inflammation, demonstrate intricate mechanisms extending beyond the respiratory system per se. Such holistic strategies identify in which ways integrating drug action with way of living interventions can synergistically enhance quality of life in respiratory disease (Keusch et al., 2017).

6.2.1. How Bronchodilators Work?

The respiratory system in humans depends upon the smooth performance of the bronchial tubes, which might get constricted or inflamed as a result of several diseases like asthma COPD. For relieving symptoms related to the constriction of the bronchial tubes, bronchodilators are utilized as a chief pharmacological management. These medications most often act by relaxing the smooth muscle covering the airways, thus dilating the bronchial tubes and allowing for freer airflow in and out of the lungs (Figure 6.8). This action is especially important during acute respiratory attacks when airway constriction impairs oxygenation. By acting at specific receptors on bronchial muscles—beta-2 adrenergic receptors or muscarinic receptors—bronchodilators block signals leading to contraction directly, improving respiratory function and patient comfort (Beeh et al., 2015). The clinical utility of bronchodilators is illustrated by combination therapies such as the fixed-dose combination of tiotropium and olodaterol, which have become well recognized in the treatment of COPD. Tiotropium is a long-acting muscarinic antagonist that inhibits acetylcholine-induced bronchoconstriction, while olodaterol is a long-acting beta-2 adrenergic agonist that causes relaxation of the muscles by acting through cyclic AMP-mediated pathways. The dual mechanism brings about not only improvements in lung function but also decreases in dyspnea and the use of rescue medication. Clinical trials with more than 15,000 patients demonstrate that this combination is more effective than monotherapies, such as improved exercise capacity and lower rates of exacerbation, suggesting a synergistic therapeutic effect in bronchodilation (Brusselle et al., 2019). In addition to short-term relief of symptoms, bronchodilators play a role in maintaining long-term respiratory health by reducing the frequency and severity of exacerbations in chronic lung disease.

For instance, sustained bronchodilation by drugs such as tiotropium and olodaterol sustains airway patency for prolonged periods of time, reducing inflammation-induced airway closure. Such extension of airway patency not only enhances quality of life but also facilitates improved physical activity and overall pulmonary rehabilitation outcomes. Furthermore, the route of administration, e.g., a soft mist inhaler, maximizes drug deposition in the lungs, maximizing clinical effects. Therefore, bronchodilators form a core part of pulmonary pharmacotherapy, acting by receptor-specific mechanisms to restore and sustain airway function and prevent disease progression (Beeh et al., 2015; Brusselle et al., 2019).

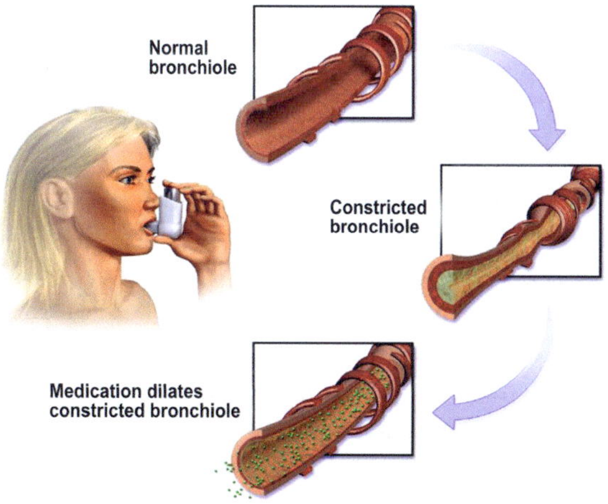

Figure 6.8. Bronchodilators work.

Source: Wikimedia Commons. (n.d.). *Bronchodilators.* https://upload.wikimedia.org/wikipedia/commons/e/e3/Bronchodilators.png.

6.2.2. The Role of Corticosteroids in Inflammation Reduction

The cascade of physiological events initiated by respiratory infections tends to end in severe inflammation, which can worsen tissue damage and compromise pulmonary function. Corticosteroids, which are synthetic analogs of endogenous glucocorticoids, have been extensively investigated for their strong anti-inflammatory properties and have become a cornerstone in the treatment of inflammatory respiratory diseases (Figure 6.9). They achieve their effect through the regulation of gene expression to suppress pro-inflammatory cytokines including interleukins and tumor necrosis factor-alpha, which modulates the dampening of immune response. They also extend their effect towards stabilization of lysosomal membranes and inhibition of capillary permeability that cumulatively reduce leukocyte infiltration and edema in lung tissues. This drug therapy helps in mitigating symptoms, avoiding airway remodeling, and enhancing general respiratory function in conditions that involve chronic or acute inflammation (Hu et al., 2020). Current clinical use of corticosteroids in respiratory medicine has been highlighted by the recent outbreak of SARS-CoV-2, which provokes a strong inflammatory response commonly termed a cytokine storm. This hyperinflammatory reaction is a primary cause of lung injury and respiratory failure in COVID-19. By dampening this excessive immune activation, corticosteroids limit alveolar cell damage and reduce systemic inflammatory markers, thereby reducing inflammation and improving outcomes. Corticosteroid therapy has been shown in trials to reduce mortality and mechanical ventilation requirements among severe cases, though timing and dose are key variables. It is noteworthy that corticosteroids reduce inflammation-induced lung injury but do not curb viral replication directly, requiring adjunctive antiviral therapy for overall viral respiratory disease management (Hu et al., 2020). Even with their therapeutic utility, corticosteroids are to be used cautiously because of their extensive immunosuppressive effects and risk for adverse effects. Excessive or long-term administration may compromise host defense mechanisms, enhancing susceptibility to secondary infections and impairing liver function, particularly in the presence of pre-existing hepatic disease or in patients on hepatotoxic drugs. Liver enzyme monitoring is mandatory, as corticosteroid-induced changes in hepatic metabolism can enhance liver stress in critically ill respiratory patients. In addition, their function of modulating systemic inflammation calls for a balancing of the inhibition of injurious immune responses against maintaining sufficient defense against infection. The incorporation of corticosteroids into respiratory drug therapy thus calls for careful management based on individual patient profiles and disease severity to maximize reduction of inflammation without sacrificing immune competency (Bertolini et al., 2020).

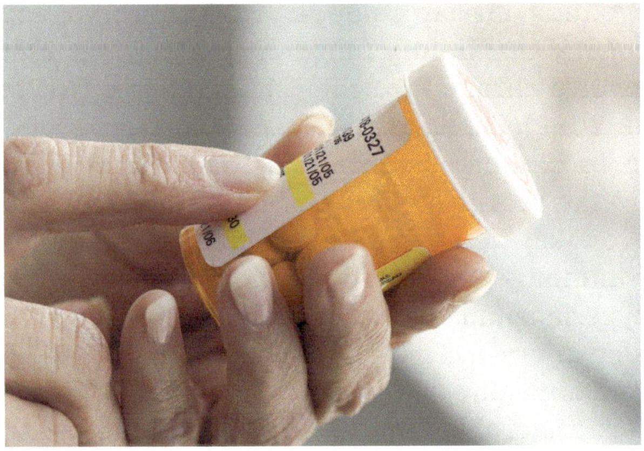

Figure 6.9. Role of corticosteroids in inflammation reduction.

Source: Milan2099 / Getty Images. (n.d.). *200514339-001*. Verywell Health. https://www.verywellhealth.com/thmb/q6moqjQoZJ0yzHw4gzZH6L4Hb4o=/1500x0/filters:no_upscale():max_bytes(150000):strip_icc()/200514339-001-56aae5c75f9b58b7d00912be.jpg.

6.2.3. Antihistamines and Their Effect on Mucus Production

Respiratory conditions are frequently treated by targeting several symptoms, such as hypersecretion of mucus, which can be worsening discomfort and inhibit the function of airways. Antihistamines play an important role in this treatment, as they counteract histamine H1 receptors, thus reducing the inflammatory reaction responsible for causing mucus hypersecretion. While most commonly known as being effective in managing the allergic symptoms of nasal congestion and sneezing, antihistamines also affect secretory mechanisms of the respiratory mucosa. Through the inhibition of histamine-induced glandular stimulation, these medications are able to reduce the amount and viscosity of mucus secretions, thus allowing for enhanced mucociliary clearance. This pharmacological action plays an important role in symptom relief in allergic rhinitis and chronic sinusitis, demonstrating thetherapeutic utility of antihistamines in respiratory medicine. The balance between mucus production and mucociliary function is a fine relationship important to ensuring respiratory health. Agents that modify mucus properties without affecting ciliary function are especially useful. Studies with nasal epithelial models have shown that some treatments, by lowering mucin concentration, do not negatively impact ciliary frequency of beating; indeed, some therapies can improve mucociliary clearance and phagocytic function (Servi et al., 2019). These results emphasize the therapeutic promise of antihistamines and analogs to maximize mucus rheology and clearance, thus enhancing airway hygiene without sacrificing the native defense mechanisms of the respiratory epithelium. Such sophisticated effects are critical in the management of chronic respiratory diseases, wherein the mucus stagnation can result in secondary infection and prolonged inflammation. As the population base changes to more older people, respiratory diseases marked by overproduction of mucus will grow substantially (Apter et al., 2010). The elderly tend to have changes in nasal physiology and immune system functioning, which enhance the effect of mucosal inflammation and hypersecretion of mucus. This epidemiological trend makes it imperative that antihistamine therapy is developed specifically in response to the specific pathophysiologic changes occurring in elderly patients. Balancing therapeutic effects in this age group requires, in addition to managing allergy-stimulated mucin production, managing age-dependent alterations in mucosal barrier properties. Therefore, continued research towards optimizing antihistamine effect and safety within elderly populations remains important for offsetting the epidemic of respiratory illnesses within this compromised group.

Test Your Knowledge

1. How do corticosteroids help in allergic inflammation?
2. How do antihistamines help in allergic rhinitis?

6.3. Common Respiratory Conditions Treated with Drugs

Learning Outcome

1. Asthma
2. Chronic Obstructive Pulmonary Disease (COPD)
3. Allergic Rhinitis

Respiratory diseases tend to present via intricate pathological processes that profoundly compromise lung function and gas exchange, requiring an advanced pharmacological strategy for optimal management. Such frequently treated respiratory diseases include asthma and COPD, two conditions that are both marked by airway inflammation and bronchoconstriction (Figure 6.10). Treatment involves bronchodilators, including beta-agonists and anticholinergics, which allow airway relaxation, in addition to corticosteroids to counteract inflammation. Moreover, conditions such as pneumonia and acute bronchitis often call for antibiotic treatment if bacterial cause is established. Also noteworthy, drug regimens have to be individualized to treat comorbid factors, for example, thrombosis risk in severe respiratory disease, for instance, in COVID-19 patients where anticoagulants are now essential adjuvants in treating pulmonary complications (Wichmann, 2020). Identifying the heterogeneity of respiratory disorders enables clinicians to use focused drug treatments that maximize patient benefit while keeping the risk of adverse effects low. Furthermore, viral respiratory infections represent a difficult therapeutic challenge because of their high rate of morbidity and risk of proclivity to rapid progression to respiratory failure. Drugs such as antiviral agents, including neuraminidase inhibitors for influenza, have been shown effective if provided early in the course of illness onset. Yet, the novel disease caused by the coronavirus disease (COVID-19) has added unprecedented challenges to the treatment protocols of drugs with a specific emphasis on preventing the inflammatory cascade and thromboembolic complications augmenting respiratory failure. Observational evidence emphasizes that add-on treatments such as corticosteroids and anticoagulants play a critical role in the treatment of severe disease and mortality control among patients admitted to hospitals (Wichmann, 2020). This dynamic changing therapeutic context illustrates how pharmacologic measures adapt in a dynamic way to the pathophysiology of novel respiratory infections and underscores the importance of continued clinical research. Critically ill patients with severe respiratory impairment are often in need of aggressive medical therapy, where pharmacologic treatment forms an essential part of support therapy. Mechanical ventilation and supplemental oxygen therapy are often supplemented by medication that targets underlying disease pathophysiology and complications like bacterial superinfection, hypercoagulability, and organ dysfunction. Recent studies of hospitalized COVID-19 patients show incidences of comorbidities such as hypertension and diabetes, making respiratory management complicated and necessitating simultaneous management. Such cases require multidisciplinary management of drug administration, ranging from the optimal use of anticoagulants against venous thromboembolism, antibacterial drugs to prevent secondary infection, and immunomodulators to check hyper-inflammatory states. Consequently, therapeutic regimens must be individualized to balance efficacy with safety in managing critical respiratory illnesses.

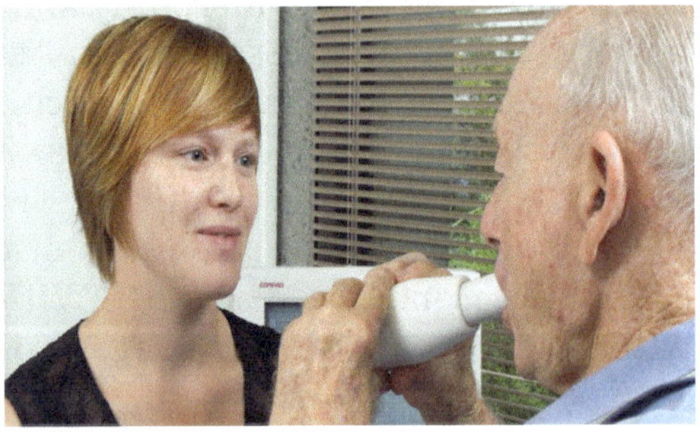

Figure 6.10. Common respiratory conditions treated with drugs.

Source: America's Best Care Plus. (2016). *Screen Shot 2016-05-07 at 3.13.27 PM.* https://americasbestcareplus.com/wp-content/uploads/2016/05/Screen-Shot-2016-05-07-at-3.13.27-PM.png.

6.3.1. Asthma

Respiratory diseases frequently necessitate the employment of pharmacological therapies to provide symptom relief and enhanced lung function, with asthma being one of the most common chronic diseases necessitating chronic treatment. Asthma (Figure 6.11) is defined by airway inflammation, bronchoconstriction, and hyperresponsiveness, resulting in coughing, wheezing, and breathlessness. The intricacy of its pathophysiology makes drug treatment complex and multifaceted and mainly depends on bronchodilators and anti-inflammatory drugs. Bronchodilators, including beta-2 adrenergic agonists, have a quick action by relaxing airway smooth muscle, offering symptomatic relief during an acute exacerbation. Corticosteroids, on the contrary, work to suppress underlying inflammation and avoid recurrence of crisis. These modalities of treatment highlight the significance of targeted therapy in maintaining airway patency, relieving symptoms, and decreasing hospitalization, thereby representing the pivotal role of pharmacological management in managing chronic respiratory illness like asthma. In treating asthma, the foundation of treatment lies heavily with inhaled corticosteroids (ICS), which considerably decrease chronic airway inflammation and inhibit exacerbations. The drug group affects gene expression in order to repress pro-inflammatory cytokines, enhancing lung function over time. The leukotriene receptor antagonists are an add-on therapy by opposing arachidonic acid-derived inflammatory mediators responsible for bronchoconstriction and mucus production. Considering asthmas heterogeneous phenotypes, individualized drug regimens enhance clinical efficacy, reflecting the need for patient-targeted therapeutic approaches. Additionally, novel biologic agents with precision targeting specific immune mechanisms, such as immunoglobulin E (IgE) or interleukin-5 (IL-5), have extended the therapeutic horizon for severe asthma. These developments reflect continued attempts to optimize respiratory medications, combining immunomodulatory strategies with traditional bronchodilators and corticosteroids for improved symptom control and quality of life. The management of asthma has relevant considerations in common with the patterns of pharmacological response registered in the respiratory infections and other respiratory complications. For instance, the overuse of antimicrobials in upper respiratory tract viral infections can lead to systemic effects as well as excess exposure to drugs, a trend registered in the recent public health emergencies (Rachina et al., 2022). Although antibiotics are not involved in the therapy of asthma, the interaction between acute respiratory infections and asthma exacerbations tends to make clinical decisions more complicated. Additionally, the pandemic highlighted the important role of immunomodulatory agents, such as corticosteroids, in controlling inflammation during viral adversity (Group I-S-C, 2020). These observations underpin the necessity of appropriate drug use and multimodal treatment approaches in respiratory medicine, as well as treatment for asthma taking into account not only disease pathogenesis but also systemic factors underlying respiratory health.

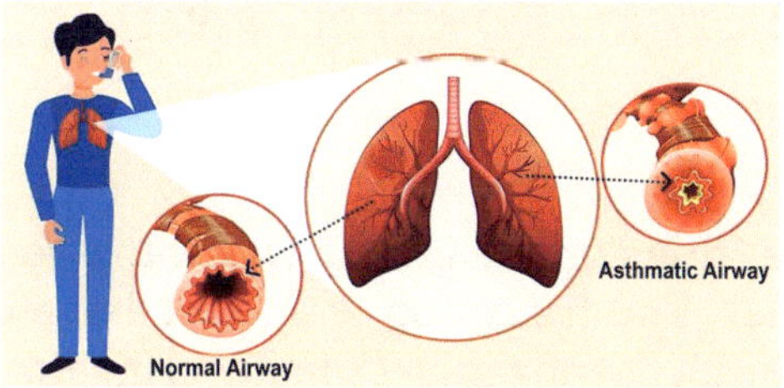

Figure 6.11. Asthma.

Source: https://duckduckgo.com/?q=Asthma&t=h_&iar=images.

6.3.2. Chronic Obstructive Pulmonary Disease (COPD)

The convergence of cardiovascular and respiratory disease brings with it difficult-to-handle challenges in patient care for patients with chronic diseases. Of these, COPD is notable, both for its respiratory manifestations, as well as for its most common association with cardiac comorbidities (Figure 6.12). The shared risk factors of smoking, inflammation, and aging further exacerbate the prognosis of patients and make the treatment regimen challenging. Of most concern is the heightened mortality due to cardiac disease in patients with COPD, at times even exceeding that of respiratory failure deaths. This combined burden requires an integrated treatment approach, where management of comorbid cardiac conditions is seen as positive, even in the context of possible drug interactions or side effects. Nevertheless, how far the survival can be extended with aggressive management of COPD and CVDs is uncertain, highlighting the importance of further research and judicious clinical decision-making (André et al., 2019). Pharmacological therapies in COPD have the objectives of symptom relief, increased lung function, and exacerbation reduction, and long-acting inhaled agents are the cornerstone of maintenance therapy. Inhaled corticosteroids (ICS) and long-acting beta2-agonists (LABAs) are most frequently used, frequently delivered in combination inhalers to increase patient compliance and therapeutic efficacy. Although the combination is frequently employed in moderate to severe asthma, the individual contribution of each remains a topic of clinical controversy. However, some research indicates that ICS essentially aim at the inflammatory aspect of COPD, while LABAs target bronchodilation, and their relative efficacy and ideal balance remain difficult to determine. The resultant uncertainty gives significant prominence to personalized treatment and regular assessment of pharmacologic regimens for maximizing respiratory outcomes without causing unwanted effects (Agarwal et al., 2011). Management of COPD with drug therapy also demands knowledge of its systemic presentation and of patients' general health status. As patients with COPD often present with comorbidities that affect drug metabolism as well as drug response, clinicians need to evaluate the risk-benefit ratio of drugs used for respiration within this larger clinical context. For example, the employment of corticosteroids may provide anti-inflammatory advantages but is also capable of making patients prone to infections or loss of bone density, especially in older age groups. Similarly, beta2-agonists, as useful bronchodilators, are likely to worsen intrinsic cardiac diseases with their systemic sympathomimetic actions. Therefore, incorporating pharmacologic treatment along with careful observation and management of comorbid illness is very important. A multidisciplinary treatment that takes into account the interaction between COPD and other chronic diseases guarantees that drug treatments for the respiratory system are safe and effective for this at-risk group (André et al., 2019).

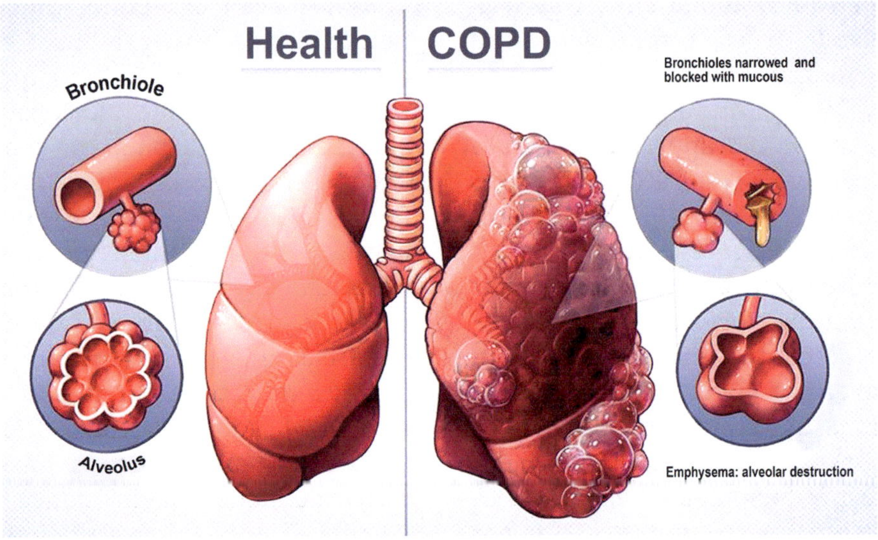

Figure 6.12. Chronic obstructive pulmonary disease (COPD).

Source: Chandigarh Ayurved Centre. (2022). *Healthy vs COPD lungs.* https://www.chandigarhayurvedcentre.com/wp-content/uploads/2022/12/HealthyvsCOPDlungs960px.jpg.

6.3.3. Allergic Rhinitis

The treatment of respiratory diseases like allergic rhinitis has transformed greatly with improvements in immune tolerance and prevention of disease approaches. The transition from an all-avoidance paradigm to a strategy for immune resilience has shown significant advantages in lowering the long-term allergic condition burden. The holistic strategy supports health by encouraging tolerance over symptom suppression alone, thus enhancing patients' quality of life. National initiatives focusing on education among healthcare providers and mass public awareness campaigns have played crucial roles in spreading this information efficiently. These efforts provide evidence that planned, population-level interventions are able to moderate the severity and frequency of allergic respiratory diseases such as allergic rhinitis through decreased unnecessary treatments and enhanced early detection and treatment of severe symptoms. These interventions not only enhance patient outcomes but also result in significant reductions in healthcare expenditure and related disability, representing a potential model for enhancing respiratory healthcare (Haahtela et al., 2021). Pharmacologic treatments continue to play a core role in the management of allergic rhinitis, targeting symptomatic relief and disease exacerbation prevention. Antihistamines, intranasal corticosteroids, and leukotriene receptor antagonists form the main classes of drugs used to suppress inflammatory reactions in the respiratory mucosa. Intranasal corticosteroids are especially useful in minimizing nasal congestion and inflammation through suppression of eosinophilic infiltration and cytokine release. Yet, long-term medication can be a source of medicalization issues, highlighting the need for balanced treatment regimens that are compatible with changing public health approaches based on immune tolerance. The application of telehealth technologies during outbreaks of respiratory disease has also become an essential adjunct in the monitoring and management of conditions such as allergic rhinitis, enabling ongoing patient care with reduced risk of exposure and burdens on healthcare systems (Monaghesh et al., 2020). This melding of pharmacologic therapy with contemporary healthcare delivery is a dynamic shift in respiratory medicine. The socioeconomic burden of allergic rhinitis goes beyond immediate medical costs, including loss of work-related productivity and reduced psychosocial well-being. Large-scale health programs have proved that integrated allergy care, including accurate diagnostics and tailored treatment, effectively prevents the development of occupational allergies and decreases emergency healthcare use. These programs emphasize the importance of multidisciplinary coordination and standardized care pathways, which improve treatment compliance and patient education. In addition, hospitalization reduction and medication dependency seen in such programs represent a two-way advantage of better patient outcomes and sustainability of the environment by reducing the carbon footprint of the healthcare system. Since allergic rhinitis frequently occurs along with other respiratory conditions, drug regimen optimization within the integrated care models is crucial for comprehensive management of respiratory conditions and reduction of the overall public health load (Haahtela et al., 2021).

Test Your Knowledge

1. Define Chronic Obstructive Pulmonary Disease (COPD).
2. How do antihistamines help manage allergic rhinitis symptoms?

6.4. Side Effects of Respiratory Drugs

Learning Outcome

1. Short-Term Side Effects
2. Long-Term Side Effects
3. Drug Interactions with Other Medications

Administration of respiratory medications, although unavoidable in the treatment of many pulmonary diseases, is frequently a delicate balance between therapeutic efficacy and toxicity (Figure 6.13). Bronchodilators, corticosteroids, and sedatives are some examples of medications that affect several body systems outside of the lungs. Sedatives administered in respiratory therapy, especially in critical care with mechanical ventilation, are associated with the risk of respiratory depression, hypotension, and change in mental status. Aged individuals are particularly susceptible because of age-related changes in pharmacokinetics and comorbid illnesses potentiating these risks. Choosing the right sedative with an optimal safety profile is thus essential in order to avoid complications and enhance outcomes. A subtle appreciation of each drug's effect on respiratory and cardiovascular function allows clinicians to optimize treatments better. Such tailored management is consistent with current evidence focusing on prudent use of sedatives in high-risk populations to prevent adverse respiratory effects (Paschoal et al., 2025). Sedatives are not the only drugs that have adverse respiratory effects but also antiepileptic drugs that indirectly impact pulmonary function. A number of anti-seizure drugs, although acting primarily on neurological mechanisms, have been found to have both direct and indirect effects on lung homeostasis. Some of them can induce respiratory depression or hypersensitivity reactions and cause complications such as infections or organized pulmonary pathology. Additionally, some antiepileptic drugs cause pulmonary artery hypertension, further complicating respiratory function. The drugs can also have protective profiles, including anti-inflammatory and immunomodulatory effects that reduce asthma airway remodeling. It is important to understand this double nature, particularly when tending to patients who have simultaneous neurological and respiratory conditions, since the respiratory side effects could demand close observation to avoid dire complications (Butera et al., 2024). The drive to enhance respiratory drug safety calls for continued advances in both clinical practice and pharmacology. Side effects transcend direct respiratory symptoms and also encompass systemic effects like cardiovascular instability and immune reactions that complicate management. In surgical and critical care environments, where sedation is commonly used, the process of selection must take into consideration heterogeneous patient-specific factors, such as age, comorbidities, and the expected duration of sedation. Evidence favors that individualized sedation practices, guided by systematic clinical trials and observational evidence, minimize incidence of respiratory compromise and other adverse effects. Therefore, education of clinicians and multidisciplinary management are crucial in achieving the best therapeutic benefits with minimum side effects. This strategy fits into the larger trend towards precision medicine in respiratory therapy, focusing on minimizing drug-induced morbidity by using individualized intervention (Paschoal et al., 2025).

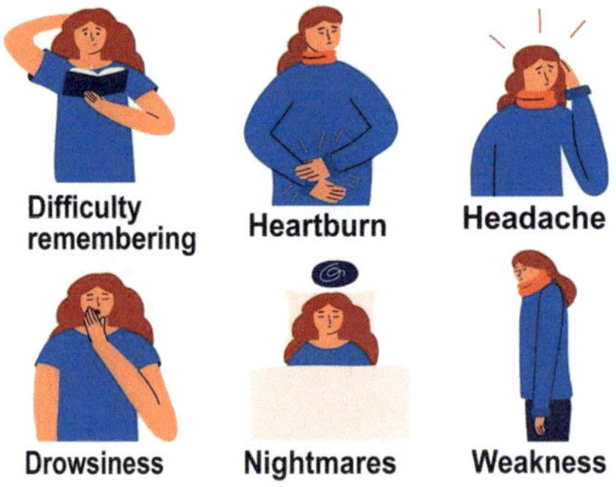

Figure 6.13. Side effects of respiratory drugs.

Source: Savich, A. (n.d.). *Infographics of Side Effects From New Drugs: The Girl Suffers From Heartburn, Headache, Weakness*. Vecteezy. https://static.vecteezy.com/system/resources/previews/012/901/133/non_2x/infographics-of-side-effects-from-new-drugs-the-girl-suffers-from-heartburn-headache-weakness-hand-drawing-illustration-vector.jpg.

6.4.1. Short-Term Side Effects

Utilization of drugs that affect the respiratory system frequently requires special consideration of their direct physiological effects, especially in relation to short-term side effects. These side effects have a strong bearing on patient compliance and overall treatment success. Bronchodilators, for example, which are frequently used for the treatment of asthma and COPD, can induce sudden-onset side effects such as tachycardia, tremor, and nervousness. These side effects are the result of the systemic absorption of beta-agonists that cause stimulation of beta-adrenergic receptors outside the lungs and influence cardiac and skeletal muscle tissue. Such side effects, as much as they are temporary, can masquerade or accentuate pre-existing comorbidities and render clinical management challenging. Furthermore, corticosteroids, despite their potency in suppressing airway inflammation, can cause oral thrush or dysphonia soon after drug administration. Identification and management of these acute side effects are crucial to the preservation of therapeutic gains from being offset by side effects during the initial treatment phase (Amaducci et al., 2018). Opioid analgesics, commonly used to treat pain in respiratory diseases or procedures, are infamous for inducing rapid respiratory side effects that complicate patient management. Respiratory depression is one of the most serious short-term adverse effects, defined as decreased respiratory rate and depth, that may lead to hypoxemia if not immediately treated. This is opioid-mediated through its interaction with mu-opioid peptide (MOP) receptors in brainstem centers that regulate respiration. Interestingly, more recently developed bifunctional agents, including the MOP/nociception opioid peptide (NOP) receptor agonist BU10038, have been examined for their analgesic effects with reduced respiratory side effects. These medications seem to preserve respiratory function at analgesic doses, unlike traditional opioids such as morphine or oxycodone, which suppress respiratory drive early in treatment (Cami-Kobeci et al., 2019). Such development would be a landmark in the control of respiratory complications of opioid treatment. In addition, short-term respiratory adverse effects of pharmacologic agents are not confined to bronchodilators and opioids. Anticholinergic drugs, used commonly to alleviate bronchospasm, produce direct effects like dryness of the mouth and throat irritation, which, though seemingly innocuous, can lead to coughing and fleeting airway discomfort. Certain inhaled treatments paradoxically cause bronchoconstriction, particularly in hyperresponsive subjects, making the first part of treatment more complex and necessitating careful surveillance. In addition, systemic adverse effects such as hypotension or arrhythmias from specific drug groups have indirect effects on breathing by decreasing oxygen supply. These acute reactions highlight the need for thorough patient evaluation during the start of respiratory treatments, seeking to reconcile therapeutic benefits with tolerable short-term side effects in order to maximize patient outcomes and compliance (Amaducci et al., 2018).

6.4.2. Long-Term Side Effects

Long-term administration of drugs acting on the respiratory system frequently evokes questions about their safety profiles over long periods of time, particularly in terms of organ function and systemic responses. Although these drugs seek to enhance pulmonary function and restore symptoms, long-term use occasionally results in complications like muscle impairment, cardiovascular stress, or disturbances in the immune system. For example, some of the therapies employed in PAH have shown improvement in exercise tolerance and quality of life but require close monitoring because of possible adverse effects such as arrhythmia or respiratory infection. The difficulty of managing these side effects is compounded by patients' propensity to overestimate their physical tolerance, which could worsen cardiac complications if exercise regimens are not closely monitored in specialized environments. This underscores the imperative need to combine medical therapy with rehabilitation by specialized centers to maximize benefits and reduce long-term hazards (Keusch et al., 2017). The cardiovascular system is especially susceptible to the long-term adverse effects of respiratory medications, as seen in the management of patients with advanced heart failure undergoing inotropic therapy. Regular or chronic drug treatment can place undue stress on cardiac function, and resulting complications may sometimes require hospitalization. For instance, intermittent infusion of levosimendan, a calcium sensitizer in the treatment of advanced heart failure, is under investigation to establish their safety and efficacy in limiting acute exacerbations without worsening long-term cardiac problems. Implications of such research emphasize the importance of properly weighing therapeutic gains against possible cumulative cardiovascular side effects in utilizing drugs that indirectly affect respiratory well-being by modulation of cardiac function (García-González et al., 2013). In addition, the interaction among respiratory and systemic organ systems requires attentiveness to long-term side effects of respiratory medicines, with these side effects potentially cascading outside the lungs. Chronic inflammation, immune dysregulation, and skeletal muscle weakness can result from long-term drug exposure, which in turn can negatively affect patients' overall functional status and quality of life. The evidence shows that specialty rehabilitation programs designed for patients with respiratory diseases such as PAH not only enhance physical performance but also reduce psychological burden associated with disease and treatment. These multidisciplinary interventions are required to treat both the direct and indirect long-term consequences, providing holistic care that goes beyond the immediate control of respiratory symptoms (Keusch et al., 2017).

6.4.3. Drug Interactions with Other Medications

The judicious handling of drugs that act on the respiratory system is necessary because of the intricate interaction between such drugs and other medications a patient might be on (Figure 6.14). Polypharmacy, which is frequently prevalent in patients with chronic respiratory diseases like asthma or COPD, predisposes to drug interactions. For instance, bronchodilator beta-agonists may interact with beta-blockers to treat CVDs and decrease therapeutic response or increase respiratory symptomatology. Also, metabolism of respiratory medication can be altered by co-medications influencing cytochrome P450 enzymes, resulting in toxic buildup or decreased therapeutic effect. With such complexity, clinicians need to carefully evaluate patients' drug histories to avoid risks. This is exacerbated in certain areas where self-medication and illicit drug use are common, raising the risk of adverse interactions and overdose (Curtis et al., 2009). The increase in self-medication for respiratory illnesses raises additional issues regarding unreported drug interactions. Patients often take over-the-counter medications or herbal supplements in addition to prescribed drugs, without reporting these to their physicians. Such practices are of considerable concern, especially when one takes into account that most herbal medicines or adjuvant treatments possess inadequately characterized pharmacokinetics and pharmacodynamics. This limited knowledge can cause unforeseen interactions, modifying the respiratory medication's action or initiating side effects. Furthermore, the absence of strong clinical studies on these therapies restricts evidence-based advice to safely incorporate them with mainstream respiratory medications. Hence, open communication between clinicians and patients is imperative in ensuring the effective management of drug regimens, since the risk of interaction is heightened within the framework of self-managed treatment modalities (Kilgore et al., 2010). Beyond self-treatment, pharmacodynamic and pharmacokinetic interactions between drugs impacting respiratory function call for continuous surveillance. Corticosteroids, commonly employed to treat inflammation in asthma and COPD, have been reported to affect the metabolism of diverse drugs by enzyme induction or inhibition, raising fear of systemic side effects when used in combination with drugs like antifungals or antivirals. Concomitant administration of various inhaled drugs can also lead to additive adverse cardiac effects, particularly if sympathomimetic agents are combined with other stimulants. Drug interaction issues apply to acute situations like overdose situations precipitated by the unforeseen combination of respiratory drugs with CNS depressants. Preventive measures such as patient education and personalized pharmacovigilance are critical in avoiding these risks and maximizing therapeutic outcomes in respiratory drug regimens (Curtis et al., 2009; Kilgore et al., 2010).

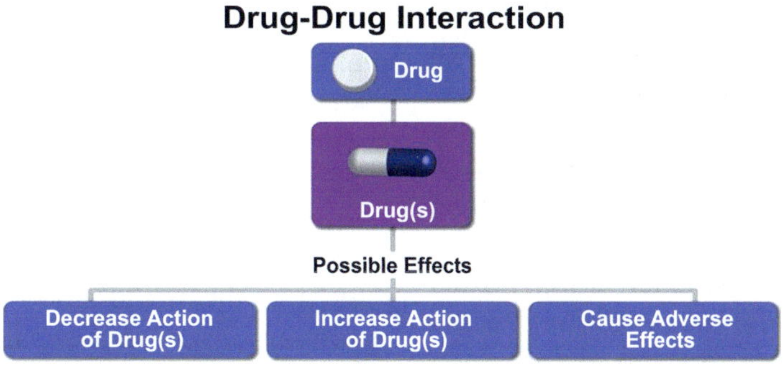

Figure 6.14. Drug interactions with other medications.

Source: U.S. Department of Health and Human Services. (n.d.). *Drug-Drug Interaction.* Clinical Info HIV.gov. https://clinicalinfo.hiv.gov/sites/default/files/glossaries/images/Drug-Drug-Interaction-800.jpg.

Test Your Knowledge

1. What is a drug–drug interaction?
2. How does long - term side effects drugs acting?

6.5. Impact of Drug Abuse on the Respiratory System

Learning Outcome

1. Effects of Recreational Drugs
2. Consequences of Smoking and Vaping
3. Long-Term Health Implications

The interaction among different substances and the physiological consequences usually unveils complex results, especially in the respiratory system. Drug abuse, defined by the excessive or undue use of substances, has strong negative impacts on respiratory functions. Smoking of drugs like cocaine, heroin, and methamphetamines can lead to acute bronchospasm, pulmonary edema, and chronic inflammation of the airways. The chronic exposure to harmful substances damages the structural framework of the alveoli and airway epithelium, resulting in reduced lung function and vulnerability to infection. In addition, the change in respiratory drive caused by narcotics also leads to hypoventilation and respiratory depression, which may be lethal. These associations need to be comprehended to effectively design interventions customized to mitigate morbidity due to respiratory complications as a result of substance abuse. Substance abuse also worsens underlying respiratory disease, tending to complicate their treatment and outcomes. For example, asthmatic or COPD patients who abuse drugs have increased airway reactivity and frequency of exacerbations. These drugs can impair mucociliary clearance and local immune function, predisposing to bacterial colonization and chronic inflammation. The smoking of drugs is especially likely to elevate the risk for respiratory infection and carcinogenesis based on inhalation of the combustion products into the lungs. Furthermore, abused drugs' systemic effects compromise host defense, which produces opportunistic diseases like tuberculosis and pneumonia. Such complexities reveal drug abuse's interference with the process of respiratory disease progression and its need for the combined clinical treatments that will focus on treating addiction and respiratory conditions at the same time.

Tackling the consequence of drug abuse on respiratory function requires robust policy intervention and strengthened clinical approaches. Existing public health agendas demand standardized measurement tools and surveillance systems to provide stronger estimates of the extent and severity of respiratory disease in drug-abusing groups. Emphasis on responsible use policies, infection control, and early diagnosis can by far reduce deleterious effects, particularly when made responsive to socioeconomic and demographic factors. One Health integration, taking into account human, animal, and environmental health sectors, can enable holistic solutions for drug abuse-related respiratory morbidity (Aarestrup et al., 2015). Further, enhancing research protocols, such as strict participant screening and standardization of control groups as suggested in clinical sleep studies, can sharpen knowledge on how impaired respiratory function presents in substance-affected individuals (Beattie et al., 2015). Combined, these actions are essential to reducing the respiratory health burden caused by drug abuse.

6.5.1. Effects of Recreational Drugs

Recreational drugs' interaction with the human body is complex, as illustrated by their mixed influence on the respiratory system, which frequently makes diagnosis and treatment more difficult (Figure 6.15). Most drugs classified as sympathomimetic agents, both synthetic and naturally occurring compounds, activate the sympathetic nervous system via various mechanisms, either by directly stimulating adrenergic receptors or indirectly by enhancing endogenous catecholamine levels. This stimulation can provoke respiratory alterations, such as bronchial smooth muscle relaxation or, conversely, bronchospasm, depending on the agent and dose used. Additionally, the recent identification of trace amine-associated receptors (TAARs) has revealed other pathways by which these sympathomimetics cause their respiratory actions, leading to a reevaluation of previously underappreciated toxicological hazards. The toxicological profile of natural sympathomimetic compounds, traditionally thought to be safe, has shown a multitude of toxic respiratory effects, highlighting the importance of having a different understanding of their pharmacodynamics and toxicology (Costa et al., 2022). Although the majority of natural recreational drugs are used for their stimulant effects, they pose serious respiratory threats that transcend mere sympathetic stimulation. One glaring instance is khat (*Catha edulis*), a herbal stimulant extensively utilized in areas of East Africa and the Arabian Peninsula. Its active alkaloids cathinone, cathine, and norephedrine are its main active agents that act as amphetamine analogues, generating not just increased alertness and energy but also different systemic problems. The respiratory effects of long-term khat consumption come as one facet of its complex toxic effects, comprising cardiovascular tension and possible neurological implications that secondarily disrupt lung capacity. Furthermore, the psychostimulant-induced effects can aggravate underlying respiratory ailments like asthma, by heightening airway hyperreactivity. The widespread availability of khat beyond its traditional use regions underscores a growing public health concern regarding chronic respiratory toxicity linked to this natural sympathomimetic (Bárbara Silva et al., 2022). Beyond isolated compounds, recreational drugs frequently exert cumulative and complex effects on respiratory physiology, often through intertwined systemic pathways. Sympathomimetic drugs, be they synthetic such as cocaine or natural such as ephedra derivatives, can cause tachypnea, impaired gas exchange, and increased bronchial inflammation, all of which impair lung function. Chronic administration also facilitates maladaptive respiratory responses such as airway remodeling and increased infectibility. These pathologies are not so much pharmacological curiosities but have important clinical implications when abusers are exposed to polydrug regimens that enhance respiratory burden. Such interaction supports the need for systematic toxicological research on respiratory endpoints, demonstrating the fine yet significant impact recreational sympathomimetics exert upon airway physiology and systemic homeostasis (Costa et al., 2022).

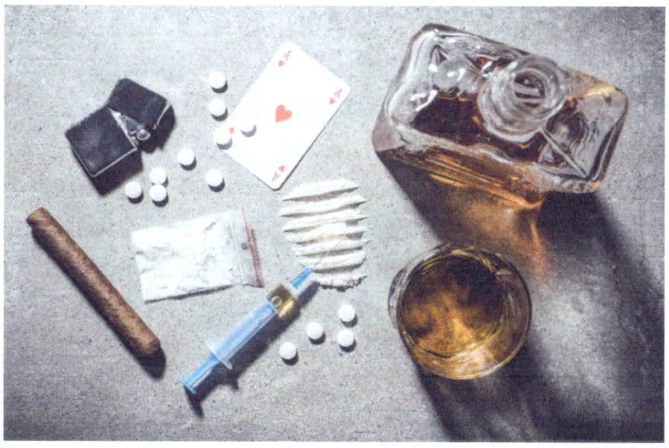

Figure 6.15. Effects of recreational drugs.

Source: WhiteSands Treatment. (2017). *Top 7 Most Abused Recreational Drugs.* https://whitesandstreatment.com/wp-content/uploads/2017/05/Top-7-Most-Abused-Recreational-Drugs-1.jpg.

6.5.2. Consequences of Smoking and Vaping

The smoking and vaping of substances deliver a complex mix of particulate matter into the respiratory system and heavily impact lung health. Studies have shown that the aerosols given off by electronic tobacco cigarette (EATC) alternatives like IQOS®, GLO®, and JUUL® are comprised primarily of particles less than one micrometer in size. These ultrafine particles have access to penetrate deeply into pulmonary tissues, enhancing the respiratory burden. While the EATCs release fewer indoor particulate matter emissions than traditional tobacco cigarettes, the levels are still high relative to normal outdoor concentrations, particularly during exhalation. The extensive variability in particle emissions is a function of device type and user behavior. Such findings emphasize that vaping is not without respiratory risks, as exposure to high concentrations of fine and ultrafine particulate matter can exacerbate lung inflammation and potentially contribute to chronic respiratory conditions (Avino et al., 2020). Understanding the appeal of vaping among youth is critical when assessing its long-term respiratory consequences. Adolescents have increasingly embraced e-cigarettes, initially marketed as cessation tools, but now widely used for recreational purposes. This trend is a concern for public health, as most of the young users are not aware of the health hazards of nicotine and inhalation of vapor. The addictive properties of e-vapor products expose the developing lungs to chemical substances that can negatively affect normal respiratory function. In addition, early use of vaping can predispose adolescents to eventual smoking or chronic pulmonary disease. Health care workers advocate for all-around strategies to stem the vaping epidemic in youth populations to avoid long-term respiratory system harm and nicotine addiction (Sisson et al., 2020). The general effects of smoking and vaping are not limited to individual health but also reach public and environmental health. Indoor air quality is significantly degraded when cigarettes or electronic nicotine delivery systems are employed, which enhances bystander exposure risks. High particulate matter from e-cigarettes poses challenges to current regulatory systems, as the health consequences of these emissions are partially unknown. Repeated inhalation of nicotine and related chemicals via smoke or vapor causes oxidative stress and inflammation in respiratory tissues, promoting COPD and bronchitis disease. Thus, the harmful effects of vaping and smoking (Figure 6.16) on respiratory health require immediate legislative measures to restrict use in the community setting and decrease community-level health risks (Avino et al., 2020).

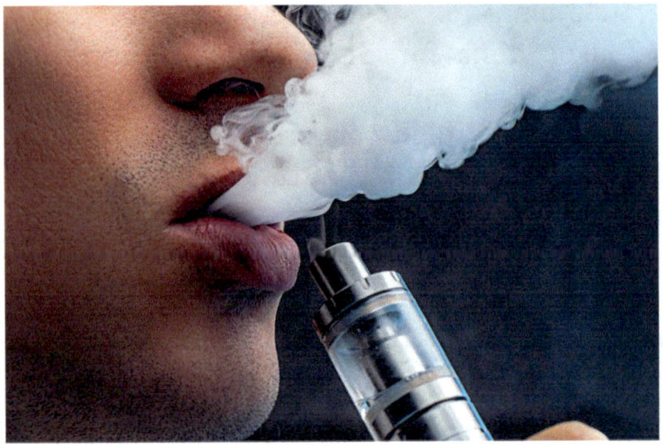

Figure 6.16. Consequences of smoking and vaping.

Source: Bigstock. (n.d.). *Close-Up Young Man Vaping Electronic Cigarette*. Incredible Things. https://incrediblethings.com/wp-content/uploads/2020/06/bigstock-Close-up-Young-Man-Vaping-E-303717082.jpg.

6.5.3. Long-Term Health Implications

The complexity of the respiratory system renders it particularly vulnerable to the long-term consequences of pharmacological intervention. Many drugs designed to alleviate respiratory conditions, such as corticosteroids or beta-agonists, while effective short-term, can induce systemic changes that affect overall health. Prolonged steroid use, for example, may suppress immune function, increase the risk of osteoporosis, and cause metabolic disturbances. In addition, chronic use of these drugs can cause tolerance, requiring increased doses that worsen side effects. Aside from the effects of individual drugs, the interaction between the autonomic nervous system (ANS) and respiratory function is instrumental in determining long-term health consequences. The modulation of cardiorespiratory coherence across various emotional states implies that respiratory medications, through the modulation of autonomic balance, may have an effect on psychological health and cardiovascular health as well, pointing towards an integrated system-wide effect (Crawford et al., 2015). Additionally, long-term pharmacological modulation of the respiratory system needs to be viewed in the context of changing treatment modalities, especially in oncological environments where immune-based therapies have become common. Medications like checkpoint inhibitors or chimeric antigen receptor (CAR) T-cell therapies, while revolutionary in the treatment of cancer, possess distinct respiratory toxicities such as pneumonitis, which can present as one of immune-related adverse events. Such complications have the potential to result in chronic pulmonary inflammation or fibrosis and significantly impair respiratory function with passage of time. Management of these side effects frequently involves delicate balancing of therapeutic effectiveness against possible respiratory toxicity, highlighting the need for longitudinal monitoring and adaptation of treatment regimens to avoid irreversible damage (Brém et al., 2020). Aside from drug-induced physiological alterations, the psychological consequences of prolonged respiratory drug use should not be overlooked. Cardiorespiratory coherence disruptions associated with stress and emotional dysregulation, modified by respiratory therapy, can create a cycle of adverse health effects. Changes in autonomic tone not only modulate respiratory parameters but also have an effect on mood disorders and stress levels, which play a key role in chronic respiratory disorders. Therapeutic strategies like mindfulness and pranayama have been proposed to counteract such effects, underlining the requirement of integrated treatment strategies that target physical as well as emotional aspects. This bio-psycho-social approach is crucial to ascertain and control the long-term health consequences of drugs acting on the respiratory system (Crawford et al., 2015).

Test Your Knowledge

1. What are the cardiovascular effects of chronic smoking?
2. How can recreational drugs affect cardiovascular health?

6.6. Current Research and Developments

Learning Outcome

1. New Drug Therapies for Respiratory Conditions
2. Advances in Inhalation Technology
3. Future Directions in Respiratory Pharmacology

Improvements in drug delivery systems have profoundly altered the scene of respiratory therapeutics over the last few years. Conventional systemic drug administration is usually plagued with issues concerning narrow efficacy and adverse side effects as a result of the broad dispersion of pharmacological agents. Recent research focuses on the formulation of inhalation therapies, especially for inflammatory lung disorders like asthma and COPD, where local deposition of the drug maximizes therapeutic effects with minimal systemic exposure (Figure 6.17). Among these advances, dry powder inhalers (DPIs) have drawn considerable interest due to breath-activated release, convenience to the user, and provision for delivering high-dose formulations. The optimization of DPI design and formulation has been a key area of emphasis to maximize particle size, stability, and lung deposition, which all impact clinical efficacy. These advances are a promising direction toward precision medicine in respiratory therapy, providing a better balance between efficacy and safety in the treatment of complex pulmonary diseases (Amir et al., 2024). Concurrent with advances in drug delivery, molecular studies have revealed fundamental knowledge of the cellular derangement responsible for respiratory diseases, leading the way for the development of new targeted treatments. Increasing evidence underlines the significance of mitochondrial quality control pathways in diseases such as COPD, lung cancer, and idiopathic pulmonary fibrosis. Mitochondrial regulation, through mechanisms such as energy metabolism through pathways such as mitophagy, biogenesis, and fusion/fission dynamics, is critical in maintaining cellular homeostasis and responding to oxidative stress and inflammation. Deviations in these processes lead to disease process through the enhancement of apoptosis and cellular senescence. This disrupts lung tissue integrity. Striking key molecules of mitochondrial quality control, such as PINK1, PRKN, DRP1, and PGC1-α, is a hopeful therapeutic approach to stop or reverse pathogenic processes, although the intricacies of these processes need to be better understood to create targeted pharmacological agents (Liu et al., 2023). In spite of these hopeful leads, there remain difficulties in translating research into clinically useful treatments for respiratory illness. The complex interplay of mitochondrial functions required for physiological processes renders the design of therapeutics to modulate these pathways with minimal adverse effects challenging. Added to this is the consideration of drug delivery systems through inhalation, which, although beneficial, encounter challenges in patient compliance, device variability in design, and formulation stability across various environmental conditions. Continuing research is becoming more centered on transcending these challenges by combining multidisciplinary technologies, such as nanotechnology, pharmacogenomics, and bioengineering, to customize respiratory therapies according to individual patient characteristics. Further investigation of DPI technologies combined with mitochondrial-targeting agents has great potential for enhancing disease prognosis, paving the way for the development of personalized and more effective respiratory therapies (Amir et al., 2024; Liu et al., 2023).

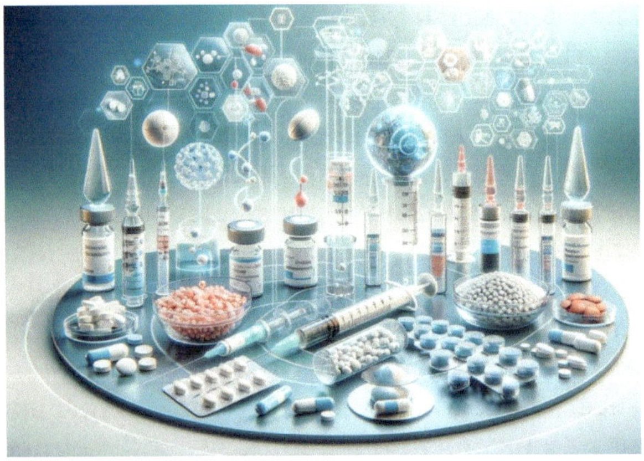

Figure 6.17. Current research and developments.

Source: Say Media. (n.d.). *Advancements and Diversity in Drug Delivery Systems.* https://images.saymedia-content.com/.image/t_share/MjAzNTI0Mjc0Njg4ODk0MzAw/advancements-and-diversity-in-drug-delivery-systems.jpg.

6.6.1. New Drug Therapies for Respiratory Conditions

The recent developments in the management of respiratory disorders have intensified focus on the design of targeted drug delivery systems, promising greater therapeutic benefits with less systemic side effects. Conventional systemic treatment regularly encounters the limitation of poor efficacy and the occurrence of generalized adverse effects within non-target organs. Inhalation treatments, especially those using DPIs, have emerged as an advanced option through the prospect of localized delivery to the lung tissue itself. This strategy not only permits immediate onset of action but also reduces systemic exposure and toxicity. DPI formulation refinement emphasizes precision, where optimal particle size and dispersibility are ensured to achieve maximum lung deposition. These developments mirror a wider shift towards personalized medicine in respiratory treatment, where drug delivery systems are designed to suit the specific needs of individual patients, enhancing compliance and clinical outcome. The changing scenario in pulmonary drug delivery supports the role of better managing chronic inflammatory ailments such as COPD and asthma (Amir et al., 2024). The experience of the pandemic of COVID-19 highlighted glaring challenges in disease management of respiratory infections, the development of multi-drug resistance being a striking one, to complicate disease management in the intensive care setup. The increased rates of secondary bacterial and fungal infections have underlined the urgent necessity for new approaches in therapy targeted both at the primary viral pathology and complications resulting from it. In the pandemic, there have been notable alterations in the environment of microbes where rises in resistance among strains of *Klebsiella pneumoniae* and *Acinetobacter baumanii* demand vigilant attention toward stewardship and development of new antimicrobials. These results underscore the need to combine microbiological monitoring with clinical pharmacology to inform rational use of antibiotics and infection control practices. As such, novel drug therapies are being developed not only to fight respiratory diseases directly but also to prevent resistance emergence by maximizing drug spectra and mechanisms of action (Malkova et al., 2023). New developments in respiratory pharmacotherapy increasingly involve the use of molecular and immunological understanding to create medicines that interfere with the underlying inflammatory and fibrotic processes that are typical of most chronic lung diseases. New agents designed to target particular immune pathways are designed to inhibit airway inflammation more specifically while maintaining lung tissue function. Such treatments try to interrupt the pathologic cycles of inflammation and remodeling in conditions such as idiopathic pulmonary fibrosis and ARDS. Concurrently, combination therapies with both anti-inflammatory and antifibrotic actions are promising for disease modification, not just symptom control. These advances are facilitated by advances in drug delivery platforms, including inhalable biologics and nanoparticles, that improve drug stability and targeted pulmonary deposition. As these new generations of therapeutics move through phases of clinical trial, they stand as the gold standard to change the treatment paradigms aligned with the complex biology of respiratory diseases (Amir et al., 2024; Malkova et al., 2023).

6.6.2. Advances in Inhalation Technology

Respiratory drug delivery innovations have revolutionized the treatment of pulmonary disorders with improved therapeutic efficacy and decreased systemic side effects. Inhalation technology has emerged with advances in aerosol science, formulation chemistry, and device engineering to maximize drug deposition in the lungs (Figure 6.18). New DPIs and pressurized metered-dose inhalers feature breath-activated release mechanisms with enhanced patient compliance and dosage precision. Additionally, the innovation of vibrating mesh nebulizers enables more effective aerosol production and penetration to the lungs, which is advantageous for patients with serious respiratory diseases. These advancements demonstrate an increased appreciation of pulmonary pharmacokinetics, with an emphasis on targeted delivery to alveolar regions where rapid absorption takes place. This change not only improves clinical results in the case of conditions like asthma and COPD but also serves to confront newly rising challenges with respect to pulmonary hypertension by making administration of vasodilatory treatment more effective and patient-centered delivery methods (Humbert et al., 2022). Clinical consequences of these technological advancements are most specific within the confines of viral respiratory infections that affect cardiovascular as well as respiratory systems.

The recent COVID-19 pandemic has highlighted the need for inhalation devices capable of delivering antiviral and anti-inflammatory drugs directly to affected lung tissue with high accuracy and low systemic exposure (Tomasz et al., 2020). Since infection with SARS-CoV-2 affects not only the respiratory epithelium but also cardiovascular function, formulations that allow localized drug delivery may prevent complications like acute respiratory distress syndrome and myocardial damage. In addition, inhalation technology designed for rapid onset and dose titration enables clinicians to adjust therapy in real time according to disease severity. Monitoring drug delivery and lung deposition increases therapeutic monitoring, and these inhalation modalities become invaluable tools in the management of complex respiratory pathologies with systemic implications (Tomasz et al., 2020). Directions of future technology in inhalation concern incorporating digital health elements to deliver personalized treatment and enhance compliance. Intelligent inhalers with sensors and wireless connectivity allow monitoring of usage habits, inhalation technique, and drug delivery parameters, offering data-driven solutions for patient and healthcare provider information. Digital technology underpins precision medicine strategies in respiratory management, streamlining drug regimens dependent on patient response and lifestyle.

Moreover, nanoparticle carrier advances and liposome formulation for inhalation also advance sustained release and selective cellular uptake in the pulmonary system. These advances also promise to increase therapeutic indices while reducing side effects. Therefore, new inhalation technologies are a cornerstone advance in pharmacotherapy of pulmonary system disease through marrying sophisticated drug delivery to modern digital health models (Humbert et al., 2022).

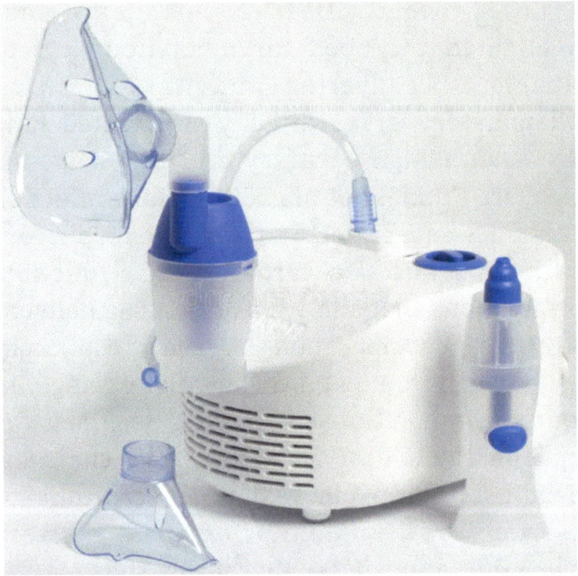

Figure 6.18. Advances in inhalation technology.

Source: Dreamstime. (n.d.). *Kiev, Ukraine - September: Nebulizer Omron Inhalation Device Isolated on White Background.* https://thumbs.dreamstime.com/b/kiev-ukraine-september-nebulizer-omron-inhalation-device-isolated-white-background-159362378.jpg.

6.6.3. Future Directions in Respiratory Pharmacology

Pharmacological advances in respiratory pharmacology are increasingly centered on elucidation of cellular and molecular processes underlying the efficacy and toxicity of drugs (Figure 6.19). More recent studies have emphasized the role of mitochondrial dysfunction as a critical mechanism underlying drug-caused cellular injury, an issue relevant to cardiac but possibly also respiratory tissues. Interventions that address mitochondrial well-being, like the use of melatonin, have been promising in modulating oxidative stress and apoptosis, which has the potential to be translated to the protection of lung cells against pharmacologic and environmental toxins. By optimizing drug design to include mitochondrial-protective drugs or adjunctive therapies that maximize cellular metabolism, new respiratory drugs could minimize side effects while maximizing therapy. Such strategies highlight the necessity for multidisciplinary research, beyond the usual symptomatic relief to mechanisms-based treatments that maintain cellular function in conditions such as COPD and asthma (Ganeshan et al., 2019). Prostanoid's therapeutic promise marks a promising advance in treating PAH and perhaps other respiratory diseases that involve vascular remodeling and inflammation. Prostacyclin analogs with vasodilatory, antiplatelet, and antiproliferative activities provide multifunctional advantages that are likely to be more effective than existing monotherapies. New formulations and delivery systems for prostanoids are being developed to enhance patient compliance and targeting specificity, which are essential for the management of chronic respiratory diseases. Additionally, intensifying studies on prostanoids may uncover new mechanisms to treat related illnesses with endothelial dysfunction and abnormal pulmonary vascular tone. The incorporation of prostanoids-based therapies into wider respiratory pharmacological approaches is indicative of a trend towards interventions that aim at both hemodynamic and cellular abnormalities (Korokin et al., 2018). In the future, the combination of pharmacogenomics and personalized medicine is expected to reshape respiratory pharmacology by adapting drug regimens to unique genetic and phenotypic profiles. This strategy has the potential to reduce side effects and enhance drug activity in heterogeneous respiratory diseases like asthma and idiopathic pulmonary fibrosis. Improvements in biomarker discovery and high-throughput screening will enable the creation of targeted therapies that not only reduce symptoms but also alter disease progression at the molecular level. Furthermore, the increasing knowledge of drug-induced mitochondrial toxicity promotes the reevaluation of current drugs and informs the development of new compounds with better safety profiles. The convergence of mechanistic understanding, new drug classes, and personalized strategies promises a future in which respiratory pharmacology can provide more targeted, effective, and safe treatment regimens (Ganeshan et al., 2019; Korokin et al., 2018).

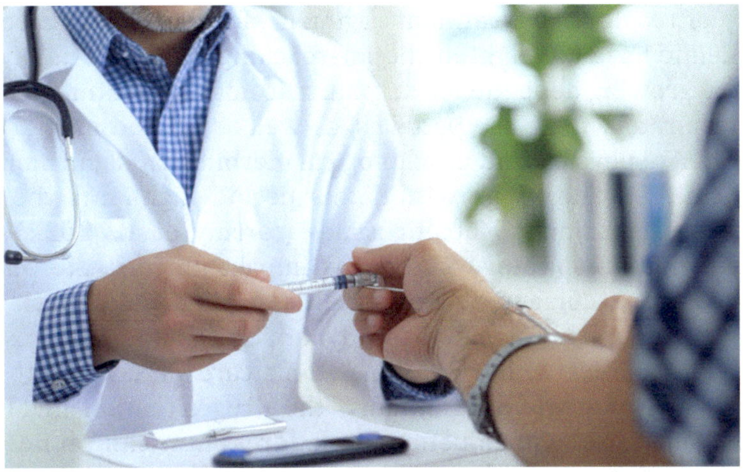

Figure 6.19. Future directions in respiratory pharmacology.

Source: Medium. (2023). *Future Directions in Respiratory.Pharmacology. https*://miro.medium.com/v2/resize:fit:1021/1*zvFTUOSXHPNYxhri_F1PWw.png.

Test Your Knowledge

1. Name one digital inhaler technology used for monitoring adherence?
2. What is the role of combination therapies in future respiratory disease management?

SUMMARY

The intricate interaction between drug treatment and respiratory system performance identifies important opportunities and challenges for the optimization of patient management. Throughout the discussion, it has been apparent that drugs used to treat respiratory diseases, including bronchodilators, corticosteroids, and antibiotics, need to be administered with meticulous attention to individual patient characteristics in order to optimize efficacy and limit side effects. The new role played by adjunct devices like health cards in enabling swift and precise exchange of information among healthcare providers further highlights the significance of holistic care in acute respiratory situations. These communication improvements enable earlier interventions by respiratory therapists, nurses, and pharmacists, ultimately leading to enhanced patient outcomes in emergency settings. These systemic improvements emphasize that the future of respiratory pharmacotherapy is more than just the drugs themselves, but also holistic approaches that enhance the safety and efficacy of respiratory treatment regimens. Furthermore, recent global events such as the COVID-19 pandemic have highlighted the far-reaching implications of respiratory diseases on public health and the growing dependence on pharmacological treatments. The pandemic led to a reconsideration of respiratory drug use patterns, as well as related mental health medicines, to manage the double burden of physical and psychological morbidity. A significant rise in psychotropic prescriptions among children and teens within this period highlights the interdependence of respiratory disease control and mental health issues (Jérémy et al., 2024). These observations highlight the extent to which respiratory pathogens impact not just the pulmonary system but the wider context of healthcare demand, where a multidisciplinary approach to drug delivery and tracking is required. An understanding of these dynamics ensures that respiratory medication is incorporated wisely in context within overall patient care paradigms to optimize treatment compliance and therapeutic outcome. In summary, the drug situation involving the respiratory system requires ongoing appraisal and adjustment to address new clinical needs. Improvements in pharmacologic drugs in conjunction with more effective healthcare communication aids signify a paradigm shift towards more individualized and effective respiratory care. Though the effectiveness of respiratory medications is still at the forefront, attention must also be given to situational factors like comorbidities, patient education, and psychosocial determinants brought to light by pandemic data (Jérémy et al., 2024). Clinical practice and future research should aim for innovations that not only enhance drug action but also promote interdisciplinary practice, patient safety, and access to treatment that is equitable. By tackling these complicated issues, healthcare systems can more effectively control respiratory diseases and enhance patient quality of life overall.

Summary of Key Points

The respiratory apparatus is vulnerable to a range of pharmacologic agents used to treat or mitigate diseases like asthma, COPD, and respiratory infections. These medications exert their effects through various mechanisms, such as bronchodilation, anti-inflammatory action, and mucolytic properties, to enhance airflow and gas exchange. Beta-agonists, for instance, activate adrenergic receptors to cause bronchodilation with fast relief from bronchospasm. By contrast, corticosteroids suppress airway inflammation more slowly, but they control chronic symptoms and prevent exacerbations. Knowledge of the particular action and use of these medications is important in maximizing therapeutic benefit, particularly with the intricate interplay of symptoms and underlying pathologies in respiratory disorders. A treatment approach that is multifaceted underscores the significance of individualized pharmacotherapy in managing both acute attacks and chronic disease management. Apart from their desired effects, medications affecting the respiratory pathway are usually accompanied by inherent side effects and hazards that need to be weighed against their therapeutic index. For example, though beta-agonists reverse bronchoconstriction, their absorption into the general circulation can induce tachycardia and trembling and thus complicate treatment in cardiovascular comorbid patients. Corticosteroids, despite their potent anti-inflammatory properties, induce immunosuppression as well as disturbances in metabolism and require judicious dosing regimens. Furthermore, antibiotic drugs employed to fight respiratory infections should be carefully administered to avoid resistance and maintain microbial equilibrium. These aspects become progressively important in public health contexts since drug abuse and excessive use of pharmacotherapies have effects on population health trends for substance abuse and chronic diseases (Authors et al., 2019). Thus, continuous monitoring and education of the patient continue to be key elements of respiratory drug treatment. New evidence also confirms the hurdles encountered in providing optimal respiratory care in different healthcare systems, especially in rural or underserved areas where access to expert healthcare professionals can be lacking. The effectivity of drugs influencing the respiratory tract relies not only upon their pharmacological characteristics but also upon appropriate administration as well as observation. Studies have highlighted deficiencies in healthcare delivery models where undertrained personnel may lack the capacity to provide consistent and comprehensive care (Eskeland et al., 2025). Such gaps can lead to suboptimal treatment adherence and poor patient outcomes, emphasizing the need for integrated health strategies that address both drug availability and healthcare infrastructure. Overall, the summary of key points reveals that while pharmacological interventions remain central to managing respiratory diseases, their success depends on a confluence of appropriate drug selection, side effect management, and systemic healthcare support.

KEY TERMS FROM THIS CHAPTER

- Mechanisms of Action
- Treatment compliance
- Nevertheless
- Chronic respiratory diseases
- Health integration
- Patient compliance
- Developments
- Respiratory System
- Antihistamines
- Respiratory System
- Emergency healthcare
- Pharmacologic
- Allergic Rhinitis

CRITICAL THINKING QUESTIONS

1. **The primary mechanism of action of corticosteroids in asthma is?**
   a. Bronchodilation
   b. Inhibition of histamine release
   c. Anti-inflammatory action
   d. Stimulation of β2-receptors
2. **Which of the following drugs is a leukotriene receptor antagonist used in asthma management?**
   a. Cromolyn sodium
   b. Montelukast
   c. Ipratropium
   d. Theophylline
3. **Ipratropium bromide is classified as a?**
   a. β2-agonist
   b. Leukotriene inhibitor
   c. Muscarinic antagonist
   d. Corticosteroid
4. **Theophylline toxicity is most likely associated with which of the following?**
   a. Hypoglycemia
   b. Narrow therapeutic index
   c. Anticholinergic effects
   d. Beta-blocker use
5. **Which inhaled corticosteroid is commonly used for long-term control of asthma?**
   a. Budesonide
   b. Tiotropium
   c. Salbutamol
   d. Montelukast

Short Answer Questions

1. Describe the classification of Types of Drugs Affecting the Respiratory System with examples?
2. What is Include their mechanism, indications, and side effects?
3. What is Common Respiratory Conditions Treated with Drugs?
4. Describe the mechanism of action, therapeutic uses, and side effects of anticholinergic drugs in COPD?
5. Which of Impact of Drug Abuse on the Respiratory System?
6. Here is a Current Research and Developments in drugs affecting the respiratory system?

Answer to Critical Thinking Questions

1. (c) 2 (b) 3. (c) 4. (b) 5. (a)

REFERENCES

1. Aarestrup, F. M., Aarestrup, A., Ahuja, S., Aidara-Kane, A., Zumla, A., Allegranzi, B., & Allegranzi, S. (2015). Exploring the evidence base for national and regional policy interventions to combat resistance. *Core*. https://core.ac.uk/download/36779210.pdf.
2. Agarwal, R., Anderson, M., Appleton, S., Barnes, P. J., Borgstrom, L., Boyd, J., et al. (2011). Inhaled corticosteroids versus long-acting beta-agonists for chronic obstructive pulmonary disease (Review). *Core*. https://core.ac.uk/download/10674735.pdf (accessed on 9 May 2025).
3. Al Harbi, Z. N. S., Al Harbi, M. B., Yami, Y. S., Al Anazi, A. A. A., Al Anazi, F. F. I., Al Mutairi, F. Q., Al Otaibi, S. M., Al Dawood, S. A., & Al Harbi, M. L. H. (2025). The role of health cards in emergency response: Enhancing respiratory care, nursing, and pharmacist support in public spaces: A literature review. *International Journal of Development Research, 15*(1), 67439–67442. https://www.semanticscholar.org/paper/0bda22abeff47b876da56e29e4629758c722122e (accessed on 9 May 2025).
4. Alicia Elvira Cruz Jiménez, L., Quintanar Vera, L., & Lujan-Montelongo, J. A. (2021). An overview of antivirals for treating lower respiratory tract infections. *Journal of the Mexican Chemical Society*. https://www.semanticscholar.org/paper/c0621f171441e9bf0b777efe17a78e3dede53713 (accessed on 9 May 2025).
5. Altman, R., Anonymous, M., Arthurs, F., Aubier, A., Bailey, M., Barnes, P., Bateman, E., et al. (2009). Regular treatment with salmeterol and inhaled steroids for chronic asthma: Serious adverse events. *Core*. https://core.ac.uk/download/9537051.pdf (accessed on 9 May 2025).
6. Amaducci, S., Bacci, E., Baldacci, S., Bartoli, et al. (2018). Inhalation therapy in the next decade: Determinants of adherence to treatment in asthma and COPD. *Core*. https://core.ac.uk/download/152415584.pdf (accessed on 9 May 2025).
7. Ambra Butera, M., Pirrone, M., Accetta, A. S., Consoli, C., Nicotera, A., & Turriziani, L. (2024). Unraveling the impact: Pulmonary side effects of anti-seizure medications. *Current Respiratory Medicine Reviews*. https://www.semanticscholar.org/paper/d842301be4b821fca6dd3ec84fd4ef61dc8adf9e (accessed on 9 May 2025).
8. André, S., Areias, V., Boléo-Tomé, J. P., Cardoso, et al. (2019). COPD and cardiovascular disease. *Core*. https://core.ac.uk/download/225163131.pdf (accessed on 9 May 2025).
9. Apter, A., Cervin, A., Greiner, A., Gruver, A., Kalpaklioglu, A., Mediaty, A., Rogkakou, A., et al. (2010). Rhinitis in the geriatric population. *Core*. https://core.ac.uk/download/pdf/8419413.pdf.
10. Authors, N. (2019). *Growing Up in Ireland: Key Findings—Cohort '98 at 20 Years Old in 2018/19 (No. 2): Physical Health and Development*. Economic and Social Research Institute. https://core.ac.uk/download/286731407.pdf (accessed on 9 May 2025).
11. Avino, P., Biondi Zoccai, G., Cammalleri, V., Frati, G., et al. (2020). Impact of electronic alternatives to tobacco cigarettes on indoor air particulate matter levels. *Core*. https://core.ac.uk/download/322821270.pdf.
12. Baiardini, I., Bosnic-Anticevich, S., Braido, F., Carter, V., et al. (2016). "Trying, but failing": The role of inhaler technique and mode of delivery in respiratory medication adherence. *Core*. https://core.ac.uk/download/77051903.pdf (accessed on 9 May 2025).

13. Bär, S., Räber, I., Koskinas, K., Schlapbach, C., & Räber, L. (2022). Transient injection site reaction to alirocumab during immune system activation: A case series. *European Heart Journal: Case Reports, 6.* https://www.semanticscholar.org/paper/a2229fe114eccc49c82a9d7a9eb18f9f85615987 (accessed on 9 May 2025).

14. Beattie, L., Biello, S. M., Espie, C. A., Kyle, S., et al. (2015). How are normal sleeping controls selected? A systematic review of cross-sectional insomnia studies, and a standardized method to select healthy controls for sleep research. *Core.* https://core.ac.uk/download/42359012.pdf (accessed on 9 May 2025).

15. Beeh, K. M., Cazzola, M., Price, D., Roche, W., & others. (2015). Assessing the clinical value of fast onset and sustained duration of action of long-acting bronchodilators for COPD. *Pulmonary Pharmacology & Therapeutics, 31*, 68–78. https://core.ac.uk/download/30435639.pdf (accessed on 9 May 2025).

16. Beltran Paschoal, J. F., Santos, I. P., Malaquias, D. M., de Freitas, K. C., Leão, M. E. B., Silva, A. C., da Silva, K. L., et al. (2025). Comparative analysis of the best drug of choice for sedation in a surgical procedure in elderly patients: Pros and side effects of sedatives. *Journal of Anesthesia.* https://www.semanticscholar.org/paper/04fed51def341c6feb9a4c7efec75f092c6236ea (accessed on 9 May 2025).

17. Bertolini, A., van de Peppel, I. P., Bodewes, F. A. J. A., Moshage, H., Fantin, A., Farinati, F., Fiorotto, R., et al. (2020). Abnormal liver function tests in patients with COVID-19: Relevance and potential pathogenesis. *Hepatology, 72*(6), 1864–1872. https://doi.org/10.1002/hep.31480.

18. Blondonnet, R., Simand, L. A., Vidal, P., Borao, L., Bourguignon, N., Morand, D., Bernard, L., et al. (2022). Design and rationale of the Sevoflurane for Sedation in Acute Respiratory Distress Syndrome (SESAR) randomized controlled trial. *Journal of Clinical Medicine, 11* https://www.semanticscholar.org/paper/1266e40c899081083abaabb657d42a1492d7c6a5 (accessed on 9 May 2025).

19. Brém, E., Koyfman, A., & Long, B. J. (2020). Oncologic emergencies: Immune-based cancer therapies and complications. *Core.* https://core.ac.uk/download/305124082.pdf.

20. Brusselle, G., Derom, E., & Joos, G. (2019). The once-daily fixed-dose combination of olodaterol and tiotropium in the management of COPD: Current evidence and future prospects. *Therapeutic Advances in Respiratory Disease, 13,* 1–24. https://core.ac.uk/download/237011606.pdf (accessed on 9 May 2025).

21. Cami-Kobeci, G., Czoty, P. W., DeLoid, H. B., Ding, F., et al. (2019). BU10038 as a safe opioid analgesic with fewer side effects after systemic and intrathecal administration in primates. *Core.* https://core.ac.uk/download/287581729.pdf (accessed on 9 May 2025).

22. Connors, G., Gould, K., King, S., Lenoir-Wijnkoop, V., et al. (2019). Does probiotic consumption reduce antibiotic utilization for common acute infections? A systematic review and meta-analysis. *Core.* https://core.ac.uk/download/323070509.pdf.

23. Costa, V. M., Grando, L. G. R., Milandri, E., Nardi, J., Teixeira, P., Mladěnka, P., Remião, F., et al. (2022). Natural sympathomimetic drugs: From pharmacology to toxicology. *Biomolecules, 12.* https://www.semanticscholar.org/paper/4eb77f95a85553c9cbfd32f38fc255a2db12fec1 (accessed on 9 May 2025).

24. Couturas, J., Jost, J., Schadler, L., Bodeau, N., Moysan, V., Lescarret, B., Olliac, B., et al. (2024). Impact of the COVID-19 health crisis on psychotropic drug use in children and adolescents in

France. *Child and Adolescent Psychiatry and Mental Health, 18*. https://www.semanticscholar.org/paper/b18fb28b4a0a655a9ec0ab16d57c8a0b0497a744 (accessed on 9 May 2025).

25. Crawford, M. W., & Jerath, R. (2015). How does the body affect the mind? Role of cardiorespiratory coherence in the spectrum of emotions. *Core*. https://core.ac.uk/download/131207333.pdf (accessed on 9 May 2025).

26. Curtis, M., & Guterman, L. (2009). *Overdose Prevention and Response: A Guide for People Who Use Drugs and Harm Reduction Staff in Eastern Europe and Central Asia*. Open Society Institute. https://core.ac.uk/download/pdf/11869816.pdf (accessed on 9 May 2025).

27. De Servi, B., & Piqué i Clusella, N. (2019). Rhinosectan® spray (containing xyloglucan) on the ciliary function of the nasal respiratory epithelium: Results of an *in vitro* study. *Allergy, Asthma & Clinical Immunology, 14*, 41. https://core.ac.uk/download/211868394.pdf (accessed on 9 May 2025).

28. Dowdy, R. A. E., Forgy, S., Hefnawi, O., & Neimar, T. A. (2023). A review of current oral sedation agents for pediatric dentistry. *Anesthesia Progress*. https://www.semanticscholar.org/paper/2d7b2d3da1cbd1a10d759624a480d7cff05feac6 (accessed on 9 May 2025).

29. Eskeland, G. S., Lewis, M., & Traa-Valerezo, X. (2025). Challenging El Salvador's rural health care strategy. *Core*. https://core.ac.uk/download/pdf/6616034.pdf (accessed on 9 May 2025).

30. Ganeshan, T. K. (2019). Investigating the protective role of the natural hormone melatonin in reducing drug-induced cardiotoxicity in the therapy of chronic diseases. https://core.ac.uk/download/287605215.pdf (accessed on 9 May 2025).

31. García-González, M., Mora-Martín, M., López-Fernández, S., López-Díaz, J., Martínez-Sellés, M., Romero-García, J., Cordero, M., et al. (2013). Rationale and design of a randomized, double-blind, placebo-controlled multicenter trial to study efficacy, safety, and long-term effects of intermittent repeated levosimendan administration in patients with advanced heart failure: LAICA study. *Cardiovascular Drugs and Therapy, 27*, 573–579. https://www.semanticscholar.org/paper/99b84b34e6fe67dfa599c9069e4518c083c11c15 (accessed on 9 May 2025).

32. Guzik, T. J., Mohiddin, S., Dimarco, A., Patel, V., Savvatis, K., Marelli-Berg, F. M., Madhur, M. S., et al. (2020). COVID-19 and the cardiovascular system: Implications for risk assessment, diagnosis, and treatment options. *Cardiovascular Research, 116*, 1666–1687. https://doi.org/10.1093/cvr/cvaa106.

33. Haahtela, T., Valovirta, E., Saarinen, K., Jantunen, J., Lindström, I., Kauppi, P., Laatikainen, T., et al. (2021). The Finnish Allergy Program 2008-2018: Society-wide proactive program for change of management to mitigate allergy burden. *Journal of Allergy and Clinical Immunology, 148*, 319–326.e4. https://doi.org/10.1016/j.jaci.2021.03.037.

34. Hou, K., Wu, Z. X., Chen, X. Y., Wang, J. Q., Zhang, D., Xiao, C., Zhu, D., et al. (2022). Microbiota in health and diseases. *Signal Transduction and Targeted Therapy, 7*. https://doi.org/10.1038/s41392-022-00974-4.

35. Hu, B., Guo, H., Zhou, P., & Shi, Z. L. (2020). Characteristics of SARS-CoV-2 and COVID-19. *Nature Reviews Microbiology, 19*, 141–154. https://doi.org/10.1038/s41579-020-00459-7.

36. Humbert, M., Kovács, G., Hoeper, M. M., Badagliacca, R., Berger, R. M. F., Brida, M., Carlsen, J., et al. (2022). 2022 ESC/ERS guidelines for the diagnosis and treatment of pulmonary hypertension. *European Respiratory Journal, 61*, 2200879. https://doi.org/10.1183/13993003.00879-2022.

37. ISI-SENAI-CIMATEC Group, & Development and Innovation Laboratory of Butantan (2020). Therapies against COVID-19: A running to a treatment. *Journal of Bioengineering and Technology Applied to Health*. https://www.semanticscholar.org/paper/c85af25528f7679ec6fcc9012ee65739f4074555 (accessed on 9 May 2025).

38. Keusch, S., Turk, A., Saxer, S., Ehlken, N., Grunig, E., Ulrich, S., & On behalf of the Swiss Society of Pulmonary Hypertension. (2017). Rehabilitation in patients with pulmonary arterial hypertension. *Swiss Medical Weekly, 147*, w14462. https://www.semanticscholar.org/paper/35adc0ee9d0e1616d95d950e09ea69d2c9a7247f (accessed on 9 May 2025).

39. Kilgore, D., & Najm, W. (2010). Common respiratory diseases. https://core.ac.uk/download/323075715.pdf.

40. Korokin, M. V., Korokina, L. V., Pokopejko, O. N., Zhernakova, T. A., et al. (2018). Principles of pharmacological correction of pulmonary arterial hypertension. https://core.ac.uk/download/161831436.pdf (accessed on 9 May 2025).

41. Liu, J., Wang, J., Xiong, A., Zhang, L., Zhang, Y., Liu, Y., Xiong, Y., et al. (2023). Mitochondrial quality control in lung diseases: Current research and future directions. *Frontiers in Physiology, 14*. https://www.semanticscholar.org/paper/37cb0727f39a6443f566d1d05710334a75a7e866 (accessed on 9 May 2025).

42. Malkova, O. G., Mashaeva, O. G., Sobetova, G. V., Orlov, A. V., Rakhimov, R. T., Vtyurina, G. V., Kistankina, M. V., et al. (2023). Assessing changes in the pattern of healthcare-associated infectious agents in intensive care units during a novel coronavirus infection pandemic (COVID-19). *Ural Medical Journal*. https://www.semanticscholar.org/paper/a4f890d39fcb7d2f007f0b1a3f5c79287a66c0dd (accessed on 9 May 2025).

43. Monaghesh, E., & Hajizadeh, A. (2020). The role of telehealth during the COVID-19 outbreak: A systematic review based on current evidence. *BMC Public Health, 20*, 1–9. https://doi.org/10.1186/s12889-020-09301-4.

44. Murray, C. J. L., Ikuta, K. S., Sharara, F., Swetschinski, L. R., Robles Aguilar, G., Gray, A. P., Han, C., et al. (2022). Global burden of bacterial antimicrobial resistance in 2019: A systematic analysis. *The Lancet, 399*(1035), 629–655. https://doi.org/10.1016/s0140-6736(21)02724-0.

45. Rachina, S., Kozlov, R., Kurkova, A., Portnyagina, U., Palyutin, S., Khokhlov, A., Reshetko, O., et al. (2022). Antimicrobial dispensing practice in community pharmacies in Russia during the COVID-19 pandemic. *Antibiotics, 11*. https://www.semanticscholar.org/paper/d008d3a4d13447318ca52a4ea29452317d3e1e0c (accessed on 9 May 2025).

46. Richardson, S., Hirsch, J. S., Narasimhan, M., Crawford, J. M., McGinn, T., Davidson, K. W., Barnaby, D. P., et al. (2020). Presenting characteristics, comorbidities, and outcomes among 5700 patients hospitalized with COVID-19 in the New York City area. *JAMA, 323*, 2052. https://doi.org/10.1001/jama.2020.6775.

47. Silva, B., Soares, J., Rocha-Pereira, C., Mladěnka, P., Remião, F., & Oemonom Researchers (2022). Khat, a cultural chewing drug: A toxicokinetic and toxicodynamic summary. *Toxins, 14*(16). https://www.semanticscholar.org/paper/16d570928ce2b125f2554e34c271f16ae1a67213 (accessed on 9 May 2025).

48. Sisson, J. (2020). The effects and implications of vaping on the youth population. https://core.ac.uk/download/304169056.pdf (accessed on 9 May 2025).

49. Symes, R., Keddie, S. H., Walker, J., McKeever, T., Ahmad, S., Arnold, D., Evans, C. M., et al. (2025). Estimating the disease burden of respiratory syncytial virus (RSV) in older adults in England during the 2023/24 season: A new national hospital-based surveillance system. https://www.semanticscholar.org/paper/46cc949c37444336e0b7469239dc7b20ec447f14 (accessed on 9 May 2025).

50. Tamboli, A. R., Yadav, V. D., Nadaf, S., Nivekar, V. V., Salve, K. S., Tamboli, E., & Nalawade, A. M. (2024). Exploring the frontier of inhalation therapy: A review of dry powder inhalers for precision management of inflammatory lung diseases. *BIO Integration*. https://www.semanticscholar.org/paper/c231f50b4c0e6f3dca299f657a1a5011fe3b1adb (accessed on 9 May 2025).

51. Thachil, J. (2020). The versatile heparin in COVID-19. *Journal of Thrombosis and Haemostasias, 18*(6), 1020–1022. https://doi.org/10.1111/jth.14821.

52. Visrodia, P., Ramireddy, A., Chugh, H., Reinier, K., Uy-Evanado, A., Jui, J., & Chugh, S. (2021). Abstract 11767: Mechanisms of nighttime sudden death: Arrhythmogenic potential of central nervous system-affecting medications. *Circulation*. https://www.semanticscholar.org/paper/c15579aa8e35c5453125eefbfafb13741ead8d62 (accessed on 9 May 2025).

53. Visseren, F. L. J., Mach, F., Smulders, Y. M., Carballo, D., Koskinas, K. C., Bäck, M., Bénétos, A., et al. (2021). 2021 ESC guidelines on cardiovascular disease prevention in clinical practice. *European Heart Journal, 42*(36), 3227–3337. https://doi.org/10.1093/eurheartj/ehab484.

54. Wichmann, D. (2020). Autopsy findings and venous thromboembolism in patients with COVID-19. *Annals of Internal Medicine, 173*, 1030–1030. https://doi.org/10.7326/l20-1206.

55. Zhou, X., Huang, T., Pan, H., Du, A., Wu, T., Lan, J., Song, Y., et al. (2024). Bioinformatics and system biology approaches to determine the connection of SARS-CoV-2 infection and intrahepatic cholangiocarcinoma. *PLOS ONE, 19*. https://www.semanticscholar.org/paper/408a667bfc672a4d5ad25737becce3bde28b1b68 (accessed on 9 May 2025).

DRUGS AFFECTING THE CENTRAL NERVOUS SYSTEM

7

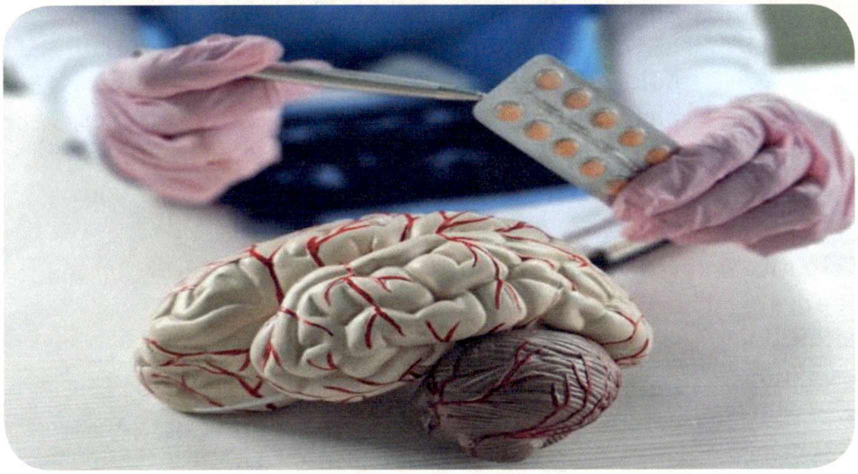

LEARNING OBJECTIVES

After studying this chapter, you will be able to:

1. Explain Types of Drugs Affecting the CNS
2. Define Mechanisms of Action
3. Identify the Short-Term Effects of CNS Drugs
4. Explore Long-Term Effects of CNS Drugs
5. Discuss the Treatment and Rehabilitation
6. Define of Societal Implications

Introduction

The human body functions through the interaction of intricate systems, which perform specialized roles to ensure general health and wellness. Of all the systems in the body, the central nervous system (CNS) plays a vital role in controlling the functions of the body, integrating sensory information, and coordinating actions. This integrated system, comprising the brain and spinal cord, governs cognition, emotion, and movement. With its importance, any change in CNS activity has the potential to significantly affect the physical and psychological well-being of an individual. Pharmacological substances that target this system—the CNS drugs—find themselves with an enormous range of uses, ranging from therapeutic medication of neurological illnesses to mood modification and behavior adjustment (Figure 7.1). It is essential to study these drugs, their modes of action, and their effects as a way to further medical science and enhance the outcome of patient care. Biomedical breakthroughs have underlined the CNS as an integral target for all types of pharmacological treatments considering its involvement in wide-ranging pathologies. Neuroactive medications will affect the proportion of neurotransmitters, enhancing or blocking synaptic action and consequently the neural circuitries. The therapy covers a continuum of drugs and treatments including analgesics, anesthetics, and psychiatric medications targeting diseases of the mind. The capacity to control CNS activity has also come with its own set of challenges, including dependency and negative side effects, highlighting the need for thorough research in drug development and clinical use. Current research highlights the interconnectivity of the CNS with other physiological systems, including the gut microbiota via the gut-brain axis, which can affect drug metabolism and efficacy in neurological therapy (Silva et al., 2020). This new perspective provides promise for creative therapeutic approaches that incorporate systemic physiological knowledge. In addition, the effect of drugs on the CNS goes beyond individual health and reaches societal and economic levels.

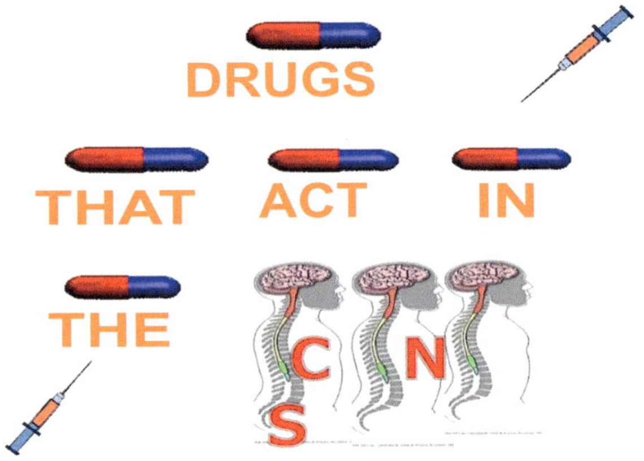

Figure 7.1. Drugs affecting the central nervous system (CNS).

Source: https://cdn.slidesharecdn.com/ss_thumbnails/pharmarprt-141004201926-conversion-gate02-thumbnail-4.jpg?cb=1412454054.

As the population ages globally, CNS-related diseases, such as neurodegenerative diseases and mental disorders, are on the increase, placing a pressing need on the need for effective pharmaceutical treatments. Predictive models of healthcare indicate that specific interventions will mitigate the increasing burden of such conditions, improve quality of life, and save healthcare costs (Bray et al., 2024). Research into CNS drugs is therefore not only a scientific pursuit but also a matter of public health urgency. Ongoing research and development hold the potential for greater insight into CNS pharmacology, refinement of drug safety profiles, and ultimately towards more effective treatment of disorders that deeply impact millions globally.

Definition of the Central Nervous System (CNS)

Appreciation of the intricate nature of the human body requires consideration of its composite systems, particularly those in charge of dealing with and integrating vital functions. Most notable among them is the central nervous system (CNS), the master regulatory structure that coordinates sensory input and motor output (Figure 7.2). The CNS is mainly composed of the brain and spinal cord, which constitute a highly complex network that regulates cognition, emotion, and physiological reactions. This system serves as the body's control center, deciphering messages from both the external and internal world to ensure homeostasis and facilitate purposeful behavior. The CNS's characteristic cellular structure, comprising neurons and glial cells, facilitates its function of information integration quickly and efficiently, thus underscoring its critical role in general human health and behavior. Becoming even more specialized anatomically and functionally, the CNS is heavily networked to the periphery yet remains dissimilar from peripheral structures. The CNS processes tremendous amounts of sensory input and formulates a correct response either automatically or in conjunction with feedback control via other systems. Data receipt, integration into a signal, and output of motion represent the essential operations of the CNS conducted in an enveloped structure within a cranium and spinal column. This encapsulation guarantees the CNS is shielded from damage, highlighting its paramount significance in survival and functionality.

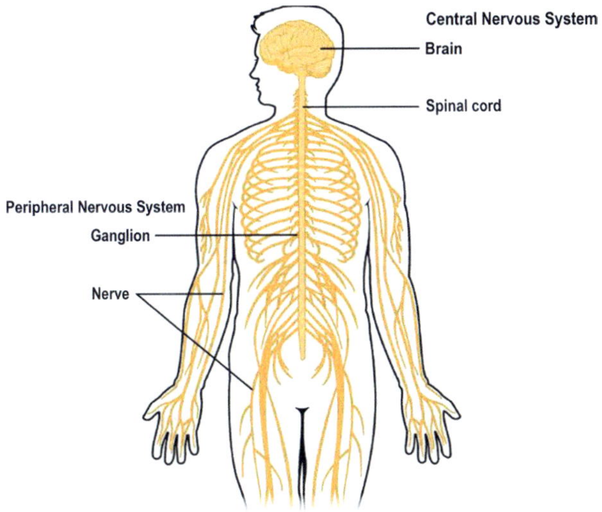

Figure 7.2. Central nervous system (CNS).

Source:

OpenStax. (n.d.). *Overview of nervous system.* Wikimedia Commons. https://upload.wikimedia.org/wikipedia/commons/d/d3/1201_Overview_of_Nervous_System.jpg.

Further, recent studies reveal its dynamic interconnection with other body systems, including the microbiota-gut-brain axis, to highlight bidirectional communication pathways that impact neurological and immune function (Hou et al., 2022; John et al., 2019). From the pharmacological viewpoint, the CNS is a principal target for several drugs designed to alter neurological function either to return balance or change mental states. Drugs that traverse the BBB enter the CNS by interacting with the neurotransmitters and receptors that are part of central processing, and thus they can influence consciousness, mood, sensation of pain, and motor function. It is vital to comprehend the subtlety of CNS anatomy and physiology for the creation of therapeutics capable of treating neurological disease effectively with minimal side effects. This also demonstrates how changes in CNS function can be due not just from injuries or genetic influences but also from changes in microbiota composition and systemic inflammation, aspects that are ever more prevalent in neuropharmacology and CNS drug discovery (Hou et al., 2022; John et al., 2019).

Importance of Studying Drugs Affecting the CNS

Identifying the intricate effects of pharmaceuticals on the CNS is critical in moving forward the development of medicine and patient success. The CNS controls an overwhelming majority of physical processes, such as motor coordination and mental capabilities, and plays a key area in which interventions could take hold to relieve various conditions, like neurodegenerative diseases, psychiatric illnesses, and neurological traumas. Without extensive research, the subtle mechanisms by which such drugs act are not well understood, and hence may lead to suboptimal efficacy or side effects. In addition, the CNS's specialized protective barriers, like the BBB, pose obstacles to drug delivery, requiring breakthroughs based on in-depth pharmacological studies. Therefore, the investigation of CNS-active drugs is essential for the development of safer, more efficacious treatments capable of tackling the intricate pathophysiology of CNS disorders. The increasing incidence of neuropsychiatric and neurodevelopmental disorders further emphasizes the relevance of CNS-acting drug research. Disorders like autism spectrum disorder (ASD) are increasingly known to have not just genetic but also immunological and environmental factors, offering complex challenges in treatment. Studies on how CNS drugs influence immune responses and neuroinflammation provide promising directions for the management of such disorders. For instance, anti-inflammatory compounds such as resveratrol and palmitoylethanolamide have shown promise in mitigating ASD symptoms by acting on neuroimmune mechanisms, underlining the relationship between the CNS and systemic mechanisms in disease expression (Heidari et al., 2021).

Through the comprehension of these intricate interactions, pharmacological studies can make progress toward focused therapies that correct underlying immunological impairments, thus enhancing quality of life in affected individuals and diminishing dependence on symptomatic management alone. In addition to neurodevelopmental disorders, research into CNS drugs has critical implications for management of global health issues, most notably the load of cancer and its neurological side effects. Cancer mainly impacts peripheral organs, yet numerous patients present with CNS symptoms like cognitive deterioration or neuropathic pain that are commonly related to either disease or therapy.

Research directed towards CNS pharmacology can result in measures that counteract these harmful effects and increase patient comfort and function. Furthermore, the incidence of cancer globally is anticipated to expand significantly, further enforcing the necessity for interventions favoring CNS health among cancer survivors (Bray et al., 2024). Researching CNS drugs can therefore not only lead to direct therapies of CNS diseases but also to holistic treatment of multifaceted conditions with neurological symptoms, highlighting the general societal and medical importance of this research area.

7.1. Types of Drugs Affecting the CNS

Learning Outcome

1. Stimulants
2. Depressants
3. Hallucinogens

The heterologous group of drugs affecting the CNS acts by controlling neuron activity through a variety of mechanisms, resulting in broad therapeutic and psychoactive impacts (Figure 7.3). Among these drugs, depressants like benzodiazepines and barbiturates act by potentiating the inhibitory neurotransmitter gamma-aminobutyric acid (GABA), leading to sedation, anxiolysis, and muscle relaxation. On the other hand, stimulants like amphetamines and methylphenidate raise synaptic levels of excitatory neurotransmitters like dopamine and norepinephrine, leading to increased alertness and attention. Opioids are another significant class, which act on specific receptors in the CNS, mainly to control pain perception and cause euphoria. The sophistication of their actions in the brain makes selective targeting critical to limit side effects. Innovations like the creation of graphene-based nanomaterials indicate promise towards more targeted drug delivery systems with the potential to transform therapeutic responses by attaining targeted release and reducing systemic toxicity (Cellot et al., 2021). The complexities of drug delivery to the CNS are greatly controlled by the presence of the blood–brain barrier (BBB), a crucial protective interface responsible for controlling the flow of materials between the blood and brain tissue. This selective barrier maintains the homeostasis of the brain through regulation of the flow and efflux of ions, nutrients, and pharmacological drugs. But its protective function presents immense problems for successful CNS pharmacotherapy since most drugs cannot permeate through the BBB to the body at concentrations that are therapeutically relevant. Disruption of the BBB is implicated in numerous neurological disorders, which makes both the pathology and treatment protocols more complex. Knowledge of the cellular elements and processes preserving BBB integrity and biomarkers reflecting its permeability is vital for the formulation of CNS-active drugs capable of traversing this barrier safely and effectively to achieve their pharmacological actions (Kadry et al., 2020). Aside from traditional CNS drugs, the development in nanotechnology advances the concept of designing new drug carriers that would revolutionize pharmacological treatment in neurological diseases. Graphene nanomaterials are an emerging frontier in this area, providing tunable platforms that can penetrate the CNS with high specificity. Functionalization of these nanomaterials with drug molecules or targeting ligands is envisioned to provide controlled release of drugs directly at the sites of disease within the brain. This method has the potential to increase therapeutic efficacy while minimizing systemic side effects, especially in sensitive patient populations like children. The capacity to control the physical and chemical features of these nanodevices points toward a breakthrough direction in precision medicine, in a position to surpass present constraints on CNS medication transport and treatment efficacy (Cellot et al., 2021).

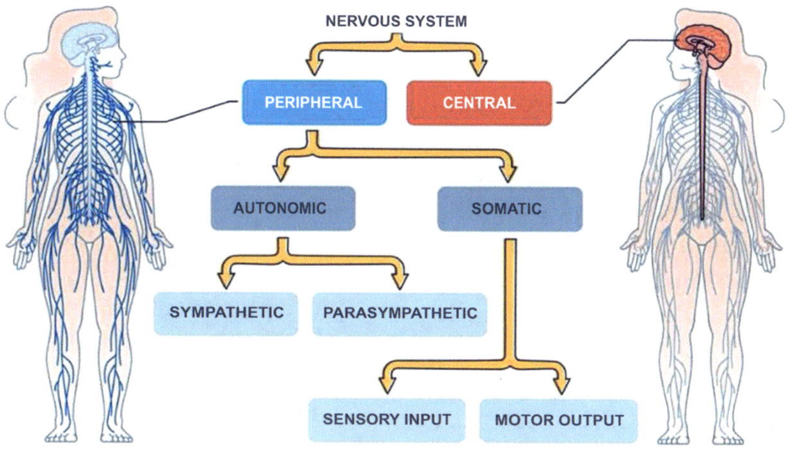

Figure 7.3. Types of drugs affecting the CNS.

Source: Illinois Recovery Center (2023). *Central Nervous System.* https://illinoisrecoverycenter.com/wp-content/uploads/2023/09/Central-Nervous-System-3-1024x768.jpg.

7.1.1. Stimulants

The acute physiological consequences shared in the course of substance use are generally associated with changes in the activity of the sympathetic nervous system. One of the most important elements in such occurrences is increased release of catecholamines like norepinephrine and epinephrine, which induce most of the somatic effects seen, such as increased heart rate, blood pressure, and body temperature changes. These effects are not peripheral but also contribute significantly to the central nervous system's (CNSs) modulation of mood and perception, leading to the typical euphoria and intoxication produced by stimulant drugs. Stimulants act upon the brain's monoaminergic systems, influencing neurotransmitters such as dopamine, serotonin, and norepinephrine by binding to receptors and modulating synaptic signals. Current theories propose that the drugs might also be bio transformed into endogenous catecholamines in the body, amplifying their neuromodulatory actions and reinforcing their addictive potential (Paul, 2021). This suggestion has far-reaching consequences for comprehending how stimulants affect the CNS beyond conventional pharmacological models. The *in vivo* conversion of stimulants to catecholamines could redefine our understanding of the biochemical mechanisms of substance abuse and dependence. Such conversion could be responsible for the sudden onset of stimulating effects and the strong psychological rewards that contribute to drug addiction. Tracking labeled stimulant precursors through state-of-the-art analytical methods such as liquid chromatography-mass spectrometry provides a good lead to prove this hypothesis and deconvolute the bioconversion dynamics. The knowledge expansion on such a molecular basis may feed back into developing new, more productive therapeutic measures in reducing stimulant addiction through modifying these metabolic routes (Paul, 2021). While determining the neurochemical effect of the stimulants is significant, the greater significance of the mechanism by which stimulants exert influence over other bodily systems needs to be seen. The sympathetic response induced by stimulants parallels the physiological stress reactions that the body typically experiences in response to acute danger or exercise. This common mechanism also points to the potential risks of long-term use of stimulants, including cardiovascular stress and disruption of homeostatic mechanisms. Identifying stimulants within the broader context of CNS-acting drugs highlights the need for further research into their multifaceted mechanisms of action, as well as systemic implications of abuse. Such a detailed understanding is essential for informing clinical guidelines and public health policy, particularly in light of the complex interplay between therapeutic applications and the liability to abuse inherent in many psychoactive substances (Paul, 2021).

7.1.2. Depressants

The pharmacological modulation of CNS activity is commonly associated with depressants, a drug class that decreases excitability of neurons and slows down the workings of the brain. Such agents are responsible for sedation, muscle relaxation, anxiolysis, as well as analgesia, thus playing an important role both in clinical situations as well as in traditional medicinal practice. Plant-derived natural compounds have been the source of significant CNS depressants (Figure 7.4) throughout history; e.g., the Holarrhena antidysenterica stem extracts showed considerable analgesic and CNS depressant effects in model systems. Varying solvent extracts of this plant showed dose-dependent locomotor inhibition activity and pain reduction responses, pointing toward their possible applications in treating pain and anxiety disorder conditions (Md. Haque et al., 2018). These observations highlight the need to explore plant sources for new depressant agents and to further elucidate their mechanisms in the modulation of CNS pathways. Clinical use of depressants requires careful consideration of their pharmacokinetics and pharmacodynamics, since these drugs interact in a complex manner with several neurotransmitter systems and metabolic pathways. Cannabinoids, despite their structural differences from traditional depressants, have CNS depressant effects because of their action on neurotransmission. Delta-9-tetrahydrocannabinol (THC) and cannabidiol (CBD), major cannabinoids, exhibit different psychoactive and analgesic effects, requiring individualized administration techniques to reduce risks and enhance therapeutic efficacy. The metabolism of cannabinoids in the liver also makes them difficult to use since enzyme interactions will change the metabolism of other CNS depressants prescribed at the same time, e.g., clobazam. These interactions have the potential to cause additive or synergistic sedation, emphasizing the need for careful dose titration and monitoring of patients to prevent toxicity and adverse effects (Lucas et al., 2018). Awareness of these dynamics is critical to safe incorporation of cannabinoid-based therapies into CNS depressant regimens. The risk of adverse effects and drug interactions is always a concern when prescribing CNS depressants, particularly in susceptible groups like the elderly or those with comorbidities. The additive depressant action of taking several agents together increases risks of cognitive impairment, respiratory depression, and cardiovascular instability and highlights the need for individualized treatment strategies. The paucity of pharmacologic data on more recently introduced plant-derived depressants and cannabinoids warrants a start low and go-slow approach with an emphasis on incremental dose changes and close clinical monitoring. This is critical to balance symptom relief against safety, especially considering the differences in bioavailability, metabolism, and patient sensitivity. Future studies should focus on large-scale clinical trials to clarify the pharmacological profiles of novel depressants to allow optimized and safer use in CNS disorder management paradigms (Lucas et al., 2018; Md. Haque et al., 2018).

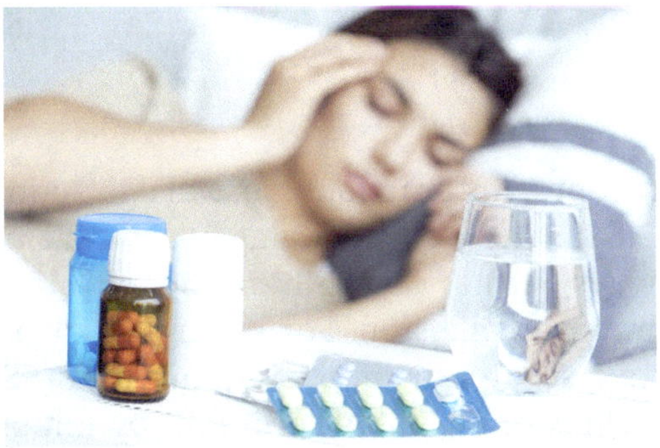

Figure 7.4. Depressants central nervous system (CNS).

Source: https://encrypted-tbn0.gstatic.com/images?q=tbn:ANd9GcQjWsHYs1cjhKr8IWV6-Qr6DDHa_yp2a8vFgA&s.

7.1.3. Hallucinogens

The CNS is strongly affected by a variety of psychoactive drugs, of which hallucinogens have a special place because of their ability to modify perception, thought, and mood (Figure 7.5). They mainly affect serotonergic neurotransmission, particularly through the modulation of the 5-HT2A receptor, which results in changed sensory perceptions and even extreme modifications of consciousness. Unlike depressants or stimulants, hallucinogens may cause vivid visual and auditory distortions without usually leading to dependence or withdrawal phenomena characteristic of other CNS drugs. Nevertheless, the variety of psychological effects is great, ranging from euphoric to horrifying, depending on individual and environmental conditions. This subtle interaction in the CNS highlights the complexity of hallucinogen pharmacodynamics and the danger of unpredictable psychotic attacks in abuse. Analyzing the abuse liability of agents acting on the CNS entails vigilant examination of their receptor affinity and central versus peripheral effects. Studies on agents such as difelikefalin, a selective kappa-opioid receptor agonist with restricted CNS penetration, have found a low risk for abuse from negligible psychoactive effects, such as hallucinogenic activity. In clinical trials of recreational polydrug abusers, difelikefalin showed only slightly higher positive effects than placebo and no worthwhile hallucinogenic events, indicating little probability of central abuse (Megan et al., 2021). These results emphasize the significance of receptor selectivity and blood-brain barrier (BBB) penetration in assessing the hallucinogenic and abuse liability of CNS-active agents, which can influence both therapeutic uses and regulatory guidelines. Outside of classical hallucinogens, it is important to keep in mind that other CNS-acting medications can cause neuropsychiatric side effects that are similar to hallucinogenic effects. Certain antiviral drugs, for example, have been associated with varied CNS toxicities, such as psychosis and perceptual disturbances, because they act on neurotransmitter systems like serotonin and GABA receptors. Interestingly, drugs such as efavirenz have affinities for serotonin receptors and monoamine oxidase enzymes, resulting in subjective effects that are similar to those caused by psychedelic hallucinogens such as lysergic acid diethylamide (LSD) (Zareifopoulos et al., 2020). These toxic effects highlight the wide range of CNS-drug interactions, showing that not only traditional hallucinogens but also other pharmacological categories can affect sensory processing and mental states through intricate neurochemical mechanisms.

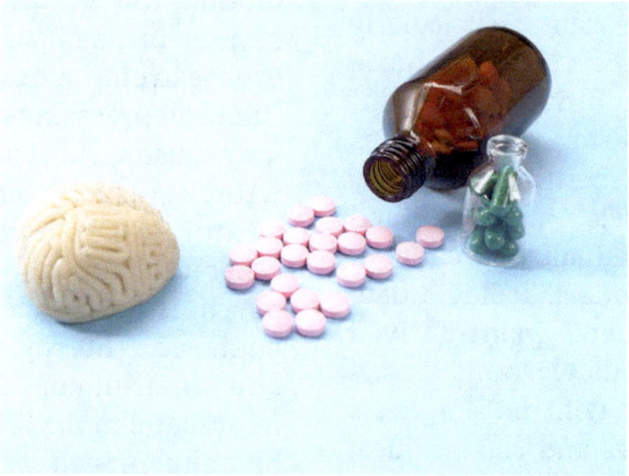

Figure 7.5. Hallucinogens.

Source: AToN Center. (2021). How are hallucinogens taken? https://atoncenter.com/wp-content/uploads/2021/01/how hallucinogens-taken-aton-center.jpg.

Test Your Knowledge

1. Give one example of a central nervous system (CNS).
2. What is a CNS depressant and how does it affect neuronal activity?

7.2. Mechanisms of Action

Learning Outcome

1. Neurotransmitter Interactions
2. Receptor Binding
3. Impact on Neuronal Firing

The complex mechanisms involved in the CNS reaction to pharmacologic agents represent an intricate interplay of cellular communication and receptor interaction. Most drugs acting on the CNS function by modifying neurotransmitter pathways, either by reinforcing or blocking synaptic transmission. For example, drugs like selective serotonin reuptake inhibitors (SSRIs) raise levels of available serotonin by inhibiting its resorption, hence changing mood and cognition. In the same way, antipsychotic drugs tend to be antagonists at dopamine receptors, decreasing overactive dopaminergic activity that is involved in conditions such as schizophrenia. Other than neurotransmitter modulation, certain

CNS medications impact intracellular signaling cascades or ion channel operation, resulting in alterations in neuronal excitability and synaptic plasticity. These varied mechanisms reflect the complex strategies used to restore or redirect neural activity, stressing the need for insight into both systemic and molecular targets within the intricate architecture of the brain. New work in neurodegenerative diseases demonstrates the widening reach of CNS drug mechanisms, especially concerning microglial function. TREM2, the receptor mainly found on microglia, represents an expanding target that affects disease pathology by controlling immune responses and removal of neurotoxic factors. Its action in controlling microglial proliferation, phagocytosis, and inflammatory signaling represents a novel mechanism as opposed to conventional neurotransmitter-based approaches. Interfering with TREM2 represents a novel opportunity for Alzheimer's disease (AD) treatment through amplification of the brain's intrinsic ability to eliminate aberrant proteins and induce neuronal survival, changing perhaps the course of disease instead of just treating its symptoms. Grasping such cellular mechanisms broadens the therapeutic toolset and provides a more sophisticated strategy for CNS drug development beyond symptomatic pharmacologic regimens (Li et al., 2023). This interaction between the CNS and peripheral influences also determines the pharmacological profile, as can be inferred from recent studies on Parkinson's disease. Changes in intestinal flora have been correlated with Parkinson's pathophysiology via mechanisms of neuronal transmission and neuroinflammation. Medications acting on the CNS can indirectly affect disease progression by altering gut microbiota, which subsequently imparts effects on the immune system and neuronal communication in the brain. Furthermore, several anti-Parkinsonian medications have differential activities on the intestinal bacterial communities, which could be responsible for their therapeutic efficacy or side effects. The discovery of this gut-brain axis adds another layer of mechanism, where microbial regulation is coupled with neuropharmacology. This paradigm highlights the need for integrated strategies in CNS drug development taking into account central and peripheral mechanisms to maximize therapeutic outcomes (Chen et al., 2021).

7.2.1. Neurotransmitter Interactions

The complexity of neuronal communication is based on the interaction of multiple neurotransmitters within the CNS. Such chemical messengers do not function alone; rather, they inhibit and modulate one another's activity to ensure synaptic balance and neural network function. Drugs acting on the CNS tend to target individual neurotransmitter systems in order to change this complex balance, perhaps facilitating or suppressing synaptic transmission. For instance, the addictive nature of nicotine stems from its action on nicotinic acetylcholine receptors and the release of neurotransmitters like dopamine, which is central to reward mechanisms and addiction mechanisms. The activation of kinases such as CaMKII and ERK also illustrates how neurotransmitter signaling cascades continue beyond simple receptor activation to impact synaptic plasticity, underlying learning and memory mechanisms that drugs interfere with (Jia et al., 2021). A further complexity comes from the CNS-peripheral systems bidirectional dialogue, particularly in the brain-gut axis. This system aggregates neuroendocrine, immune, and neural signals, and serves to demonstrate the manner in which neurotransmitter activity is modulated not only intrinsically in the brain but also through external influences such as the gastrointestinal (GI) microbiome. Neuroactive substances like serotonin and dopamine, which are made or regulated by gut microbes, have the ability to greatly influence CNS homeostasis by crossing the BBB or activating vagal pathways. Such effects regulate neuroinflammatory processes and immune events associated with injury and disease states. Thus, pharmacological regulation of neurotransmitters has an impact beyond the synaptic cleft, involving systemic well-being and neuroimmune interaction (Wojciech Dąbrowski et al., 2020). Elucidation of neurotransmitter interactions is central to the discovery of therapeutic agents against the CNS, particularly against addiction and neuroinflammatory disorders (Figure 7.6). Intracellular kinases-controlled complex dopamine and acetylcholine signaling pathways provide potential therapeutic targets for modulation of maladaptive plasticity induced by long-term drug exposure. In addition, the identification of the role of neuroactive substances derived from the gut provides windows into CNS disorder treatment from a whole-body approach, treating both the central and the peripheral factors affecting neurotransmission. Further study of these signaling networks and their pharmacological regulation continues to hold the promise of leading to treatments that restore neurochemical balance, prevent addiction, and control neuroinflammation, improving CNS-related disorder outcomes (Jia et al., 2021; Wojciech Dąbrowski et al., 2020).

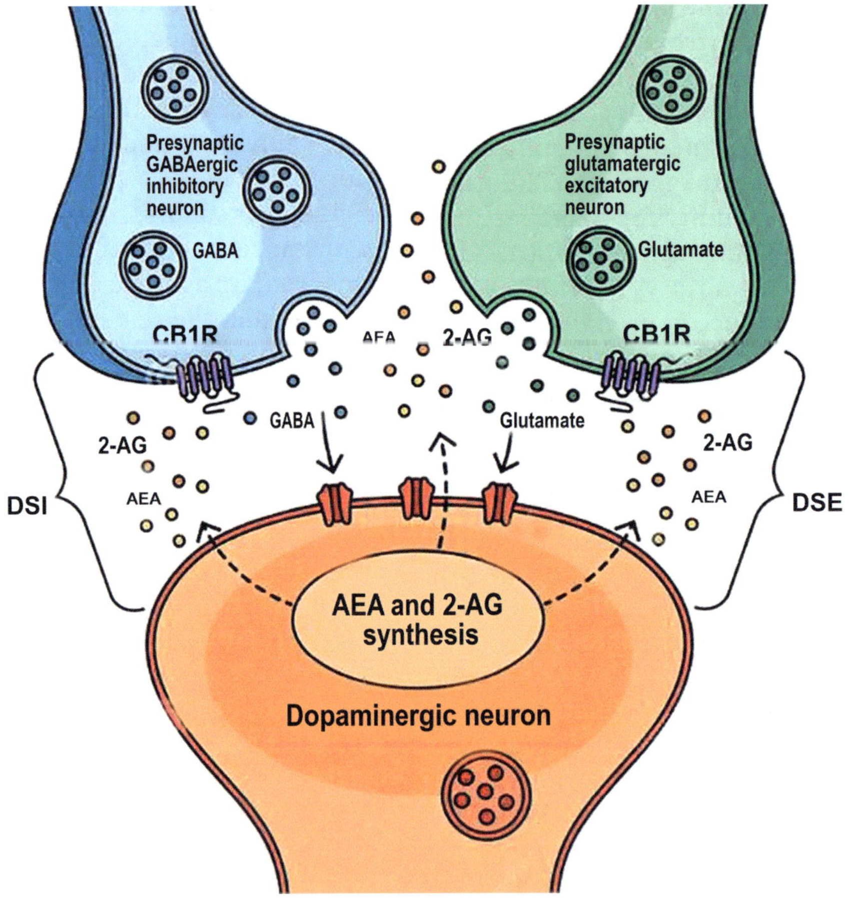

Figure 7.6. Neurotransmitter interactions.

Source: **Pokusay, A.** (n.d.). *Neurotransmitter interactions diagram: Cannabinol and Neuron Structure.* Dreamstime. https://thumbs.dreamstime.com/z/neurotransmitter-interactions-diagram-science-neurotransmitter-interactions-cannabinol-neuron-structure-brain-cell-diagram-292130654.jpg?w=768.

7.2.2. Receptor Binding

The complex interaction between drugs and receptor sites forms the basis for most pharmacological actions seen within the CNS. Neurotransmitters GABA modulate neuronal excitability via receptor binding and have an impact on a vast variety of physiological responses. Drugs that interact with these receptors tend to be agonists, antagonists, or modulators, thus modifying receptor activity to mediate therapeutic or toxic effects. For instance, GABAergic neurotransmission is largely mediated by GABAA and GABAB receptors that have different pharmacodynamic profiles. GABAA receptor modulation by barbiturates or benzodiazepines increases inhibitory signaling and forms the basis for the treatment of conditions like anxiety and epilepsy. All these receptor interactions must be fully comprehended in order to advance the construction of drugs that achieve maximum efficacy while suppressing side effects, thus highlighting the necessity of studying receptor subtypes and allosteric binding sites for precise tailoring of treatments within the CNS (Jazvin et al., 2015). CNS depressants illustrate the intricate pharmacology of receptor binding, especially with endogenous substances like gamma-hydroxybutyrate (GHB). Being a metabolite of GABA, GHB binds significantly with GABAB receptors, acting as neurotransmitter as well as neuromodulator and imparting its sedative and euphoric effects. Its therapeutic application in the treatment of narcolepsy and alcohol withdrawal demonstrates how receptor binding is used for medicinal advantage. However, its narrow therapeutic window and potential for abuse stem from its profound influence on receptor activity, which affects neuronal communication critically. The rapid conversion of GHB precursors and swift pharmacokinetics further complicate clinical management and forensic detection, underlying challenges in monitoring receptor-binding drugs that possess dual roles as medicines and substances of abuse (Busard et al., 2014). Receptor binding selectivity and subtype specificity continue to be paramount in CNS drug design, considering the multiplicity of receptor isoforms and their disparate distributions. Action on unique receptor conformations can maximize therapeutic effects while minimizing untoward effects commonly experienced with broad-spectrum drugs. Such is clearly illustrated for drugs that act on the GABAA receptor complex, where multiple allosteric sites provide chemically unique ligands with fine-tuned modulatory capability. Novel research is becoming more dedicated to the development of subtype-selective ligands that take advantage of such receptor heterogeneities to deliver improved efficacy for the treatment of neuropsychiatric disease without the sedation, tolerance, and dependence that are so typical of non-selective drugs. Such developments hold out a new era in CNS pharmacotherapy by specifically aligning receptor interaction to pathophysiology of particular conditions (Jazvin et al., 2015).

7.2.3. Impact on Neuronal Firing

The drug modulation of neuronal firing, which involves activity in the CNS, is indicative of a subtle interaction between the pharmacological drugs and the patterns of intrinsic neural activity. Firing rates and patterns of neuronal activity are pivotal for encoding sensory information, governing cognition, and ensuring homeostasis in CNS circuits. Pharmacological drugs such as opioids bind to certain subtypes of receptors on neurons, especially in pathways involved in pain processing, thus causing changes in neuronal excitability and firing rates. Morphine, for instance, elicits analgesia through reduction of neuronal discharge by inhibiting neurotransmitter release at synaptic endings. However, long-term administration interferes with the normal patterns of discharge by virtue of neuroadaptations involving changes in gene expression and synaptic plasticity, which can lead to tolerance, dependence, and even neurotoxicity. These interruptions are the perfect illustration of how sustained alterations in neuronal firing underlie the dualistic character of some CNS drugs to deliver both therapeutic and maladaptive effects (Mehrabi et al., 2024). Research using human induced pluripotent stem cell (iPSC)-derived neurons has enhanced the understanding of how neuromodulators essential for CNS function impact neuronal firing patterns. Neurotransmitters like serotonin, acetylcholine, and noradrenaline, which vary throughout the sleep–wake cycle, cause dose-dependent increases in synchronized burst firings in dopaminergic neurons. This action highlights the sensitivity of neuronal networks to chemical modulation and the significance of these neuromodulators in sustaining rhythmic firing necessary for cognitive processing and behavioral states. Moreover, slow-wave sleep-like low-frequency electrical stimulation induces a transient reduction of firing frequency and burst synchrony in glutamatergic neurons, indicative of long-term depression-like events that decrease the efficacy of synapses. The results establish a mechanistic paradigm for how drug-induced modification of neuromodulatory processes can reorganize neuronal firing patterns and synaptic connections within CNS networks (Yokoi et al., 2019). Insight into drug effects on neuronal firing is not limited to acute pharmacodynamics but includes changes in network-level plasticity and synchronization that affect CNS function long-term. The capacity of drugs to produce long-term changes in firing rate and synaptic efficacy can disrupt neural circuitry, appearing as cognitive impairment, emotional dysregulation, or neurodegeneration. For example, repetitive stimulation protocols that regulate firing rates can selectively downregulate large synaptic contacts but not the global network, demonstrating a selective reorganization of firing patterns that drugs can manipulate or interfere with. These plasticity mechanisms are important in both therapeutic interventions, such as recovery promotion in neuropsychiatric disorders, and drug-induced neurotoxicity pathogenesis. Proper regard of these firing-associated effects is thus critical for maximizing CNS drug efficacy and avoiding unwanted consequences (Mehrabi et al., 2024; Yokoi et al., 2019).

Test Your Knowledge

1. What is a neurotransmitter and how does it transmit signals in the CNS?
2. How do CNS stimulants affect neuronal firing rates?

7.3. Short-Term Effects of CNS Drugs

Learning Outcome

1. Changes in Mood and Behavior
2. Cognitive Impairments
3. Physical Effects on the Body

Administration of CNS drugs typically produces a variety of short-term physiological and behavioral effects that are essential for both therapeutic activity and side effect profiles. These effects may occur with rapid onset following drug exposure, consistent with direct modulation of neurotransmitter systems, receptor function, or intracellular signaling cascades. For example, some drugs used to treat neurodegenerative diseases can affect memory and cognition by days of initiating treatment, as revealed from experimental models mimicking disease states. Valproic acid has been shown to have potential in improving deficits in short-term memory in studies of streptozotocin-induced cognitive impairment, indicating that CNS medications are capable of initiating quick neurobehavioral changes through modulation of crucial enzymes in brain insulin signaling pathways (Sorial et al., 2025). These temporary modifications emphasize the significance of knowing the molecular mechanisms of CNS agents, even while their more extended effects remain to be clarified. Short-term effects of CNS drugs beyond cognitive modulation often extend to neuroendocrine systems, in which hormonal change may result as a direct function of drug action. This is most clearly seen in disease-altering treatments for autoimmune CNS conditions, including multiple sclerosis, where thyroid function has been found to change shortly following the initiation of therapy. In studies monitoring thyroid hormone concentrations and autoantibody titers for six months, marked changes in free T3, free T4, and thyroid-stimulating hormone (TSH) levels in the early months of therapy are seen, reflecting an acute endocrine reaction to CNS-directed medications (Dalas et al., 2023). These temporary endocrine changes underscore the need for monitoring of systemic effects in initial stages of treatment, since they may impact patient well-being and potentially guide optimization of dosing or drug choice. Behaviorally, CNS drugs may produce rapid action on anxiety, locomotion, and general neuroactivity, affecting patient responsiveness and safety profiles. Experimental animal models show that blockade of certain enzymes involved in neurodegenerative mechanisms not only affects cognitive functions but also causes changes in anxiety-like behaviors within hours following drug treatment. The rapidity of such effects indicates that CNS medications can influence neural networks outside of traditional neurotransmission and thereby influence epigenetic processes, histone modification, and associated molecular systems (Sorial et al., 2025). Clinically, such quick behavioral modulation requires caution in relation to side effects and potentially directs clinicians to manage therapeutic benefit versus tolerability. Therefore, transient CNS drug effects are a complicated phenomenon with neurochemical, endocrine, and behavioral aspects necessary for thorough drug analysis.

7.3.1. Changes in Mood and Behavior

The complex interaction between neurotransmitters within the CNS controls mood and behavior, and a disruption created through pharmacological actions can create extreme psychological impact. Pharmacological substances acting on neurotransmitter systems, especially serotonin, may lead to alterations of mood from relieving depressive illness to undesirable blunting or irritability. The maternal brain is a prime example of this subtle interplay, in which modulation of serotonin is crucial not just for normal mood regulation but also for caregiving and aggression-related behaviors in the postpartum period. Pharmacological treatments like SSRIs act on this system to treat maternal psychiatric illnesses, illustrating how changes in mood and behavior can be therapeutically mediated through neurochemical mechanisms. Yet, the subtlety of the serotonergic system's role in various behaviors highlights the intricacy of anticipating drug impact on mood and behavioral outcomes, especially in susceptible populations (Li et al., 2019). The pharmacotherapy of depression in the CNS also demonstrates how drug-altered mood and behavior are associated with neurochemical and neurotrophic processes. While classical antidepressants mainly increase monoamine neurotransmitters such as serotonin and noradrenaline, their therapeutic effects are temporally delayed, underscoring neurobiological adaptations more than straightforward neurotransmitter replacement. Depression has been found to be associated with structural brain alterations, and most prominently, neuronal loss in limbic areas of the brain, including the hippocampus, which is involved in emotion and cognition. Treatment drugs that increase brain-derived neurotrophic factor (BDNF) levels can enhance neurogenesis and synaptic plasticity, functions regarded as crucial in the recovery of normal mood regulation. Therefore, behavioral alterations after antidepressant treatment go beyond momentary chemical changes; they involve long-term neuroplastic transformations that support recovery from mood disorders (Dom Bínguez et al., 2011). Behavioral alterations caused by drugs acting on the CNS go beyond mood management and can occur in the form of changes in social interaction, cognition, and emotional reactivity. Pharmacological treatment variability in individual responses exposes that behavioral results vary depending on several factors such as baseline neurochemical states and neural circuit integrity. For instance, whereas SSRIs enhance mood in numerous patients, in other patients, they can precipitate anxiety or agitation, which demonstrates a complex, sometimes contradictory impact on behavior. In addition, sudden drug discontinuation may lead to depressive symptom relapse or the appearance of new behavioral problems, illustrating the significance of familiarity with drug action temporal dynamics. These findings necessitate ongoing study of neurochemical and structural behavior substrates aimed at creating increasingly accurate CNS-directed agents that decrease mood-related unfavorable side effects while increasing therapeutic impact (Dom Bínguez et al., 2011; Li et al., 2019).

7.3.2. Cognitive Impairments

Cognitive impairments tend to occur as secondary, often unwanted effects of pharmacological interventions on the CNS, specifically in patient groups that are already at risk due to organic disease. Chronic kidney disease (CKD) patients are a good case in point, as they tend to take complicated medication schedules involving psychotropic drugs, opioids, corticosteroids, and anticholinergic drugs. Although these pharmacotherapies are necessary to treat comorbidities, they have been associated with negative impacts on cognition. The alteration of intact cognitive function could be due to mechanisms like vascular injury, disruption of the blood–brain barrier, and the buildup of uremic toxins, which result in increased sensitivity to neurotoxic action. It is essential to know the interplay between CKD and CNS-drugs in order to maximize therapeutic regimens and reduce cognitive impairment in this vulnerable population (Hafez et al., 2023). Outside chronic disease settings, cancer survivors reflect another important area where CNS-active medications produce cognitive deficits. Chemotherapy-induced cognitive impairment, commonly referred to as chemo brain, reflects the neurotoxic effects of traditional and novel cancer treatment. Such medications have the potential to trigger a spectrum of neurological side effects that compromise cognitive processes like memory, attention, and speed of processing. The multifactorial nature of mechanisms involved comprises direct neurotoxicity, immune-mediated toxicity, and peripheral neurotoxicity indirectly disrupting central cognitive function. Notwithstanding oncological advances, viable curative or prophylactic measures for chemotherapy-induced cognitive impairment are yet to be found, emphasizing the necessity of ongoing research with a focus on neuroprotection and symptom control (Alberti et al., 2022). The general significance of drug-induced cognitive impairments includes patient quality of life, clinical decision-making, and healthcare costs related to the management of CNS side effects. Cognitive impairment due to pharmacological treatment hinders functional independence and social integration, possibly augmenting the overall disease burden. This emphasizes the need for close monitoring and cautious prescribing, especially for drugs with established anticholinergic or GABAergic activity that preferentially impact cognitive function. Future studies should aim at identifying drug-specific neurotoxic mechanisms and biomarkers of cognitive susceptibility. This would enable personalized treatments that achieve efficacy while maintaining minimum cognitive side effects, hence enhancing the overall patient outcomes in CNS-directed pharmacotherapy (Alberti et al., 2022; Hafez et al., 2023).

7.3.3. Physical Effects on the Body

The complex interaction between the CNS and the overall physiological condition of the body is significantly affected by drugs acting on neural mechanisms. Such pharmacological agents tend to create a cascade of physical effects that extend beyond changes in cognition or emotion, having a direct effect on functions of the body such as motor control, cardiovascular functions, and respiratory patterns. For example, some CNS depressants can produce diminished muscle coordination and decreased reflexes, whereas stimulants can produce elevated heart rate and blood pressure, reflecting the wide range of physical effects. Such interaction of neural modulation and peripheral body responses underscores the need for a complete understanding of how CNS-acting medications disrupt homeostasis. These disruptions have physical consequences on health, such as the possibility of long-term tissue injury or systemic stress, highlighting that the physical consequences are not second order but part of the drug's overall action. Behind these physical symptoms lies the growing acceptance of the microbiota-gut-brain axis, demonstrating another aspect of how CNS drugs can impact the body. The gut microbiome, a sophisticated collective of microbes, talks back and forth with the CNS via immune signals, metabolic processes, and neural pathways such as the vagus nerve. Changes in the composition of the microbiota—either through drug interactions or by other external causes—can modulate neurochemical homeostasis, immune activity, and even neurodevelopmental processes. CNS drugs can, therefore, affect physical health indirectly by altering this microbiota-gut-brain axis, in turn potentially causative of a range of conditions from metabolic diseases to neurodegenerative disease. This axis demonstrates the multidimensional nature of drug action, wherein physical effects include not just immediate neural effects but also systemic biologic interactions that remain to be explained (John et al., 2019). The progress of drug delivery systems, especially lipid-based nanocarriers, has further made physical effects more complex and potentiated in response to CNS-active agents. These carrier systems enhance drug solubility and stability, with the potential for more effective penetration of the BBB and site-specific release in neural tissues. The physical properties of these carriers, including particle size and distribution uniformity, have a crucial impact on drug bioavailability and systemic toxicity, thereby controlling both intended therapeutic and unwanted physical effects on the body. Optimization of parameters such as size and polydispersity index allows for more accurate dosing and reduces side effects, enhancing overall treatment efficacy. Hence, the characterization and design of these lipidic delivery systems are crucial in exploiting the physical effects of CNS drugs in a safe and controlled manner, connecting pharmaceutical innovation with patient-focused care (Danaei et al., 2018).

Test Your Knowledge

1. How do CNS stimulants affect mood and behavior?
2. How does the CNS regulate body temperature?

7.4. Long-Term Effects of CNS Drugs

Learning Outcome

1. Dependency and Addiction
2. Neurological Damage
3. Mental Health Disorders

A comprehension of the long-term effects of drugs on the CNS involves an investigation of developmental vulnerabilities, especially during prenatal periods. The prenatal period is a window of vulnerability when the CNS is extremely sensitive to external factors. The disturbances caused by drugs given during pregnancy can result in structural and functional changes not only in the brain but also in other CNS elements like the retina. These alterations can impact neuronal, glial, and vascular components, compromising retinal tissue maturation and even resulting in permanent visual impairments. These long-term effects highlight the manner in which early exposure to CNS-active medications can reorganize neural development, elevating the risk of neuropsychiatric and sensory disorders in offspring, which has implications for the need for preventive interventions and early intervention protocols to reduce harmful effects (Baptista et al., 2024). Furthermore, long-term use of CNS medicines in adults is problematic on account of their potential to pass through the BBB and build up in neural tissue. For example, drugs such as dolutegravir, which are used widely in antiretroviral therapy, have been associated with a range of CNS-associated adverse effects when administered chronically. These range from subtle cognitive impairment to frank psychiatric abnormalities that result in discontinuation. Variability in patient response necessitates vigilant pharmacovigilance and continuous clinical monitoring to detect and control potential drug-induced neurotoxicity or functional impairment during long-term drug exposure. This vigilance is paramount to optimizing treatment regimens and guaranteeing patient safety with extended treatment periods (Jakimiuk et al., 2023). Additionally, chronic exposure to CNS drugs may induce neuroadaptive changes, affecting not just therapeutic efficacy but also the risk of dependency as well as withdrawal syndromes. The long-term effects of such medications may consist of changes in neurotransmitter systems, receptor sensitivities, and neural circuits, all of which alter brain homeostasis. This neuroplasticity, although sometimes in favor of drug efficacy, may paradoxically cause tolerance or worsen underlying neurological disease if not effectively controlled. Knowledge of these intricate interactions is needed for maximizing treatment regimens and preventing harmful effects, underscoring the value of personalized care regimens and more research into the mechanisms for long-term CNS drug effects. This integrative view is vital for maximizing therapeutic benefit while protecting neural health.

7.4.1. Dependency and Addiction

The delicate balance of brain function is largely dependent on the exact control of cerebral blood flow, coordinating metabolic demand with nutrient supply and waste elimination. Such regulation is crucial in ensuring neuronal health and function. When drugs that act on the CNS are administered, they tend to break this delicate balance, tending to produce a different brain activity and perpetuating drug-taking behavior. These disruptions are essential in dependency and addiction development, as the brain becomes accustomed to external agents through adjustments in neurotransmitter systems and cerebral perfusion. The neurochemical alterations that result from these disruptions can weaken judgment and self-control, leading to compulsive seeking of drugs that is typical of addiction (Claassen et al., 2021). Therefore, the physiological basis for addiction encompasses not just neurotransmitter disturbance but also the compromised regulatory functions of the brain's metabolic demands, emphasizing the intricate characteristics of dependency among CNS disorders. Neurohormonal processes also play an important role in susceptibility to addiction, with particular peptides exhibiting multifunctional roles in brain behavior and function alteration. Of these, glucagon-like peptide-1 (GLP-1) has been of interest as a result of its varied neuroprotection and modulatory actions. GLP-1 affects reward behavior, learning, and memory—functions deeply associated with dependency and addiction. Through the modulation of neurotransmitter systems and decreased inflammatory and apoptotic reactions, GLP-1 reduces several of the neurotoxic effects of chronic drug exposure, holding potential therapeutic opportunity for the treatment of addiction (Timo et al., 2019). Knowledge of the interaction between GLP-1 and other like molecules with CNS pathways improves our understanding of the neurobiology of addiction and creates opportunities for pharmacological interventions addressing both the metabolic and behavioral components of drug dependence. Drug addiction is the result of an interplay between biological susceptibilities and environmental exposure in which repeated exposure to drugs inscribes pathological habits into the CNS. Addiction occurs as the brain reward system gets hijacked, where the dopamine signaling cascades get disrupted and enhanced drug craving and withdrawal signs show up on stopping. Further, the chronicity of addiction is supported by changed cerebral blood flow patterns and metabolic requirements, highlighting the physiological adaptations that fuel dependency. Therapeutic intervention must thus target these multi-layered modifications by re-establishing homeostatic brain function as well as repairing compromised neurovascular coupling (Claassen et al., 2021). By combining metabolic, neurochemical, and behavioral factors, a broader strategy for the treatment of addiction can be formulated focusing on prevention as well as recovery in CNS-disordered disorders.

7.4.2. Neurological Damage

The complex interplay between the CNS and drugs has deep-seated implications for neurological well-being. Some drugs, therapeutic as they are, might cause neurological harm incidentally by various mechanisms such as neuroinflammation, apoptosis of neurons, and interference with synaptic function. The gut-brain axis is one such important neurochemical pathway that can be targeted by external substances like probiotics and paraprobiotics. These microorganisms affect the CNS through modifying gut microbial content, which in turn can aggravate or improve neuropsychiatric symptoms. Of note, probiotics have exhibited potential in lessening neuropsychiatric disorders through restoration of gut homeostasis and modulation of neuroinflammatory pathways. Nevertheless, safety remains an issue, particularly in vulnerable individuals, with more research required to explore safer alternatives such as paraprobiotics. Elucidation of such interactions underscores the therapeutic potential for microbial-based treatments to prevent drug-induced neurological injury, demonstrating the intricate relationship between systemic therapies and CNS health (Mudaliar et al., 2024). The off-target side effects of pharmacotherapies transcend targeted disease pathways and emerge as severe neurological injury, most notably in the peripheral and CNSs. Immune-checkpoint inhibitors (ICIs), which are becoming more common in oncology, present a dramatic case where desired immune activation against neoplasia can have harmful consequences on nerve function. ICIs have been linked to a range of neurological side effects, such as peripheral neuropathies and myopathies. A reported case presented with acute onset muscular weakness and sensory impairment after pembrolizumab, necessitating immunomodulatory treatment and drug withdrawal. This case highlights the susceptibility of neural tissues to drug-induced immune dysregulation and the need for early clinical identification and intervention to avoid irreversible injury. The neurologic impairments resulting from ICIs highlight that therapeutic effectiveness must be weighed against careful monitoring for neurotoxicity (Çakar Arman et al., 2023). Neurological impairment associated with drug-induced damage to the CNS can present as irreversible cognitive, motor, and sensory impairments, making disease treatment and patient outcome challenging. Underlying mechanisms are diverse and involve immune-mediated neuropathology, metabolic derangement, and perturbation of neuronal connectivity. Proinflammatory effects induced by some drugs may promote chronic neuroinflammation that modifies brain plasticity and function. This is especially relevant since the CNS has limited regenerative capacity. Also, the development of neurotoxic profiles in certain immunotherapies and psychiatric drugs calls for a thorough assessment of risk factors, such as genetic susceptibility and comorbidities. Refinery technologies like electromyography and nerve conduction tests are preciously useful in picking up on early neural involvement, allowing timely therapeutic modifications. Finally, prevention and neuroprotection against drug-induced damage need an integrated knowledge of drug action, patient vulnerabilities, and new neuroprotective modalities (Çakar Arman et al., 2023; Mudaliar et al., 2024).

7.4.3. Mental Health Disorders

External factors have a significant psychological and cognitive effect on the prevalence and management of mental health conditions. As an example, the COVID-19 pandemic worsened pre-existing psychiatric disorders while evoking novel mental health issues in the general population. The overwhelming spread of the virus and the subsequent preventive measures such as quarantine, social isolation, and interrupted medical services increasingly contributed to anxiety, depression, and insomnia symptoms across the world. Pre-existing psychiatric patients deteriorated in part because of access hurdles for day-to-day care, shortages of medications, and increased fear of infection. These interruptions emphasize the precarious balance involved in treating mental illnesses in contexts of widespread crisis. Telemedicine and virtual platforms, in addition, have become indispensable in closing the gap in care delivery, even though their uptake is below optimal levels among some patient cohorts (Zhou et al., 2020). This setting characterizes the interaction between CNS stressors and mental illness, highlighting the need for adaptive CNS-directed pharmacotherapies as well as models of healthcare delivery. Neuropharmacologic treatments directed against mental illness commonly represent multifaceted pathophysiologic processes within the CNS. Chemotherapeutic drugs, being life-saving in cancer, also characterize the fragility of the adult CNS, since they can cause cognitive dysfunction mimicking that found in neurodegenerative and psychiatric disorders. For example, chemo brain—a term describing chemotherapy-induced cognitive decline—shares mechanistic overlaps with neuroinflammation, synaptic dysfunction, and impaired neurogenesis commonly implicated in mental illnesses such as depression and anxiety. These overlapping cellular pathways involve disruptions in neurotransmitter balance, dendritic spine density, and neurotrophic support, which contribute to the cognitive and emotional symptoms observed clinically. Knowledge of these pathophysiological intersections is essential for the creation of CNS medications that not only alleviate primary psychiatric symptoms but also address secondary cognitive impairments generated by systemic therapies (Lien et al., 2020). This emphasizes the significance of creating pharmacological agents that possess neuroprotective functions in order to boost mental health outcomes. Pharmacological treatments' interaction with CNS function requires thorough consideration of drug mechanisms and their chronic impact on mental health. Numerous psychiatric drugs regulate neurotransmitter mechanisms like serotonin, dopamine, and glutamate to improve symptoms of illness like depression, schizophrenia, and bipolar disorder. Nevertheless, long-term use of such drugs can change neural plasticity and immune function in the brain, at times yielding negative cognitive and emotional consequences. Synthesizing findings from neurodegenerative and neurooncological studies has enabled a better understanding of how systemic drugs affect CNS cellular mechanisms, such as microglial activation and oxidative stress pathways. Such an understanding underpins a precision medicine strategy in psychiatry, individualizing drug choice and dosing according to neurobiological profiles. Progressing this paradigm has the potential to increase efficacy and decrease the burden of mental illness while lessening the collateral CNS effect of systemic pharmacotherapies (Lien et al., 2020; Zhou J et al., 2020).

Test Your Knowledge

1. What is neurological damage?
2. Give an example of a drug-induced side effect affecting mental health?

7.5. Treatment and Rehabilitation

Learning Outcome

1. Detoxification Processes
2. Behavioral Therapies
3. Pharmacological Interventions

The complexity of CNS disorder treatment necessitates multi-domain treatments beyond simple drug usage. CNS drugs typically need adjunctive treatment and rehabilitation to ensure maximum patient benefit, particularly with injury or long-term neurological disorders. Neuroprotectants, promising in preclinical models, tend to fall short of promise in the clinic because of the intricate secondary mechanisms provoked by injury. These secondary events include inflammation, excitotoxicity, and cell death cascades that need to be addressed by targeted therapies committed to preserving the integrity of vulnerable neuronal tissue and keeping functional neural networks intact. Rehabilitation strategies designed to enhance neuroplasticity complement medication programs by promoting adaptive neural reorganization. This approach highlights the importance of the integration of pharmacological treatments with physical interventions to facilitate restitution of motor and cognitive function, thus representing a holistic approach to CNS repair and restoration of function. Recent advances in CNS injury treatment modalities highlight the benefits of combined therapeutic approaches that address both intrinsic neuronal disabilities and extrinsic inhibitory conditions that restrict regeneration. Cell transplantation therapies, for instance, have advanced to the level of incorporating stem cell–derived neural progenitors that not only replace lost or damaged cells but also secrete neurotrophic factors that are accountable for neuronal survival and axon growth. Success with these therapies is dependent in part on the regulation of the pathological post-injury microenvironment infested with many inhibitory molecules such as chondroitin sulfate proteoglycans (CSPGs). Enzyme treatment of

CSPGs, along with immune modulation and activation of intrinsic growth mechanisms, has yielded improved functional results in animal models. The combined effect of these measures provides a permissive environment for axonal regeneration and circuit reconstruction essential to overall rehabilitation. In CNS disorder treatment complicated by thromboembolism and coagulopathies, pharmacological therapy must be carefully weighed in the treatment and rehabilitation paradigm. Current evidence gives highest priority to anticoagulant therapy in preventing secondary sequelae such as fatal venous thromboembolism in severe CNS diseases, which can greatly influence patient prognosis and rehabilitative capacity (Wichmann, 2020). The therapeutic window, however, remains uncertain and needs individualized treatment regimens and close clinical monitoring. Meanwhile, rehabilitation regimens tailored to the patients' shifting neurological status ensure functional independence and quality of life after treatment. These viewpoints foster interdisciplinary collaboration between pharmacological management and rehabilitative interventions for the treatment of neurological deficits as well as system comorbidities inherent to CNS disorders (Wichmann, 2020).

7.5.1. Detoxification Processes

The drug metabolism involving action on the CNS involves sophisticated detoxification mechanisms that are predominantly active in the liver. These mechanisms transform lipophilic chemicals into more hydrophilic metabolites, facilitating easier excretion as well as reducing toxicity. Phase I reactions, usually by cytochrome P450 enzymes, introduce reactive or polar functional groups to the drug molecules, thereby altering their structure. Phase II reactions, which come afterward, conjugate such metabolites with endogenous molecules such as glucuronic acid or sulfate to increase solubility. Biotransformation is vital in order not to cause extended activity of CNS-active drugs and the buildup which could lead to neurotoxicity or overdose. The careful balance established by these pathways is the foundation for safe pharmacologic use, and the importance of achieving metabolic diversity in individuals that can influence drug effectiveness and side effects. Subsequent to bio transformation, excretion of detoxified metabolites depends significantly on renal and biliary systems as major elimination routes. In the case of chronic exposure or overdose of drugs, such systems could get overworked and might necessitate the application of medical interventions such as augmented elimination techniques. Additionally, the body's ability to modulate inflammatory responses during detoxification is vital, as activation of the immune system will contribute to CNS damage; for instance, Toll-like receptor 4 (TLR4) participates in inflammatory signaling mediation of toxic agents and pathogens that are involved in neurodegeneration (Ciesielska et al., 2020). Modulation of these immune responses has a therapeutic target in reducing collateral damage during the process of detoxification, stressing the intricateness of maintaining CNS homeostasis despite pharmacological insults. Guidelines for the clinical practice management of detoxification among patients with CNS-acting medication involve conservative tracking of dose, duration, and patient-risk factors to forestall undesirable sequelae such as opioid use disorder or overdose (Dowell et al., 2022). These recommendations emphasize the necessity of multidisciplinary treatment, including pharmacological information along with patient factors to optimize detoxification effectiveness. Balancing acts involved here include not just cleansing the system of noxious materials but ensuring adequate CNS function and quality of life. Understanding the process of detoxification in these words brings into focus the importance of judicious prescribing and ongoing research to maximize detox operations in an effort to safely and effectively reverse CNS drug therapy.

7.5.2. Behavioral Therapies

The intricate interaction of neurochemical processes and behavior is the critical frontier in formulating an understanding of how drugs interact with the CNS. Behavioral treatments, when combined with pharmacologic management, constitute a synergistic approach to modifying deviant neural pathways and maximizing therapeutic responses. Such synergy is perhaps best demonstrated in the control of sexual behavior, where psycho-emotional and neuroendocrine factors blend. For instance, the pharmacological effect of neuropeptides that have the ability to modulate inhibitory and excitatory neurotransmitter balances on a very small scale illustrates how CNS-targeting can redefine behavioral response. Such drug compounds, in the process of modulating GABA and dopamine-based mechanisms, highlight the place of an integrated framework that weighs drug therapy and behavioral modification intervention, hinting at the potential to optimize patient outcomes within clinical intervention (Kozlov, 2023). In the field of clinical practice, the combination of the use of behavioral therapies with CNS-acting drugs has been quite effective in the treatment of neurological diseases such as epilepsy. The administration of antiepileptic drugs like lamotrigine shows not only a direct effect on seizure control but also a beneficial effect on cognitive and behavioral functions. In the majority of instances, patients can fare well on combination therapy modalities that address the physiological and psychological components of the illness, which contributes to general treatment efficacy. The tolerability and safety profile of these drugs is significant, particularly when one anticipates improvement in neurobehavioral symptoms. The integration of behavioral therapies with pharmacotherapy forms the basis of an integrated model of care that employs neurochemical stabilization to support positive behavioral adaptations and thus maintain remission of seizure activity and enhance quality of life (Мухин et al., 2020). In addition, behavior therapies with drugs that act on CNS pathways have far-reaching implications for the management of neuropsychiatric disorders. Interventions that attempt to rewire pathological patterned behavior are supplemented by medication with a capability to fine-tune neurotransmitter function, governing mood, drive, and cognitive control processes. This two-track approach is increasingly being viewed as possessing the capability to induce enduring behavioral change by targeting both the biochemical and psychosocial substrates of illness. Therefore, patient-centered strategies combining pharmacological innovation with evidence-based behavioral modification are an optimistic model for improving adherence, reducing symptom severity, and ultimately realizing therapeutic remission in a range of CNS disorders (Kozlov, 2023; Мухин et al., 2020).

7.5.3. Pharmacological Interventions

Pharmacological treatments in the CNS are faced with severe challenges owing mainly to the limiting nature of the BBB. The physiological barrier significantly controls molecular movement in a strict manner, protecting neural tissue at the expense of interfering with the efficacy of therapeutic drugs. The majority of CNS conditions such as Alzheimer's disease and brain tumors do not receive appropriate treatment because the majority of drugs cannot effectively pass through this barrier. Current advances have revolved around innovative delivery strategies, including targeted ultrasound to briefly perturb the BBB, innovative physicochemical forms of drugs, and intranasal routes. These techniques are aimed at increasing the bioavailability of drugs within the brain without restricting systemic toxicity. Creating adequate CNS drug delivery systems is highly important because present invasive approaches suffer from considerable undesirable effects and moderate potency. Extended research into these targeted delivery methods holds the promise of overcoming the physiological barriers imposed by the BBB (Ursula, 2025). Complex neurological diseases require pharmacologic agents that not only reach the brain but also promote neuroregeneration and synaptic integration. Neurogenesis and neuritogenesis, which are integral to neuronal development and repair, are regulated by endogenous modulators such as neurotrophic molecules and by exogenous pharmacologic agents. Agents like SSRIs and atypical antipsychotics exhibit differential efficacy based on genetic, epigenetic, and gender-specific mechanisms. Additionally, new evidence suggests the possible role of agents on BDNF pathways and peroxisome proliferator-activated receptor gamma agonists in modulating CNS repair mechanisms. By integrating an understanding of these neurobiological processes into drug design, therapeutic efficacy and specificity can be enhanced, paving the way for therapies that not only alleviate symptoms but also restore neural function (Sebastian et al., 2024). Nanotechnology is a paradigm-shifting frontier in pharmacotherapy for CNS disease through the delivery of targeted drugs and support in the regeneration of neural tissue. Gold nanoparticles have also been found to induce hippocampal neurogenesis and promote neurite outgrowth, critical to reconstruct neural networks disrupted by neurodegenerative diseases. Recent nanomaterials like quantum dots and nanolayered double hydroxides facilitate drug penetration across the BBB and provide support for neuronal outgrowth. However, the influence of gender-dependent biological parameters on the safety and efficacy of nanomedicine is yet to be thoroughly studied. Resolution of these differences can optimize targeted CNS therapies and amplify clinical responses. Integrating nanotechnology progress with a feeling of appreciation of uniqueness can revolutionize pharmacological strategies to CNS pathology (Sebastian et al., 2024).

Test Your Knowledge

1. Name one common type of behavioral therapy?
2. What is a pharmacological intervention in clinical practice?

7.6. Societal Implications

Learning Outcome

1. Economic Costs of Drug Abuse
2. Impact on Public Health
3. Legal and Ethical Considerations

The complex interplay between health impacts on society and the increasing use of drugs acting upon the CNS must be examined in detail. CNS drugs predominantly focus on managing symptoms of neurodegenerative disorders, psychiatric conditions, and pain disorders, diseases that are augmented by an age-ing population worldwide. As the demographic trend continues, the social burden cost with CNS-related illnesses rises, contributing to healthcare services as well as economic productivity. Additionally, CNS drugs indirectly work on public health problems, like increased risk of cardiovascular disease, with partially lifestyle-driven determinants that are entangled with neurologic well-being. Such fineness points to the need for holistic healthcare strategies that address both neurological and systemic health dangers, affirming the priority of prevention as much as cure in public policy. Equitable access to the interventions remains paramount in an attempt to reduce discrepancies in health outcomes, a goal made difficult by differing social determinants influencing drug use and disease progression both. Beyond the confines of direct clinical fields, drugs targeting the CNS have significant social structure implications and for the dynamics of mental health as well. Optimal treatment of diseases such as Alzheimer's and Parkinson's not only improves quality of life at the individual level but also reduces caregiver burden and societal economic costs of long-term care. The path to accelerated aging and neurological disease obfuscates the distinctions between them, and thus a sophisticated understanding of the biological mechanisms of aging as well as their modulation through pharmacological interventions is required. Breakthroughs in geroscience mean the assault on common molecular processes would forestall or enhance a range of age diseases simultaneously, presenting desperately needed ways of extending health span and counteracting the accumulated society burden of such disorders (Franceschi et al., 2018). Thus, CNS medication development and use must consider their broader role within models of aging pathways and public health, as well as how disease manifestation and biological aging are interrelated. Because the health systems are under increasing pressure from older people with complex CNS disorders, policy must evolve to address the social implications of drug use in a holistic way. Control and sales of CNS-affecting drugs raise ethical concerns regarding access, risk of addiction, and potential abuse, all having implications for social justice and public health. Specifically, vulnerable individuals experiencing accelerated senescence or co-morbidities of chronic disorders are best cases in point of the need for precision medicine approaches integrating genetic, environmental, and lifestyle factors to leverage therapeutic effectiveness. Merging data infrastructures to monitor drug effect and disease trends, specifically cardiovascular and neurological co-morbidities, will aid evidence-based policymaking. Systemic reforms such as these are needed to reduce health disparities, improve early detection, and promote preventive strategies that align healthcare resource planning with the shifting demographic and epidemiological environment (Franceschi et al., 2018; N/A, 2020).

7.6.1. Economic Costs of Drug Abuse

The consequences of drug abuse are much broader than individual health, with severe economic consequences that beset society at large. Health care systems have major costs in the treatment of drug-related conditions that are aimed directly at the CNS, like overdoses, chronic conditions, and psychiatric disease. These are augmented by increased rates of hospitalization, prolonged periods of recovery, and requirements for sophisticated medical treatment. A case in point is opioid abuse, which necessitates extensive medical treatment and repeated extended use of highly potent drugs to minimize withdrawal or neurologic dysfunction. Furthermore, indirect costs associated with lost productivity and decreased workforce activity are a major economic burden. Addicts experience diminished cognitive and functioning capabilities, thus impacting labor stability and economic productivity. These combined direct and indirect expenses underscore the heavy financial burden of drug abuse upon the health care and social support system. Placing additional financial burden on the cost of drug abuse is the additional strain on public resources, especially on law enforcement and social welfare agencies. Chemical dependency often comes with an increased crime rate, such as property offenses and violent offense, yielding more calls for police service, judicial proceedings, and imprisonment expenses. Allocation of resources in these areas deprives other critical public services, creating community-level fiscal strain. In addition, social welfare programs incur additional costs as drug-addicted families require aid, treatment for rehabilitation, and shelter. These varied needs show how neurological impairment caused by addiction is not only confined to healthcare spending but seeps into social structures in subtle ways. Addressing these issues requires multi-dimensional policy interventions incorporating prevention, treatment, and social reintegration to minimize cascading budgetary effects. In the face of the complexities of drug abuse care, clinical practice guidelines emphasize optimal pain relief to prevent opioid dependence, which significantly contributes to the economic burden related to CNS drug abuse. The 2022 CDC guidelines encourage judicious use of opioids, careful dosing, and rigorous assessment of patient risk factors to avert the development of opioid use disorder. These recommendations are intended not only to enhance therapeutic benefit but also to reduce the incidence of adverse events, including addiction and overdose, that generate staggering treatment and societal costs. By promoting safer pain management, clinicians can reduce the incidence of drug-induced neurological impairment and associated economic costs to patients and public health systems. Hence, evidence-based prescribing is one such measure that can be utilized for curbing the tremendous economic burden caused by drug abuse on the CNS.

7.6.2. Impact on Public Health

The widespread availability of CNS medications, particularly those accessed without medical supervision, poses severe threats to public health systems worldwide. Such medications, ranging from prescription medications to recreational drugs and uncontrolled supplements, can induce a variety of adverse health impacts ranging from mild cognitive impairment to severe psychiatric disorders. Uncontrolled consumption has a tendency to yield variable dosage and undefined interactions, thus complicating diagnosis and treatment. In addition, the social cost gets transmitted beyond simplistic individual health to crime, emergency medical cost, and lengthy disability benefit networks. Such as these complications render surveillance, prophylactic education, and controls more essential in minimizing the potential harm, but not stifling access to necessary therapeutic substances (Dando et al., 2003). Identification of these factors is valuable to public health practitioners attempting to develop evidence-based interventions that reduce harm and encourage safer drug use among populations. Epidemiologic studies highlight that the intersection of CNS-acting drugs and mental illness represents a particular urgent public health concern. Psychiatric manifestations caused by certain substances—such as mood changes, anxiety, hallucinations, and addictions—adversely worsen the overall mental well-being of populations, generally complicating underlying psychiatric illnesses. This applies more so to individuals who take sexual enhancement medications that contain such active compounds as yohimbine, maca, horny goat weed, and Ginkgo biloba, which have been reported to cause such adverse psychological effects. The uncontrolled access of these drugs on the internet permits their unrestricted sale, which calls for enhanced clinical awareness and enhanced public education on the potential risks these drugs entail (Chillemi et al., 2014). Their treatment requires the coordinated effort of healthcare providers, control agencies, and policymakers to safeguard the vulnerable population. Going beyond individual-level health consequences, CNS-altering drugs have profound effects on broader societal and economic dimensions of public health systems. Chronic management of drug-induced neuropsychiatric disorder is frequently enormously resource-intensive and adds to health system pressures exacerbated by other long-term illnesses. Furthermore, the incapacitation resultant from drug dependency can reduce workforces' productive capacity and enhance dependency ratios, ultimately affecting economic stability. The clandestine and cyber-based distribution networks of the majority of psychoactive substances further complicate enforcement and prevention, hence undermining the effectiveness of public health interventions. Therefore, comprehensive measures such as surveillance, regulation, education, and community protection are important to enhance the negative effect of these drugs on health in the population (Chillemi et al., 2014). These need to be sensitive to emerging trends in drugs and grounded in continuous studies to properly respond to public health concerns.

7.6.3. Legal and Ethical Considerations

The crossroads of legal principles and medical innovation is an onerous intersection, particularly in the case of drugs acting on the CNS. Neurologically-based therapies, promising therapeutic benefits, raise significant ethical questions about autonomy, consent, and the potentiality of coercion, particularly in the criminal justice arena. Attempting to reconcile a desire to treat offenders and also respect individual cognitive liberty is a nuanced challenge. Doctors who are dealing with CNS-active medications must navigate such problems while ensuring patient safety and dignity. The ever-changing nature of neuroscientific treatments calls for continuous ethical scrutiny to prevent abuse and ensure human rights protection. Practitioner experience stresses walking the tightrope of combining expert practice with maintaining ethics, highlighting the requirement for effective legal frameworks to facilitate medical innovation without compromising human dignity (Whitaker et al., 2018). This dispute reflects the broader public debate over the inclusion of cutting-edge interventions within mainstream legal and moral systems. Palliative care also identifies the radical legal and ethical issues surrounding CNS-active drugs, particularly in palliative care. Decisions to administer life-shortening drugs bring up moral concerns with regard to patient autonomy, quality of life, and the sanctity-of-life principle. Physicians usually encounter dilemmas where the reason behind CNS drug use has immense ethical significance, especially when treatments lower life expectancy. Patient, family, and multi-professional team contributions in making such judgments help ensure ethical values are upheld, despite varied beliefs about assisted dying. Notably, religious values and beliefs determine medical choices, reflecting the advanced interaction among ethical guidelines and legal boundaries in CNS pharmacotherapy for terminal care (Seale et al., 2009). This complexity underscores the necessity for sincere ethical deliberation in the use of CNS drugs whose effect takes hold outside the relief of symptoms. Moreover, vulnerable groups like the elderly and mentally impaired present unique challenges to the legal and ethical handling of CNS-active medications. Their compromised capacity for providing informed consent raises issues concerning autonomy and prevention from exploitation or abuse. Legal codes need to offer these persons protection for their rights while facilitating necessary medical therapy to alleviate suffering. Ethical concerns rise when CNS drugs impact cognition or behavior, and they can be potentially disrupting freedom of the individual or modifying the self. The role of neuropharmacological advances demands that physicians, legal experts, and ethicists work together to develop standards that prioritize patient welfare without violating ethics (Seale et al., 2009; Whitaker et al., 2018). These efforts are crucial to maintaining public trust and guaranteeing CNS-related treatments are administered wisely within societal morality and legal responsibility.

Test Your Knowledge

1. How do chronic diseases influence public health systems?
2. What are the legal responsibilities of healthcare providers in managing CNS drugs?

SUMMARY

The intricacies of the CNS and its vulnerabilities to a plethora of disorders create a need for a sophisticated approach to pharmacological interventions. The progresses in developing medications that aim the CNS have generated encouraging data toward controlling signs and modifying the evolution of illness in chronic disease such as diabetes mellitus complications and multiple sclerosis, especially. Present treatments that entail disease-modifying drugs minimize exacerbation occurrences while enhancing functionality levels in the patients but serve at the same time to reveal a need to reach a compromise among therapeutic efficiency versus possible detrimental impacts. Ongoing research on drug mechanism and patient-individualized response is crucial to optimize treatment paradigms and create more effective, safer CNS-targeted drugs, ultimately enhancing the quality of life of patients (McGinley et al., 2021; Zhou et al., 2019). In addition, natural products have become promising assets in CNS drug discovery because of their multi-target pharmacological activity. For example, ginsenoside Rb1 from Panax plants illustrates how phytoactive plant compounds can influence intricate pathophysiological processes, including oxidative stress, inflammation, and insulin resistance, involved in CNS-associated metabolic and vascular derangements. This presents the widening vistas of CNS pharmacotherapies beyond the traditional synthetic compounds and implies that combining phytochemicals with well-established drugs could improve efficacy with decreased side effects. Such integration requires strong clinical and mechanistic research to fully explain synergistic effects and maximize dosing for CNS treatments (Zhou et al., 2019). In conclusion, the current state of drugs that influence the CNS highlights marked progress with mixed blessings. Optimal treatment of CNS disorders encompasses not just alleviation of symptoms but also the modulation of basic pathological processes to halt or avert progression. Disease-modifying drugs in diseases such as multiple sclerosis exhibit significant decreases in relapse rates and lesion formation but must be closely monitored for side effects (McGinley et al., 2021). At the same time, new medicines with origins in nature have promise to supplement current treatments by exerting multiple-mode biological effects (Zhou et al., 2019). Future studies ought to focus on individualized medicine strategies, integrating pharmacogenetics and new drug candidates, to drive CNS therapeutics, eventually improving patient outcomes and decreasing the social cost of neurological disorders.

Summary of Key Points

The clinical profile of drugs acting on the CNS is dominated by an intricate interaction between pharmacodynamics and pharmacokinetics that affect clinical effects. The drugs modulate neurotransmitter mechanisms, thus affecting synaptic transmission as well as neural excitability. The modulation produces diverse effects from sedation to stimulation, analgesia, or neuroprotection. Knowledge of these mechanisms is crucial for maximizing drug efficacy and reducing side effects, particularly because CNS-active drugs need to penetrate the BBB in order to act. Furthermore, accuracy in describing experimental techniques, as highlighted in recent research protocols, maximizes the reliability and reproducibility of preclinical findings employed in the development of CNS drugs, which is important for the advancement of therapeutic interventions (Percie et al., 2020). Such high-level scientific reporting guarantees transparent recording of findings pertinent to CNS pharmacology to ensure effective bench-to-bedside translation. Current developments in neuropharmacology highlight the importance of oxidative stress and mechanisms of cell death in the pathology targeted by CNS medications. Interestingly, the identification of ferroptosis, a controlled mechanism of cell death initiated by iron accumulation and lipid peroxidation, has revealed new pathways for neurodegenerative disease and brain injury understanding. CNS drugs with the ability to modulate ferroptosis could provide neuroprotection through increased antioxidant capacity and decreased reactive oxygen species in neuronal cells. Inhibition of these molecular cascades has potential to reduce conditions like stroke or neurodegeneration, where oxidative injury plays a crucial role. The current investigation into ferroptosis mechanisms and pharmacological targeting, therefore, constitutes a field in CNS therapeutics with therapeutic opportunities for new intervention (Li et al., 2020). Overall, the major points concerning drugs impacting the CNS point to the need for an interdisciplinary approach that combines pharmacological understanding, strict scientific standards, and new mechanistic information. Successful CNS drugs will need to prove specific action along neural pathways in spite of physiological barriers and avoiding toxicity. The compliance with extensive experimental reporting guidelines guarantees that study results are still reproducible and informative, establishing a solid ground for clinical use (Percie et al., 2020). At the same time, new molecular targets like ferroptosis-related pathways present promising opportunities for innovative treatments of neuroprotection and disease modification (Li et al., 2020). All these aspects constitute the modern paradigm for further CNS drug development and enhanced patient outcomes.

KEY TERMS FROM THIS CHAPTER

- Central nervous system (CNS)
- Drug delivery systems
- Patient safety
- Neuronal communication
- Neurodegenerative
- Pharmacokinetics
- Neuropsychiatric
- Physiological
- Pharmacotherapy
- Drugs Affecting
- Neurodevelopmental
- Health care systems

CRITICAL THINKING QUESTIONS

1. **Which of the following is a selective serotonin reuptake inhibitor (SSRI)?**
   a. Amitriptyline
   b. Fluoxetine
   c. Diazepam
   d. Phenelzine
2. **Levodopa is used in the treatment of Parkinson's disease because it?**
   a. Inhibits dopamine receptors
   b. Is a dopamine receptor agonist
   c. Crosses the blood-brain barrier and is converted to dopamine
   d. Prevents dopamine degradation in the periphery
3. **Which of the following is a typical antipsychotic drug?**
   a. Risperidone
   b. Haloperidol
   c. Olanzapine
   d. Quetiapine
4. **Which of the following drugs is used to treat absence seizures?**
   a. Phenytoin
   b. Carbamazepine
   c. Ethosuximide
   d. Valproic acid
5. **What is the mechanism of action of morphine?**
   a. Dopamine receptor antagonist
   b. GABA receptor agonist
   c. Opioid receptor agonist
   d. Serotonin reuptake inhibitor

Short Answer Questions

1. Here is the main types of drugs affecting the Central Nervous System (CNS) examples?
2. What is Mechanisms of Action?
3. Describe the short-term effects of drugs acting on the central nervous system?
4. Discuss the principles of treatment and rehabilitation in central nervous system (CNS) disorders?
5. What do you Societal Implications?

Answer to Critical Thinking Questions

1. (b) 2 (c) 3. (b) 4. (c) 5. (c)

REFERENCES

1. Akram, M., Iqbal, M., Daniyal, M., & Khan, A. U. (2017). Awareness and current knowledge of breast cancer. *Biological Research, 50*(1), Article 33. https://doi.org/10.1186/s40659-017-0140-9.
2. Alberti, P., Salvalaggio, A., Argyriou, A. A., Bruna, J., Visentin, A., Cavaletti, G., & Briani, C. (2022). Neurological complications of conventional and novel anticancer treatments. *Cancers, 14*(24), 6088. https://doi.org/10.3390/cancers14246088.
3. Alzheimer's Association. (2023). 2023 Alzheimer's disease facts and figures. *Alzheimer's & Dementia, 19*, 1598–1695. https://doi.org/10.1002/alz.13016.
4. Anirud, U. A. (2025). Overcoming the blood-brain barrier, strategies and advances in therapeutic delivery: A literature review. *Undergraduate Research in Natural and Clinical Science and Technology (URNCST) Journal*. https://www.semanticscholar.org/paper/13782b8012d131eb6a1c31c0f808939649776a7c (accessed on 9 May 2025).
5. Baptista, F., & Ambrósio, A. F. (2024). Tracing the influence of prenatal risk factors on the offspring retina: Focus on development and putative long-term consequences. *European Journal of Clinical Investigation*. https://www.semanticscholar.org/paper/8fa173f1e5c3317ed3b4a1401f1d5114d0e782f7 (accessed on 9 May 2025).
6. Berrocoso Domínguez, E. M., Borges, G., Micó Segura, J. A., & Neto, et al. (2011). Neurotrophins role in depression neurobiology: A review of basic and clinical evidence. https://core.ac.uk/download/161360632.pdf (accessed on 9 May 2025).
7. Bray, F., Laversanne, M., Sung, H., Ferlay, J., Siegel, R. L., Soerjomataram, I., & Jemal, A. (2024). Global cancer statistics 2022: GLOBOCAN estimates of incidence and mortality worldwide for 36 cancers in 185 countries. *CA: A Cancer Journal for Clinicians, 74*, 229–263. https://doi.org/10.3322/caac.21834.
8. Busardò, F. P., & Jones, A. W. (2014). GHB pharmacology and toxicology: Acute intoxication, concentrations in blood and urine in forensic cases and treatment of the withdrawal syndrome. *Current Neuropharmacology, 13*, 47–70. https://doi.org/10.2174/1570159x13666141210215423.
9. Çakar Arman, K., Kamaci, İ., Orhan Kocasoy, E., Durmuş, H., & Parman, Y. (2023). Pembrolizumab-induced peripheral nervous system damage: A combination of myositis/myasthenia overlap syndrome and motor axonal polyneuropathy. *Ideggyógyászati Szemle, 76*(11, 12), 422–426. https://www.semanticscholar.org/paper/8df4903079f196e2f93d3b5540154414f544a767 (accessed on 9 May 2025).
10. Cellot, G., Franceschi Biagioni, A., & Ballerini, L. (2021). Nanomedicine and graphene-based materials: Advanced technologies for potential treatments of diseases in the developing nervous system. *Pediatric Research, 92*, 71–79. https://doi.org/10.1038/s41390-021-01681-6.
11. Chen, Z. J., Liang, C., Yang, L., Ren, S. M., Xia, Y., Cui, L., Li, X., et al. (2021). Association of Parkinson's disease with microbes and microbiological therapy. *Frontiers in Cellular and Infection Microbiology, 11*, Article 619354. https://doi.org/10.3389/fcimb.2021.619354.
12. Chillemi, E., Schifano, F., Martinotti, G., Di Giannantonio, M., Corazza, O., Santacroce, R., & Cellek, S. (2014). Sexual enhancement products for sale online: Raising awareness of the

psychoactive effects of yohimbine, maca, horny goat weed and ginkgo biloba. https://core.ac.uk/download/29841888.pdf (accessed on 9 May 2025).

13. Ciesielska, A., Matyjek, M., & Kwiatkowska, K. (2020). TLR4 and CD14 trafficking and its influence on LPS-induced pro-inflammatory signaling. *Cellular and Molecular Life Sciences, 78*, 1233–1261. https://doi.org/10.1007/s00018-020-03656-y.

14. Claassen, J. A. H. R., Thijssen, D. H. J., Panerai, R. B., & Faraci, F. M. (2021). Regulation of cerebral blood flow in humans: Physiology and clinical implications of autoregulation. *Physiological Reviews, 101*, 1487–1559. https://doi.org/10.1152/physrev.00022.2020.

15. Cryan, J. F., O'Riordan, K. J., Cowan, C. S. M., Sandhu, K. V., Bastiaanssen, T. F. S., Boehme, M., Codagnone, M. G., et al. (2019). The microbiota-gut-brain axis. *Physiological Reviews, 99*, 1877–2013. https://doi.org/10.1152/physrev.00018.2018.

16. Dąbrowski, W., Siwicka-Gieroba, D., Kotfis, K., Zaid, S., Terpiłowska, S., Robba, C., & Siwicki, A. K. (2020). The brain-gut axis—Where are we now and how can we modulate these connections? *Current Neuropharmacology, 19*(12), 1164–1177. https://doi.org/10.2174/1570159x18666201119155535.

17. Dalas, E., Hamad, M., & Taha, M. (2023). Assessment of thyroid functions in multiple sclerosis patients treated with disease modifying therapies. *AL-Kindy College Medical Journal.* https://www.semanticscholar.org/paper/6ef4562ede027f570447b931839a43cc34eae61d (accessed on 9 May 2025).

18. Danaei, M., Dehghankhold, M., Ataei, S., Hasanzadeh Davarani, F., Javanmard, R., Dokhani, A., Khorasani, S., et al. (2018). Impact of particle size and polydispersity index on the clinical applications of lipidic nanocarrier systems. *Pharmaceutics, 10*, 57. https://doi.org/10.3390/pharmaceutics10020057.

19. Dando, M. R. (2003). *The Danger to the Chemical Weapons Convention from Incapacitating Chemicals*. https://core.ac.uk/download/6159.pdf.

20. Dowell, D., Ragan, K., Jones, C. M., Baldwin, G., & Chou, R. (2022). CDC clinical practice guideline for prescribing opioids for pain—United States, 2022. *MMWR Recommendations and Reports, 71*, 1–95. https://doi.org/10.15585/mmwr.rr7103a1.

21. Fitzgerald, P. J. (2021). Many drugs of abuse may be acutely transformed to dopamine, norepinephrine and epinephrine *in vivo*. *International Journal of Molecular Sciences, 22*(19), 10706. https://doi.org/10.3390/ijms221910706.

22. Franceschi, C., Garagnani, P., Morsiani, C., Conte, M., Santoro, A., Grignolio, A., Monti, D., et al. (2018). The continuum of aging and age-related diseases: Common mechanisms but different rates. *Frontiers in Medicine, 5*. https://doi.org/10.3389/fmed.2018.00061.

23. Griffin, J. M., & Bradke, F. (2020). Therapeutic repair for spinal cord injury: Combinatory approaches to address a multifaceted problem. *EMBO Molecular Medicine, 12*. https://doi.org/10.15252/emmm.201911505.

24. Hafez, G., Małyszko, J., Golenia, A., Klimkowicz-Mrowiec, A., Ferreira, A. C., Arıcı, M., Bruchfeld, A., et al. (2023). Drugs with a negative impact on cognitive functions (Part 2): Drug classes to consider while prescribing in CKD patients. *Clinical Kidney Journal, 16*, 2378–2392. https://doi.org/10.1093/ckj/sfad239.

25. Haque, M. A., Haque, M. A., & Islam, M. A. U. (2018). Evaluation of analgesic and central nervous system depressant effects of *Holarrhena antidysenterica* stem on Swiss albino mice model. *Bangladesh Pharmaceutical Journal, 20*(2), 205–212. https://doi.org/10.3329/bpj.v20i2.37887.

26. Heidari, A., Rostam-Abadi, Y., & Rezaei, N. (2021). The immune system and autism spectrum disorder: Association and therapeutic challenges. *Acta Neurobiological Experimentalize, 81*, 249–263. https://doi.org/10.21307/ane-2021-023.

27. Hou, K., Wu, Z. X., Chen, X. Y., Wang, J. Q., Zhang, D., Xiao, C., Zhu, D., et al. (2022). Microbiota in health and diseases. *Signal Transduction and Targeted Therapy, 7*. https://doi.org/10.1038/s41392-022-00974-4.

28. Jakimiuk, A., Piechal, A., Wiercińska-Drapało, A., Nowaczyk, A., & Mirowska-Guzel, D. (2023). Central nervous system disorders after use of dolutegravir: Evidence from preclinical and clinical studies. *Pharmacological Reports, 75*, 1138–1151. https://www.semanticscholar.org/paper/c9a4eb2e834b42dabc3580148d6a3723e2cfabc1 (accessed on 9 May 2025).

29. Jazvinšćak Jembrek, M., & Vlainić, J. (2015). GABA receptors: Pharmacological potential and pitfalls. *Current Pharmaceutical Design, 21*, 4943–4959. https://doi.org/10.2174/1381612821666150914121624.

30. Jia, W., Kawahata, K., Cheng, A., & Fukunaga, K. (2021). The role of CaMKII and ERK signaling in addiction. *International Journal of Molecular Sciences, 22*(6), 3189. https://doi.org/10.3390/ijms22063189.

31. Kadry, H., Noorani, B., & Cucullo, L. (2020). A blood–brain barrier overview on structure, function, impairment, and biomarkers of integrity. *Fluids and Barriers of the CNS, 17*. https://doi.org/10.1186/s12987-020-00230-3.

32. Kozlov, P. (2023). Regulation of female sexual behavior and possibilities of drug therapy. *Meditsinskiy Sovet = Medical Council*. https://www.semanticscholar.org/paper/4a13bf0cb6d7f75d232546989f55d73164b82b92 (accessed on 9 May 2025).

33. Li, J., Cao, F., Yin, H., Huang, Z., Lin, Z., Mao, N., Sun, B., et al. (2020). Ferroptosis: Past, present and future. *Cell Death and Disease, 11*. https://doi.org/10.1038/s41419-020-2298-2.

34. Li, M., Lonstein, J. S., & Pawluski, J. L. (2019). Serotonin and motherhood: From molecules to mood. https://core.ac.uk/download/286364516.pdf (accessed on 9 May 2025).

35. Li, Y., Xu, H., Wang, H., Yang, K., Luan, J., & Wang, S. (2023). TREM2: Potential therapeutic targeting of microglia for Alzheimer's disease. *Biomedicine & Pharmacotherapy, 165*, 115218. https://doi.org/10.1016/j.biopha.2023.115218.

36. Lucas, C., Galettis, P., & Schneider, J. (2018). The pharmacokinetics and the pharmacodynamics of cannabinoids. *British Journal of Clinical Pharmacology, 84*, 2477–2482. https://doi.org/10.1111/bcp.13710.

37. McGinley, M., Goldschmidt, C., & Rae-Grant, A. (2021). Diagnosis and treatment of multiple sclerosis. *JAMA, 325*(8), 765–765. https://doi.org/10.1001/jama.2020.26858.

38. Mehrabi, A., Lashtoo Aghaee, B., & Farrokhfar, S. (2024). The effects of morphine administration on the central nervous system (CNS): Advantages and disadvantages. *Neuroscience Research Notes*. https://www.semanticscholar.org/paper/af3263ee7dd9e32c8b31ce145660ba47bfbf90a1 (accessed on 9 May 2025).

39. Mudaliar, S. B., Poojary, S. S., Prasad, A. B., & Mazumder, N. (2024). Probiotics and paraprobiotics: Effects on microbiota-gut-brain axis and their consequent potential in neuropsychiatric therapy. *Probiotics and Antimicrobial Proteins, 16*(6), 1440–1464. https://www.semanticscholar.org/paper/57abd1384a1f573d7718a86868b32f7f0f1e436b (accessed on 9 May 2025).

40. Müller, T. D., Finan, B., Bloom, S. R., D'Alessio, D. A., Drucker, D. J., Flatt, P. R., Fritsche, A., et al. (2019). Glucagon-like peptide 1 (GLP-1). *Molecular Metabolism, 30*, 72–130. https://doi.org/10.1016/j.molmet.2019.09.010.

41. Nguyen, L. D., & Ehrlich, B. E. (2020). Cellular mechanisms and treatments for chemo brain: Insight from aging and neurodegenerative diseases. *EMBO Molecular Medicine, 12*. https://doi.org/10.15252/emmm.202012075.

42. Organization for Economic Co-operation and Development. (2020). *Is Cardiovascular Disease Slowing Improvements in Life Expectancy?* https://doi.org/10.1787/47a04a11-en.

43. Percie du Sert, N., Ahluwalia, A., Alam, S., Avey, M. T., Baker, M., Browne, W. J., Clark, A., et al. (2020). Reporting animal research: Explanation and elaboration for the ARRIVE guidelines 2.0. *PLOS Biology, 18*(7), e3000411. https://doi.org/10.1371/journal.pbio.3000411.

44. Seale, C. (2009). Hastening death in end-of-life care: A survey of doctors. *Social Science & Medicine, 69*(11), 1659–1666. https://core.ac.uk/download/20572783.pdf (accessed on 9 May 2025).

45. Sebastian, A., Shanmuganathan, M., Tripathy, C., Chakravarty, S., & Ghosh, S. (2024). Understanding neurogenesis and neurogenesis via molecular insights, gender influence, and therapeutic implications: Intervention of nanomaterials. *ACS Applied Bio Materials*. https://www.semanticscholar.org/paper/6268e3eeb3c6971352ed1df0f88355b479838641 (accessed on 9 May 2025).

46. Shram, M. J., Spencer, R. H., Qian, J., Munera, C., Lewis, M. E., Henningfield, J. E., Webster, L. R., et al. (2021). Evaluation of the abuse potential of difelikefalin, a selective kappa-opioid receptor agonist, in recreational polydrug users. *Clinical and Translational Science, 15*(3), 535–547. https://doi.org/10.1111/cts.13173.

47. Silva, Y. P., Bernardi, A., & Frozza, R. L. (2020). The role of short-chain fatty acids from gut microbiota in gut-brain communication. *Frontiers in Endocrinology, 11*, Article 25. https://doi.org/10.3389/fendo.2020.00025.

48. Sorial, M. E. S., Abdelghany, R. M., & El Sayed, N. S. (2025). Modulation of the cognitive impairment associated with Alzheimer's disease by valproic acid: Possible drug repurposing. *Inflammopharmacology, 33*, 2083–2094. https://www.semanticscholar.org/paper/09683a0e955201d06dbc8913d5149fdf2189f780 (accessed on 9 May 2025).

49. Whitaker, H. N. (2018). Attitudes on medical ethics of criminal neurointerventional treatment. https://core.ac.uk/download/213462108.pdf (accessed on 9 May 2025).

50. Wichmann, D. (2020). Autopsy findings and venous thromboembolism in patients with COVID-19. *Annals of Internal Medicine, 173*, 1030. https://doi.org/10.7326/l20-1206.

51. Yokoi, R., Okabe, M., Matsuda, N., Odawara, A., Karashima, A., & Suzuki, I. (2019). Impact of sleep–wake-associated neuromodulators and repetitive low-frequency stimulation on human iPSC-derived neurons. *Frontiers in Neuroscience, 13*, Article 760. https://www.semanticscholar.org/paper/f56a6057748971933435596e2bf99b0d93970eff (accessed on 9 May 2025).

52. Zareifopoulos, N., Lagadinou, M., Karela, A., Kyriakopoulou, O., & Velissaris, D. (2020). Neuropsychiatric effects of antiviral drugs. *Cures, 12*(7), e9536. https://doi.org/10.7759/cureus.9536.

53. Zhou, J., Liu, L., Xue, P., Yang, X., & Tang, X. (2020). Mental health response to the COVID-19 outbreak in China. *American Journal of Psychiatry, 177*, 574–575. https://doi.org/10.1176/appi.ajp.2020.20030304.

54. Zhou, P., Xie, W., He, S., Sun, Y., Meng, X., Sun, G., & Sun, X. (2019). Ginsenoside Rb1 as an anti-diabetic agent and its underlying mechanism analysis. *Cells, 8*(3), 204. https://doi.org/10.3390/cells8030204.

55. Мухин, К. Ю., & Пылаева, О. А. (2020). Эффективность и переносимость прегабалина (лирика) у больных эпилепсией (обзор литературы). https://www.semanticscholar.org/paper/be54f93dc9e7e6ad59c626070fc2ce60109c374a (accessed on 9 May 2025).

DRUGS AFFECTING THE GASTROINTESTINAL SYSTEM

8

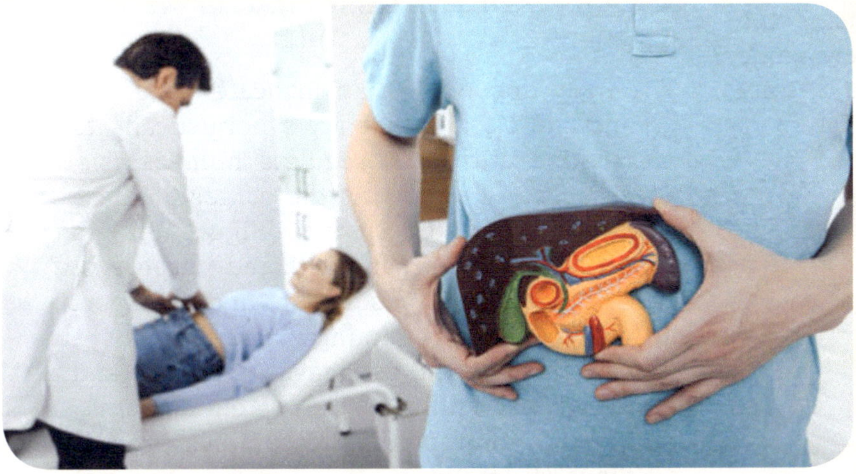

LEARNING OBJECTIVES

After studying this chapter, you will be able to:

1. Explain Types of Drugs Affecting the Gastrointestinal System
2. Define Mechanisms of Action
3. Explain about Common Gastrointestinal Disorders Treated by Drugs
4. Understand Side Effects of Gastrointestinal Drugs
5. Define Drug Interactions
6. Explain about Patient Considerations

Introduction

The simplicity of the human gastrointestinal (GI) system makes it incredibly challenging to build efficient pharmaceutical interventions. Conventional in vitro two-dimensional cultures and animal models have long been used to examine the impact of drugs on the GI tract; however, these are often unable to model accurately human physiological conditions. This lack of similarity leads to unreliable predictions of drug efficacy and possible side effects in clinical trials. New technologies like organ-on-chip and micro physiological systems offer novel platforms that more accurately reproduce the human GI environment, improving the predictive value of preclinical testing. The technologies allow for a more precise exploration of disease mechanisms and drug interactions in the GI tract, ultimately leading to the expedited development of targeted therapeutics with enhanced safety profiles (Monteduro et al., 2023). Oral drug administration is the most prevalent route for delivering drugs, simply because of convenience and compliance on the part of the patient. Yet, lipophilic drugs, i.e., drugs soluble in fats, face extreme barriers to accessing satisfactory oral bioavailability. The water microenvironment of the GI tract restricts dissolution of such molecules, leading to poor absorption and inconsistent pharmacokinetics. Resolution of these issues requires advanced formulation techniques aimed at shielding lipophilic drugs until they arrive at the sites of absorption in the intestine. Advances in drug delivery technologies, such as encapsulation techniques and the employment of bile acids, show significant potential for enhancing the stability, permeation, and ultimately therapeutic effectiveness of lipophilic drugs in the GI tract (Wagle et al., 2020).

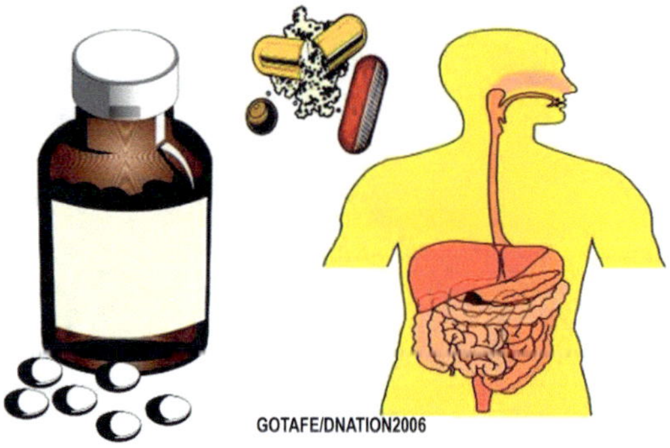

Figure 8.1. Drugs affecting the gastrointestinal (GI) system.

Source: Annick. (2014, September 2). *Drugs Affecting the Gastrointestinal Tract.* SlideServe https://image2.slideserve.com/3824024/drugs-affecting-the-gastrointestinal-tract-n.jpg.

Comprehensive drug studies on the GI system (Figure 8.1) increasingly utilize new experimental models that combine microfluidic devices with multi-organ simulations to mimic complex physiological interactions. These platforms allow for accurate control of drug testing environments, enabling real-time monitoring of drug transport, metabolism, and pharmacodynamic responses. Moreover, the intersection of material science and biomedical engineering has increased the ability of *in vitro* models to include living tissue and vascular structures, mimicking human GI function precisely. This interdisciplinary concept not only progresses drug development procedures but also highlights the role of personalized medicine through enabling personalized therapeutic screening representative of variability in response to drugs on an individual basis (Monteduro et al., 2023).

Definition of the Gastrointestinal System

The body depends on an intricate system of organs and tissues that act synergistically to metabolize nutrients, regulate homeostasis, and dispose of waste. At the center of these functions is the GI system (Figure 8.2), a complex array of organs with the purpose of enabling digestion, absorption, and transport of food material. Beginning in the oral cavity, passing through the esophagus, stomach, and intestines, and ending at the rectum and anus, this system choreographs a complex process of digested material. Its elements are not only charged with mechanical and chemical digestion of food but also have critical functions in immune protection and metabolic control. This multifactorial role of the GI tract is particularly pertinent when one considers the pharmacodynamics of drugs acting upon this system, since shifts in microbial composition or epithelial function can heavily impact drug efficacy and safety. The functionality of the GI system is greatly impacted by its resident microbiota, which ferments nondigestible dietary fibers to create short-chain fatty acids (SCFAs) like acetate, propionate, and butyrate. These metabolites play an important role in intestinal homeostasis as signaling molecules via select G-protein-coupled receptors on immune, endocrine, and epithelial cells. SCFAs not only feed colonocytes but also influence epigenetic landscapes and systemic immunity, demonstrating their wide-ranging physiological effects. Additionally, shifts in the microbiota, induced by diet or therapeutic compounds, can potentially change SCFA production and hence influence intestinal and systemic health. Appreciation of these dynamics is essential for drug development and management of GI drugs, as therapeutic interventions increasingly take into account microbiome interactions to maximize clinical efficacy (Bart van der Hee et al., 2021). The evolution of drug delivery systems has embraced the complexity of the GI tract, with nanomedicine as a promising route to increase treatment specificity and efficacy. Nanoscale engineering of therapeutic molecules enables targeted delivery and controlled release, reducing systemic side effects and enhancing bioavailability.

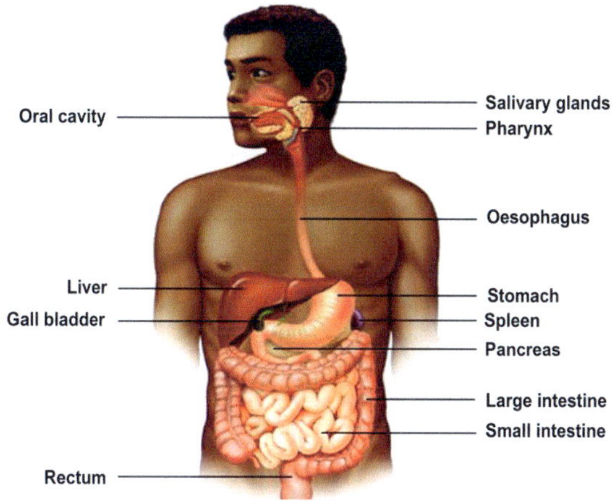

Figure 8.2. Gastrointestinal system the human body.

Source: Virtual Medical Centre. (n.d.). *Gastrointestinal Anatomy Diagram*. HealthEngine. https://healthinfo.healthengine.com.au/uploads/VMC/Anatomy/gastro/gastro_450.jpg.

This is especially relevant to GI diseases, in which localized drug action can minimize damage to off-target tissues and enhance patient compliance. Nano-delivery platforms may be engineered to survive the aggressive gastric environment, interact with unique cell types, or manipulate microbiota composition, illustrating an optimized approach to GI therapeutics. As research continues to unfold, the incorporation of nanotechnology not only enhances existing drug paradigms but also provides avenues for new interventions in multifaceted GI diseases (Patra et al., 2018).

Overview of Drugs Affecting the Gastrointestinal System

The multifactorial nature of GI diseases requires a heterogeneous array of pharmacological treatments directed toward modulating disparate physiological processes in the GI tract. GI drugs can be classified broadly according to their mechanism of action and therapeutic targets (Figure 8.3). These include acid suppressants like proton pump inhibitors (PPI) and H2 receptor antagonists, which are mainly employed for the management of acid-related disorders like gastroesophageal reflux disease (GERD) and peptic ulcers. Prokinetic agents also increase GI motility, promoting the transit of contents in the digestive tract and are useful in conditions with delayed gastric emptying. Antiemetics, antidiarrheals, and laxatives play symptomatic functions, assisting the body's natural mechanisms by alleviating nausea, managing diarrhea, or provoking bowel movements, respectively. In addition, novel therapies aimed at specific inflammatory pathways are becoming increasingly popular, as the new knowledge of GI pathophysiology and the necessity for targeted treatment modalities emerge. One important class of drugs with broad applications in GI practice is glucocorticoids. These drugs, with their powerful anti-inflammatory and immunosuppressive actions, have been used successfully to treat a number of inflammatory conditions, including those of the GI tract. Though glucocorticoids induce marked symptomatic relief by modulating the behavior of inflammatory cells and production of cytokines, their therapeutic use is tempered by a variety of side effects that precludes prolonged usage. Research now centers on improving the therapeutic index of glucocorticoids, with a focus on increasing efficacy while reducing side effects. Developments like chemical modifications and site-specific delivery systems, such as nanoformulations, reflect the advances in drug design to achieve the best results in GI inflammatory diseases, calling for a more targeted use of these old but potent drugs (Sybille et al., 2021). Along with traditional therapies, another emerging area in GI pharmacology includes the modulation of cell death pathways like ferroptosis, an iron-catalyzed oxidative cell death process. Recent findings show that induction or inhibition of ferroptosis could be central to the pathogenesis of GI disorders, particularly in scenarios such as tumor initiation, ischemia-reperfusion injury, and inflammatory bowel disease. The complex interplay between ferroptosis and lipid peroxidation points to therapeutic opportunities for preventing oxidative damage in GI tissues. Pharmacological compounds that modulate ferroptotic mechanisms hold great hope for future treatments, as they work to restore cellular homeostasis and avoid progressive tissue damage. This emerging discipline underlines the kinetic nature of drug development in the GI tract with a focus on the need to continue research that will better inform molecular mechanisms and translate them to effective clinical regimens (Li et al., 2020).

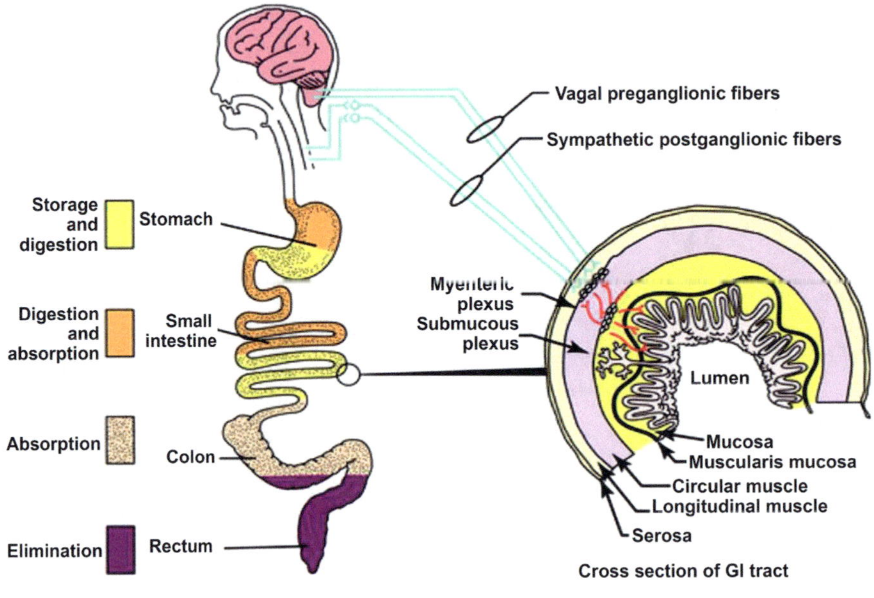

Figure 8.3. Drugs affecting the gastrointestinal system.

Source: Basic Medical Key. (2016). *Drugs Affecting the Gastrointestinal System.* https://basicmedicalkey.com/wp-content/uploads/2016/06/B9780323053747000185_gr1.jpg.

Importance of Understanding Drug Effects on Gastrointestinal Health

The complex interplay between GI health and drugs highlights the need for sophisticated consideration of pharmacological effects on this system. Most drugs, in attempting to treat systemic or local disorders, unintentionally modify the subtle microbial ecology or gut physiology. For example, some drugs may dysregulate the intestinal populations of symbiotic bacteria that are vital for SCFAs production necessary for promoting intestinal homeostasis and immune regulation. A drug-induced imbalance can result in unfavorable effects like inflammation or disturbed nutrient absorption, possibly aggravating or even precipitating GI diseases. Comprehending these alterations due to drugs is vital for maximizing therapeutic benefits and preventing unwanted complications, particularly because alterations in the intestinal environment have systemic consequences that are not limited to the GI tract (Bart van der Hee et al., 2021). Such awareness is basis in creating safer drugs and tailored treatment regimens that maintain GI health. In addition, drug action on the GI tract also reaches higher order signaling mechanisms that include host receptor activation and epigenetic modulation. Certain drugs have the ability to alter the synthesis or function of microbial metabolites like SCFAs, which play a central role in regulating gene expression via epigenetic mechanisms such as histone acetylation and deacetylation. These adaptations play a critical role in modulating inflammation and preserving the structural integrity of the intestinal epithelium. An altered balance due to drug actions can then impair such regulatory processes, leading to pathologies like inflammatory bowel disease or colorectal cancer. A thorough understanding of these interactions allows clinicians and researchers to better predict drug effects and to develop novel targeted interventions, such as adjunctive treatments like prebiotics and probiotics to reestablish microbial balance and support mucosal integrity (Bart van der Hee et al., 2021). Such multifaceted understanding increases the potential to prevent and treat GI adverse effects effectively. The growing industries of probiotics and prebiotics underscore the changing strategies to reverse the adverse GI effects of drugs. These microbiome-altering interventions hold the promise to restore healthy bacterial communities and enhance the production of metabolites that maintain gut barrier integrity, immune modulation, and metabolic homeostasis. With the emergence of new probiotic strains and prebiotic molecules, their potential to reverse drug-induced dysbiosis and intestinal inflammation is increasingly receiving attention. Implementation of this understanding into clinical practice requires not only understanding the background microbiological and pharmacological interactions but also understanding regulatory and quality assurance issues related to such products. Finally, knowledge of drug effects on GI health enables patient-specific therapeutic strategies based on microbiota-targeted therapies to enhance patient outcomes and mitigate the impact of GI complications due to pharmacotherapy. This integrative approach is crucial in contemporary medicine's quest to maximize both the effectiveness and safety of treatment.

8.1. Types of Drugs Affecting the Gastrointestinal System

Learning Outcome

1. Antacids and Their Role in Neutralizing Stomach Acid
2. Proton Pump Inhibitors (PPI) and Their Mechanism of Action
3. Laxatives and Their Use in Treating Constipation

Therapeutic treatment of gastrointestinal (GI) disorders involves a broad range of drugs with mechanisms of action against varying pathophysiological characteristics (Figure 8.4). Acid-suppressing agents like proton pump inhibitors (PPIs) and H_2 receptor antagonists are central to inhibiting gastric acid output, thus treating conditions such as gastroesophageal reflux disease (GERD) and peptic ulcers. The effectiveness of these drugs lies in their capacity to block proton pumps or histamine receptors, which offer symptomatic improvement and enable mucosal healing. In addition, prokinetic drugs enhance GI motility, reversing delayed gastric emptying and enhancing peristalsis in the context of gastroparesis. Laxatives are widely applied in the treatment of constipation, with varying effects ranging from stool softening to causing intestinal motility stimulation. Antidiarrheal drugs such as loperamide, on the other hand, retard intestinal transit and minimize loss of fluid. Each category of these drugs has a specific role in the management of individual GI functional disturbances as well as considerations for side effects and chronic use. Pharmacological interventions now increasingly involve more advanced microbiome-targeted therapies that take advantage of the gut's complex microbial community to manage GI disease. Probiotics and prebiotics are exemplary of this class, attempting to restore and regulate intestinal microbiota equilibrium. Probiotics, viable beneficial microorganisms, may benefit colonic health and immune homeostasis by competing with pathogens, improving barrier function, and communicating with host immune cells. Prebiotics, undigestible fibers, selectively stimulate the growth of these beneficial bacteria, thus influencing the production of short-chain fatty acids (SCFAs) that impact metabolism and inflammation. New developments highlight new microbiome-modulating agents like synbiotics and postbiotics, which hold promise in precision medicine and personalized nutrition. Yet, the intricacy of probiotic and prebiotic mechanisms, including host interactions and strain-specific effects, requires intensive research to best exploit their therapeutic potential (Cunningham et al., 2021).

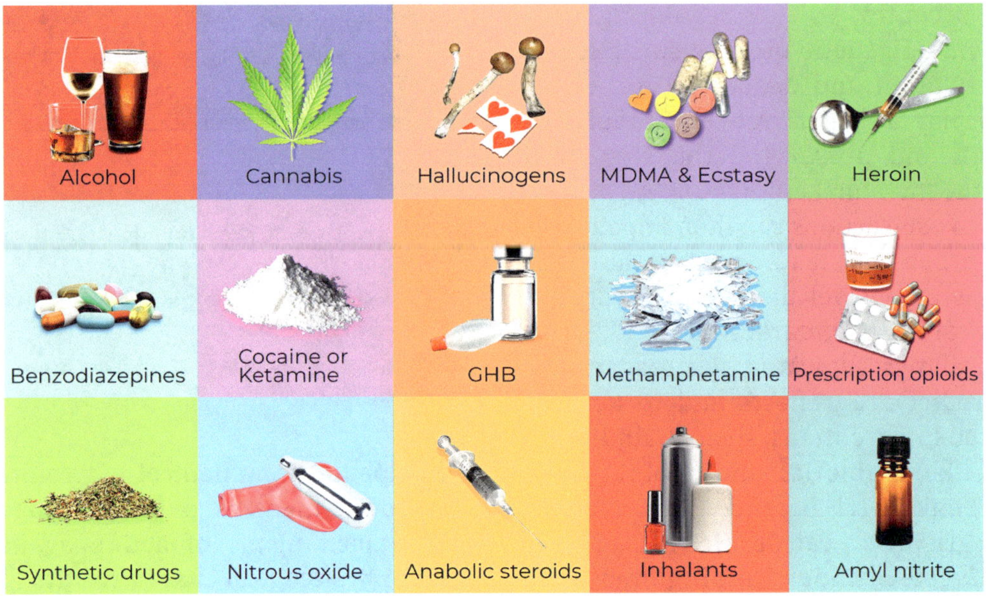

Figure 8.4. Types of drugs affecting the gastrointestinal (GI) system.

Source: Health NSW. (n.d.). *Types of Drugs Affecting the Gastrointestinal (GI) System.* https://yourroom.health.nsw.gov.au/Families/PublishingImages/Pages/AOD-information/About-drugs-banner.png.

These new methods complement conventional drug approaches by incorporating microbial ecology as a therapeutic target in GI health. Apart from conventional and microbiome-directed therapy, biologics and immunomodulators are now indispensable for the control of chronic GI conditions such as inflammatory bowel disease (IBD). Drugs such as tumor necrosis factor (TNF) inhibitors, integrin receptor antagonists, and interleukin blockers act through modulation of inappropriate immune mechanisms leading to mucosal inflammation and tissue injury. These medications can induce and sustain remission, vastly enhancing the quality of life of the patient and decreasing the dependency on corticosteroids and surgery. The immunosuppressive action of these drugs requires vigilant monitoring to avoid complications like infections. Current studies, including information regarding systemic effects due to infectious disease such as COVID-19, emphasize the necessity of an understanding of immune system interactions in the GI tract, particularly in susceptible populations. Together, these treatments reflect increasing sophistication in GI disease treatment with a focus on individualized approach combining efficacy and safety with patient-specific considerations.

8.1.1. Antacids and Their Role in Neutralizing Stomach Acid

The human GI tract is provided with several defense mechanisms to ensure homeostasis in spite of constant exposure to severe conditions like low pH and digestive enzymes. Yet, overproduction or excessive acidity of gastric juice frequently results in discomfort and disorders like acid reflux and peptic ulcers. Under such conditions, the function of antacids becomes crucial in symptom relief by chemically neutralizing excess stomach acid. Antacids have alkaline ingredients like magnesium hydroxide, calcium carbonate, or sodium bicarbonate, which act on hydrochloric acid in the stomach to produce neutral salts and water. This not only increases the gastric pH but also decreases mucosal irritation, resulting in immediate symptomatic relief. Their action is different from other GI drugs like PPIs or H_2 receptor antagonists, whose acid production is decreased slowly. Antacids are therefore acute therapeutic drugs in the control of acid-mediated GI distress. Although effective in alleviating symptoms, antacids need to be employed cautiously because of possible systemic actions and interaction with other drugs. The swift neutralization of stomach acid may change the pH-dependent drug absorption of some drugs, like antibiotics and antifungals, which may decrease their bioavailability and efficacy. In addition, long-term use of antacids with aluminum or magnesium ions may lead to electrolyte imbalance or constipation, respectively. Proper patient instruction regarding the dosing and timing of antacid use is necessary to prevent these complications. Also, although antacids may neutralize acid, they cannot treat underlying pathologic conditions leading to acid hypersecretion or mucosal injury. This limitation underscores the value of multimodal treatment strategies, such as lifestyle change and pharmacologic therapy directed at acid formation or mucosal defense (Meryl et al., 2022). Outside of symptom control, a grasp of the wider context of GI health provides the value of specific pharmacotherapy in avoiding complications secondary to acid-related disease. Chronic acid excess also causes GI mucosal erosion, making patients susceptible to ulcers and bleeding that might require more aggressive acid-suppressing drugs or protectants. Additionally, a fine balance between acid neutralization and maintaining normal digestive functions has to be preserved to prevent compromising nutrient absorption or inducing secondary disease states. Proper use of antacids, thus, is a critical part of an integrated therapeutic approach to maximize GI function and avoid chronic morbidity. Clinical practice evidence increasingly highlights ongoing monitoring of treatment effectiveness and safety, highlighting the importance of well-informed prescribing similar to the vigilance needed in the management of other systemic illnesses such as osteoporosis (Meryl et al., 2022) where continuous monitoring guarantees positive outcomes.

8.1.2. Proton Pump Inhibitors (PPI) and Their Mechanism of Action

Control of gastric acid output is central to ensuring digestive health and avoiding ulcerative disease states. The mechanism depends primarily on the action of the hydrogen-potassium adenosine triphosphatase enzyme, better referred to as the proton pump, found in the parietal cells lining the stomach. PPIs target this enzyme specifically to irreversibly inhibit the terminal step in acid production, leading to a dramatic and long-lasting suppression of gastric acidity (Figure 8.5). PPIs inhibit the exchange of hydrogen ions for potassium ions by covalently bonding to cysteine residues on the pump.

This action makes PPIs different from other acid-suppressing medications, like H2-receptor antagonists, that only inhibit histamine-mediated stimulation instead of the actual acid secretion, thus increasing the clinical effectiveness of PPIs in the treatment of GERD and peptic ulcers. After administration, PPIs get absorbed into the circulation system and then accumulate within the acidic surroundings of the secretory canaliculi of parietal cells, where they get activated. This acid-promoted prodrug activation is crucial to their pharmacological action, since only in their active state do PPIs have a specific affinity for the proton pumps. Because of this need for acid-activated prompting, the administration of PPIs is generally recommended prior to meals to synchronize with peak proton pump activity. Once activated, the covalent inhibition continues until new proton pump synthesis is achieved, which implies acid-suppressive activity lasts longer than the plasma half-life of the drug.

The sustained inhibition is consistent with once-daily dosing regimens and aids patient compliance and efficient control of acid-related disorders. Although they have advantages, the powerful acid suppression by PPIs requires guarded clinical use because of long-term effects on gastric physiology (Dowell et al., 2022). Their clinical use goes beyond their acid-suppressive effect, and they have varied therapeutic uses such as the treatment of GERD, Zollinger-Ellison syndrome, and cure of *Helicobacter pylori* infections when combined with antibiotics. The specificity and efficacy of PPIs render them essential in minimizing mucosal injury from excess acid. Chronic gastric acid suppression, though, can modify nutrient absorption and the GI microbiota, and concerns regarding heightened infection susceptibility and deficiency are raised. The balance between therapeutic efficacy and risk of long-term PPI use continues to be studied, prompting clinicians to prescribe these drugs wisely. Future developments seek to optimize PPI pharmacodynamics in order to reduce side effects with preserved efficacy, emphasizing the evolving character of drugs acting on the GI system and their continuous improvement in clinical therapeutics (Alexander et al., 2022).

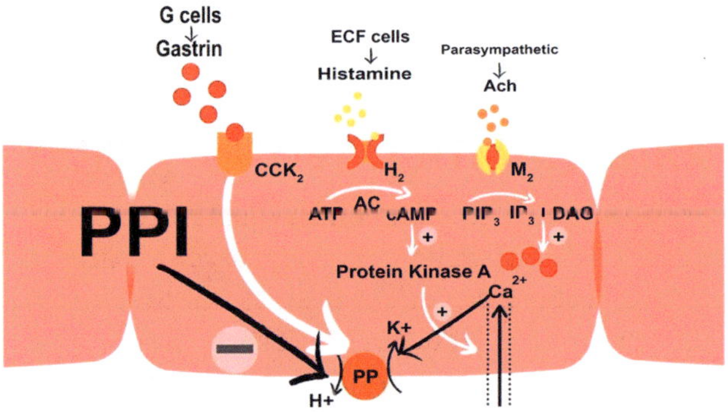

Figure 8.5. Proton pump inhibitors and their mechanism of action.

Source: YouTube. (n.d.). *Proton Pump Inhibitors and Their Mechanism of Action.* https://i.ytimg.com/vi/ffX39qu5yqk/maxresdefault.jpg.

8.1.3. Laxatives and Their Use in Treating Constipation

Diagnosis and treatment of constipation demand a thorough knowledge of its etiology and physiological mechanisms. Constipation is defined by decreased frequency of bowel movements, hard defecation, or sensation of incomplete evacuation, which usually results from defective colonic transit or defecation mechanics dysfunction. Therapeutic interventions thus seek to correct these particular dysfunctions to normalize bowel function.

Pharmacologic therapy, particularly laxatives, has emerged as a more prominent role in the treatment of constipation since they can produce bowel movements through several mechanisms that include increasing stool bulk, making stool consistency softer, or initiating colonic motility. Clinicians have to individualize laxative options based on patient profiles, especially taking into account comorbidities and symptom severity, to provide effective and safe symptom alleviation without risk of adverse effects due to long-term administration or misuse (Gardiner et al., 2016). Among pharmacologic therapies, the role of laxative use is central in both the general and specialized patient with constipation. Laxatives have varying mechanisms of action: bulk-forming laxatives augment fecal bulk, osmotic laxatives bring in water to the colon to laxate stools, stimulant laxatives stimulate intestinal motility, and stool softeners decrease stool hardness. This range of agents enables clinicians to choose laxatives appropriate for patient-specific pathophysiology and symptomatology. Particular attention should be given in patients with opioid-induced constipation, a frequent complication of chronic opioid exposure that drastically compromises quality of life. Standard laxatives do not always fully treat this condition, so targeted therapies to reverse opioid receptor-mediated bowel dysfunction are needed (Gardiner et al., 2016).

New developments have brought about peripherally acting μ-opioid receptor antagonists as a new generation of agents that are specifically created to reverse opioid-induced bowel dysfunction without sacrificing analgesia. In contrast to traditional laxatives, such antagonists preferentially block μ-opioid receptors within the GI tract without penetrating the blood-brain barrier (BBB), thereby avoiding the detrimental effect on opioid analgesic activity. Drugs like Alvi Mopan, methylnaltrexone, and naloxegol have demonstrated efficacy in clinical trials, though available studies differ in their endpoints and quality, precluding definitive comparisons of efficacy. In spite of these drawbacks, these medications are a significant step forward in the management of complicated constipation that occurs secondary to opioid treatment, highlighting the multifaceted nature of pharmacological management of GI motility disorders.

Test Your Knowledge

1. How do proton pump inhibitors (PPIs) work in the GI system?
2. What is the primary function of antacids in the gastrointestinal system?

8.2. Mechanisms of Action

Learning Outcome

1. How Antacids Alter Gastric pH Levels?
2. The Role of Proton Pump Inhibitors (PPIs) in Reducing Acid Secretion
3. The Physiological Effects of Laxatives on Bowel Movement

Comprehension of therapeutic actions of drugs in the GI tract necessitates an extensive examination of their mechanism of action, which determines how these drugs interact with cellular and molecular targets to yield clinical effects (Figure 8.6). Most GI drugs exert their effects through modulation of secretory processes, for example, inhibition of proton pumps for inhibition of gastric acid secretion or blockade of histamine H2 receptors on parietal cells. This interference selectively stops the excess acid formation, hence easing symptoms for disorders such as peptic ulcers. Others achieve this through facilitation of motility by activation of muscarinic receptors, which advances organized contractions and enables transit. These interventions highlight the subtle equilibrium sustained by physiological enzymes and receptors, and the manner in which selective pharmacologic intervention aids restoration of GI homeostasis to ultimately enhance the quality of life of the patient while preventing systemic side effects (Visseren et al., 2021).

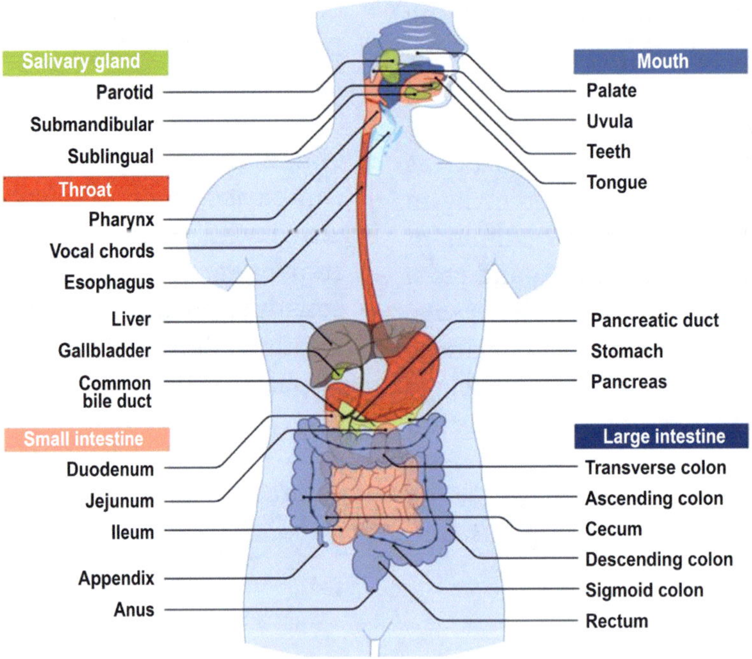

Figure 8.6. Mechanisms of action.

Source: Medical News Today. (2022). *Digestion Process.* https://post.medicalnewstoday.com/wp-content/uploads/sites/3/2022/06/1958689-Digestion_1296x1296-body-1-1024x1024.png.

Besides receptor modulation, some types of GI drugs produce their effects through modification of intracellular signaling cascades and ion channel operation, which are indispensable to the integrity of the mucosal barrier and to the control of smooth muscle tone. Laxatives, for instance, tend to stimulate the secretion of water into the bowel through the activation of chloride channels, leading to the softening of stools and relaxation of bowel movements. On the other hand, antidiarrheals could inhibit gut motility by binding to opioid receptors within the enteric nervous system (ENS), slowing down hypermotility and fluid secretion. These mechanisms emphasize the intricacy of GI pharmacotherapy and the need for mechanistic specificity to attain the intended therapeutic aim without hindering absorption or inducing side effects (Visseren et al., 2021). New research highlights the value of deciphering drug mechanisms beyond receptor binding, especially in inflammatory and infectious processes within the GI tract. Specific phytochemicals and new agents hold promise by regulating oxidative stress and inflammatory signaling pathways, reducing mucosal injury and enhancing tissue repair. Additionally, with the interaction between GI function and systemic infections like viral pathogens, there is increasing interest in drugs that modulate molecular pathways engaged in both viral replication and host immune responses. Research into these mechanisms is essential for the development of novel treatments that improve antiviral defense without compromising GI health, thus demonstrating the multidimensional nature of mechanisms involved in GI pharmacology.

8.2.1. How Antacids Alter Gastric pH Levels?

The delicate balance of gastric acidity is of vital importance for digestive physiology, as it affects enzyme activity and microbial defense within the stomach. The normal secretion of hydrochloric acid, mainly by parietal cells, ensures a very acidic environment with a pH of usually 1.5 to 3.5, which is necessary for protein denaturation and activation of pepsinogen to pepsin. Antacids, as therapeutic chemicals, act by directly neutralizing this gastric acid, raising the pH of the stomach towards an alkaline state (Figure 8.7). This neutralization is brought about chemically by several active ingredients such as magnesium hydroxide, aluminum hydroxide, calcium carbonate, or sodium bicarbonate reacting with hydrochloric acid to produce water and other neutral salts. By raising gastric pH, antacids reduce symptoms of acid indigestion and gastroesophageal reflux, highlighting their importance in treating GI disorders as part of the larger picture of drugs that act on the GI system. The effectiveness of antacids in changing gastric pH levels depends on their quick onset of action and buffering capacity, which may differ depending on their formulation and individual patient considerations. On intake, these substances dissociate to give off hydroxide ions or carbonate ions that chemically react with hydrogen ions in the gastric lumen to decrease free acid concentration. This rapid neutralization alters the stomach environment, affecting not only symptomatic relief but also physiological responses like gastric emptying and mucosal protection. Yet, the magnitude and duration of pH rise are determined by dose, administration frequency, and patient-specific acid secretion rate. In addition, elevating the pH can have unintended consequences on the GI microbiota and patterns of drug absorption, demonstrating the intricate balance between antacid administration and GI homeostasis (Bergan et al., 2021). Such factors underscore the necessity of individualized therapeutic approaches in real-world clinical practice. Whereas antacids successfully increase gastric pH, this change has potential to affect drug metabolism and GI health more widely, requiring accurate clinical scrutiny. Raising the stomach's pH decreases acid-dependent breakdown of some drugs, having the potential to enhance their bioavailability, but causing others that need an acid environment for best absorption to become less soluble. Besides that, pH change can advance alteration of gut microbiota with shifted microbial niches leading to dysbiosis or susceptibility to infections. Utilization of antacids is correlated with variation of the gut-lung axis as well as with immune function alterations, noting the systemic role of these medicines over gastric control (Bergan et al., 2021; Hufnagl et al., 2020). Thus, knowledge of antacids' mechanistic impact on gastric pH and their interactions at the systemic level continues to be central in maximizing their utility in GI pharmacotherapy.

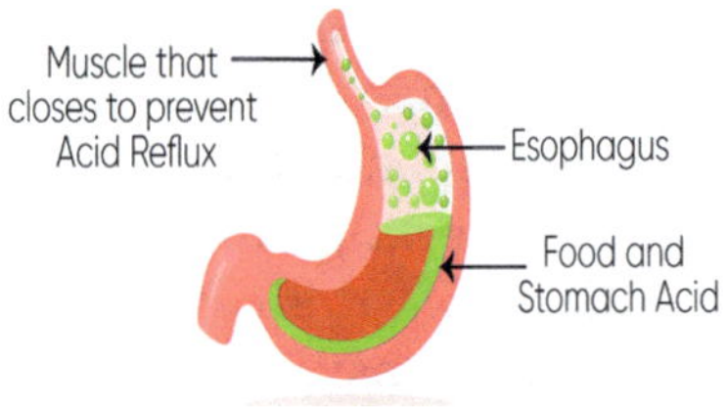

Figure 8.7. Antacids alter gastric pH levels.

Source: Teachoo. (n.d.). *Pharmacology in the Digestive System.* https://external-content.duckduckgo.com/iu/?u=https%3A%2F%2Fd1avenlh0i1xmr.cloudfront.net%2Fa92f8417-bdc7-4457-8968-de7f9d63ecd4%2Fph-in-digestive-system-teachoo.jpg&f=1&nofb=1&ipt=667d06ef84b7310b06e69a3b3ccd4fcbc890078c09a7f2c136c6a54ddbd6f53d.

8.2.2. The Role of Proton Pump Inhibitors (PPIs) in Reducing Acid Secretion

The GI system depends upon a fine equilibrium of protection and secretion to perform its function and integrity. Among the numerous secretions, the gastric acid takes a central place in digestion as well as protection against microbes. Excessive secretion of acid leads to diseases like GERD, peptic ulcer, and Zollinger-Ellison syndrome. PPIs have come to be a specific therapeutic remedy by irreversibly blocking the H+/K+ ATPase enzyme on the parietal cells lining the stomach. The blockage successfully curtails the release of hydrogen ions, causing a significant reduction in gastric acidity. The effectiveness of PPIs in the management of acid hypersecretion not only facilitates mucosal healing but also brings symptomatic relief, thus making them cornerstone drugs in GI pharmacotherapy. The mode of action of PPIs revolves around their selective inhibition of the proton pumps that secrete acid within the stomach. In contrast to H_2 receptor blockers or antacids, PPIs inhibit acid secretion at the last and limiting step, providing a more significant and long-lasting decrease in gastric acidity. This pharmacodynamic feature translates into enhanced clinical efficacy in the treatment of acid-related disorders. Additionally, due to their capacity to sustain a more alkaline pH within the gastric lumen, PPIs promote ulcer and erosion healing, along with shielding susceptible tissue from damage. Gastric acidity modulation by PPIs has distal impact on GI microbiota and immune interactions that could exert effects on systemic health, a factor worthy of further exploration (Agustín et al., 2019; Hou et al., 2022). Chronic use of PPIs should be considered with caution owing to possible changes in GI homeostasis outside the realm of acid suppression. Chronic acid inhibition may affect the gut-liver axis by changing microbial structure and the intestinal barrier, components central to systemic immunity as well as metabolic control (Agustín et al., 2019). Such alterations highlight the need for prudent PPI prescription, weighing treatment benefits against risks like microbiota dysbiosis and heightened infection susceptibility. In spite of these reservations, clinical use of PPIs continues to be invaluable because of their strong acid-reducing activity, thereby ameliorating symptoms and encouraging mucosal protection in acid-peptic conditions. Continued investigations continue to sharpen knowledge on their systemic actions and pave the way for individualized treatment approaches in GI therapeutics.

8.2.3. The Physiological Effects of Laxatives on Bowel Movement

The mechanism of bowel movement is a sophisticated physiological process with cooperative muscular contractions and fluid exchange within the GI tract. Any interruptions in the process are frequently reflected as constipation, in the form of infrequent or hard defecation and the sensation of incomplete evacuation. Laxatives are pharmacologic substances used to reduce these symptoms through the modulation of bowel activity (Figure 8.8). Their physiological actions are diverse depending on the laxative type but mostly aim at accelerating colonic transit and relaxing stool consistency to enable easier passage. Laxatives can act through different mechanisms such as stimulating intestinal motility, promoting intestinal secretions, or adding bulk to stool, finally encouraging defecation. Therapeutic knowledge about these mechanisms is crucial to deliver effective treatment, particularly in cases with comorbidities, which can undermine normal bowel action (Gardiner et al., 2016). Administering laxatives impacts bowels through distortion of the physiology of the rectum and the colon. Stimulant laxatives, for instance, trigger contraction of peristalsis at the direct action on the intestinal wall, and they increase movement of fecal content within the large intestine at a higher velocity. On the other hand, osmotic laxatives produce their effect through the attraction of water into bowel lumen, moistening the stool and filling it, inducing reflex peristalsis thereafter. Bulk-forming laxatives add mass to stool by imbibing water, rendering defecation effective without inducing stringent contractions. These diverse actions correct various causes of constipation and are chosen according to severity and nature of bowel dysfunction. Clinicians must have an understanding of these physiological effects in order to appropriately individualize treatment and prevent possible negative consequences like dehydration or dependency (Gardiner et al., 2016). Although constipation is prevalent GI complaint that occurs in a large proportion of the general population, the physiological nuances underlying treatment make laxative use controversial and requires proper consideration. Severe or chronic constipation may result in complications like fecal impaction or secondary fecal soiling, both of which complicate bowel function and are psychologically significant. The physiological intervention offered by laxatives is not only to restore bowel movement but also to enhance the quality of life as a whole by removing discomfort and preventing further GI disturbance. Nonetheless, indiscriminate utilization of laxatives may injure bowel reflexes and result in dependency, which points to the need for evidence-based prescribing. Comprehensive knowledge of the physiological actions of laxatives is thus central to the effective management of constipation in different patient populations.

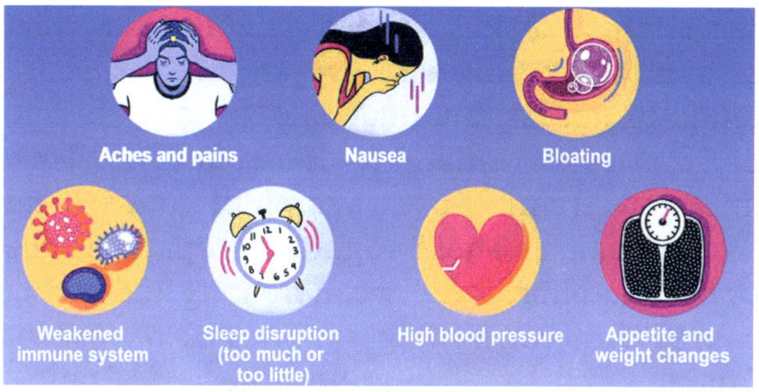

Figure 8.8. The physiological effects of laxatives on bowel movement.

Source: Verywell Mind. (n.d.). *Physical Effects of Depression.* https://www.verywellmind.com/thmb/AsSC4Qkz0mcLvxbbREQxWu4pTxI=/1500x1000/filters:fill(ABEAC3,1)/physical-effects-of-depression-1066890_final-88d54295f77e42d6acce6f096bec1da0.gif.

Test Your Knowledge

1. What is the main physiological effect of laxatives on the gastrointestinal system?
2. What is the primary mechanism by which antacids alter gastric pH?

8.3. Common Gastrointestinal Disorders Treated by Drugs

Learning Outcome

1. Gastroesophageal Reflux Disease (GERD) and Its Treatment Options
2. Peptic Ulcers and the Role of Medication in Management
3. Irritable Bowel Syndrome (IBS) and Pharmacological Interventions

GI conditions include a spectrum of diseases with significant effects on patient quality of life, for which varied pharmacologic treatment is required. Among them, GERD is very common, described by the retrograde flow of stomach acid into the esophagus producing heartburn and possible mucosal injury. PPIs are the drugs of choice to suppress gastric acid secretion, allowing mucosal healing and relief of symptoms. Likewise, peptic ulcer disease tends to necessitate dual therapy of PPIs and antibiotics to eliminate *Helicobacter pylori* infection, treating both symptom control and disease cause. These regimens represent the precise equilibrium between treating underlying causes and controlling symptoms, a precept fundamental to GI pharmacotherapy. Clinical practice guidelines highlight individualized treatment regimens to maximize outcomes, with stress on evidence-based therapeutics to treat GI system disorders (Visseren et al., 2021). IBD, such as Crohn's disease and ulcerative colitis, poses complicated therapeutic challenges because of its autoimmune pathophysiology and chronic GI tract inflammation. Pharmacologic therapy focuses mainly on the reduction of inflammation and remission maintenance. Amino salicylates, corticosteroids, and immunomodulators constitute the first pharmacologic strategy, manipulating the immune response to decrease intestinal inflammation. More recently, biologic agents that target specific cytokines and immune pathways, including anti-TNF agents, have significantly enhanced patient outcomes by allowing targeted immunosuppression. In addition, newer treatment modalities using immunotherapy in addition to angiogenesis inhibitors have demonstrated efficacy in adjacent GI cancers, showing the changing dynamics of drug therapy and research in the field (Richard et al., 2020). Such newer modalities indicate the necessity for continued drug development innovation in treating complicated GI diseases. Functional GI disorders, including IBS, present special therapeutic challenges because they have a multifactorial etiology with changes in motility, visceral hypersensitivity, and psychosocial aspects. Pharmacologic management primarily focuses on relief of symptoms, with measures such as antispasmodics to decrease bowel cramps, laxatives and antidiarrheals to normalize bowel habits, and selective serotonin reuptake inhibitors (SSRIs) to treat concomitant mood disorders and influence gut-brain interaction. Customization of treatment is important, considering patient variation in symptom patterns and severity. In addition, the blending of pharmacologic and non-pharmacologic strategies represents an overall approach to treating these disorders efficiently, highlighting the value of patient-focused care conforming to up-to-date clinical guidelines in GI therapeutics (Visseren et al., 2021).

8.3.1. Gastroesophageal Reflux Disease (GERD) and Its Treatment Options

Challenging GI disorders usually demand sophisticated knowledge of their pathophysiology and individualized therapeutic strategies. GERD is a prime example of such complexity, since it constitutes the abnormal retrograde flow of stomach contents into the esophagus, causing mucosal injury and considerable distress (Figure 8.9). Although transient lower esophageal sphincter relaxations normally control reflux events, hiatal hernias and delayed gastric emptying are among the factors that can enhance this condition. The differentiation from sporadic gastroesophageal reflux to GERD is important, as the latter involves ongoing symptoms or complications like esophagitis. The clinical dilemma is in properly identifying alarming features such as weight loss, bleeding, or persistent emesis, which can require more invasive diagnostics and more aggressive treatment. Early recognition and treatment are essential to prevent complications like esophageal strictures, particularly in high-risk groups such as pediatrics. Pharmacologic improvement has greatly improved GERD management, with emphasis put on acid suppression for the purpose of reducing mucosal damage and symptomatology. Histamine-2 receptor antagonists (H2RAs) used to be the first-line drugs initially, their mechanism being the blockage of H_2 receptors on the gastric parietal cells to lower acid output. Nevertheless, clinical practice and recent case studies have shown minimal effectiveness of H2RAs in patients with alarm features or severe reflux, such as hiatal hernia, among others. PPIs have now become the foundation of drug treatment because of their strong and prolonged acid suppression mediated by irreversible inhibition of the H+/K+-ATPase pump. Additionally, novel agents like potassium-competitive acid blockers (P-CABs) provide speedy onset and powerful acid control, promising a novel option or adjunct in refractory situations. Choosing appropriate acid-suppressive treatment should be evidence-based and tailored, bearing in mind that poor initial treatment may expose the patient to complications (Sattaru et al., 2025). Aside from pharmacological treatment, some GERD patients need to undergo surgery, particularly if medical management is inadequate or complications such as esophageal stricture occur. Laparoscopic fundoplication is a procedure used to restore the integrity of the lower esophageal sphincter so it can mechanically prevent reflux. It is especially appropriate when anatomical defects, such as hiatal hernia, are involved in pathogenesis. In addition, adjunctive surgical procedures like gastrostomy and endoscopic balloon dilation satisfy nutritional demands and treat established strictures, allowing recovery and enhanced quality of life. The multifaceted treatment strategy for GERD mirrors its common relationship with systemic diseases like diabetes mellitus, which can complicate GI motility and symptom control (Sattaru et al., 2025). Comprehensive management therefore consists of a blend of pharmacologic, surgical, and supportive therapy based on the severity and cause of the disease.

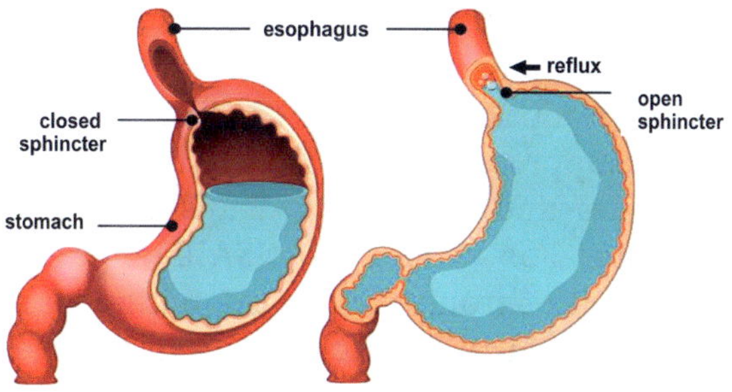

Figure 8.9. Gastroesophageal reflux disease (GERD).

Source: Fortis Healthcare. (2024). *Fortis Blog Banner.* https://www.fortishealthcare.com/drupal-data/styles/blog_detail/azblob/2024-01/Fortis%20Blog%20Banners_05-01-2024_%5B%204%20%5D_0.jpg?itok=7Go_k-eC.

8.3.2. Peptic Ulcers and the Role of Medication in Management

The human GI tract is extremely vulnerable to disturbances induced by numerous factors, such as bacterial infections, lifestyle factors, and drug side effects. Of these disturbances, peptic ulcers pose a major clinical problem, with breaks in the mucosal lining of the stomach or duodenum. The etiology of peptic ulcers is frequently caused by *Helicobacter pylori* infection or long-term use of nonsteroidal anti-inflammatory drugs (NSAIDs), which weaken mucosal protective mechanisms. Management of peptic ulcers involves an integrated strategy, with medication having a central role. Pharmacological treatment aims to suppress gastric acid, facilitate mucosal healing, and eliminate *H. pylori*, if seen. PPIs and histamine H_2-receptor antagonists are the first-line treatments, decreasing acid production substantially. Antibiotics are also included for bacterial elimination, hence addressing the causative etiology instead of solely managing symptoms. This drug treatment approach has significantly reduced adverse effects like perforation and bleeding, enhancing the quality of patients' outcomes within the larger perspective of GI medications. The drug treatment strategy to control peptic ulcers must account not just for acid suppression but also the health status of patients and additional drugs they might be taking. For opioid or NSAID-dependent patients with chronic pain, caution is necessary in evaluating the balance between analgesic requirements and GI safety (Dowell et al., 2022). This is important since opioids, though useful for pain, will perpetuate GI motility disorders, while NSAIDs are responsible for directly causing mucosal damage. New evidence points towards the promise of adjunct therapy, such as nutraceuticals like black cumin (*Nigella sativa*), which has anti-inflammatory and cytoprotective activities (Md. Hannan et al., 2021). These agents can potentially supplement standard medications by reducing oxidative stress and inflammation in the mucosa, though clinical use is investigational. Therefore, treatment regimens for peptic ulcers need to be personalized, taking into account pharmacodynamic principles and potential herb-drug interactions to maximize healing and reduce side effects. Newer developments highlight the need for a holistic, patient-oriented approach to the management of peptic ulcers, beyond acid suppression to the optimization of diet, smoking, and stress. Adherence to medication is crucial when multidrug therapy for *H. pylori* is employed. pylori eradication, since suboptimal courses can promote resistant bacterial strains and recurrent ulceration. Researchers have also highlighted the contribution of oxidative stress and immune modulation to ulcer healing, where agents acting on these pathways may be used as future therapeutic adjuncts (Md. Hannan et al., 2021). In clinical practice, vigilance for adverse reactions, including nutrient malabsorption or drug-induced toxicity, continues to be important. The convergence of innovative pharmacological understandings with pre-existing therapeutic algorithms mirrors the interactive nature of GI drug management with a focus on efficacy and safety to minimize peptic ulcer disease burden in the larger context of GI pharmacotherapy (Dowell et al., 2022).

8.3.3. Irritable Bowel Syndrome (IBS) and Pharmacological Interventions

The challenge in managing GI disorders stems from their multifactorial etiologies, which frequently imply complex interactions among motility, visceral sensitivity, and psychosocial determinants. With IBS, the lack of definite organic pathology makes diagnosis and treatment challenging, requiring emphasis on symptomatic improvement and quality of life enhancement (Figure 8.10). Pharmacotherapy of IBS is therefore intended to address targeted symptoms like diarrhea, constipation, or pain, with varied drugs affecting motility, secretion, and sensory pathways. Such an individualized strategy highlights the necessity of assessing patient profiles on a case-to-case basis in order to ensure maximal therapeutic effectiveness since manifestations of IBS show marked variability. While non-pharmacological strategies remain vital, integrating appropriate drug therapies can significantly modulate symptom severity and frequency, highlighting the need for ongoing research in effective, patient-specific management. Central to recent advances in IBS treatment is the recognition of the gut microbiota's role in GI health and disease. Microbial dysbiosis has been implicated in altered gut motility, immune activation, and visceral hypersensitivity, all hallmark features of IBS. Pharmacological treatments are increasingly taking this relationship into account, with drugs like probiotics looking to rebalance microbial populations, thereby improving symptoms. Moreover, antibiotics like rifaximin have been used to abate bacterial overgrowth caused by IBS, but worries regarding resistance and long-term side effects modify their application. This is an expanding knowledge of microbiota-host relationships that guides the design of new therapies that extend beyond the management of symptoms to alter pathogenic mechanisms underlying the disease, aligning also with general trends in gastroenterology to utilize microbiome science for therapeutic gain (Hou et al., 2022).

These developments hold the promise of more effective and sustained treatment of IBS. The heterogeneity of IBS continues to present challenges in clinical management, even with advances in pharmacotherapy, usually requiring a multidisciplinary strategy. Today's medications comprise antispasmodics, laxatives, antidiarrheals, and central neuromodulators that target different symptom clusters. Antidepressant use, for instance, indicates the significance of the brain-gut axis in the pathophysiology of IBS, influencing visceral pain and psychosocial comorbidities. However, drug effectiveness may be compromised by patient heterogeneity and side effect profiles, thus emphasizing the use of tailored treatment approaches. Furthermore, IBS usually co-occurs with other systemic disorders, which underscores the importance of an integrated approach combining pharmacologic therapy with lifestyle and psychological treatments. This multidisciplinary model of care is imperative considering the chronic and recurring character of IBS symptoms, as seen in the treatment of other chronic multisystem illnesses (Andrew et al., 2022).

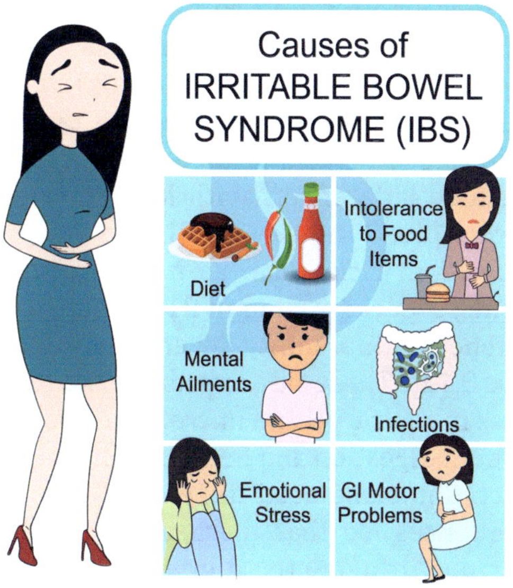

Figure 8.10. Irritable bowel syndrome (IBS) and pharmacological interventions.

Source: The GI Docs (2023). *Irritable Bowel Syndrome (IBS) and Pharmacological Interventions.* https://thegidocs.com/wp-content/uploads/2023/06/IBS1.jpg.

Test Your Knowledge

1. What is GERD and its primary pathophysiology?
2. What is Irritable Bowel Syndrome (IBS) and its main characteristics?

8.4. Side Effects of Gastrointestinal Drugs

Learning Outcome

1. Common Side Effects Associated with Antacids
2. Potential Risks of Long-Term Use of Proton Pump Inhibitors (PPIs)
3. Adverse Effects of Laxatives on Digestive Health

Drugs that act on the GI system are frequently administered in a delicate balance between therapeutic and adverse effects. Most GI drugs, including PPIs and antacids, while useful for the treatment of acid-related disorders, have unintended side effects with long-term usage. For example, long-term PPI use has been implicated in risks such as malabsorption of nutrients, especially vitamin B12 deficiency, and heightened vulnerability to enteric infections (Figure 8.11). These side effects are the result of changes in gastric pH and microbiota, which then affect both digestion and immune function in the GI tract. Clinicians need to be mindful of these consequences, so that therapeutic maneuvers do not unwittingly create other health issues, particularly in susceptible groups like the elderly. Close monitoring of patients and regular monitoring of the drug need are part of reducing side effects attributed to GI pharmacotherapy (Visseren et al., 2021). In addition to the direct biochemical changes provoked by GI drugs, systemic conditions can also occur, attesting to the multidimensional action of such drugs. As an illustration, opioid analgesics, commonly used in treating abdominal pain, are known to cause acute constipation through decreased GI motility and disturbances in ENS function. This side effect, also known as opioid-induced bowel dysfunction, can be associated with considerable patient distress and may necessitate adjunctive pharmacologic interventions or lifestyle changes to control. Likewise, some medications used to manage functional GI disorders can cause dry mouth, blurred vision, and urinary retention as a result of their diffuse inhibitory effects on parasympathetic nervous function. These systemic presentations underscore the need for overall patient education on the possible side effects of GI drugs as well as enhance the need for individualized treatment approaches taking into account efficacy as well as safety profiles (Visseren et al., 2021). Further, upcoming environmental considerations might alter the GI side effect profiles of drugs, making the clinical picture even more complex.

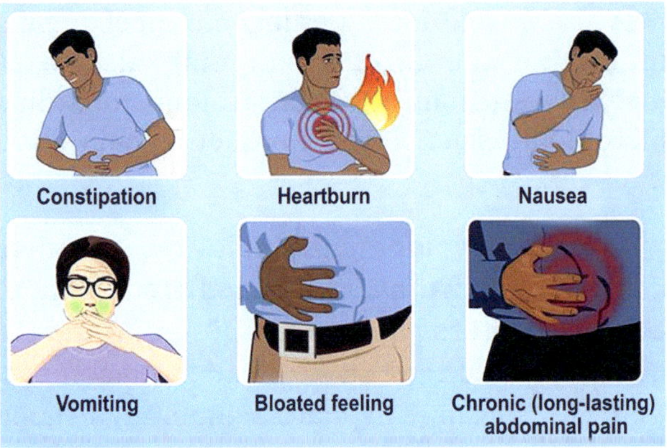

Figure 8.11. Side effects of gastrointestinal (GI) drugs.

Source: You and Constipation. (n.d.). *Diagnosing OIC: OIC—Most Common Digestive System Side Effect of Opioids.* https://external-content.duckduckgo.com/iu/?u=https%3A%2F%2Fwww.youandconstipation.org%2Fen-cnstp%2Fslides%2Fdiagnosing-oic-oic-most-common-digestive-system-side-effect-of-opioids%2Fcpt03-slides-m8_slide_04%24jpg&f=1&nofb=1&ipt=102c231b36566080cafe6b2c512033f5eb5be83b5426163a5af000691afbe99c.

Recent investigations have focused attention on the occurrence of microplastics within human tissues, including the GI tract, and raised concerns about their interaction with drugs taken orally. While the direct impact of microplastics on drug absorption and metabolism is not yet fully understood, their accumulation within human tissues could in theory change the pharmacokinetics or induce inflammatory reactions that enhance drug side effects. This convergence of environmental toxins and pharmacology highlights a new aspect to the understanding of GI drug safety and efficacy. Future studies should aim at exploring the possible implications of such environmental exposures in patients receiving pharmacological therapy for GI disorders to maximize therapeutic benefit.

8.4.1. Common Side Effects Associated with Antacids

The antacid is therapeutically used extensively in the treatment of conditions associated with hypersecretion of gastric acid, like GERD and peptic ulcer. Though these drugs are effective, they tend to bring about numerous side effects, which need cautious deliberation on the part of healthcare practitioners. Among the most common complaints from patients taking antacids are GI disturbances in the form of constipation or diarrhea. This difference is primarily based on the individual active component of the antacid preparation. For instance, aluminum-based antacids are more frequently related to constipation, while those based on magnesium are likely to cause a laxative effect. These dual effects are a result of the effect of these components on motility in the intestine and absorption of fluid, notching the intricacy of relatively simple treatments in the GI tract. In addition to mechanical effects on bowel habits, antacids may impact systemic electrolyte balance, occasionally leading to disturbances such as hypercalcemia or hypophosphatemia. Prolonged use of calcium carbonate-based antacids has been known to contribute to an elevated calcium level in the blood, posing risks such as kidney stone formation and, in rare cases, milk-alkali syndrome. In addition, phosphate binding by aluminum antacids may cause hypophosphatemia with resultant effects on bone metabolism and neuromuscular function. Systemic effects of such emphasize the need for monitoring intake, particularly among at-risk groups such as the elderly, patients with renal dysfunction, or individuals on concomitant medications altering renal excretory mechanisms. Such interaction again adds to the complexity of the safety profile of antacids, reflecting the interlinked nature of GI treatment and metabolic homeostasis in general. Aside from direct GI and metabolic effects, antacid use may also affect the pharmacokinetics of other drugs being taken concomitantly, thus modifying therapeutic effects. Most antacids increase gastric pH, which in turn may change the solubility and absorption of drugs that need acidic environments, like some antifungals and iron supplements. Some antacid ingredients' chelation property can also decrease the bioavailability of antibiotics like tetracyclines and fluoroquinolones. Such interactions require proper timing and patient education to counteract harmful clinical effects. Within the general picture of drugs on the GI system, the identification and management of common antacid side effects are essential in optimizing patient treatment and preventing unintended health outcomes (Bárbara et al., 2022; Divitiis et al., 2016).

8.4.2. Potential Risks of Long-Term Use of Proton Pump Inhibitors (PPIs)

New pharmacologic agents have transformed the treatment of acid-related diseases, but their safety profile must be reevaluated on an ongoing basis. PPIs, introduced in the early 1990s, have become the mainstay of treatment for GERD and peptic ulcer disease. Prolonged PPI use, however, has invited growing attention because of possible side effects (Figure 8.12). Recently, PCABs have emerged as substitutes, possibly alleviating some issues associated with long-term PPI treatment. In spite of such progress, approved use of PPIs continues to be accompanied by dangers that go beyond their desired therapeutic effects, demonstrating the need for careful scrutiny and analysis of emerging evidence to obtain an accurate picture of long-term implications (Jankovic et al., 2024). In clinical practice, the rising rate of PPI prescriptions has occurred ahead of the thorough understanding of their long-term safety. Although PPIs suppress gastric acid secretion effectively, their prolonged usage has been followed by numerous systemic complications. To note, in addition to burgeoning evidence linking PPI use for long durations with increased vulnerability towards renal and liver diseases, CVD, as well as decline in cognitive performance, including dementia,. These interactions are compounded further by enhanced susceptibility to infections in both respiratory and GI tracts due to suppression of natural microbial defenses by acid suppression. Furthermore, extended acid inhibition has been shown to interfere with absorption of essential nutrients, possibly resulting in deficiencies that compromise overall health. This array of risks highlights the pharmacodynamics complexity of PPIs and warrants continued research into duration of dose and appropriate patient selection (Hoque, 2024). Effective treatment of acid-related disorders involves reconciling therapeutic benefit with avoiding possible harm from extended drug exposure. To counter the risks of long-term PPI therapy, physicians must critically justify continued therapy, regularly reviewing treatment need and reducing dosage and duration where possible. While research to alter PPI molecular forms or create new agents for enhancing safety profiles is ongoing, present strategies focus on patient-targeted treatment and careful observation for adverse effects. Through the combination of evidence-based prescribing and keen surveillance, healthcare practitioners can avoid complications like nutrient malabsorption, increased susceptibility to infection, and organ system impairment, thus maximizing patient outcomes while minimizing unnecessary healthcare expenditure and morbidity (Hoque, 2024).

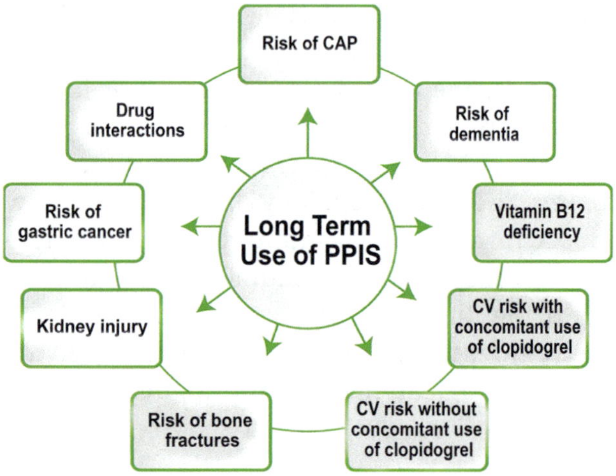

Figure 8.12. Potential risks of long-term use of proton pump inhibitors (PPIs).

Source: https://assets.cureus.com/uploads/figure/file/860769/article_river_99bb40a09f2b11eeb08c99b936289449-graph-13.png.

8.4.3. Adverse Effects of Laxatives on Digestive Health

Use of laxatives to treat constipation is common, but long-term or inappropriate use can cause negative consequences on bowel well-being (Figure 8.13). A major issue is the establishment of dependence, with the normal motility of the bowel reduced because the bowel has been over-stimulated with laxatives. This can lead to long-term constipation, ironically making the original symptom worse and requiring increased doses to produce the same effect. Additionally, some of these laxatives, particularly those that include magnesium salts or bulk-forming agents, are not sufficiently effective in patients with underlying ailments like chronic kidney disease (CKD) and may lead to the precipitant electrolyte disturbances or dehydration. These imbalances can also worsen GI function and overall systemic health. Furthermore, induction of disturbed gut flora and mucosal integrity by certain laxatives may trigger damage or inflammation, highlighting the imperative of careful, tailored therapeutic approaches (Ri et al., 2023). In addition to physiological dependence, use of laxatives risks causing negative changes in intestinal mucosa and absorption mechanisms. Certain stimulant laxatives, if abused, can trigger inflammatory changes and mucosal damage to the epithelial lining, which can impair nutrient uptake and alter the microbiome equilibrium. Such a change in gut ecology has far-reaching effects, such as increased susceptibility to infections or worsening of GI conditions like irritable bowel syndrome (IBS). Osmotic laxatives can also trigger fluid shifts that lead to bloating, cramping, and discomfort, sometimes even worsening constipation symptoms or triggering diarrhea. Complications like electrolyte disturbances, i.e., hypokalemia, may have systemic effects by influencing neuromuscular function, including GI tract function. Such multi-dimensional effects emphasize the precaution in prescribing laxatives and the long-term safety (Ri et al., 2023). Due to the potential dangers with traditional laxatives, focus has increased towards the application of herbal and plant-based formulations as therapeutic options. Several medicinal herbs provide fiber content and bioactive constituents that ensure bowel normality without the severe side effects seen with chemical laxatives. Despite their long history of use and seemingly benign profile, herbal medicines' laxative potential must undergo intense clinical analysis to determine efficacy, dosage, and safety limits. Current data indicate that species like *Aloe barbadensis* and *Cassia angustifolia* possess promising laxative properties with fewer negative effects on gut physiology. However, variability in herbal formulations and absence of standardized formulations create a problem for their incorporation into conventional treatment. The trend toward botanical remedies highlights an urgent need for well-designed research studies to learn more about their impact on gastrointestinal health and to ascertain patient safety.

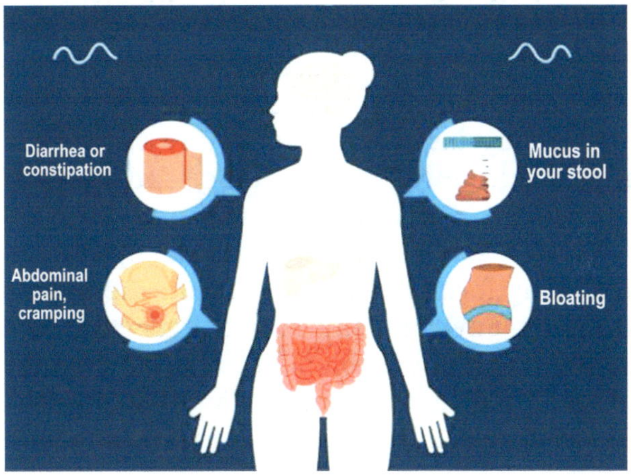

Figure 8.13. Adverse effects of laxatives on digestive health.

Source: Everyday Health. (n.d.). *How Irritable Bowel Syndrome Affects the Digestive Tract.* https://images.everydayhealth.com/images/seo-graphic-content-initiative/eh---how-irritable-bowel-syndrome-affects-the-digestive-tract--seo-graphics-gs.png?sfvrsn=3427287d_3.

Test Your Knowledge

1. What are proton pump inhibitors (PPIs) and their primary function?
2. Name one common side effect of proton pump inhibitors (PPIs).

8.5. Drug Interactions

Learning Outcome

1. Understand hotel maintenance management and its impact
2. Perform preventive maintenance
3. Discuss about breakdown maintenance

The GI system is important in the metabolism and absorption of drugs taken orally, and therefore, it is especially susceptible to sophisticated drug interactions (Figure 8.14). When more than one medication is taken together, their biochemical interaction can modify therapeutic effects, affect drug bioavailability, and intensify side effects. For example, some drug delivery systems, i.e., chitosan/alginate nanoparticles, are being formulated to withstand the hostile stomach environment and trigger targeted delivery within the colon. These products tune the physicochemical environment inside the GI tract, possibly exhibiting interaction with concomitantly administered drugs as well as a change in absorption patterns. These interactions and their tendency to stick to intestinal mucosa can extend retention time of the drug, increasing interaction at the site of absorption and modifying pharmacokinetics (Li et al., 2022). Also, drug-GI system interaction is not limited to absorption alone but also systemic effects through metabolically mediated processes controlled by enzymes in the gut. Some GI medications can impact cytochrome P450 enzymes and transporters like P-glycoprotein, causing either inhibition or induction of metabolizing functions. As a result, co-administration with other drugs that are metabolized through these pathways can result in decreased effectiveness or enhanced toxicity. Additionally, medications impacting GI motility and pH can modify the solubility and rate of dissolution of other drugs, further adding to interactions. Knowledge of these multifactorial actions is necessary to maximize pharmacotherapy and avoid unexpected clinical outcomes in patients on multi-drug therapy. Apart from local GI effects, drug interactions with GI agents have other systemic consequences, including cardiotoxicity. Certain drugs employed in the treatment of GI disorders have molecular mechanisms in common with cardiotoxic drugs affecting mitochondrial function, cell signaling, and cardiac contractility. This overlap enhances the risk for adverse cardiac events, particularly when used in combination with other drugs known to impact cardiac electrophysiology or function (Mamoshina et al., 2021). Therefore, clinicians need to extensively weigh the possibility of drug interactions both within the GI tract and their systemic consequences. Holistic assessment of drug-drug interactions (DDIs) is crucial in minimizing adverse events and providing safe and effective therapeutic regimens for GI disorders.

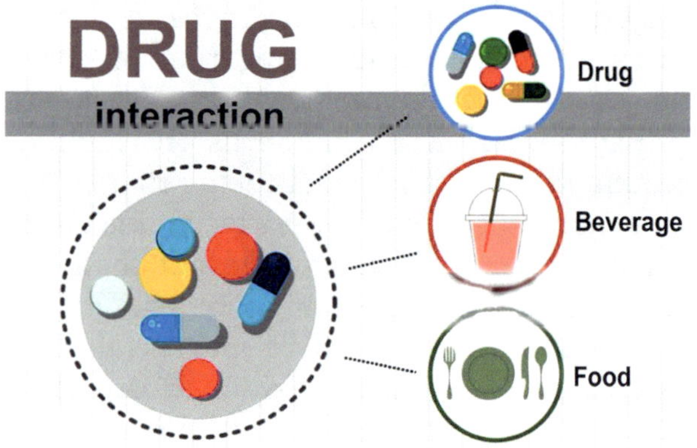

Figure 8.14. Drug interactions.

Source: iStock. (n.d.). *Drug Interaction Infographic for Medical Concept.* https://media.istockphoto.com/id/1415937731/vector/drug-interaction-infographic-for-medical-concept-vector.jpg?s=1024x1024&w=is&k=20&c=FLQ2mjEE4C96Qi_xfn3h4YZwRGNwczapCxRRe7eThDY=.

8.5.1. How Antacids Can Affect the Absorption of Other Medications

The interaction of antacids with concomitantly taken drugs is a significant consideration in the treatment of patients with GI disease. Antacids act mainly by neutralizing gastric acid, raising the pH in the stomach. Such a shift in the gastric pH can have a dramatic impact on the solubility and ionization of medications that must have an acidic environment to be best absorbed. For example, drugs like ketoconazole and some calcium channel blockers have their bioavailability reduced when they are coadministered with antacids. The increase in gastric pH may impair the dissolution of these drugs, hence lowering plasma concentrations to subtherapeutic levels and reducing clinical activity. Also, the chelation mechanism where antacids chelate on drugs like tetracyclines and fluoroquinolones to give insoluble complexes that do not get absorbed. These pharmacokinetic interactions highlight the importance of precise timing and monitoring when antacids are administered together with other drugs to prevent unwanted therapeutic effects. In addition to pH-dependent mechanisms, antacids can affect drug absorption kinetics by altering gastric emptying and intestinal transit time. Through modification of the GI environment, antacids can alter drug release profiles, resulting in fluctuation in peak plasma levels and time to onset of action. Narrow therapeutic index drugs, including digoxin and levothyroxine, are most vulnerable to these changes, which may put patient safety at risk. Additionally, the systemic impact of antacids, like metabolic alkalosis due to bicarbonate-based preparations, can alter renal drug clearance and electrolyte status. These physiological alterations have a secondary effect on the pharmacodynamics of drugs, particularly on drugs undergoing renal elimination. Therefore, comprehension of the complex impact of antacids on GI as well as systemic parameters is critical for maximizing drug therapy in practice (Do et al., 2022). In clinical practice, the effects of drug absorption changes due to antacids require thorough patient education and therapeutic surveillance. Practitioners should be able to foresee possible interactions, modifying dosage regimens or choosing alternative medications as needed. For instance, a gap of at least two hours between antacid intake and affected drugs can prevent absorption interference. The use of non-absorbable antacid preparations may also limit systemic complications. Caution should be taken in groups with impaired renal function or polypharmacy, where the risk of adverse interaction increases. Inclusion of multidisciplinary practices involving pharmacists' suggestions and patient education increases compliance and therapeutic response. Ultimately, acknowledging the complexities of antacid-drug interactions contributes to safer, more effective management strategies within the broader context of drugs affecting the GI system (Meryl et al., 2022).

8.5.2. Interactions Between Proton Pump Inhibitors (PPIs) and Anticoagulants

The intricate pharmacological environment of GI drugs demands special attention to drug interactions, especially between anticoagulants and PPIs (Figure 8.15). Both are frequently used to treat disparate yet frequently co-morbid illnesses, with PPIs solely preventing acid-related diseases and anticoagulants used to avoid thromboembolism. But their concomitant administration is fraught with problems due to different drug metabolism and absorption mechanisms. PPIs can influence the gastric pH, potentially affecting the solubility and bioavailability of certain oral anticoagulants. This alteration may lead to suboptimal anticoagulation, increasing the risk of thrombotic events or, conversely, bleeding complications. It is crucial to understand the interaction between these drug mechanisms to optimize therapeutic regimens, especially in elderly patients with comorbidities, where accurate dosing of anticoagulants and GI tract protective effects have to be balanced carefully (Alexander et al., 2022). Clinically, PPI-anticoagulant interaction usually necessitates careful monitoring to prevent adverse outcomes. For instance, certain DOACs show pH-dependent solubility, which PPIs can reduce, thus lowering plasma concentrations and the effect of medications. By contrast, PPIs themselves have been found to be involved in altering the expression of cytochrome P450 enzymes, enzymes playing essential roles in metabolic clearance of warfarin and other vitamin K antagonists. Such interaction may cause increased anticoagulant activity, with enhanced risk for GI bleeding—a considerable clinical issue in that anticoagulants by themselves subject patients to hemorrhagic hazards. Since these drugs are often given together, especially in patients who are at risk for both peptic ulcer disease and thromboembolic episodes, a judicious understanding of their interaction assists clinicians in the individualization of therapy and stresses the relevance of evidence-based recommendations (Cosentino et al., 2019). Recommendations for the concurrent management of PPI and anticoagulant therapy highlight the importance of individualized risk-benefit evaluation, considering the patient's clinical setting, comorbidities, and potential DDIs. Although PPIs have a protective role versus anticoagulant-induced GI mucosal injury, the nonselective use of PPIs could have the opposite unintended effect, either by rendering an anticoagulant less effective or by increasing adverse effects. The general consensus is to closely monitor coagulation parameters and GI symptoms and adjust therapy accordingly to avoid both thromboembolic and bleeding complications. Health care professionals need to remain aware of the latest scientific evidence and clinical guidelines and use professional judgment adapted to each patient to maximize outcomes. This dynamic strategy ensures that therapeutic maneuvers in the GI system not only maintain symptom control but also ensure systemic safety in intricate pharmacotherapy regimens (Cosentino et al., 2019).

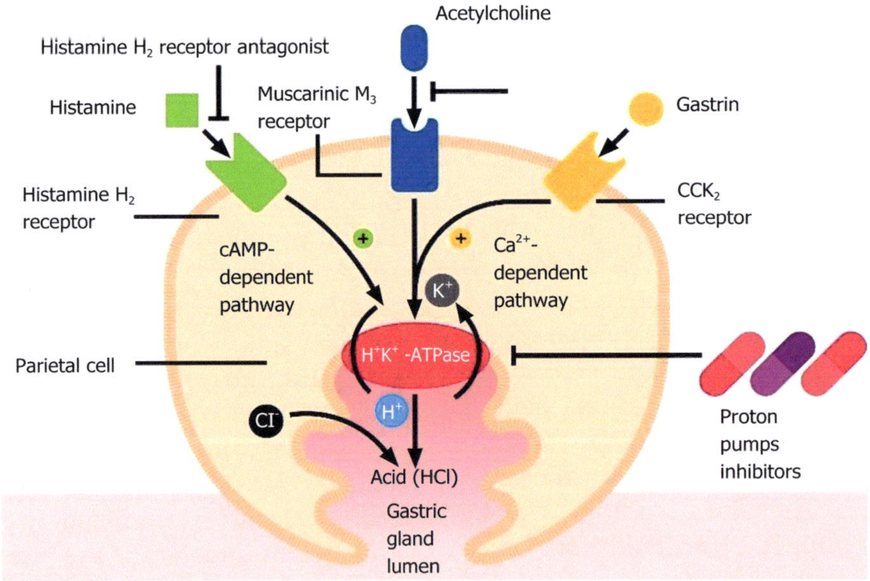

Figure 8.15. Interactions between proton pump inhibitors (PPIs) and anticoagulants.

Source: WJCC. (n.d.). *Interactions Between Proton Pump Inhibitors (PPIs) and Anticoagulants.* https://external-content.duckduckgo.com/iu/?u=https%3A%2F%2Ff6publishing.blob.core.windows.net%2Fedae4e66-c2ab-4b48-a87e-8c595e2fa734%2FWJCC-9-2763-g001.png&f=1&nofb=1&ipt=c1d7612ca590b5feb97b35c5db4d1235b5e721cb57744323b9f70fffc4cb3cfe.

8.5.3. The Impact of Laxatives on the Efficacy of Other Treatments

The complex coordination of GI motility may be seriously affected by the administration of laxatives, which, though essentially devised to treat constipation, may incidentally also change the pharmacokinetics of other drugs. Laxatives, for example, hasten intestinal transit time and thereby reduce the drug's window of absorption that is necessary for maximal uptake since optimal drug take-up depends on prolonged contact with the mucosal surface. This change may reduce the bioavailability of some orally administered drugs, thus compromising their effectiveness. In addition, certain laxatives cause electrolyte disturbances or alteration of GI pH, further influencing solubility and stability of drugs within the intestinal tract. Physicians must thus take into account the timing and nature of laxative treatment when administering drugs to treat GI or systemic disease to prevent compromising therapeutic success. In patients who are being treated for chronic pain with opioid drugs, concurrent use of laxatives presents a complicating factor. Opioid-induced constipation is typically treated with laxatives, but the consequent changes in bowel function can affect the efficacy of peripherally acting μ-opioid receptor antagonists intended to block opioid-induced bowel dysfunction without affecting analgesia (Baratta et al., 2017). The simultaneous use of laxatives and such antagonists is best done with titration because the laxatives can potentiate or mask the effect of the drug, thereby making clinical outcomes complicated. Owing to patient variability and lack of standardized procedures for their combined use, such interactions continue to be important areas for study in order to optimally manage pain and GI function simultaneously. In addition to pharmacodynamic interactions, the psychological and physiological settings in which laxatives are being taken influence the effectiveness of other treatments as well. GI symptoms that vary in relation to stress, as in IBS, can cause patients to use laxatives to self-medicate, which can mask or interfere with intended therapies (Zammit et al., 2009). The cyclical nature of the diarrhea and constipation, along with fluctuating symptoms driven by stress, makes therapeutic regimens difficult and patient compliance challenging. Laxative ingestion in such patients can relieve the symptoms in the short term but also has the potential to mask the diagnosis or reduce the efficacy of drugs aimed at treating pathophysiologic mechanisms. Therefore, a multidisciplinary approach coupling behavioral management and pharmacologic intervention is needed to optimize the treatment outcome in such patients.

Test Your Knowledge

1. How can laxatives affect the absorption of orally administered drugs?
2. What precautions should be taken when combining GI motility drugs with other treatments?

8.6. Patient Considerations

Learning Outcome

1. Importance of Consulting Healthcare Providers Before Use
2. Factors Influencing Drug Choice for Gastrointestinal Issues
3. Patient Education on the Proper Use of Gastrointestinal Drugs

Patient care in the case of drugs that influence the GI system has to start with an understanding of the complex nature of GI diseases. Symptoms like nausea, vomiting, diarrhea, and abdominal pain tend to overlap with signs of infectious diseases, including viral infections like COVID-19, which have been seen to affect the digestive tract. The susceptibility of the GI system to viral infection underscores the need for adequate patient workup prior to starting pharmacologic therapy. Thus, for example, recent data point towards the detection of viral RNA in GI secretions and feces, suggesting possible fecal-oral transmission mechanisms (Gu et al., 2020). This calls for increased awareness to prevent mistaken attributions of drug- or disease-induced side effects for viral-induced GI symptoms. Therefore, clinicians need to incorporate comprehensive patient histories and laboratory data when deciding on GI drug treatments, so that therapies will not aggravate root infectious processes or suppress important symptoms necessitating different management approaches. The pharmacokinetics and pharmacodynamics of GI drugs may be highly variable among patients based on the presence of comorbid conditions, viral infections, and immune status. The effect of SARS-CoV-2 on liver function and bile duct integrity, for instance, highlights the necessity to assess liver function tightly when GI medications are being prescribed since compromised hepatic metabolism can affect drug clearance and enhance the risk of toxicity (Gu et al., 2020). Special populations, such as the elderly, children, pregnant women, or immunocompromised individuals, need specialized therapeutic regimens to optimize adverse effects reduction and maintain efficacy. Monitoring parameters should involve levels of liver enzymes, coagulation parameters, and markers of systemic inflammation, in view of the systemic impact that GI disease and infection may provoke.

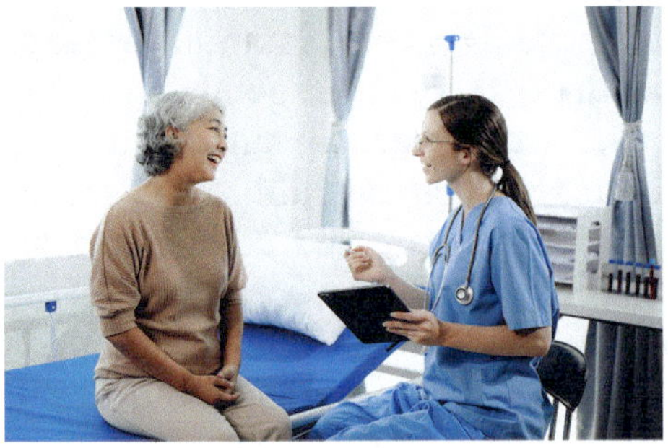

Figure 8.16. Patient considerations.

Source: Flearning Studio. (2024). *How to Improve Patient Education.*

Additionally, possible drug interactions with antiviral or adjuvant treatments call for multistakeholder management by specialists and pharmacists to ensure optimal dosing and minimize unintended effects, thus increasing patient safety and treatment efficacy. Patient education and compliance are essential parts of managing GI disorders with pharmacologic therapy. Due to the systemic effects of GI symptoms that may be associated with infectious causes, patients need to be made aware of the urgency of reporting worse or new symptoms like severe diarrhea, abdominal discomfort, or unforeseen bleeding early. The potential of asymptomatic viral shedding and GI infection in conditions such as COVID-19 also underscores the importance of adherence to rigorous hygiene procedures in order to avoid transmission, which should be reinforced in addition to medication instructions (Gu et al., 2020). Psychological intervention might be required to manage anxiety over GI symptoms coinciding with infectious disease manifestations. Finally, individual care plans must take into account patient environment, support systems, and capacity to follow complicated therapeutic regimens so that drug use influencing the GI tract is safe, effective, and consistent with the patient's total health context (Figure 8.16).

8.6.1. Importance of Consulting Healthcare Providers Before Use

The intricate interactions in the GI system require a judicious use of drugs, especially since most drugs have the potential to significantly affect digestive function. The GI tract's fine balance of microbiota, enzymatic activity, and mucosal integrity can be upset by inadmissible drug use, causing negative effects like malabsorption, changed motility, or mucosal damage. With this complexity, self-treatment with GI medications in the absence of professional advice may worsen underlying disease or initiate unforeseen complications. Medical professionals have the knowledge to perform comprehensive assessments, taking into account patient history, concomitant medication, and particular gastrointestinal disorders (Figure 8.17). Such an informed evaluation guarantees that prescribed medication is consistent with the patient's individual physiological and pathological setting, thus maximizing therapeutic benefit and reducing harm. Such meticulous consultation is necessary to prevent drug interactions and side effects that may undermine GI health and general well-being. Patients with concurrent health conditions, such as CVDs or hormonal disorders, highlight the urgent need for consultation with healthcare providers prior to the initiation of GI drug therapy. Some drugs that impact the digestive system can interact adversely with chronic disease treatments, possibly lowering efficacy or enhancing toxicity. High-risk populations, such as pregnant females or those with underlying metabolic disturbances, are placed at increased risk when taking GI drugs without prescription guidance. Clinicians are better positioned to counterbalance the benefits and risks through the use of customized prescriptions, considering possible interactions and contraindications. Such practice fits into the burgeoning paradigm of personalized medicine, where therapies are made individualized in order to foster safety and efficacy. Not consulting healthcare practitioners may thus result in undetected contraindications and lost opportunities for safer, evidence-based options, hence diminishing patient safety and quality of care (Raffaelli et al., 2023).

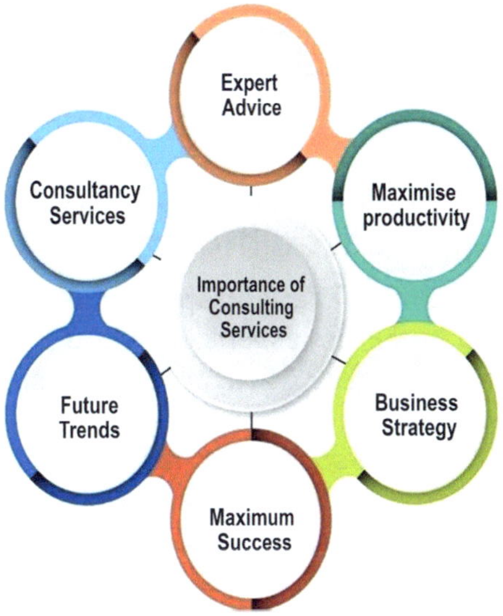

Figure 8.17. Importance of consulting healthcare providers.

Source: Enterprise Wired. (2024). *Importance of Consulting Services for New Businesses.* https://enterprisewired.com/wp-content/uploads/2024/10/1.1-Importance-of-Consulting-Services-for-New-Businesses.jpg.

In addition, the changing environment of drug innovations targeting GI disorders requires current information and professionalism when choosing and handling drugs. Evidence-based clinical practice guidelines highlight the need for healthcare professionals to stay updated with developments in drug therapy, based on research findings and patient-centered outcomes. Proper healthcare consultation supports compliance with such guidelines, leading not only to symptom management but also to the prevention of complications such as nutrient deficiencies or GI malignancies in the long term. In addition, providers enable education regarding lifestyle changes and complementary interventions that optimize pharmacologic treatment effectiveness. Consultation with professionals guarantees that patients are provided with holistic care including both pharmacological and holistic, minimizing the potential for suboptimal therapy and ensuring enhanced quality of life. Therefore, consulting healthcare professionals prior to the administration of GI drugs is an indispensable cornerstone of safe and effective care (Teede et al., 2023).

8.6.2. Factors Influencing Drug Choice for Gastrointestinal Issues

Consideration of patient-specific issues in a subtle manner is essential while choosing medication to treat GI disorders. Physiological alterations that occur due to age significantly affect drug absorption, metabolism, and excretion, thus changing pharmacokinetics and pharmacodynamics in the GI tract. In elderly individuals, especially with polypharmacy and comorbidities, a vigilant approach to prescribing is needed since these increase the potential for drug-related adverse effects (ADRs). There is evidence that the GI tract is often impacted by ADRs, which contribute to a high percentage of complications in elderly patients undergoing treatment (Dagnew et al., 2024). As such, clinicians are required to evaluate comorbidities, hospitalization history, and body composition, including overweight status, in order to prevent risks and maximize therapeutic outcomes. The complexity of the patient's profile highlights the imperative necessity of individualized drug selections in treating GI disorders. Infectious and inflammatory disorders, with those caused by systemic diseases, add an extra layer of complexity to drug choice in GI disorders. The COVID-19 pandemic of recent years brought viral pathology and GI involvement into the spotlight, with various histopathological changes like gastritis, ulceration, and mucosal edema seen in affected patients (Geramizadeh et al., 2024). This only underscores the need to take infections and hepatic disease into account when selecting pharmacologic agents. Medications should not only be chosen for their potency but also for their safety profiles to prevent provoking liver and GI tract injury. Treatment should be tailored to the pathophysiological setting, such as possible viral etiology or ischemic damage, to provide a rational strategy for therapeutic actions in GI care. The healthcare environment and history of previous medication exposure influence drug selection for GI conditions dramatically. Hyper polypharmacy and rehospitalization have also been found to be significant drivers in the generation of ADRs, especially in the case of elderly patients (Dagnew et al., 2024). This points to the significance of reviewing recent medication use and possible DDIs to avert cumulative toxicity within the GI tract. In addition, the diversity of GI pathologies calls for close attention to drug classes that are implicated in side effects; for example, antibiotics and anticoagulants are frequently implicated in GI complications (Dagnew et al., 2024). Successful drug choice thus demands thorough consideration of the clinical situation, prior therapeutic history, and the likelihood of pharmacologically induced GI injury so as to prevent both efficacy and safety in treatment regimens.

8.6.3. Patient Education on the Proper Use of Gastrointestinal Drugs

Optimal therapeutic outcome is a cornerstone using GI drugs when prescribing (Figure 8.18). Instructing patients on the proper administration, timing, and dosage of these medications increases adherence and reduces possible adverse effects. For instance, patients should know the instructions for taking PPIs before meals to achieve maximum acid suppression or the need for hydration in osmotic laxative use. Additionally, open communication about potential side effects and which symptoms need to be seen by a doctor makes patients active participants in their treatment regimens. Healthcare workers should also highlight the importance of taking full courses, particularly for antibiotics used to treat GI infections, to avoid resistance and relapse. Individualized education interventions, taking patients' literacy levels and cultural backgrounds into account, lead to greater understanding and recall of information. A formal patient education strategy, therefore, optimizes drug efficacy while minimizing the risk of complications and enhancing general GI well-being. In addition to drug-delivery mechanics, patient education needs to address lifestyle and food factors impacting GI drug effectiveness. Patients taking antacids or H_2-receptor antagonists need to be instructed on minimizing foods or activities that stress acid reflux or ulcers, including spicy foods, alcohol, and smoking. Furthermore, it is imperative that patients are educated on how GI drugs may interact with other medications or supplements they use to avoid negative effects. For example, teachers ought to emphasize how some antacids can interfere with the absorption of other medications, which requires proper dosing intervals. Additionally, patients who receive opioids for GI motility disorders need to be educated on identifying constipation signs and the role of dietary fiber and exercise in controlling these side effects efficiently. Such full-fledged education helps patients value the complexity of GI treatment, leading to safer and more efficient use of drugs (Evans et al., 2021). In the case of complicated GI diseases, ongoing patient education is critical to modifying treatment regimens according to patient response.

Providers should instruct patients to report any unusual symptoms or failure to improve in a timely fashion so that therapy can be adjusted on time. In chronic illnesses necessitating prolonged drug therapy, like inflammatory bowel disease, patients need to be taught about medication compliance and follow-up measures, such as regular laboratory studies. In addition, patients must be educated about risks posed by self-medication or dose adjustment without medical advice, which may result in complications or drug resistance. Incorporation of educational resources and follow-up visits is pivotal in enhancing retention of knowledge and resolving impending issues. Highlighting shared decision-making enhances patients as active partners for their care, improving clinical outcomes and treatment satisfaction for GI disorders (Alexander et al., 2020).

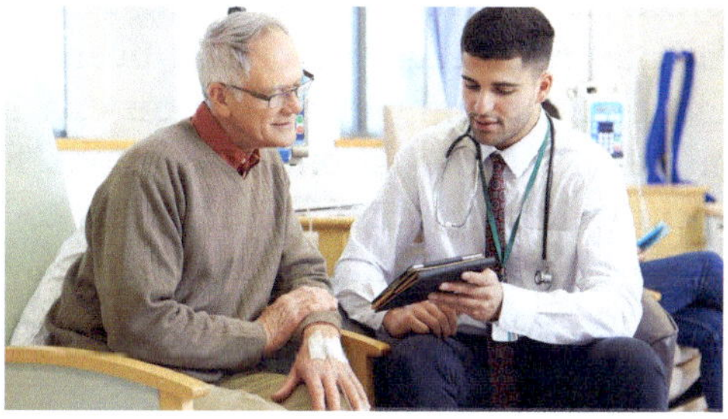

Figure 8.18. Patient education.

Source: Guideway Care. (n.d.). *The Importance of Patient Engagement and Education.* https://guidewaycare.com/wp-content/themes/yootheme/cache/d3/the-importance-of-patient-engagement-and-education-d302a8ee.jpeg.

Test Your Knowledge

1. What role does the side effect profile play in selecting a GI drug?
2. How can a healthcare provider help prevent adverse drug reactions?

SUMMARY

The complex interaction between drug therapy and the GI tract necessitates ongoing assessment to maximize therapeutic effects with minimum side effects. Different drug agents acting on GI disorders or taken concomitantly for systemic illness frequently affect the condition of the gut, affecting the microbiota, motility, and mucosal integrity. Studies of novel formulations, including synbiotic protein supplements, identify the therapeutic potential of interventions that not only meet primary clinical objectives but also enhance GI balance. For example, the creation of a high-protein supplement with probiotics and prebiotics shows great promise in improving gut microbiota composition, enhancing beneficial SCFA production, and overall gut health in athletes. This implies that drug therapies may be optimized to include supportive GI actions, eventually leading to enhanced patient well-being and resistance against drug-induced dysbiosis (Keawyok et al., 2025). Similarly, identification of ADRs on the GI tract is equally significant, which continue to represent a common and significant complication in practice. Research on chemotherapeutic drugs highlights the rate and severity of GI ADRs like nausea, vomiting, and mucositis, that significantly reduce patients' quality of life. Full understanding of the side effects by healthcare professionals will allow them to apply preventive interventions, dose regimens, and supportive care for reducing discomfort and enhancing treatment adherence. Additionally, using validated measures of ADR causality and patient-reported outcomes allows for customized management strategies. This holistic approach not only tackles the direct GI effects of drugs but also enhances overall clinical results and patient satisfaction in extended treatment regimens (Krishnarajan et al., 2021). In summary, a multidisciplinary approach to drugs on the GI system is important for the promotion of therapeutic efficacy and patient well-being. Combining new nutritional supplements that promote gut microbiota with careful surveillance and control of drug-induced GI adverse effects is a prime example of this overall approach. Promoting synergy between pharmacological treatment and healthy gut function can help clinicians maximize the efficacy and tolerability of treatments in various patient populations. Future work must continue to investigate new formulations and accurate management techniques to prevent GI toxicity, maximize microbiome balance, and ultimately enhance patient outcomes. Such endeavors highlight the critical role of the GI system as both a target and a mediator in drug therapy, justifying continued clinical and scientific interest in this area (Keawyok et al., 2025; Krishnarajan et al., 2021).

Summary of the Impact of Drugs on the Gastrointestinal System

The GI tract is particularly susceptible to the actions of many drugs because of its large surface area, heterogeneous cellular composition, and intricate interactions with the gut microbiota and immune cells. Pharmacologic agents tend to modify GI physiology both directly and indirectly, affecting motility, secretion, absorption, and local immune responses. For example, antibiotics may interfere with the balance of commensal bacteria, like lactobacilli, which would otherwise contribute to digestion, vitamin production, and pathogen colonization prevention. Although these microbes tend to support gut health, some strains have been linked to negative effects, particularly in immunocompromised hosts, highlighting the intricacy of drug-microbiome interactions (Antony, 2024). In addition, certain drugs affect epithelial integrity and immune signaling, possibly aggravating inflammatory bowel diseases or predisposing to infections. Therefore, knowledge of these complex mechanisms becomes necessary for the optimal drug therapy and prevention of GI complications. Neuroimmune dialogue in the GI tract is an important aspect wherein drugs could affect gut function and health. Recent studies have outlined the manner in which activation of particular neuronal populations influences local immune cell subsets, modulating inflammatory and homeostatic processes. Activation of nociceptive Trpv1-expressing neurons, for instance, has been found to control regulatory T cells (Tregs) via neuropeptide signaling that involves calcitonin gene–related peptide. Such neuroimmune interactions can modulate tolerance to microbiota of the gut and to pathogens, and these can be targeted or nontargeted by pharmacologic agents (Zhu et al., 2024). Neuroactive drugs as well as certain analgesics can thus exert downstream immunological effects in the GI environment. Understanding these neuroimmune interactions deepens the picture of drug effects beyond traditional pharmacokinetics and underscores the value of integrated gut-brain-immune axis thought. Lastly, the effects of drugs on the GI tract extend to their effects on microbial communities and the resulting immune reactions, which tend to be interdependent. Probiotic supplementation, while safe and in most cases beneficial, needs to be given careful thought due to the risk of pathogenicity in susceptible individuals, highlighting the precarious balance within gut communities (Antony, 2024). In addition, the modulation or activation of specific neuronal circuits by drugs can alter immune cell kinetics such as T helper cells and macrophages, which can influence inflammation and tissue healing (Zhu et al., 2024). All these interactions demonstrate a full network with an intricate web where drug actions are facilitated through multidirectional mechanisms with the participation of the microbiome, nervous system, and immunity. As a result, therapeutic interventions involving the GI tract require an integrative strategy that addresses not only the primary pharmacological effects but also their wider biological consequences.

KEY TERMS FROM THIS CHAPTER

- Gastrointestinal (GI)
- drug interactions
- Medications
- Pharmacologic agents
- Physiological
- Polypharmacy
- Pharmacodynamic
- Healthcare practitioners
- Patient Considerations
- Clinicians
- Gastrointestinal System
- GI drug
- Gastrointestinal Drugs
- Pharmacologic
- Patient safety

CRITICAL THINKING QUESTIONS

1. **Which of the following drugs is a proton pump inhibitor (PPI)?**
   a. Ranitidine
   b. Sucralfate
   c. Omeprazole
   d. Metoclopramide
2. **Which drug is commonly used as an antiemetic due to its dopamine antagonistic action?**
   a. Loperamide
   b. Metoclopramide
   c. Ondansetron
   d. Ranitidine
3. **Which of the following agents is used as a mucosal protective agent in peptic ulcer disease?**
   a. Omeprazole
   b. Sucralfate
   c. Famotidine
   d. Misoprostol
4. **Loperamide is primarily used for the treatment of?**
   a. Constipation
   b. Vomiting
   c. Diarrhea
   d. Gastric ulcers
5. **Misoprostol is contraindicated in?**
   a. Elderly patients
   b. Peptic ulcer disease
   c. Pregnancy
   d. GERD

Short Answer Questions

1. Here are the types of drugs affecting the gastrointestinal (GI) system, categorized by drug classes and their functions?
2. What is a Mechanisms of Action of Drugs Affecting the Gastrointestinal System?
3. Explain about the topic of Common Gastrointestinal Disorders Treated by Drugs?
4. Which gastrointestinal drug is known to cause extrapyramidal side effects?
5. Discuss the mechanism and consequences of drug interactions caused by antacids?
6. Why should prolonged use of proton pump inhibitors (PPIs) be monitored in elderly patients Considerations?

Answer to Critical Thinking Questions

1. (c) 2 (b) 3. (b) 4. (c) 5. (c)

REFERENCES

1. Albillos, A., De Gottardi, A., & Rescigno, M. (2019). The gut–liver axis in liver disease: Pathophysiological basis for therapy. *Journal of Hepatology, 72*(3), 558–577. https://doi.org/10.1016/j.jhep.2019.10.003.
2. Alexander, G. C., Stoller, K. B., Haffajee, R. L., & Saloner, B. (2020). An epidemic in the midst of a pandemic: Opioid use disorder and COVID-19. *Annals of Internal Medicine, 173*, 57–58. https://doi.org/10.7326/M20-1141.
3. Antony, B. (2024). Lactobacilli—Probiotic as well as an uncommon pathogen: Current status regarding the "two sides of the same coin." *SBV Journal of Basic, Clinical and Applied Health Science.* https://www.semanticscholar.org/paper/a9cb264e5cb2343efcdbce5b4c52f0220a7293e3 (accessed on 9 May 2025).
4. Baratta, J. L., Grant, A. E., McNulty, S. E., & Schwenk, E. (2017). The efficacy of peripheral opioid antagonists in opioid-induced constipation and postoperative ileus: A systematic review of the literature. https://core.ac.uk/download/155271457.pdf (accessed on 9 May 2025).
5. Bergan, S., Brunet, M., Hesselink, D. A., Johnson-Davis, K. L., Kunicki, P. K., Lemaître, F., Marquet, P., et al. (2021). Personalized therapy for mycophenolate: Consensus report by the International Association of Therapeutic Drug Monitoring and Clinical Toxicology. *Therapeutic Drug Monitoring, 43*, 150–200. https://doi.org/10.1097/ftd.0000000000000871.
6. Cosentino, F., Grant, P. J., Aboyans, V., Bailey, C. J., Ceriello, A., Delgado, V., Federici, M., et al. (2019). 2019 ESC guidelines on diabetes, pre-diabetes, and cardiovascular diseases developed in collaboration with the EASD. *European Heart Journal, 41*, 255–323. https://doi.org/10.1093/eurheartj/ehz486.
7. Cunningham, M., Azcárate-Peril, M. A., Barnard, A., Benoit, V., Grimaldi, R., Guyonnet, D., Holscher, H. D., et al. (2021). Shaping the future of probiotics and prebiotics. *Trends in Microbiology, 29*, 667–685. https://doi.org/10.1016/j.tim.2021.01.003.
8. Dagnew, S. B., Moges, T. A., Ayele, T., Wondm, S. A., Yazie, T. S., & Dagnew, F. N. (2024). Adverse drug reactions and its associated factors among geriatric hospitalized patients at selected comprehensive specialized hospitals of the Amhara Region, Ethiopia: A multicenter prospective cohort study. *BMC Geriatrics, 24.* https://www.semanticscholar.org/paper/59cc217afe8f612a185a108dd4eb66abd2dd3a35 (accessed on 9 May 2025).
9. Divitiis, C., Arx, C., Grimaldi, A., Cicala, D., Tatangelo, F., Arcella, A., Romano, G., et al. (2016). Metronomic temozolomide as second-line treatment for metastatic poorly differentiated pancreatic neuroendocrine carcinoma. *Journal of Translational Medicine, 14*(1), Article 58. https://www.semanticscholar.org/paper/d44b82ee99ebbad94b2e315e4e77fb5151e94897 (accessed on 9 May 2025).
10. Do, C., Vasquez, P. C., & Soleimani, M. (2022). Metabolic alkalosis pathogenesis, diagnosis, and treatment: Core curriculum 2022. *American Journal of Kidney Diseases, 80*, 536–551. https://doi.org/10.1053/j.ajkd.2021.12.016.
11. Dowell, D., Ragan, K., Jones, C. M., Baldwin, G., & Chou, R. (2022). CDC clinical practice guideline for prescribing opioids for pain—United States, 2022. *MMWR Recommendations and Reports, 71*, 1–95. https://doi.org/10.15585/mmwr.rr7103a1.

12. Evans, L., Rhodes, A., Alhazzani, W., Antonelli, M., Coopersmith, C. M., French, C., Machado, F. R., et al. (2021). Surviving sepsis campaign: International guidelines for management of sepsis and septic shock 2021. *Critical Care Medicine, 49*, e1063–e1143. https://doi.org/10.1097/ccm.0000000000005337.

13. Finn, R. S., Qin, S., Ikeda, M., Galle, P. R., Ducreux, M., Kim, T. Y., Kudo, M., et al. (2020). Atezolizumab plus bevacizumab in unresectable hepatocellular carcinoma. *New England Journal of Medicine, 382*, 1894–1905. https://doi.org/10.1056/nejmoa1915745.

14. Gardiner, A., & Hilton, A. (2016). Managing constipation in adults with co-morbidities. https://core.ac.uk/download/151161237.pdf (accessed on 9 May 2025).

15. Geramizadeh, B., Yazdanparast, M., & Mahboobi, H. (2024). Gastrointestinal and liver histopathology in confirmed SARS-CoV-2 patients: A case series. *The International Journal of Gastroenterology and Hepatology Diseases.* https://www.semanticscholar.org/paper/dc841ba3c270c27bbbaeb89d72b2a2389801f0a5 (accessed on 9 May 2025).

16. Gu, J., Han, B., & Wang, J. (2020). COVID-19: Gastrointestinal manifestations and potential fecal–oral transmission. *Gastroenterology, 158*, 1518–1519. https://doi.org/10.1053/j.gastro.2020.02.054.

17. Hannan, M. A., Rahman, M. A., Sohag, A. A. M., Uddin, M. J., Dash, R., Sikder, M. H., Rahman, M. S., et al. (2021). Black cumin (*Nigella sativa* L.): A comprehensive review on phytochemistry, health benefits, molecular pharmacology, and safety. *Nutrients, 13*, 1784. https://doi.org/10.3390/nu13061784.

18. Hoque, M. (2024). Exploring and understanding adverse effect of proton pump inhibitors. *Hospital Pharmacology–International Multidisciplinary Journal.* https://www.semanticscholar.org/paper/615dc9dc50bb6aabeba9ee60dc1dee452200dd61 (accessed on 9 May 2025).

19. Horne, A. W., & Missmer, S. A. (2022). Pathophysiology, diagnosis, and management of endometriosis. *BMJ*, e070750. https://doi.org/10.1136/bmj-2022-070750.

20. Hou, K., Wu, Z. X., Chen, X. Y., Wang, J. Q., Zhang, D., Xiao, C., Zhu, D., et al. (2022). Microbiota in health and diseases. *Signal Transduction and Targeted Therapy, 7.* https://doi.org/10.1038/s41392-022-00974-4.

21. Hufnagl, K., Pali-Schöll, I., Roth-Walter, F., & Jensen-Jarolim, E. (2020). Dysbiosis of the gut and lung microbiome has a role in asthma. *Seminars in Immunopathology, 42*, 75–93. https://doi.org/10.1007/s00281-019-00775-y.

22. Jankovic, K., Gralnek, I., & Awadie, H. (2024). Emerging long-term risks of the use of proton pump inhibitors and potassium-competitive acid blockers. *Annual Review of Medicine.* https://www.semanticscholar.org/paper/840db73c9bf5fffa477a73a4ec0731c51a92f0fb (accessed on 9 May 2025).

23. Kakiuchi, T., Obata, S., Koji, A., Minematsu, N., Fuchigami, M., Fukuta, A., Tajiri, T., et al. (2024). Case report: The importance of early intervention for gastroesophageal reflux disease caused by hiatal hernia. *Frontiers in Pediatrics, 12.* https://www.semanticscholar.org/paper/c6b4800f288a3802c9577ca3fc8f32cd54d1da3c (accessed on 9 May 2025).

24. Keawyok, K., & Jodnak, S. (2025). Development of high protein supplements containing symbiotic for athletes. *Bioactive Compounds in Health and Disease.* https://www.semanticscholar.org/paper/aaf71d320a333a3f801bc33fd2f152293f5ae25d (accessed on 9 May 2025).

25. Krishnarajan, D., Sivasakthi, K., Ariyamol, R., Kumar, D., & Varghese, S. (2021). A prospective observational study of chemotherapy-induced adverse drug reaction and the quality of life in cancer patients in a tertiary care hospital. *Journal of Cancer Research and Therapeutics, 17,* 530–536. https://www.semanticscholar.org/paper/29327ad87913b0dab57522a7f3a0e917325e5b36 (accessed on 9 May 2025).

26. LeBoff, M. S., Greenspan, S. L., Insogna, K., Lewiecki, E. M., Saag, K. G., Singer, A., & Siris, E. S. (2022). The clinician's guide to prevention and treatment of osteoporosis. *Osteoporosis International, 33,* 2049–2102. https://doi.org/10.1007/s00198-021-05900-y.

27. Lévy, É., Delvin, E., Marcil, V., & Spahis, S. (2020). Can phytotherapy with polyphenols serve as a powerful approach for the prevention and therapy tool of novel coronavirus disease 2019 (COVID-19)? *AJP Endocrinology and Metabolism, 319,* E689–E708. https://doi.org/10.1152/ajpendo.00298.2020.

28. Li, J., Cao, F., Yin, H., Huang, Z., Lin, Z., Mao, N., Sun, B., et al. (2020). Ferroptosis: Past, present and future. *Cell Death and Disease, 11.* https://doi.org/10.1038/s41419-020-2298-2.

29. Li, S., Zhang, H., Chen, K., Jin, M., Vu, S. H., Jung, S., He, N., et al. (2022). Application of chitosan/alginate nanoparticle in oral drug delivery systems: Prospects and challenges. *Drug Delivery, 29,* 1142–1149. https://doi.org/10.1080/10717544.2022.2058646.

30. Lyon, A. R., López-Fernández, T., Couch, L. S., Asteggiano, R., Aznar, M. C., Bergler-Klein, J., Boriani, G., et al. (2022). 2022 ESC guidelines on cardio-oncology developed in collaboration with the European Hematology Association (EHA), the European Society for Therapeutic Radiology and Oncology (ESTRO), and the International Cardio-Oncology Society (IC-OS). *European Heart Journal, 43*(42), 4229–4361. https://doi.org/10.1093/eurheartj/ehac244.

31. Mamoshina, P., Rodríguez, B., & Bueno-Orovio, A. (2021). Toward a broader view of mechanisms of drug cardiotoxicity. *Cell Reports Medicine, 2,* 100216. https://doi.org/10.1016/j.xcrm.2021.100216.

32. Marks, S. L., Kook, P. H., Papich, M. G., Tolbert, M. K., & Willard, M. D. (2018). ACVIM consensus statement: Support for rational administration of gastrointestinal protectants to dogs and cats. *Journal of Veterinary Internal Medicine, 32,* 1823–1840. https://doi.org/10.1111/jvim.15337.

33. Monteduro, A. G., Rizzato, S., Caragnano, G., Trapani, A., Giannelli, G., & Maruccio, G. (2023). Organs-on-chips technologies–A guide from disease models to opportunities for drug development. *Biosensors and Bioelectronics, 231,* 115271. https://doi.org/10.1016/j.bios.2023.115271.

34. N/A. (2021). *Constipation.* https://core.ac.uk/download/478104861.pdf (accessed on 9 May 2025).

35. Patra, J. K., Das, G., Fraceto, L. F., Campos, E. V. R., Rodriguez-Torres, M. del P., Acosta-Torres, L. S., Díaz-Torres, L. A., et al. (2018). Nano-based drug delivery systems: Recent developments and future prospects. *Journal of Nanobiotechnology, 16.* https://doi.org/10.1186/s12951-018-0392-8.

36. Raffaelli, B., Rubio-Beltrán, E., Cho, S.-J., De Icco, R., Labastida-Ramírez, A., Onan, D., Ornello, R., et al. (2023). Health equity, care access and quality in headache–Part 2. *The Journal of Headache and Pain, 24,* Article 99. https://doi.org/10.1186/s10194-023-01699-7.

37. Ragusa, A., Svelato, A., Santacroce, C., Catalano, P., Notarstefano, V., Carnevali, O., Papa, F., et al. (2020). Plasticenta: First evidence of microplastics in human placenta. *Environment International, 146*, 106274. https://doi.org/10.1016/j.envint.2020.106274.

38. Reichardt, S. D., Amouret, A., Muzzi, C., Vettorazzi, S., Tuckermann, J., Lühder, F., & Reichardt, H. M. (2021). The role of glucocorticoids in inflammatory diseases. *Cells, 10*, 2921. https://doi.org/10.3390/cells10112921.

39. Ri, R., Park, S. Y., & Camilleri, M. (2023). Constipation in patients with chronic kidney disease. *Journal of Neurogastroenterology and Motility, 29*, 428–435. https://doi.org/10.5056/jnm23133.

40. Sattaru, K., Madhu, M. T., Singh, J. K., Kandi, V., Gupta, A., Ca, J., Balaji, O., et al. (2025). A comprehensive review of the effects of diabetes mellitus on the gastrointestinal system. *Cures, 17.* https://www.semanticscholar.org/paper/d1562b23b6449d94cf41e0391ca85d570ceb1c81 (accessed on 9 May 2025).

41. Silva, B., Soares, J., Rocha-Pereira, C., Mladěnka, P., & Remião, F. (2022). Khat, a cultural chewing drug: A toxicokinetic and toxicodynamic summary. *Toxins, 14*(1), Article 1. https://www.semanticscholar.org/paper/16d570928ce2b125f2554e34c271f16ae1a67213 (accessed on 9 May 2025).

42. Teede, H., Tay, C. T., Laven, J. S. E., Dokras, A., Moran, L., Piltonen, T., Costello, M., et al. (2023). Recommendations from the 2023 international evidence-based guideline for the assessment and management of polycystic ovary syndrome. *Fertility and Sterility, 120*, 767–793. https://doi.org/10.1016/j.fertnstert.2023.07.025.

43. Thiruvengadam, M., Shariati, M. A., Akram, M., Zainab, R., Daniyal, M., Bankolé, M. M., Ребезов, M., et al. (2021). Herbal medicine for the management of laxative activity. *Current Pharmaceutical Biotechnology, 23*, 1269–1283. https://doi.org/10.2174/1389201022666210812121328.

44. van der Hee, B., & Wells, J. M. (2021). Microbial regulation of host physiology by short-chain fatty acids. *Trends in Microbiology, 29*(9), 700–712. https://doi.org/10.1016/j.tim.2021.02.001

45. Visseren, F. L. J., Mach, F., Smulders, Y. M., Carballo, D., Koskinas, K. C., Bäck, M., Bénétos, A., et al. (2021). 2021 ESC guidelines on cardiovascular disease prevention in clinical practice. *European Heart Journal, 42*, 3227–3337. https://doi.org/10.1093/eurheartj/ehab484.

46. Wagle, S. R., Kovačević, B., Walker, D. P., Ionescu, C. M., Shah, U., Stojanović, G., Kojić, S., et al. (2020). Alginate-based drug oral targeting using bio-micro/nano encapsulation technologies. *Expert Opinion on Drug Delivery, 17*, 1361–1376. https://doi.org/10.1080/17425247.2020.1789587.

47. Wei, P. F. (2020). Diagnosis and treatment protocol for novel coronavirus pneumonia (trial version 7). *Chinese Medical Journal, 133*, 1087–1095. https://doi.org/10.1097/cm9.0000000000000819.

48. Zammit, E. (2009). *The Irritable Bowel Syndrome.* https://core.ac.uk/download/46602223.pdf (accessed on 9 May 2025).

49. Zhu, Y., Meerschaert, K. A., Galván-Peña, S., Bin, N. R., Yang, D., Basu, H., Kawamoto, R., et al. (2024). A chemogenetic screen reveals that Trpv1-expressing neurons control regulatory T cells in the gut. *Science, 385.* https://www.semanticscholar.org/paper/8cc3e68d4dce42d24766cb1f7f30192a194ad616 (accessed on 9 May 2025).

ANTIMICROBIAL AGENTS

9

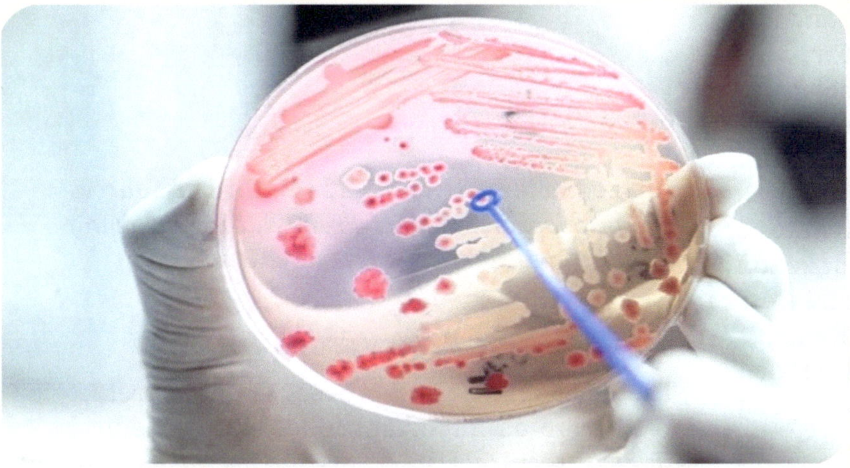

LEARNING OBJECTIVES

After studying this chapter, you will be able to:

1. List the types of antimicrobial agents
2. Discuss of mechanisms of action
3. Define spectrum of activity
4. Explore of resistance to antimicrobial agents
5. Explain the development of new antimicrobial agents
6. Identify the clinical applications

Introduction

The recurring challenge presented by infectious diseases has long required the creation of agents that can manage microbial growth and dissemination. From the early discovery of antibiotics, antimicrobial agents have transformed medicine by making it possible to treat bacterial, viral, fungal, and parasitic infections effectively. Yet, the evolutionary plasticity of microorganisms continually renders current drugs ineffective, requiring continuous innovation in antimicrobial approaches. Elucidating the biochemical and molecular basis of microbial inhibition is crucial for progress, as it can inform the development and use of novel agents that possess more favorable therapeutic properties. This multidisciplinary field includes both classical chemical antibiotics and biologically based compounds, which emphasizes the development of integrating microbiology, pharmacology, and clinical medicine to combat evolving infectious challenges in an ever-evolving and interactive way (Lorrence et al., 2021). Over the past few years, the increasing number of antimicrobial resistance

(AMR) cases has increased the pressure to discover new compounds that can bypass the defense mechanism of microbes. When pathogens develop mechanisms to resist the action of drugs that kill them, they become resistant, causing treatment failures as well as adding costs to healthcare worldwide. The crisis calls for novel solutions, and one is looking into natural products as a source of new antimicrobial molecules. Natural extracts and phytochemicals have gained renewed attention due to their diverse bioactive properties and low propensity for promoting resistance. Moreover, combining these agents with conventional drugs may enhance treatment efficacy, providing a synergistic effect that mitigates the spread of resistant strains. As a result, scientific research aims to explain their structures, biosynthesis processes, and particular mechanisms of action to design stable antimicrobials that can address today's and tomorrow's therapeutic requirements (Guglielmi et al., 2020). Essential to the creation of effective antimicrobial drugs is a good understanding of microbial physiology and the specific biochemical targets that can be targeted therapeutically (Figure 9.1). Microorganisms have structural and functional diversity, which controls susceptibility to various agents, and therefore accurate identification and targeting are essential. Development in microbiological methods, such as molecular diagnostics and susceptibility testing, allows for tailored application of antimicrobials and controls the risk of resistance emergence. Furthermore, studying how antimicrobial compounds interfere with the mechanisms of microbial viability, such as inhibiting cell wall formation, protein synthesis, or damaging nucleic acids, yields key information to streamline drug development. By synthesizing these scientific paradigms and using multidisciplinary approaches, the discipline of antimicrobial science keeps progressing towards maintaining public health in the face of continuous outbreaks of infectious disease (Lorrence et al., 2021).

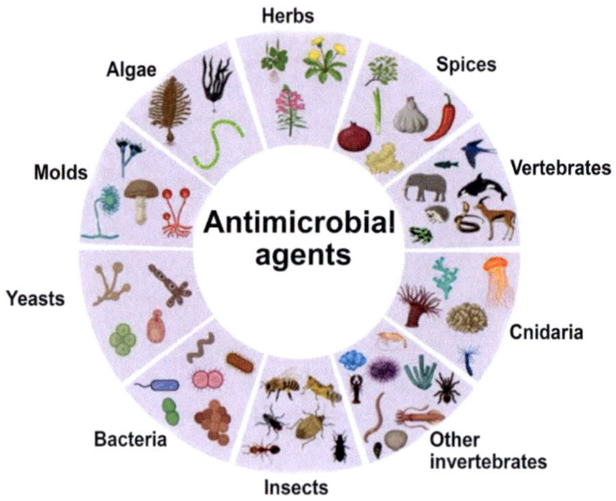

Figure 9.1. Antimicrobial agents.

Source: Sulieman, A.-M. (2023). *Diverse Sources of Antimicrobial Agents From Nature Involving Either Phytochemicals.* ResearchGate.

Definition of Antimicrobial Agents

The development and process of antimicrobial agents are an important milestone in medical science to target microorganisms that cause infection. Antimicrobial agents refer to a large group of materials that can be used to prevent or kill bacteria, viruses, fungi, or parasites. They differ from typical medications in the sense that antimicrobial agents exclusively disrupt the proliferation or activity of disease-causing microbes, ensuring better patient prognosis and disease dissemination prevention. Their effectiveness relies to a significant extent on their mechanism of action, which varies from interfering with cell wall synthesis to inhibiting protein or nucleic acid production. Their ongoing development meets the ever-evolving nature of microbial resistance, requiring agents that can both identify and characterize resistance patterns reliably to inform effective treatment protocols (Bortolaia et al., 2020). This dynamic interaction emphasizes the multifaceted nature of antimicrobial agents in clinical and research contexts. Antimicrobial agents are varied in their classification, reflecting the pathogens they target and the manner of action. In general, they can be grouped into antibiotics, antivirals, antifungals, and antiparasitic, with varying clinical applications and molecular targets. Antibiotics, for example, act mostly on bacterial infections by disrupting processes that are specific to bacterial cells, e.g., cell wall formation or ribosomal activity. Antiviral agents, on the other hand, are designed to inhibit viral replication without being toxic to host cells. This selectivity is important to avoid cytotoxicity while providing maximal therapeutic effects. Knowledge of these differences is essential when choosing an effective antimicrobial agent for treatment, as misuse can result in suboptimal results and enhanced resistance. Evidence-based guidelines, including those created for the management of sepsis, highlight the careful use of antimicrobial agents to maximize patient outcomes and minimize resistance development (Rhodes et al., 2017).

In addition to their therapeutic roles, antimicrobial agents play a vital role in public health and infection control. Their clinical implementation as a strategy decreases morbidity and mortality from infectious diseases. Yet for them to remain effective, it is critical that one not only has an understanding of the pharmacological properties but also of the genetic drivers of microbial resistance processes. Improved genomic technologies have made it possible to engineer tools such as *in silico* antibiograms, which decode whole genome sequencing data to make accurate antimicrobial susceptibility predictions (Bortolaia et al., 2020). Such advances support the capacity to individualize treatment based on the unique microbial resistance patterns, allowing for precision medicine practices. As such, the definition of antimicrobial agents has expanded beyond the chemical or biological nature of their identities to encompass their incorporation into complex diagnostic and stewardship systems.

Importance in Medicine and Public Health

The dynamic nature of infectious disease highlights the pivotal importance of antimicrobial drugs in medicine and public health (Figure 9.2). As antibiotic-resistant bacteria such as methicillin-resistant *Staphylococcus aureus* (MRSA) have grown in popularity, the world's healthcare systems are increasingly confronted with rising difficulties in successfully treating routine infections. The shrinking antibiotic development pipeline, which has been caused primarily by decreased investment by pharmaceutical companies, has exacerbated the need for other options. Conventional medicinal herbal plants offer a promising lead, since recent research demonstrates their extensive antibacterial activity against resistant bacteria, some equivalent to the action of proven antibiotics such as vancomycin. Such discoveries illustrate the double importance of antimicrobial agents: both in the treatment of clinical infection and in limiting the public health danger presented by resistant microorganisms. Further investigation of such natural products may lead to new therapeutics that meet medical needs as well as the general societal cost of drug resistance (He, 2019). Tackling AMR necessitates innovative approaches that go beyond traditional antibiotics, particularly when dealing with multidrug-resistant pathogens involved in widespread disease. For instance, the position of *Campylobacter* as the primary bacterial cause of diarrheal disease worldwide requires efficient intervention measures because severe infections frequently manifest in susceptible groups such as children and the elderly. The investigation of nanotechnology, specifically glutathione-stabilized silver nanoparticles (GSH-Ag NPs), presents promising antimicrobial activity against multidrug-resistant *Campylobacter* strains. These nanoparticles demonstrate effective bactericidal activity at relatively low doses, implying potential use in medical environments to manage infections in which conventional antibiotics are ineffective. In addition, a balance between antimicrobial efficacy and biocompatibility is still essential; continued cytotoxicity tests suggest additional investigation but also support the promise of new agents to increase public health gains by combating resistant infections (Silvan et al., 2018). Aside from their therapeutic uses, antimicrobial agents are also crucial for the overall scope of public health by inhibiting the transmission of infectious diseases. This mandate is not only limited to healthcare settings but is extended to agricultural and community settings where resistant microbes are often a common occurrence. Antimicrobial agents' effectiveness therefore directly correlates with infection control strategies, disease outbreak control, and the containment of drug-resistant microorganisms at the population level. Moreover, synergy seen upon co-administration of new drugs with current antibiotics has the potential to potentiate therapy, decrease dosing requirements, and curtail side effects, while promoting antimicrobial stewardship. Thus, the development and judicious use of antimicrobial agents are critical in sustaining their effectiveness, protecting public health infrastructure, and combating widespread threats caused by emerging microbial adversity in the 21st century (He, 2019; Silvan et al., 2018).

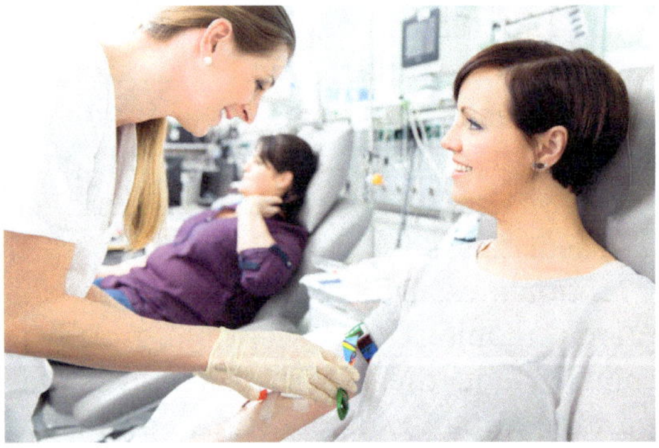

Figure 9.2. Medicine and public health.

Source: Masters Programs Guide. (2018). *Shutterstock_697455157.* https://www.mastersprogramsguide.com/wp-content/uploads/2018/02/shutterstock_697455157.jpg.

9.1. Types of Antimicrobial Agents

Learning Outcome

1. Antibiotics
2. Antifungals
3. Antivirals

The multi-faceted character of antimicrobial agents stems from their varied chemical structures and modes of action, which determine their activity against different pathogens. Of the dominant forms, polysaccharide-based nanocomposites have emerged because they can be filled with reinforcing nanoparticles such as silver, increasing mechanical strength and possessing strong antimicrobial activity (Figure 9.3). Nanocomposites are especially promising for use in food packaging, where microbial contamination can cause serious threats. Their architecture is usually in the form of an external polysaccharide network, e.g., chitosan or cellulose, with nanoscale reinforcements, while maintaining mechanisms for preventing bacterial growth by disrupting cell membranes and inducing oxidative stress. This multi-functionality not only enhances durability but also broadens the antimicrobial activity, rendering them useful substitutes or adjuncts to conventional antimicrobials. The promise of these composites suggests a shift toward materials that are both physically durable and microbially inhibitory without the use of traditional chemical antibiotics (Pal et al., 2021). The development of antibiotic-resistant bacteria has made new alternatives necessary, with bacteriocins being promising peptide-based antimicrobial compounds. These ribosomal synthesized peptides from different bacteria are of varied structures and mechanisms, such as permeabilization of the membrane, inhibition of cell wall formation, and interference in critical metabolic pathways. In contrast to broad-spectrum antibiotics, bacteriocins have the capability to provide extremely specific activity towards specific bacterial species, minimizing harm to the host microbiota. Moreover, being of natural origin and having lesser chances of developing resistance, they are good drug candidates for clinical applications. Significantly, bacteriocins can be bioengineered to optimize their stability and efficacy, making them amenable to personalized antimicrobial intervention. They also demonstrate promise for prophylactic as well as therapeutic interventions, especially in treating infections where conventional antibiotics are no longer effective because of resistance (Hols et al., 2019). In addition to conventional antibiotics and bacteriocins, antimicrobial agents include a wide range of classes such as antibiotics, heat- and proteolytic-resistant small peptides that act on lipid II in bacterial cell walls, thereby compromising membrane integrity.

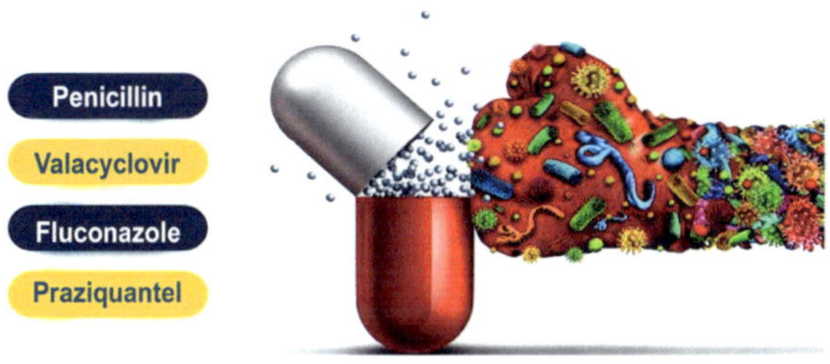

Figure 9.3. Types of antimicrobial agents.

Source: PathKind. (n.d.). *Types of Antimicrobials.* https://pathkindwebsiteprod.blob.core.windows.net/websiteprod/uploads/blogs/Types-of-Antimicrobials.jpg.

These agents, for example, nisin, have been widely used in food preservation and hold potential for clinical use because of their broad-spectrum activity and capacity to target resistant pathogens. In addition to peptides, chemical derivatization and synthetic methods allow for the generation of hybrid molecules and nanostructured composites with improved pharmacokinetics and increased antimicrobial spectra. Through integration of natural and synthetic properties, these new antimicrobials overcome limitations of traditional antibiotics such as toxicity and environmental persistence. Accordingly, the antimicrobial agent field keeps growing, incorporating natural peptides, designed molecules, and nanomaterials to fight increasing antimicrobial resistance (AMR) issues (Hols et al., 2019; Pal et al., 2021).

9.1.1. Antibiotics

The growing incidence of antibiotic-resistant bacteria is a key challenge in contemporary medicine, and the need for the discovery of novel antimicrobial agents has been emphasized. Current studies have identified the potential of plant-derived molecules as a useful adjunct or substitute for traditional antibiotics. Phytochemicals, especially polyphenols and terpenes, have shown potent antimicrobial activity, frequently by mechanisms involving the disruption of bacterial plasma membranes. Particular structural characteristics, including phenolic hydroxyl group placement and conjugation in flavonoids, determine the potency of these compounds. Furthermore, the synergistic potential between these plant agents and classical antibiotics provides avenues for furthering resistance conquest. For instance, the conjugation of phytochemicals with beta-lactam antibiotics mainly allows for the inhibition of bacterial efflux pumps, which is one of the widespread mechanisms of resistance. This integrative strategy highlights the need to develop omics technologies and network pharmacology to maximize the application of plant antimicrobials and renew current antibiotic therapy (Javier et al., 2021). Nosocomial pathogens such as *Pseudomonas aeruginosa* demonstrate the need for addressing antibiotic resistance, which the World Health Organization has classified as a priority one pathogen. This organism's capacity for developing intrinsic, adaptive, and acquired resistance mechanisms makes treatment challenging, particularly under conditions of high stress like cystic fibrosis-affected lungs. Processes like extended antibiotic therapy and augmented immune reactions enhance the pathogen's virulence and multi-drug resistance. The COVID-19 pandemic has, unfortunately, inadvertently caused AMR to escalate further due to global empirical antibiotic use and augmented application of disinfectants. Therefore, controlling such persistent pathogens requires new approaches beyond traditional antibiotics to maintain antimicrobial activity and mitigate healthcare-associated infections (Frèdi et al., 2021).

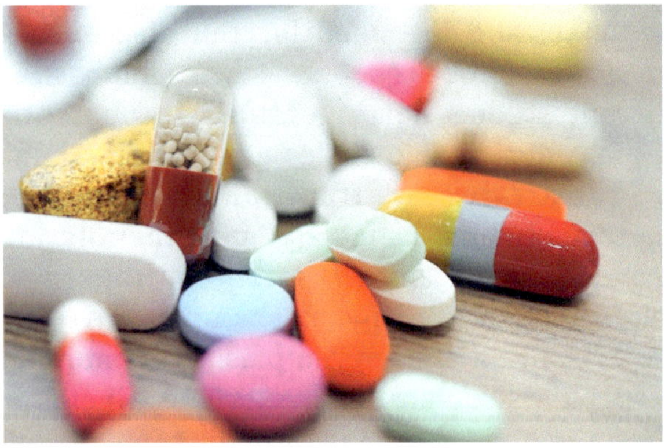

Figure 9.4. Antibiotics.

Source: https://cdn.mos.cms.futurecdn.net/JNcdr4XQV5nZoVVGgS8yRn.jpg.

In the face of increasing resistance, anti-resistance adjuvant treatments have come forward as a strategic adjunct to antibiotic therapy. These treatments aim to neutralize bacterial resistance strategies instead of targeting direct killing of pathogens, hence minimizing selective pressure and the emergence of resistance. Through the targeting of efflux pumps or pathways of biofilm formation, adjuvants can improve penetration and efficacy of antibiotics (Figure 9.4). Particularly, this method has the potential to extend the lifespan of current antibiotics, an important consideration amidst the glacial pace of new drug development. With difficulties in designing effective adjuvants and mapping microbial resistance networks, continued innovations bring a promising hope. Under such circumstances, antimicrobial stewardship needs to integrate such adjunct therapies so that the clinical efficacy of antibiotics is maintained and the development of multidrug-resistant infections is curbed (Frèdi et al., 2021).

9.1.2. Antifungals

The rise in the incidence of fungal infections, especially *Candida* species and dermatophytes, presents great challenges in clinical management through an increase in resistance to traditional antifungal agents like fluconazole. This has stimulated the investigation of new antimicrobial approaches that can counter both efficacy and safety issues. One of the notable improvements is the utilization of silver nanoparticles (AgNPs), which are prepared using environmentally benign routes based on plant extracts. These AgNPs exhibit excellent antifungal activity by interfering with the integrity of fungal cell membranes and inhibiting virulence factors such as biofilm formation and hyphal growth. Additionally, their growth inhibition in species such as Trichophyton rubrum and Microsporum canis indicates their potential as a new class of antimicrobial agents with dual advantages, including anticancer properties. This multifunctionality highlights the potential biomedical uses of such nanoparticles in the fight against resistant fungal infections and potentially reducing side effects (Badiâa et al., 2022). Chronic wounds, especially diabetic foot ulcers (DFUs), frequently contain advanced polymicrobial communities with both bacteria and fungi, making treatment challenging. Fungal infection in such wounds leads to necrosis and delays healing, but antifungal agents' role in the treatment of such infections is underemphasized. The emergence of AMR highlights the need for novel antifungal therapies with broad-spectrum activity. Endogenous antimicrobial peptides (AMPs) are attractive candidates because they are naturally present in mammalian skin and can act against a wide range of pathogens, including fungi. In addition to their potent antifungal activity, these peptides also facilitate wound healing, a critical property for the treatment of DFUs. The dual antimicrobial and repairing role of AMPs provides a strategic benefit in treating polymicrobial infections where traditional antifungals might not be effective, calling for increased research to enhance their use clinically (Jéssica et al., 2021). The establishment of antifungal treatment needs to involve mechanisms that take into account biofilm-linked resistance and modulation of virulence factors. Fungal biofilms form a strong drug penetration and immune clearance barrier, thus leading to chronic infections and relapse. These biofilms are penetrated by agents such as AgNPs, which interfere with fungal morphogenesis, effectively reducing the pathogen's capacity to form infection and resist host defenses. In turn, AMPs have potential for synergism with conventional antifungals or monotherapy by fighting fungal membranes alongside activating host immune responses. This holistic method may increase the efficiency of treatment and lower resistance emergence. Thus, progress in antifungal modalities with nanotechnology and peptide science is a turning point toward more effective antimicrobial medicines that respond to existing constraints and intricate infection mechanisms (Badiâa et al., 2022; Jéssica et al., 2021).

9.1.3. Antivirals

The ongoing risk of microbial infection has underlined the need for targeted therapeutic agents, among which antivirals have a central role (Figure 9.5). Unlike antibiotics, which are primarily employed to combat bacterial pathogens, antivirals are designed to inhibit the replication and spread of viruses in the host, ideally by interfering with specific stages of the viral life cycle such as entry, nucleic acid replication, or assembly. Synthesis of antiviral drugs requires a deep understanding of viral and host cell processes to prevent resistance and toxicity. A number of natural compounds have been the focus of recent research, for example, limonene, a monoterpene constituent of citrus rind oil, which has shown good antiviral as well as antibacterial and antifungal activity. This indicates a potential multifunctional function of such molecules for viral infection control, including new emerging diseases, by mechanisms other than conventional antivirals and which could potentially be instrumental in resolving the issue of drug resistance (Gupta et al., 2021). Complex diseases have raised interesting questions about the interplay between infection and chronic pathology and the broader implications of antiviral therapies. For instance, Alzheimer's disease (AD), traditionally characterized by amyloid-β plaques and tau protein accumulation, potentially has an infectious component, as recent studies reveal the antimicrobial activity of amyloid-β peptides suggesting a reaction against infectious pathogens. This school of thought has expanded the antiviral research agenda through the correlation of viral infections with neurodegenerative diseases, whereby pathogens could trigger or hasten disease process. The presence of compromised immune defenses in AD patients increases susceptibility to a range of infections, including viral pathogens, and hence complete antiviral regimes must be employed. Thus, the use of antivirals in combination with other antimicrobial drugs can help moderate the microbial load responsible for such multifactorial pathologies (Viga et al., 2021). The emergence of multi-pathogen infections presents a complicated challenge to antiviral treatment in the broad category of antimicrobial agents. Traditional antiviral drugs will target specific viruses, but patient outcomes demonstrate that co-infection and biofilm development complicate the process. Modern diagnostics increasingly now prefer simultaneous detection of more than one pathogen in order to devise better treatment strategies that include combinations of antiviral, antibacterial, antifungal, and anti-biofilm therapies. This general strategy aims not only to eliminate the pathogens but also reduce inflammation and immune dysregulation, potentially preventing chronic sequelae. With ongoing research, the future of antiviral agents lies in the development of broad-spectrum drugs and adjunct therapies that react to the diverse microbial milieu of acute infections as well as chronic illnesses (Viga et al., 2021).

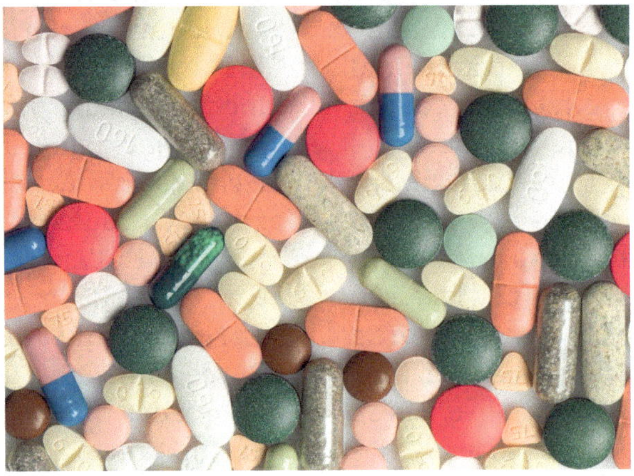

Figure 9.5. Antivirals.

Source: Contemporary Pediatrics. (2021). *Antivirals*. Sanity.io. https://cdn.sanity.io/images/0vv8moc6/contpeds/65a5790a2b4121d3cdf7c142cef7022a2521447f-1440x1080.jpg?fit=crop&auto=format.

Test Your Knowledge

1. What is antibiotics?
2. What is the primary mechanism of antiviral drugs?

9.2. Mechanisms of Action

Learning Outcome

1. Inhibition of Cell Wall Synthesis
2. Disruption of Protein Synthesis
3. Interference with Nucleic Acid Synthesis

Structural integrity and membrane function of bacterial cell membranes are of critical significance to microbial survival and are therefore critical targets for antimicrobial drugs (Figure 9.6). Certain substances, such as plant flavonoids, exert their action by destabilizing membrane organization, thus incurring bacterial death. For example, quercetin is a lipophilic flavonoid that was found to increase bacterial cell diameter and alter membrane fluidity, leading eventually to lipid bilayer destabilization. In addition to this, its selective modification of membrane domains enhances the sensitivity of bacteria to lysis without actually reaching inhibitory levels harmful to bacterial growth, offering an elegant mechanism targeting microbial membrane organization. It can displace incorporation of bacterial toxins into host cells and dampen virulence in the pathogens as well. These findings illustrate the mechanism through which membrane disorder acts as a direct antibacterial effect of flavonoids, demonstrating the potential of these natural compounds as a platform for new antimicrobial therapy (Artem et al., 2023). Other than flavonoids, phytochemicals from other fruits act differently in antimicrobial activity through multifunctional interaction with bacteria. These compounds possess a broad spectrum of antioxidant activity which not only inhibits harmful radicals but also engages in metal ion chelation, affecting bacterial metabolism. Importantly, fruit phytochemicals disrupt the bacterial cell envelope, suppresses communication processes such as quorum sensing, and disrupts gene regulation for pathogenicity.

These activities all manifest as inhibiting growth of bacteria or silencing virulence factor expression. By targeting multiple bacterial mechanisms simultaneously, fruit-derived molecules present a multilateral mechanism of action that can restrict the development of resistance and have complementary activities with conventional antibiotics (Suriyaprom et al., 2022). The variety of antimicrobial mechanisms highlights the significance of both direct and indirect mechanisms against microorganisms. Direct interference with the cell structures, e.g., membrane disruption by flavonoids, causes immediate disruption of cellular integrity, whereas indirect action, e.g., influence of gene expression by fruit phytochemicals, acts on the pathogen's ability to acquire resistance and infect. This twofold action is significant, as it expands the scope of antibacterial action and may also avert the onset of resistant strains. Additionally, the synergy between antioxidant action and antimicrobial action imparts a therapeutic advantage by protecting host cells against oxidative stress during infection. Clarity of these intricate mechanisms offers valuable information to inform the creation of more effective antimicrobial agents that leverage natural bioactive compounds, enhancing efficacy and safety profiles for clinical application (Artem et al., 2023; Suriyaprom et al., 2022).

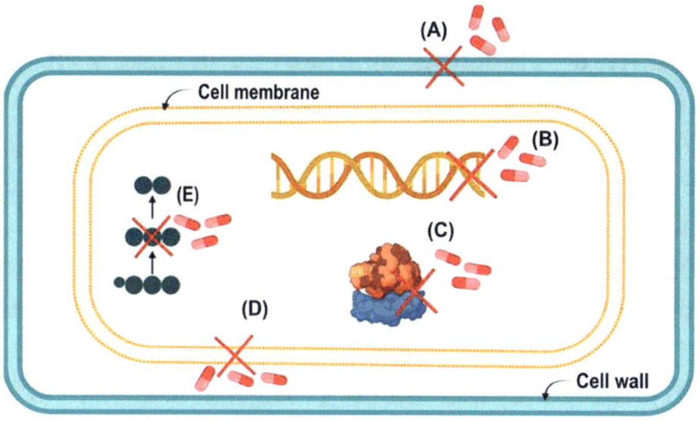

Figure 9.6. Mechanisms of action for antimicrobial agents.

Source: **A**greles, M. A., Cavalcanti, I., & Ferro Cavalcanti, I. M. (2022). *Mechanisms of Antibacterial Action of Antibiotics*. In *Synergism Between Metallic Nanoparticles and Antibiotics*. Applied Microbiology and Biotechnology. https://www.researchgate.net/publication/361148703/figure/fig1/AS:1167416046419968@1655345083100/Mechanisms-of-antibacterial-action-of-antibiotics-A-Inhibition-of-cell-wall-synthesis.png.

9.2.1. Inhibition of Cell Wall Synthesis

Bacterial cell structural integrity is primarily controlled by the intensive synthesis of the cell walls, which are the primary barrier for protection against external stress and osmotic pressure. Disruption of this synthetic pathway offers an antimicrobial effect that is highly specific, making the bacteria vulnerable and ultimately leading to cell lysis. They operate by inhibiting essential enzymes required for peptidoglycan construction, which is a significant structural element of the bacterial cell wall. This is a very useful mechanism of action given that peptidoglycan is not present in mammalian cells and serves to reduce host toxicity. The recent advances in medicinal chemistry have witnessed the development of nitrogen-heterocyclic compounds with the potency to inhibit cell wall synthesis and the ability to combat multidrug-resistant bacterial pathogens. The compounds exhibited selectivity against bacterial enzymes, which holds a promising pharmacotherapeutic target in the development of antimicrobial drugs (Solanki et al., 2025). Chemical modifications to enhance antimicrobial activity have utilized reactions such as the Mannich reaction for the synthesis of structurally divergent derivatives of higher biological activity. Mannich base derivatives synthesized from various natural products have exhibited considerable promise in inhibiting bacterial cell wall formation by targeting the enzyme targets critical to peptidoglycan biosynthesis. Their capacity to disrupt the biosynthetic pathway prevents bacterial growth and survival, presenting a multi-targeting strategy against resistant pathogens. The derivatives also possess additional mechanisms such as membrane disruption and protein synthesis inhibition, which augment their antimicrobial activity. This structural optimization is indicative of how chemical modification of established bioactive agents can yield new drugs that can counteract the problem of bacterial resistance (Siburian et al., 2025). Clinical efficacy of antimicrobials against cell wall formation relies on their ability to inhibit transpeptidases and other enzymes required for cross-linking peptidoglycan chains, thereby weakening the cell wall. Beta-lactam antibiotics are the classic drug class exploiting this mechanism; however, developing resistance necessitates searching for alternative agents. The recent literature reviewed heterocyclic nitrogenous compounds which are promising to possess potential activity through mimicking the natural substrates and competitively inhibiting enzymes. Also, their overall chemical backbones allow for fine modulation of pharmacokinetics and pharmacodynamics with a potential to evade resistance mechanisms such as beta-lactamase production. Sustained efforts in this area are essential for the production of next-generation antimicrobials that can optimally inhibit cell wall formation and suppress the growth of resistant bacteria (Solanki et al., 2025).

9.2.2. Disruption of Protein Synthesis

The battle against bacterial infections typically depends on exploiting vital differences between eukaryotic and prokaryotic cells, and disrupting protein synthesis is a central mode of action of antimicrobial drugs. Many antibiotics act by specifically inhibiting the bacterial ribosome, thereby precluding the production of essential proteins and causing inhibition of growth or cell death. This process takes advantage of structural variations between bacterial ribosomal subunits and their equivalents in human cells. Inhibitors such as aminoglycosides, tetracyclines, macrolides, and chloramphenicol bind to particular sites on the bacterial ribosome to inhibit translation at different stages—either by preventing tRNA binding, elongation, or peptide bond synthesis. The effectiveness of such agents also underscores the importance of targeting protein synthesis pathways as it allows selective toxicity against the pathogen with minimal damage to host tissues. Vigilance in appreciating mechanisms of resistance is always necessary, though, because of the possibility of adaptation by bacteria (Baran et al., 2023). Widespread use of protein synthesis inhibitors is hampered by the emergence of bacterial resistance mechanisms that counteract these drugs directly. Resistance is also maintained through ribosomal binding site mutations, enzymatic modification or breakdown of the antibiotic, and active efflux pumps reducing intracellular drug concentrations. Such adaptation not only defeats therapeutic efficacy but also plays a role in the staggering rise in multidrug-resistant strains. To circumvent these difficulties, recent advances in nanomedicine have reassuringly enhanced the delivery and potency of available antibiotics that function by inhibiting protein synthesis. Target specificity, reduced off-target toxicity, and negation of particular bacterial protective mechanisms may be conferred by particle-based delivery systems via controlled release and improved intracellular concentration. Such new approaches can restore the clinical effectiveness of current drugs and limit resistance emergence by optimizing antimicrobial exposure (Baran et al., 2023).

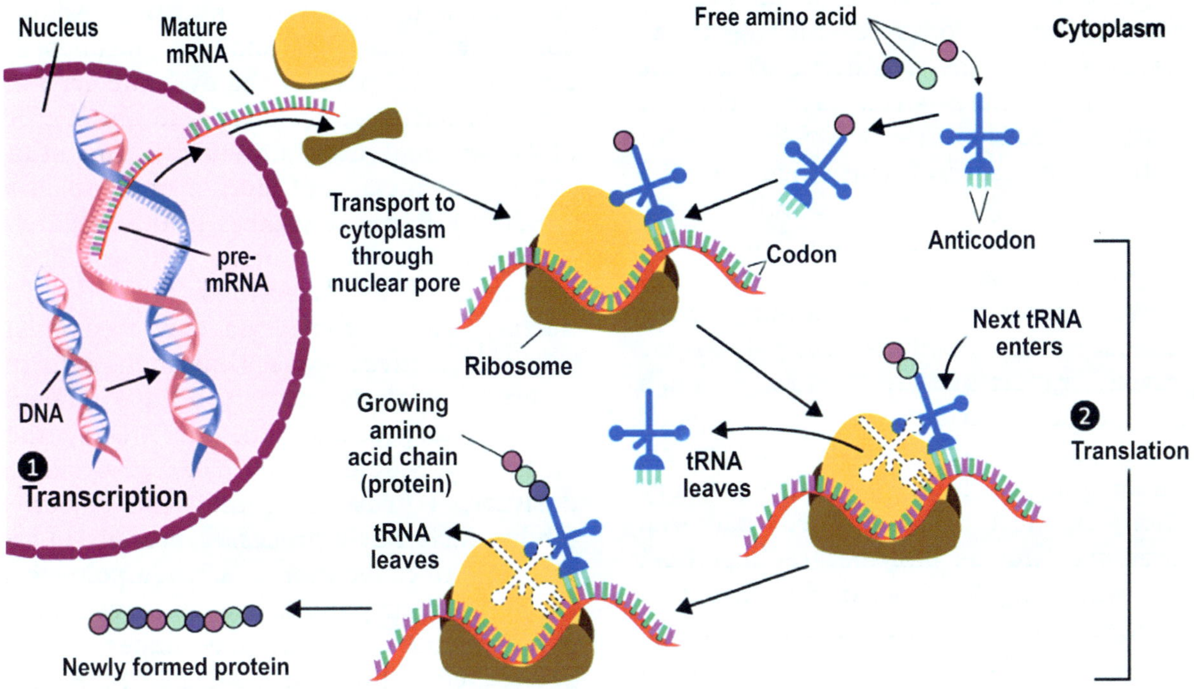

Figure 9.7. Disruption of protein synthesis.

Source: **GeeksforGeeks.** (2024). *Diagram of Protein Synthesis.* https://media.geeksforgeeks.org/wp-content/uploads/20240419102439/Diagram-of-Protein-Synthesis.png.

Furthermore, the future of protein synthesis-targeting antimicrobial agents lies in the intersection of nanotechnology and molecular pharmacology. Nanomedicine provides a platform for designing multifunctional nanoparticles that, in combination, release protein synthesis inhibitors, evade resistance mechanisms, and enable precise targeting of bacterial populations. In addition to the mere enhancement of drug bioavailability, these nanoscale carriers can be designed to be responsive to bacterial microenvironments, releasing their contents in space and time controlled release. This targeted approach not only optimizes the efficacy of antimicrobials but also reduces toxicity and collateral damage to the beneficial microbiota. Current research in these nano-based delivery systems holds colossal potential to transform the current situation of antimicrobial therapy by evading traditional mechanisms of resistance and reactivating approaches against protein synthesis inhibition (Figure 9.7).

9.2.3. Interference with Nucleic Acid Synthesis

The development of antimicrobial compounds has greatly added to the therapeutic armament at our disposal against bacterial infections, with a great variety of mechanisms intervening in basic cellular processes. Among them, interference with the synthesis of nucleic acids is a particularly strong approach. The mechanism blocks bacterial DNA and RNA replication and transcription, which are vital for survival and growth of the cell. Agents such as fluoroquinolones inhibit DNA gyrase and topoisomerase IV, which are enzymes for DNA supercoiling and unwinding during replication. Rifampin inhibits RNA polymerase to prevent transcription initiation. Through inhibition of nucleic acid synthesis, these agents effectively prevent bacteria from proliferation, thus managing the infection. The inhibitory specificity of these agents towards bacterial enzymes over human enzymes reduces host toxicity, which highlights their clinical use in the treatment of bacterial infections. Although nucleic acid synthesis inhibitors have been effective, resistance among bacteria has risen as a growing problem, complicating treatment regimens. This may develop through mutations that modify target enzymes, reducing drug affinity for binding, or horizontal gene transfer resulting in the acquisition of genes that code for alternative enzymes. Efflux pumps also facilitate elimination of antimicrobial agents before they achieve toxic intracellular concentrations, and enzymatic drug inactivation further limits effectiveness. Genetic mechanisms like transposons facilitate the spread of multidrug resistance by inserting multiple resistance genes into bacterial genomes or plasmids. Such adaptive traits portray the dynamic arms race between bacterial evolution and antimicrobial discovery that necessitates constant studies of new chemicals and mechanisms (Solanki et al., 2025). Recent advances in the research of nitrogen-containing heterocyclic compounds reveal hopeful directions for disrupting nucleic acid synthesis via new mechanisms. These derivatives possess enormous structural diversity to allow them to engage numerous bacterial targets like DNA and RNA synthesis machinery. Studies on pyrrole and pyrimidine derivatives prove that they can selectively inhibit nucleic acid processes, presenting novel solutions to conventional fluoroquinolones and rifampin. Their potential to circumvent shared mechanisms of resistance makes nitrogen heterocycles a hope for the drugs in the arsenal against multidrug-resistant strains. It not only expands antimicrobial knowledge but also encourages the development of compounds with better specificity and reduced side effects (Solanki et al., 2025).

Test Your Knowledge

1. What is the primary target of antibiotics that inhibit cell wall synthesis?
2. Why are antibiotics that block DNA/RNA synthesis?

9.3. Spectrum of Activity

Learning Outcome

1. Broad-Spectrum Antimicrobials
2. Narrow-Spectrum Antimicrobials
3. Factors Influencing Spectrum of Activity

The action of antimicrobial agents is generally measured by their spectrum of activity, which defines the range of microorganisms inhibited or killed by them (Figure 9.8). The range of this diversity may be narrow-spectrum agents against specific types of bacteria to broad-spectrum agents against a diverse range of pathogens. For example, industrial antimicrobials such as Hydritreat 2216 show broad-spectrum action by efficiently inhibiting both bacterial isolates and yeast such as *Saccharomyces cerevisiae*, and they are therefore useful for uses where overall microbial control is desired. On the other hand, agents such as Hops BetaStab XL show selectivity, mainly acting against Gram-positive bacteria. The importance of understanding the spectrum of activity lies in maximizing deployment of antimicrobials, reducing risk of resistance development, and maximizing their utilization within all settings, industrial and clinical (Gillian et al., 2025). Investigations into novel antimicrobial agents continue to extend the model of spectrum-associated efficacy.

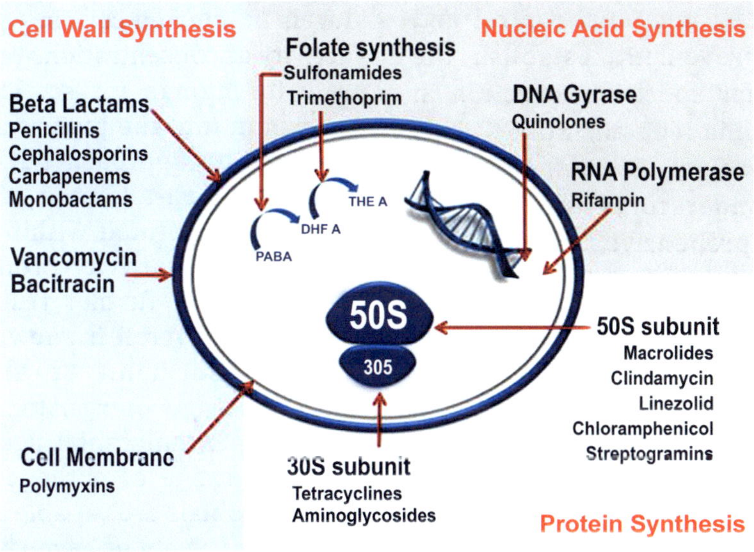

Figure 9.8. Spectrum of activity.

Source: Microbiology Class (2022). *Target Sites of Antibiotics*. https://microbiologyclass.net/wp-content/uploads/2022/12/target-sites-of-antibiotics.png.

Recent studies of ligands synthesized and coordinated to various metal ions show high biological activity against a broad range of microorganisms, including Gram-positive and Gram-negative bacteria, and fungi. These metal complexes are generally more effective as antibacterial and antifungal agents than the ligand precursors used to synthesize them due to variations in chemical stability and molecular geometry. Notably, metal-complexed compounds such as copper, palladium, and platinum complexes exhibited deep inhibitory activities against *Staphylococcus*, *Escherichia coli*, and *Candida albicans*, which demonstrate the capability of structural modification to broaden antimicrobial spectrums. Such findings present the potential of metal-ligand complexes as poly-functional agents against a range of microbial invasions (Thuraya et al., 2024). Determining the exact spectrum of activity not only informs the direct use of antimicrobial agents but also directs strategic planning and usage policy. By knowing exactly which organisms are susceptible to an individual agent, scientists can design interventions to eliminate dominant pathogens without too greatly upsetting beneficial microflora. This is especially critical in plants like sugar mills, where microbial spoilage leads to significant economic losses through sucrose damage. Broad-spectrum agents reduce the risk of single-species dominance and preserve product integrity more effectively. Additionally, cost-effectiveness analysis of antimicrobial application, balanced against the anticipated microbial control and potential yield improvement, establish the utilitarian reasons for spectrum selection in factory settings (Gillian et al., 2025). This integration of spectrum assessment with economic factors underscores the intricate importance of comprehensive antimicrobial agent analysis.

9.3.1. Broad-Spectrum Antimicrobials

The advancement of efficient antimicrobial approaches has made great strides with the incorporation of nanotechnology, especially with the application of metal nanoparticles (MNPs). Such nanoscale materials possess unique antimicrobial characteristics that maximize the performance of medical devices and drug formulations. When MNPs are used in combination with traditional antimicrobial agents like antibiotics, antifungals, or antivirals, they create conjugates that enhance drug delivery by prolonging circulation time, delivering intracellular pathogens more effectively, and stabilizing the active ingredients. This is not only an expansion of the spectrum of antimicrobial activity but also a decrease in toxicity so that less drug can be used without sacrificing therapeutic effects. The capacity of MNP conjugates to evade microbial resistance mechanisms by more than one mode of action further emphasizes their promise in the treatment of varied infections efficaciously (Ribeiro et al., 2022). Such discoveries point toward the promising potential of broad-spectrum antimicrobial treatments based on nanotechnology. When searching for broad-spectrum antiviral drugs, natural products have gained ever-growing interest because of their complex biological activities. Curcumin, a bioactive compound of turmeric root, is an example of a natural product with significant broad-spectrum antimicrobial activity. Recent research shows curcumin's effectiveness in inactivating a variety of pathogens, including the new coronavirus SARS-CoV-2. The compound's capacity to decrease viral RNA levels in infected cells suggests strong antiviral activity at concentrations previously considered safe for human intake. This not only brings curcumin into the picture as a complementary therapeutic approach but also as an off-the-shelf and well-tolerated candidate that can be easily incorporated within available regimens. Its expansive activity profile and limited side effects justify further research into its place within the overall framework of antimicrobial agents (Bormann et al., 2021). Meeting the challenge of resistant microbial strains requires antimicrobial agents that can target a broad range of pathogens. Broad-spectrum antimicrobials are capable of doing so by acting against a variety of bacteria, viruses, and fungi, thereby preventing the hazards associated with polymicrobial infections or co-infections. Increasing their therapeutic effectiveness using novel delivery platforms—e.g., nanoparticle conjugates—and through the use of natural products such as curcumin can dramatically enhance clinical outcomes. These approaches accentuate the dynamic world of antimicrobial agents in which synthetic and natural sources work together to surmount the drawback of conventional monotherapy. The interface of nanotechnology and phytochemicals is a hopeful paradigm shift towards the development of therapies that are effective and flexible, opening up the way to more holistic infection control strategies (Bormann et al., 2021; Ribeiro et al., 2022).

9.3.2. Narrow-Spectrum Antimicrobials

The tactical application of antimicrobial agents demands a subtle comprehension of their specificity in order to treat infection effectively with minimal collateral damage to helpful microorganisms. Narrow-spectrum antimicrobials (Figure 9.9), which target specific bacteria or a narrow subset of pathogens, illustrate the principle by locating treatment where it is needed without wasting action elsewhere. This selectivity minimizes disruption of the host's normal flora and consequently decreases the risk of secondary infection and AMR development. In contrast to broad-spectrum agents, which can non-selectively kill a broad range of microbes, narrow-spectrum agents do not disrupt ecological balance in the microbiome. This focused therapy is more crucial in clinical practice where the detection of the etiologic pathogen is aided by quick diagnostic methods, enabling the application of narrow-spectrum antimicrobials as an initial treatment and enhancing patient outcomes through accurate microbial elimination. Among the main benefits of narrow-spectrum antimicrobials is their lower potential for triggering resistance mechanisms over broad-spectrum counterparts. Since such agents put pressure on a restricted spectrum of microbes, the development of resistance is reduced to a minimum, thus retaining their therapeutic activity over time. Narrow-spectrum antimicrobials are especially useful in the treatment of infections due to well-established pathogens, e.g., methicillin-sensitive *Staphylococcus aureus* or specific Gram-negative rods, where specific therapy can be accurately fitted. Such specificity also results in fewer side effects, as reduced activity against commensal bacteria reduces the potential for side effects such as antibiotic-associated diarrhea or fungal superinfections. Nevertheless, clinical usefulness of narrow-spectrum antimicrobials tends to depend upon rapidity and accuracy of microbial diagnosis, highlighting the need for better diagnostic technology to maximize their use.

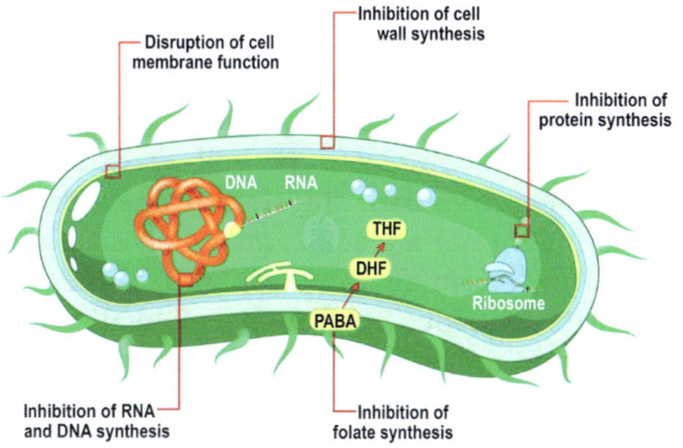

Figure 9.9. Narrow-spectrum antimicrobials.

Source: Respiratory Therapy Zone (2022). *Antibiotics Mechanisms of Action.*

Even though narrow-spectrum antimicrobials clearly have advantages, their use should be weighed against obstacles of the complexity of the infection and microbial resistance in progress. Broad-spectrum agents will be needed first in polymicrobial infections or those where it is not possible to rapidly identify, followed by narrow-spectrum medication when the offending organism has been determined. In addition, the creation of new narrow-spectrum agents involves a heavy investment in research, with the aim of targeting specific microbial processes or virulence factors without interfering with beneficial microbes. New technologies, including antimicrobial textiles and AgNP-based therapies, show potential in certain situations by providing targeted antimicrobial activity while reducing environmental footprint and resistance development (Kumari et al., 2025; Monali et al., 2025). These developments illustrate the promise of combining narrow-spectrum approaches with new delivery strategies to maximize antimicrobial activity and sustainability in both clinical and industrial applications.

9.3.3. Factors Influencing Spectrum of Activity

The success of antimicrobial agents depends largely on their spectrum of action, which is determined by intrinsic as well as extrinsic factors (Figure 9.10). Physical properties of the antimicrobial molecule, including size and solubility, determine how deeply the molecule penetrates various microbial cell walls and membranes, thus determining the broadness or specificity of the agent's action. Furthermore, the mechanism of action—whether it inhibits cell wall formation, protein synthesis, or nucleic acid replication—is important in determining the spectrum. More-broad-spectrum agents become first choices in empirical treatment because of their ability to target a variety of organisms, but their uncontrolled use can foster resistance, underscoring the conflict between therapeutic breadth and stewardship. Mechanisms like bacterial intrinsic resistance and enzymatic hydrolysis also constrain spectrum, highlighting the intricacies of optimizing antimicrobial application. External factors significantly contribute to antimicrobial spectrum via modulating accessibility and activity *in vivo*. Introductions of national guidelines like the National Action Plan (NAP) on AMR and history-making events like the COVID-19 pandemic have shifted consumption patterns, especially for broad-spectrum products. For instance, these have resulted in a reduction in oral broad-spectrum antimicrobial consumption, probably indicating changes in prescribing patterns intended to reduce resistance emergence (Goto et al., 2025). Environmental factors like pH, oxygen tension, and availability of host enzymes also influence the chemical stability and activity of antimicrobials. In addition, nanotechnology advancements have provided nanozymes with broad-spectrum activity that is more stable and less toxic, providing potential alternatives that can be designed to target specific pathogen interaction without harming normal flora (Yan et al., 2024).

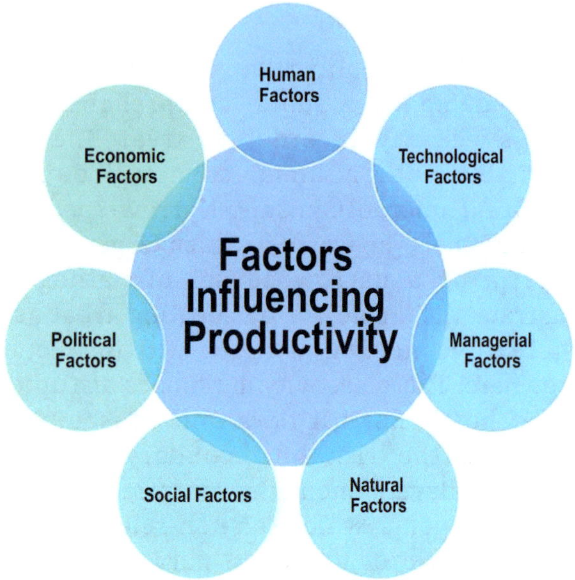

Figure 9.10. Factors influencing spectrum of activity.

Source: Business Jargons. (2022). *Factors Influencing Productivity*. https://businessjargons.com/wp-content/uploads/2022/02/factors-influencing-productivity.jpg.

Therefore, both biomedical and policy innovations largely influence spectrum dynamics. Antimicrobial design becomes increasingly sophisticated with innovations aimed at fine-tuning spectrum to fight emerging resistance and maintain host microbiota. Recent work focuses on nanozyme-derived agents that bear enzymatic mimetic function with selective targeting against bacteria, thus increasing biosafety and minimizing collateral damage to useful microbes (Yan et al., 2024). These tunable agents leverage external stimuli, including light or ultrasound, to enhance function in aggressive physiological milieus characterized by low levels of reactive oxygen species precursor substrates, enhancing efficacy against drug-resistant pathogens. Furthermore, the advent of non-redox nanozymes mitigates issues of oxidative damage and toxicity, opening possibilities for the treatment of less frequent and drug-resistant bacteria. Such developing knowledge points to the value of incorporating biochemical, physiological, and microbial aspects in maximizing spectrum of activity in order to achieve more strategic deployment of antimicrobials within clinical and public health contexts.

Test Your Knowledge

1. Give one example of a narrow-spectrum antibiotic.
2. What is one advantage of using broad-spectrum antimicrobials?

9.4. Resistance to Antimicrobial Agents

Learning Outcome

1. Mechanisms of Resistance
2. Impact of Antibiotic Misuse
3. Global Implications of Resistance

Resistance to antimicrobial agents is a multifaceted process with many determining factors, such as the pattern of use of these drugs within human therapy and animal husbandry (Figure 9.11). Evidence provides large differences in antimicrobial use among countries and sectors, which is associated with the variability that has been witnessed in levels of resistance. Studies have shown that antimicrobial application in food animals, though overall lower in volume than in humans, is directly linked with the development of resistant bacterial strains, which have the potential to cross over to human populations. This interrelated dynamic underscores the need to adopt an integrated approach to antimicrobial stewardship. Interventions targeted at diminishing the general consumption of antimicrobials have shown promise in stemming resistance, underscoring the need for judicious use in conjunction with strict infection control. These interventions are essential to counteract the ever-present menace of antimicrobial-resistant pathogens in both human medicine and agriculture. Treatment regimens for bacterial infections reinforce the difficulties AMR presents to successful treatment. For example, *Helicobacter pylori* infections have long been treated with targeted antibiotic regimens based on resistance patterns. A meta-analysis of eradication treatment proved that resistance patterns in a region have a major impact on the success rates of treatment. Alternative regimens had better eradication rates in regions with high resistance to one of the agents, suggesting that standard treatment protocols may not be effective everywhere with changing resistance patterns. This demonstrates the necessity of ongoing monitoring of antimicrobial susceptibility and individualized therapeutic strategies, which react dynamically to the changing pattern of resistance. In the absence of such initiatives, the efficacy of conventional antibiotic regimens is undermined, compromising patient outcomes and public health (Murata et al., 2020). Finally, antimicrobial resistance poses a complex challenge that requires collective action between healthcare and agricultural communities. Transfer of resistant bacteria between humans and animals illustrates the interdependency of resistance development, necessitating surveillance mechanisms that can measure the data from both groups. The heterogeneity in strength of association between antimicrobial use and resistance as a function of microbial species and drug class further adds complexity to the design of interventions. Continued effort at minimizing unjustified antimicrobial use, maximizing diagnostic capacity to deliver targeted therapy, and reinforcing infection prevention will be critical in maintaining the effectiveness of current antimicrobials. International collaboration and policy execution based on research that continues to emerge are still necessary in facing the ongoing and changing challenge presented by AMR.

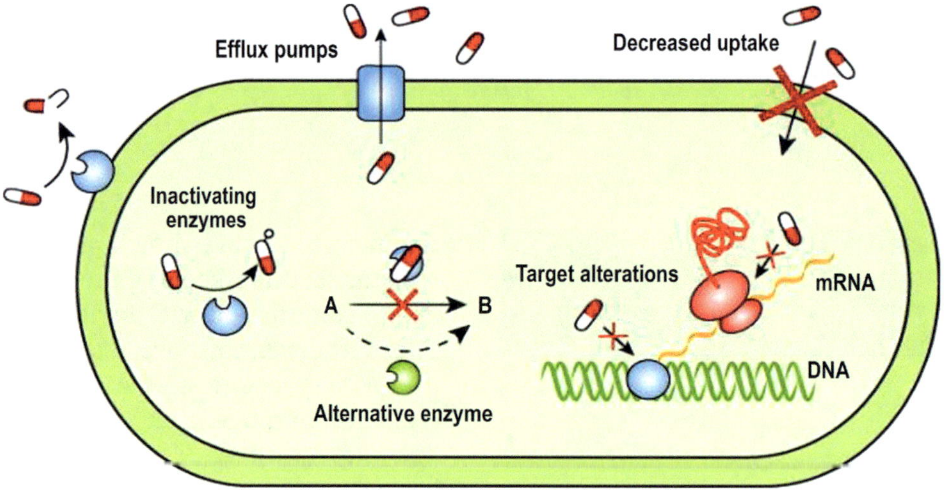

Figure 9.11. Resistance to antimicrobial agents.

Source: Gullberg, E. (2016). *Resistance Mechanisms.* REACT Group.

9.4.1. Mechanisms of Resistance

The challenge of fighting infectious diseases is further complicated by the development of mechanisms of resistance that lower the effectiveness of antimicrobial drugs. Microbes have developed various strategies to resist the lethal effects of these drugs, complicating treatment. One basic mechanism is the alteration of target sites within the microbial cell so that the antimicrobial drugs cannot bind effectively. Another widely used resistance mechanism is enzymatic degradation or alteration of the drug molecule itself, neutralizing its antimicrobial effect prior to any action. Some bacteria also utilize efflux pumps, specialized transport proteins that actively push antimicrobial agents out of the cell, lowering intracellular drug levels below the therapeutic threshold. These resistance modes, frequently seen alone or combined, require the creation of new agents that are able to penetrate them, as emphasized in new studies on molecules with dual mechanism of action meant to reduce the chances of the development of resistance (Bai et al., 2021). Added to the inherent mechanisms of resistance in microbial cells is the biofilm protective environment, a complex collection of microbes encompassed by an extracellular polymeric substance that they produce. Such a configuration not only protects constituent microorganisms physically against external attack but also establishes a microenvironment that promotes resistance. Nutrient and oxygen gradients within the biofilm result in heterogeneously metabolic states for cells, where some enter less susceptible states of dormancy specific to antimicrobials that are active against proliferating cells. Furthermore, the extracellular polymeric substance (EPS) matrix interferes with the entry of antimicrobial substances, effectively reducing their local concentration and activity. Communication systems such as quorum sensing also control resistance-associated gene expression, whereas genetic mutability in biofilms enhances adaptation. These multicategorical mechanisms account for the failure to eliminate biofilm-infected infections despite intensive antimicrobial regimens (Li et al., 2020). Counteracting AMR requires a comprehensive appreciation of these molecular and community-level defense mechanisms. New therapeutic strategies need not only to target bacterial viability but also resistance pathways and biofilm integrity. The use of multimodal antimicrobials can decrease the likelihood of resistance formation, as it is much harder for microbes to acquire resistance to multiple mechanisms. Furthermore, adjuvant therapy targeting the disruption of biofilm dispersion or interference with quorum sensing has the potential to regain the susceptibility of bacteria to the traditional agents. Finally, resistance growth prevention is dependent on responsible use of antimicrobial agents along with ongoing monitoring of developing patterns of resistance. Such approaches will prove instrumental in addressing existing and future issues presented by resilient microbial communities (Bai et al., 2021; Li et al., 2020).

9.4.2. Impact of Antibiotic Misuse

The unforeseen effects of inappropriate use of antibiotics have emerged as a vital issue in the realms of public health (Figure 9.12). Overuse and unspecific use of these medications create a pressure for selection that speeds up the development and spread of AMR between pathogenic and commensal microorganisms. This process undermines the therapeutic efficacy against infectious diseases and increases the rate of morbidity and mortality worldwide. Transmission of resistant organisms, primarily through human-to-human interaction, highlights the complex nature of problems encountered in healthcare facilities and further extends to community settings. Additionally, contributory factors include extensive antibiotic application in agriculture, particularly in livestock production, where non-therapeutic use enhances resistance development. This disseminated AMR not only puts individual patient outcomes at risk but even compromises overall healthcare structures through restricted therapeutic choices and the inflation of related costs, hence requiring immediate and concerted interventions (Md. Salam et al., 2023). The formulation of corrective measures to counter the impact of antibiotic misuse requires new and sustainable strategies that supplement current pharmacological measures. Recent studies emphasize the promise of novel antimicrobial agents based on natural sources, including essential oils, which have broad-spectrum antimicrobial activities. When these agents are incorporated into delivery systems like cyclodextrin-based tablets, they show prolonged activity against biofilm-forming pathogens causing chronic infections. Use of such environmentally friendly, biocompatible materials promises a promising adjunct or alternative to traditional antibiotics and can potentially lower selective pressure on microbial communities. In addition, natural products have the ability to combat resistant species such as *Pseudomonas aeruginosa* and *Staphylococcus aureus* by combating biofilms that naturally are resistant to antibiotic treatment. Adopting green and efficient antimicrobial approaches thus constitutes an essential aspect in the grand scheme for resistance amplification caused by antibiotic abuse (Arrais et al., 2023). Wider implications of antibiotic abuse extend into economic and societal realms, affecting both the availability of effective treatments and the durability of health systems globally. Constraints on the discovery and manufacturing of new antimicrobial drugs increase the danger posed by resistant infections, ensuring dependence on older, frequently less effective agents that may be more toxic. The resulting rise in treatment failures results in extended illness, increased transmission rates, and increased healthcare costs. Overcoming these issues necessitates extensive surveillance, strict regulation of antibiotic dispensation, and enhanced public awareness of the judicious use of such agents. Furthermore, promoting collaboration between national and global institutions is crucial to enforce the law, ensure access to quality medicines, stimulate vaccination and diagnostic innovation, and thus prevent the silent but widespread pandemic of AMR largely caused by misuse. In the absence of such coordinated action, the threat of a post-antibiotic era hangs over global health as a very real prospect (Md. Salam et al., 2023).

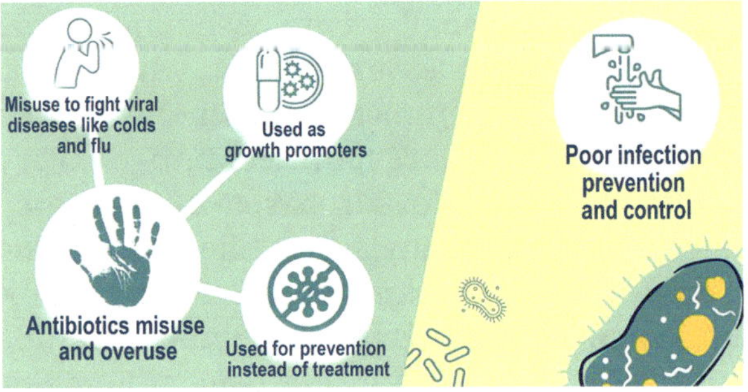

Figure 9.12. Impact of antibiotic misuse.

Source: Boehringer Ingelheim. (n.d.). *Factors Contributing to Antimicrobial Resistance.* https://www.boehringer-ingelheim.com/sites/default/files/Animal_Health/Factors%20contributing%20to%20antimicrobial%20resistance%20FINAL.png.

9.4.3. Global Implications of Resistance

The rising tide of AMR has deeply significant global implications that transcend individual patient outcomes to impact public health infrastructures and economic stability on a global scale. Healthcare systems are especially under pressure as resistant diseases, like those associated with biofilm-producing bacteria in the healthcare setting, become increasingly intractable. Such infections frequently necessitate greater doses or pairing of broad-spectrum antibiotics, accelerating resistance emergence and hindering clinical management. Further, the existence of drug-resistant organisms in healthcare environments extends patient stays and leads to higher mortality rates, fueling the strain on already strained medical facilities. As such, the development of resistant strains calls for speedy innovation in material science, such as the engineering of functionalized, nanoscale materials that can prevent biofilm growth and lower infection levels on medical devices to ease some of the pressures on healthcare systems (Bhattacharjee et al., 2023). Antimicrobial agent resistance also interferes with global economic and political circles by endangering the productivity of the workforce and escalating healthcare costs. The dependence upon effective antimicrobials supports numerous industries, from agriculture to tourism, making resistance a multi-industry problem with far-reaching consequences. The plateau in finding new antibiotics requires that new therapeutic approaches be investigated, including AMPs, which have potential due to their broad-spectrum activity and lower tendency to encourage resistance development. These peptides, which are central to innate immune defense, show promise as next-generation antimicrobial agents that are capable of targeting resistant pathogens. Their translation into standard clinical use, though, is an impediment that entails surmounting significant formulation, stability, and regulatory issues. Therefore, global resistance combat depends on aligning new therapies with harmonized policy interventions in order to reduce the growing threat to public health and economic resilience (Talapko et al., 2022). Resolution of the worldwide implications of resistance needs a multidisciplinary strategy integrating scientific progress, clinical awareness, and global collaboration (Figure 9.13). Monitoring of AMR trends needs to be strengthened worldwide to guide treatment protocols and policy, reducing misuse and overuse of available drugs. Concurrently, research to develop next-generation antimicrobial agents and materials with inherent bactericidal activity is essential to combat biofilm-related infections and resistant bacterial strains. Public campaigns and stewardship initiatives can also curtail wasteful antimicrobial use in both healthcare and community environments. The synthesis of emerging nanotechnology-based approaches with new compounds such as AMPs offers a promising avenue towards overcoming resistance. In the end, worldwide coordination and commitment to research, regulation, and training are essential to solving the intertwined health, financial, and social problems arising from AMR (Bhattacharjee et al., 2023; Talapko et al., 2022).

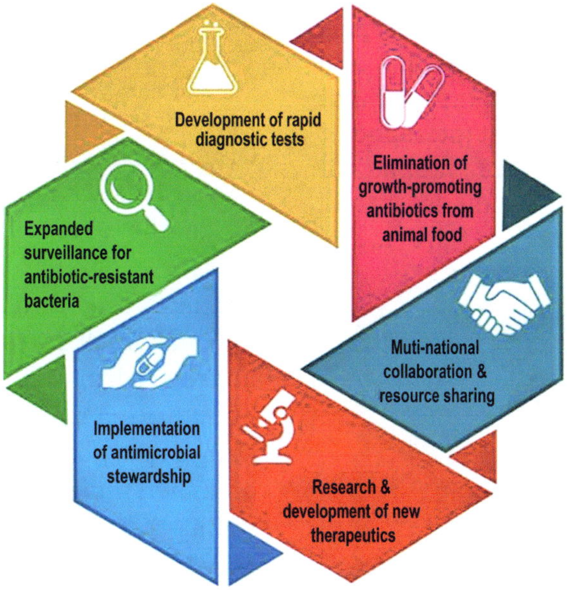

Figure 9.13. Global implications of resistance.

Source: Frontiers. (2020). *Figure 1: Pathophysiology of COVID-19-Induced Hypercoagulability*. Frontiers in Public Health. https://www.frontiersin.org/files/Articles/629120/fpubh-08-629120-HTML/image_m/fpubh-08-629120-g001.jpg.

Test Your Knowledge

1. What is antimicrobial resistance (AMR)?
2. What is the primary mechanism by which bacteria develop antimicrobial resistance?

9.5. Development of New Antimicrobial Agents

Learning Outcome

1. Challenges in Drug Development
2. Role of Biotechnology
3. Future Directions in Antimicrobial Research

Advances in computational science and biotechnology have opened up new directions for tackling the growing threat of AMR. Emerging techniques utilize genomic sequencing and proteomic profiling to reveal more insights into pathogen dynamics and drug-target interactions. The technologies provide the means to interrogate novel microbial weaknesses and potential drug targets that were not previously tractable using traditional techniques.

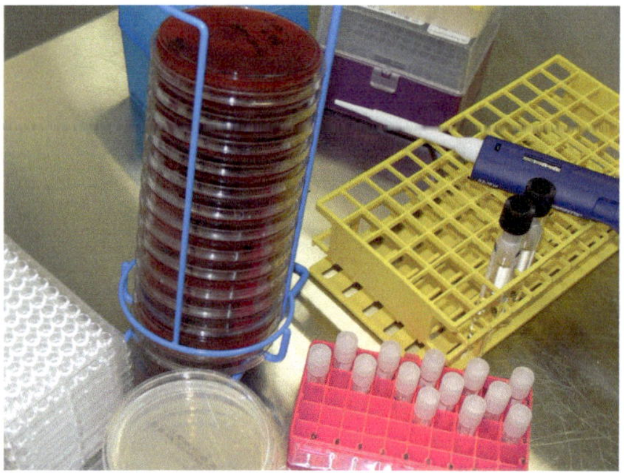

Figure 9.14. Development of new antimicrobial agents.

Source: Labspec (2018). *Lightroom*. https://www.labspec.org/wp-content/uploads/2018/11/Lightroom--1200x900.jpg.

In addition, machine learning and artificial intelligence algorithms enable high-throughput screening and drug efficacy prediction, speeding up the drug discovery process and the accuracy of candidate selection. In spite of these welcome tools, their adoption into drug development pipelines is hindered by challenges like ethical issues, data complexity, and the requirement for interdisciplinary effort to get over regulatory and practical hurdles. However, these breakthroughs represent a revolutionary paradigm change in strategies to develop antimicrobial agents that are capable of staying ahead of evolving resistant pathogens and providing more efficacious therapeutics (Thalia, 2025).

There is an increasing need to design new antimicrobial agents because drug-resistant and extensively drug-resistant bacterial strains are arising at a quickening pace and risk invalidating existing treatment modalities. The World Health Organization has estimated a dire situation where bacterial AMR could result in millions of deaths every year by 2050 if corrective measures are not adopted. In turn, scientists are adopting different innovative strategies, one of which is the prodrug strategy, which improves drug selectivity and decreases toxicity by activating compounds in the target organism. Drug repurposing and chemical derivatization of known molecules are cost-effective and time-saving avenues for finding new antimicrobial agents. Also, the incorporation of nanotechnology enhances drug delivery and bioavailability, and natural products remain a rich source of lead compounds for new drugs. Such multidimensional strategies unveil the multi-faceted but promising scenario for antimicrobial development required to meet AMR's increasing challenge (Maria et al., 2024). Even with outstanding advances, the translational gap between new discoveries and clinically accepted antimicrobials is still substantial. One of the main issues is to sustain the fine balance between efficacy, safety, and avoiding the risk of resistance emergence. Multi-disciplinary synergy integrating knowledge from molecular biology, bioinformatics, and pharmacology is critical to support rational drug design and optimize pharmacokinetics.

Besides, regulatory systems have to adapt to new technologies and streamline approval processes without jeopardizing patient safety. Public health efforts that combine surveillance with continuous research are critical in anticipating resistance patterns and modifying treatment approaches. Together, they point out that the creation of novel antimicrobial agents (Figure 9.14) is not merely an exercise in the sciences but is also a systems problem that necessitates collaboration in the sciences, policy-making processes, and across global health institutions (Maria et al., 2024; Thalia, 2025).

9.5.1. Challenges in Drug Development

The search for new antimicrobial drugs is plagued by several intricate challenges inherent in the drug development pipeline. One of the main hurdles is the versatility and optimization of extraction procedures, particularly in the case of medicinal plants. Such natural sources contain a rich diversity of bioactive molecules, but the achievement of selective and effective extracts depends on very specific and species-specific procedures. Moreover, experimental variability like variable antimicrobial susceptibility testing results further hinder the assessment of plant-derived compounds efficacy. The pharmacokinetics and pharmacodynamics of such compounds are not well studied, further constraining our knowledge of their behavior in the biological system. As such, elaborate mechanistic understandings and strict standardization are key to guaranteeing that plant extracts can be successfully applied as antimicrobial agents and further developed into clinically reasonable drugs (Vaou et al., 2021). Unless these basic difficulties are resolved, the therapeutic potential of natural products is not significantly realized in combat against pathogenic microorganisms. At the same time, traditional antimicrobial medications are also faced with inherent obstacles that further increase the problem of drug development. Most currently available agents have problems with transport through biological membranes, poor water solubility, and low oral bioavailability, reducing their pharmacological activity. In addition, toxicity and patients' lack of compliance limit their real applicability. Critically, the growing issue of microbial resistance has the potential to make existing pharmacotherapies ineffective, instilling fear of being plunged into a pre-antibiotic period. Such multifaceted liabilities call for innovative solutions not just to enhance drug efficiency but also to avoid mechanisms of resistance. Therefore, the development process needs to incorporate strategies to refine targeting specificity, stability, and safety profiles to create next-generation antimicrobials that can address current clinical needs (Spirescu et al., 2021). Emerging technologies provide exciting means to transcend various drug development challenges related to antimicrobial therapy. Nanotechnology, especially the use of polymeric nanoparticles, has multifaceted benefits, such as enhanced drug solubility, encapsulation, and targeted delivery functionalities. These nanoscale vehicles can be designed to increase biocompatibility and biodegradability while decreasing toxicity, thus solving various pharmacokinetic issues related to conventional agents. In addition, their ability to synergistically integrate therapeutic effects and attain selective killing of therapeutic microorganisms is a pivotal development. These technologies have encouraged intensive exploration of their use as drug delivery antimicrobial agents, with the potential to revolutionize treatment strategies and counteract the resistance challenge. Clinical translation of these new platforms is, however, still limited by synthesis challenges, regulatory obstacles, and the necessity for thorough safety assessments (Spirescu et al., 2021).

9.5.2. Role of Biotechnology

Recent breakthroughs in modern science have further emphasized the revolutionary influence of biotechnological techniques on medicine, particularly in the creation of antimicrobial compounds (Figure 9.15). Incorporation of biotechnology has allowed the construction of sophisticated molecular frameworks with the ability to target resistant pathogens more efficiently than conventional approaches. One such innovation is the use of boron compounds that have presented both anticancer and antimicrobial activity based on their special chemical reactivity. Boron compounds can suppress enzymes linked to drug resistance like β-lactamases, thereby restoring the effectiveness of current medicines. In addition to this, the versatility of boron can be used to enhance drug delivery systems to enable targeted treatments and minimize side effects and optimize therapeutic effects. The convergence of boron chemistry and biotechnology exhibits encouraging progress in the fight against resistant infections and highlights the pivotal role of such advanced compounds in determining the future of antimicrobial drug discovery (Gul, 2025). In addition to chemical synthesis, biotechnology further utilizes biological entities for antimicrobial use, with bacteriophages becoming a crucial resource phages, viruses that infect bacteria specifically, have come back into focus as novel antimicrobial weapons, particularly with the growing resistance to antibiotics. Their inherent capacity to lyse specific bacterial cells presents a biological specificity that eludes synthetic medicines. Additionally, their nanoscale self-assembled architectures and lack of toxicity towards humans further advance their therapeutic potential. Genetic manipulation methods also widen the realm of phage application to include the presentation of functional peptides designed for distinct bacterial targets. These developments not only renew phage therapy but also widen their application as biosensors and in tissue engineering, adding to an interdisciplinary strategy in biotechnology that pushes antimicrobial strategies beyond traditional paradigms (Kim et al., 2024). The integration of biotechnology and antimicrobial agent research enables the design of multifunctional treatment platforms that bypass the limitations of single-faceted treatment modalities. As an example, the design of boron-based compounds with dual roles in drug delivery and enzyme inhibition is a two-action strategy that can simultaneously compromise pathogens and release treatment effectively. When integrated with the targeted treatment capabilities of engineered phages, such strategies demonstrate the potential to bypass traditional methods of resistance and enhance clinical success. Biotechnology also quickens the functionalization and screening of new compounds, allowing for high-throughput discovery of good antimicrobial prospects. All together, these innovations highlight biotechnology's central importance in the history of antimicrobial agents, presenting customized, effective, and dynamic solutions to intractable infection problems (Gul, 2025; Kim et al., 2024).

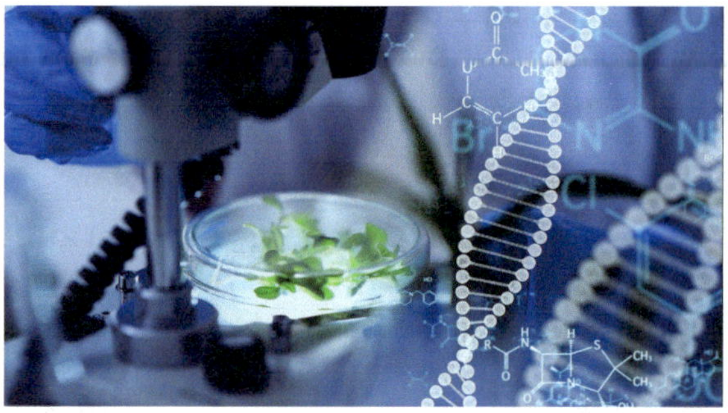

Figure 9.15. Role of biotechnology.

Source: Agritech Digest. (2024). *Role of Biotechnology. https*://agritechdigest.com/wp-content/uploads/2024/03/7xm.xyz669381.jpg.

9.5.3. Future Directions in Antimicrobial Research

With advancements in technology evolving, revolutionary research approaches have now become a possibility for antimicrobials through genomics incorporation. Improved sequencing of whole genomes in recent years has advanced insights into the mechanism of AMR and its propagation in multiple bacterial pathogens. This use of the genomic information requires identification and study to more than merely capitalize upon. Successful integration between the public health and the clinical interface is crucial to deliver actionable data that can inform treatment guidelines and infection control measures. Standardized sampling of data, analysis, and reporting according to global guidelines will further facilitate the translation of genomic data into practical interventions. Most importantly, fair access to such technologies in all parts of the world, aided by policies promoting data accessibility and interoperability, will be critical to confronting AMR on a global level. The potential for genomics-enhanced antimicrobial research therefore resides not just in technological breakthrough but also in systematic integration of these tools into public health infrastructures (Sherry et al., 2025). The increasing problem of antibiotic resistance requires looking beyond the conventional synthetic antimicrobials for alternative sources. Natural bioactive compounds from algae, including cyanobacteria and microalgae, have received a great deal of scientific interest due to their high antimicrobial activities. The algal metabolites, like polysaccharides, fatty acids, and phenolic compounds, have been found to inhibit multi-drug-resistant strains of bacteria, and new hope has emerged for transcending the current shortcomings of antibiotic therapy. A bibliometric examination pinpointed the key focus domains such as antibiotic resistance prevention, optimization of biosynthesis, and new pharmacologic findings, highlighting the multidisciplinary character of such a research field. Mechanistic investigations show that such bioactive compounds hinder bacterial growth by inhibiting vital processes such as protein synthesis inhibition and cellular membrane disruption. Optimization of biomass production and utilization of genetic engineering methodologies to improve metabolite yield is promising for large-scale and sustainable algal-based antimicrobial development (Zuorro et al., 2024). In the future, the destiny of antimicrobial research will most probably lie at the nexus of new biotechnology and holistic public health approaches. Coupling new developments in pathogen genomics with new natural product discovery has the potential to enable the production of next-generation antimicrobial agents specifically designed to better fight resistant infections. To realize maximal impact, future initiatives will need to focus on translational paradigms that link laboratory breakthroughs with bedside practice, providing timely delivery of therapy to patients while enabling surveillance of global resistance patterns. Delivery system advancements—nanotechnology and targeted drug carriers, for example—may also enhance the bioavailability and targeted activity of these agents while reducing side effects. Coupled with coordinated global data sharing, these synergistic strategies hold the promise of bringing a new age of antimicrobial agents that are effective against the complex issues of resistance, accessibility, and environmental sustainability (Sherry et al., 2025; Zuorro et al., 2024).

Test Your Knowledge

1. Which of the challenges in drug development?
2. How is biotechnology used in drug development?

9.6. Clinical Applications

Learning Outcome

1. Treatment of Infections
2. Prophylactic Use in Surgery
3. Role in Immunocompromised Patients

The development of AMPs as therapeutic drugs underscores an encouraging milestone in fighting resistant infections. These short, positively charged, amphiphilic peptides have broad-spectrum antibacterial and antifungal activity, acting as important defenders of the innate immune system. The earliest history of peptides such as polymyxins and tyrothricin established more than sixty years ago serves to emphasize the therapeutic efficacy of AMPs against mucosal infections. In more recent years, investigation has centered on uses in inflammatory dermatoses and infected wound healing, in which AMPs have been shown to exert positive influences on elimination of pathogens and healing of tissue.

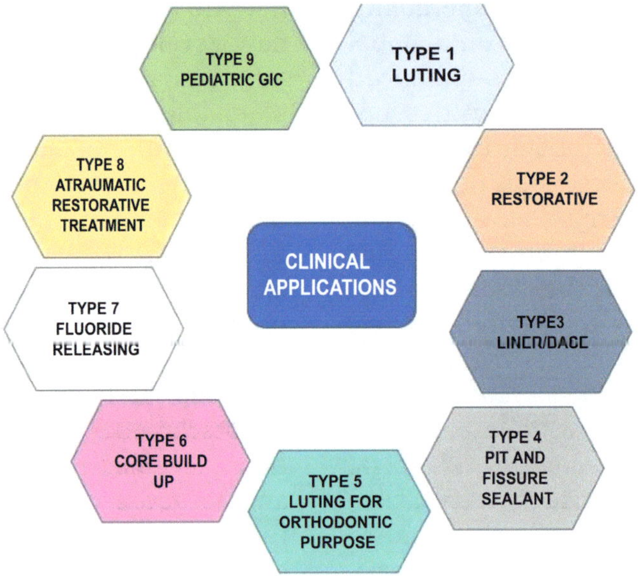

Figure 9.16. Clinical applications.

Source: Sulieman, A.-M. (2023). *Clinical Applications of GIC.* ResearchGate.

Notably, AMPs differ from conventional antibiotics in having less ability to promote microbial resistance, a significant plus in clinical environments beset by multidrug-resistant pathogens. Translational research is presently developing targeted treatments that leverage AMP properties, suggesting a paradigm shift towards new treatments that fuse basic molecular knowledge with clinical requirements (VC AM et al., 2012). Nanotechnology is another frontier in the clinical application of antimicrobial agents, and it involves designing nanoparticle-based drug delivery systems. Chitosan-alginate nanoparticles have also been recognized for their inherent antimicrobial activities, particularly against skin pathogens like *Propionibacterium acnes*, which is involved in acne vulgaris. Electron microscopy data show that the nanoparticles cause cell membrane disruption of bacteria, resulting in direct bactericidal effects. They also have immunomodulatory effects by reducing inflammatory cytokine production in infected tissues, treating both microbial and inflammatory aspects of disease. Encapsulation of traditional antibiotics such as benzoyl peroxide within such nanoparticles not only increases antimicrobial potency but also reduces cytotoxicity to host cells, thus illustrating improved safety profiles for application to the skin. Such dual-function nanoparticle systems illustrate the potential of engineering techniques to move antimicrobial treatment beyond traditional antibiotics toward better therapeutic outcomes (Blecher-Paz et al., 2013). The introduction of new antimicrobial formulations in clinical practice requires serious assessment of efficacy, safety, and potential for resistance in order to balance therapeutic gains against risks. Present clinical trials on AMPs and nanoparticle-based therapies are geared toward establishing evidence for the treatment of chronic wounds, inflammatory dermatoses, and resistant infections where traditional antibiotics are ineffective. These novel agents provide the promise of custom-made interventions minimizing systemic side effects and maximizing host tissue compatibility while maximizing local antimicrobial activity. Additionally, their capacity to avoid conventional resistance mechanisms highlights an essential role in fighting the worldwide AMR crisis. Ongoing interdisciplinary interaction between molecular biology, pharmacology, and clinical medicine will be critical in accomplishing the full potential of these advancements and in translating them into routine care procedures for a range of infectious and inflammatory conditions (Figure 9.16).

9.6.1. Treatment of Infections

Advancements in the treatment of infections have become crucial in light of the growing challenges posed by healthcare-associated infections, particularly those linked to invasive devices such as central venous catheters. Among these, central line-associated bloodstream infections (CLABSIs) are especially concerning due to their high morbidity, mortality, and economic costs. Recent clinical studies have yielded comprehensive guidelines aimed at improving prevention, diagnosis, and treatment of such infections. These guidelines not only highlight the significance of choosing proper catheter types and sites of insertion but also promote strict catheter management protocols. The incorporation of evidence-based practices guided by systematic reviews and expert consensus guarantees that healthcare professionals implement standardized practices to reduce infection risks. Therefore, the adjustment of treatment approaches in accordance with changing patterns of antibiotic resistance and the inclusion of newer antimicrobial agents becomes necessary for optimal management in critical care (Care MCSOC, 2025). Increasing risk of multidrug-resistant organisms adds to the complexity of treatment possibilities and requires new-age antimicrobial strategies. Drug-resistant organisms such as *Klebsiella pneumoniae* are of serious public health concern because they have limited sensitivity to the traditional antibiotics and have the ability to develop stable biofilms. Recent studies of AMPs like K11 have shown great potential in therapy against these resistant bacteria. K11 has not just direct antibacterial effects but synergizes with standard antibiotics, further enhancing their effects and bypassing resistance mechanisms. Further, its interference with the biofilm production that usually inhibits treatment presents a major break through in eliminating persistent and chronic infections. The stability of K11 in different physiological conditions and low resistance induction potential point to its potential as a new adjunct or alternative therapy in antimicrobial treatment (Chatupheeraphat et al., 2023). To optimize infection treatment protocols, thus, is a complex process with multiple facets balancing innovation and evidence-based clinical actions. The combination of newly synthesized agents such as K11 with conventional antibiotics can improve therapeutic results, especially when treating resistant bacterial strains in susceptible patient groups. Moreover, compliance with revised clinical guidelines guarantees uniformity and efficacy in infection control while preventing the development of resistance. As resistance patterns change, ongoing monitoring and adjustment of antimicrobial regimens become essential to ensure their clinical usefulness. Ultimately, successful treatment of infections relies on a balance between the implementation of leading-edge research, strict clinical standards, and close antimicrobial stewardship to maintain the effectiveness of available agents and enhance patient prognoses (Care MCSOC, 2025; Chatupheeraphat et al., 2023).

9.6.2. Prophylactic Use in Surgery

Prevention of surgical site infections (SSIs) is an essential challenge in clinical practice since these infections considerably undermine patient outcomes and healthcare resources. Historically, the use of antimicrobial agents as a prophylactic measure has been well documented to be effective in reducing microbial contamination during surgical procedures (Figure 9.17). The timing, selection, and dose of antibiotics are critical variables determining prophylactic effectiveness, with optimal timing being one hour before incision to ensure the highest tissue levels. Additionally, patient-specific factors—e.g., allergies, comorbidities, and local microbial resistance patterns—assume crucial roles in individualizing prophylaxis strategies to maximize benefit while avoiding risk. Although great advances have been made, indiscriminate antimicrobial usage in surgical situations has played a part in the growing danger of AMR, and hence there is a need for prudent selection and stewardship of prophylactic regimens (Dhole et al., 2023). In urological surgery, especially in prostate biopsy operations, prophylactic antibiotic administration has proven highly effective in reducing postoperative infection complications. Historically, fluoroquinolones were the stand-by for prophylaxis because of their broad spectrum of activity and desirable pharmacokinetics, but resistance patterns and regulatory constraints have required reconsideration. Current evidence from meta-analyses and systematic reviews indicates that antibiotic prophylaxis halves the risk of subsequent infection following biopsy compared with no prophylaxis, highlighting its essential role. However, long or insufficient regimens are less than optimal since evidence suggests that a minimum one-day antibiotic administration is more effective than single doses. Also, individualized prophylaxis according to rectal swab culture improves infection prevention by tackling resistance, although the strength of evidence is still low (Pilatz et al., 2020).

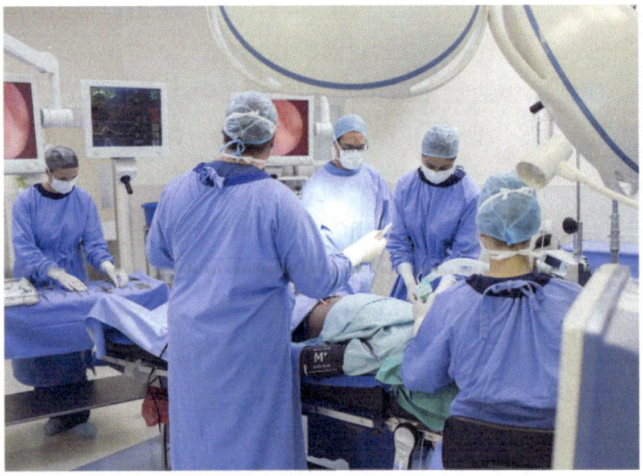

Figure 9.17. Prophylactic use in surgery.

Source: https://www.verywellhealth.com/thmb/ku9xo9T8Tu8yo5Yh0baK9DI6bDo=/1500x0/filters:no_upscale():max_bytes(150000):strip_icc()/GettyImages-5306855671-5953be875f9b584bfe98b4a3.jpg.

The changing antimicrobial prophylaxis of surgery requires new approaches beyond standard antibiotic use to maintain effectiveness and battle resistance. Among options, nonantibiotic means—such as antimicrobial instrument coating, the use of probiotics, and immunomodulatory drugs—have become attractive for their capacity to lower infectious hazards without furthering resistance emergence. In addition, combination antibiotic regimens, or intensified prophylaxis, have been promising in selected high-risk situations, but are problematic in terms of antibiotic stewardship and need to be weighed against the potential for adverse effects. Regular review of local resistance trends and compliance with evidence-based recommendations are essential to maximizing prophylactic therapies. With changing surgical practice and microbial threats, incorporating multidisciplinary approaches will be necessary for long-term infection prevention and enhanced surgical outcomes (Dhole et al., 2023; Pilatz et al., 2020).

9.6.3. Role in Immunocompromised Patients

The challenge of curing infections among immunocompromised patients lies in their vulnerability to opportunistic pathogens that hardly infect fully immunized individuals (Figure 9.18). Traditional antimicrobial treatments, although successful in most situations, prove inadequate here because drug resistance and side effects are more likely among such vulnerable individuals. Immunocompromised hosts—including HIV/AIDS, cancer patients who are being treated with chemotherapy, or organ recipients on immunosuppressive regimens—call for individualized antimicrobial methods that weigh effectiveness against safety. Newer methodologies such as radioimmunotherapy have been demonstrated to hold merit by selectively marking infected cells while causing minimal off-target damage using radionuclides including bismuth-213 and rhenium-188. This specificity not only maximizes pathogen elimination but also minimizes systemic toxicity, a major improvement in the treatment of infections in which conventional antimicrobial therapy is ineffective or contraindicated (Helal et al., 2018). Infections due to low virulent but potentially lethal pathogens, such as *Citrobacter koseri*, pose a special problem for immunocompromised patients. Neonates and those with weakened immune defenses are especially vulnerable, requiring early and effective antimicrobial therapy. The treatment strategy should be directed by accurate antimicrobial susceptibility testing to choose agents that are capable of penetrating the pathogen's resistance. Antibiotic classes such as aminoglycosides, carbapenems, cephalosporins, chloramphenicol, and quinolones are regularly used; however, developing resistance makes empirical treatment regimes more challenging. The judicious use and choice of such agents in this population highlight the value of continuous monitoring and individualized antimicrobial stewardship to maximize outcomes, prevent resistance emergence, and limit side effects in immunocompromised patients (Deveci et al., 2014).

The use of antimicrobial drugs in immunocompromised hosts goes beyond the killing of causative agents to encompass modulation of long-term infection risk and secondary complication prevention. Chronic infections and repeated antibiotic exposure in such patients raise the likelihood of multi-drug-resistant pathogens, creating a further burden on therapeutic choice. Therapies that integrate new antimicrobial modalities with traditional agents are central to managing these intricacies. Furthermore, the interaction between antimicrobial treatment and host immunity necessitates clinicians to repeatedly re-evaluate regimens to respond to changing pathogen patterns. As shown in targeted treatments such as radioimmunotherapy, combining emerging strategies has promising options to improve efficacy while limiting treatment-related risks, eventually enhancing prognosis and quality of life in immunocompromised patients (Deveci et al., 2014; Helal et al., 2018).

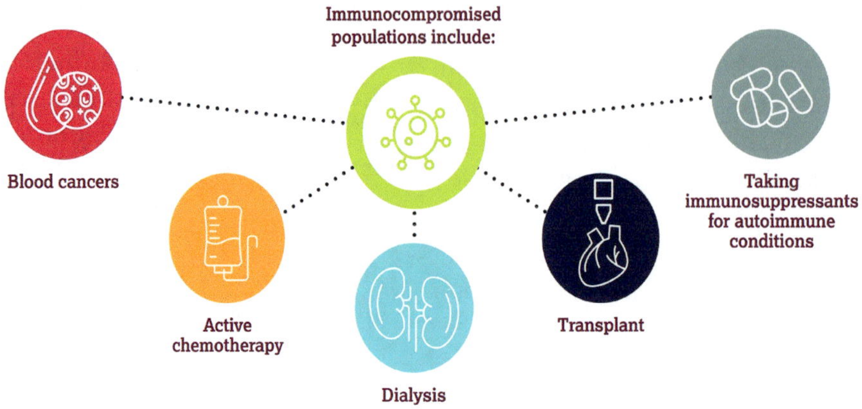

Figure 9.18. Role in immunocompromised patients.

Source: https://pbs.twimg.com/media/FJZCzuQWQAUKmrL?format=jpg&name=4096x4096.

Test Your Knowledge

1. What are potential challenges in AMP development?
2. What is Role in immunocompromised patients?

SUMMARY

The advance in knowledge on antimicrobial agents has notably accelerated through the inclusion of new approaches and an even broader diversity of compounds from more traditional antibiotics. Investigating drugs such as acetaminophen and ibuprofen, often not considered to be primarily antimicrobials by category, presents hopeful adjunctive antimicrobial effects. Their activity with essential proteins essential for microbial virulence and metabolism, notably against periodontal pathogens, shows the multiple potential applications of standard drugs. These revelations, based on *in silico* research, present opportunities for the repurposing of available drugs to fight resistant pathogens, which highlights the worth of interdisciplinary science in this research area. The changing scenario of antimicrobial compounds thus demands sustained research to properly tap these potentialities and counter the pressing necessity for efficient microbial control in a clinical environment (Jayaseelan, 2019). Concurrently, the changing emphasis on natural compounds as antimicrobial agents is a response to increasing concerns regarding the use of synthetic pesticides and microbial resistance. Tea polyphenols, for example, have shown significant activity against a range of phytopathogens, indicating their potential as sustainable and environmentally friendly alternatives in agriculture. Whereas laboratory and controlled environment experiments suggest considerable antimicrobial activity and modes of action, there is a key shortfall of field-based verifications to document these impacts at larger scales. However, the initial findings affirm the promise of such natural compounds for integrated pest management, highlighting the need to progress research from molecular understanding towards utilitarian applications in crop management (Yang et al., 2019). This strategy not only responds to consumer pressure for more secure products but is also a strategic change in the development of antimicrobial agents. Overall, the future of antimicrobial agents is the multifaceted search for synthetic and natural compounds alike, such as the repurposing of drugs and the discovery of compounds from plants. The growing insight into the molecular interactions and virulence-targeting mechanisms increases the potential to develop improved-targeted therapies and agricultural agents with fewer side effects and environmental footprint. Yet, translating these results from controlled studies to practical applications is still a major challenge that needs to be addressed through rigorous experimental validation. Therefore, a holistic strategy integrating *in silico* prediction, *in vitro* testing, and field studies is necessary to utilize the potential of novel antimicrobial agents to the fullest and manage the mounting problem of microbial resistance in an effective manner (Jayaseelan, 2019; Yang et al., 2019).

Summary of Key Points

The changing landscape of infectious disease reiterates the pivotal function of antimicrobial agents in contemporary medicine. Up-to-date epidemiological information documents a consistently high global incidence of sexually transmitted infections, such as chlamydia, gonorrhea, trichomoniasis, and syphilis, among millions each year. These diseases not only call for effective antimicrobial treatment but also emphasize the need for full-scale surveillance and current therapeutic schemes. The evidence highlights that with the progress in treatment, the rates of incidence and prevalence are still alarming, reflecting the need to improve antimicrobial stewardship and create new agents with better efficacy. Additionally, incorporating quantitative burden estimates helps estimate the effects of current antimicrobials and informs policy-making to slow down infection rates and drug resistance spread (Rowley et al., 2019). Environmental and sustainability issues are increasingly influencing the formulation of antimicrobial agents, with green synthesis leading the way as a key innovation in the field. This green approach utilizes natural biological constituents such as phytochemical-rich plant extracts to enable the synthesis of phytochemical nanoparticles with antimicrobial activity. Using such biogenic processes not only decreases environmental toxicity commonly linked with traditional chemical synthesis but also increases the biocompatibility and stability of the end products. The developments mirror a shift in paradigm that reconciles sustainability with effectiveness to promote the creation of new antimicrobial materials that reduce ecological footprint without sacrificing potent activity against pathogenic microorganisms (Singh et al., 2018). Overall, the major highlights of antimicrobial agents include both the epidemiological issue of infectious disease and the creative synthetic methods toward solving such an issue. The continued incidence of curable but endemic infection necessitates double efforts toward efficacious antimicrobial treatment and efficient surveillance systems. In parallel, the development of green synthesis approaches presents a fruitful direction for achieving safer, ecologically friendly antimicrobial agents. Combined, these findings emphasize the complex efforts needed to maintain the efficacy of antimicrobial agents in the face of emerging microbial threats and environmental sustainability needs, toward overarching strategies that balance clinical performance and sustainability objectives (Rowley et al., 2019; Singh et al., 2018).

KEY TERMS FROM THIS CHAPTER

Antimicrobial agents	Clinical applications	Public Health
Nanocomposites	Phytochemicals	Antimicrobial peptides
Nanotechnology	Chemical	Nucleic Acid Synthesis
Broad-Spectrum Antimicrobials	Polymicrobial	Mechanisms
Antimicrobial resistance (AMR)	Protein synthesis	Surgery
Antimicrobial treatment		

CRITICAL THINKING QUESTIONS

1. **The primary mechanism of action of aminoglycosides is?**
   a. Inhibition of cell wall synthesis
   b. Inhibition of protein synthesis
   c. Inhibition of DNA synthesis
   d. Disruption of folic acid synthesis
2. **Which of the following antibiotics is most effective against anaerobic bacteria?**
   a. Metronidazole
   b. Gentamicin
   c. Cephalexin
   d. Tetracycline
3. **Resistance to penicillin is commonly due to?**
   a. Increased drug absorption
   b. Efflux pumps
   c. β-lactamase production
   d. Enzyme methylation
4. **Which antimicrobial agent inhibits DNA gyrase in bacteria?**
   a. Chloramphenicol
   b. Ciprofloxacin
   c. Rifampin
   d. Streptomycin
5. **Vancomycin is primarily used to treat infections caused by?**
   a. Gram-negative bacteria
   b. Mycobacteria
   c. Gram-positive bacteria
   d. Viruses

Short Answer Questions

1. What is types of antimicrobial agents?
2. Explain about the various mechanisms by which antimicrobial agents?
3. What is meant by the spectrum of activity of an antimicrobial agent?
4. What are the major scientific and clinical challenges in developing new antimicrobial agents today?
5. Explain the key factors clinicians consider when selecting an antimicrobial agent for a patient?

Answers to Multiple choice Questions.

1. (b) 2 (a) 3. (c) 4. (b) 5. (c)

REFERENCES

1. Aljilawi, M. (2024). Antibiotic resistance in *E. coli*. *Karbala Journal of Medicine*. https://www.semanticscholar.org/paper/afd2e3f42adae935c25c3a25abf144c50c98693e (accessed on 9 May 2025).
2. Álvarez-Martínez, F. J., Barrajón-Catalán, E., Herranz-López, M., & Micol, V. (2021). Antibacterial plant compounds, extracts, and essential oils: An updated review on their effects and putative mechanisms of action. *Phytomedicine, 90*, 153626. https://doi.org/10.1016/j.phymed.2021.153626.
3. Arrais, A., Bona, E., Todeschini, V., Caramaschi, A., Massa, N., Roncoli, M., Minervi, A., et al. (2023). Thymus vulgaris essential oil in beta-cyclodextrin for solid-state pharmaceutical applications. *Pharmaceutics, 15*, 914. https://doi.org/10.3390/pharmaceutics15030914.
4. Bai, S., Wang, J., Yang, K., Zhou, C., Xu, Y., Song, J., Gu, Y., et al. (2021). A polymeric approach toward resistance-resistant antimicrobial agent with dual-selective mechanisms of action. *Science Advances, 7*(10), eabc9917. https://doi.org/10.1126/sciadv.abc9917.
5. Baran, A., Kwiatkowska, A., & Potocki, L. (2023). Antibiotics and bacterial resistance—A short story of an endless arms race. *International Journal of Molecular Sciences, 24*, 5777. https://doi.org/10.3390/ijms24065777.
6. Bhattacharjee, R., Negi, A., Bhattacharya, B., Dey, T., Mitra, P., Preetam, S., Kumar, L., et al. (2023). Nanotheranostics to target antibiotic-resistant bacteria: Strategies and applications. *OpenNano, 11*, 100138. https://doi.org/10.1016/j.onano.2023.100138.
7. Blecher-Paz, K., Champer, J., Friedman, A. J., Kim, et al. (2013). Antimicrobial and anti-inflammatory activity of chitosan-alginate nanoparticles: A targeted therapy for cutaneous pathogens. https://core.ac.uk/download/323078644.pdf.
8. Bormann, M., Alt, M., Schipper, L., van de Sand, L., Le-Trilling, V. T. K., Rink, L., Heinen, N., et al. (2021). Turmeric root and its bioactive ingredient curcumin effectively neutralize SARS-CoV-2 *in vitro*. *Viruses, 13*, 1914. https://doi.org/10.3390/v13101914.
9. Bortolaia, V., Kaas, R. S., Ruppé, É., Roberts, M. C., Schwarz, Š., Cattoir, V., Philippon, A., et al. (2020). ResFinder 4.0 for predictions of phenotypes from genotypes. *Journal of Antimicrobial Chemotherapy, 75*, 3491–3500. https://doi.org/10.1093/jac/dkaa345.
10. Bruni, G. O., Terrell, E., Klasson, K. T., & Qi, Y. (2025). Control of industrially relevant microbial isolates by antimicrobial agents: Implications for sugar factories. *Journal of Industrial Microbiology & Biotechnology*. https://www.semanticscholar.org/paper/3d464a9d678fa3d935778af4d9719afba63f72d8 (accessed on 9 May 2025).
11. Chatupheeraphat, C., Peamchai, J., Luk-in, S., & Eiamphungporn, W. (2023). Synergistic effect and antibiofilm activity of the antimicrobial peptide K11 with conventional antibiotics against multidrug-resistant and extensively drug-resistant *Klebsiella pneumoniae*. *Frontiers in Cellular and Infection Microbiology, 13*. https://www.semanticscholar.org/paper/4525025caff3df2d4ea5f0e41e31855a1137496d (accessed on 9 May 2025).
12. Chinese Society of Critical Care Medicine. (2025). Practice guideline on the prevention and treatment of central line associated bloodstream infection in 2025. *Zhonghua Wei Zhong Bing Ji Jiu Yi Xue, 37*(3), 193–220. https://www.semanticscholar.org/paper/2cd3786fe372222e47f8091dd0c4396f1d7c5a70 (accessed on 9 May 2025).

13. Da Silva, J., Leal, E. C., & Carvalho, E. (2021). Bioactive antimicrobial peptides as therapeutic agents for infected diabetic foot ulcers. *Biomolecules, 11*, 1894. https://doi.org/10.3390/biom11121894.

14. de Matos, C. M., Rauter, A. P., & de Matos, A. M. (2024). Antibacterial prodrugs to overcome bacterial antimicrobial resistance. *Pharmaceuticals, 17*. https://www.semanticscholar.org/paper/d309b7d4afe4d464e3c94add6cc842f51e420df9 (accessed on 9 May 2025).

15. Deveci, A., & Çoban, A. (2014). Optimum management of *Citrobacter koseri* infection. *Expert Review of Anti-infective Therapy, 12*, 1137–1142. https://www.semanticscholar.org/paper/3934368dffffaa762e048a58919e3b3811509a6b (accessed on 9 May 2025).

16. Dhole, S., Mahakalkar, C., Kshirsagar, S., & Bhargava, A. (2023). Antibiotic prophylaxis in surgery: Current insights and future directions for surgical site infection prevention. *Cureus*. https://doi.org/10.7759/cureus.47858.

17. Essghaier, B., Toukabri, N., Dridi, R., Hannachi, H., Limam, I., Mottola, F., Mokni, M., et al. (2022). First report of the biosynthesis and characterization of silver nanoparticles using *Scabiosa atropurpurea* subsp. maritima fruit extracts and their antioxidant, antimicrobial, and cytotoxic properties. *Nanomaterials, 12*, 1585. https://doi.org/10.3390/nano12091585.

18. European Centre for Disease Prevention and Control (ECDC), European Food Safety Authority (EFSA), & European Medicines Agency (EMA). (2021). Third joint inter-agency report on integrated analysis of consumption of antimicrobial agents and occurrence of antimicrobial resistance in bacteria from humans and food-producing animals in the EU/EEA. *EFSA Journal, 19*. https://doi.org/10.2903/j.efsa.2021.6712.

19. Goto, R., Inose, R., Koizumi, R., Sawada, K., Ishikane, M., Ohmagari, N., & Muraki, Y. (2025). Evaluation of the influence of the National Action Plan on antimicrobial resistance and the COVID-19 pandemic on the consumption of broad-spectrum antimicrobial and anti-methicillin-resistant *Staphylococcus aureus* agents. *Biological & Pharmaceutical Bulletin, 48*(4), 415–421. https://www.semanticscholar.org/paper/3283e556bbe51e0dac28f776b129a04b0d046774 (accessed on 9 May 2025).

20. Green, L. H., & Goldman, E. (2021). *Practical Handbook of Microbiology*. CRC Press eBooks. https://doi.org/10.1201/9781003099277.

21. Guglielmi, P., Pontecorvi, V., & Rotondi, G. (2020). Natural compounds and extracts as novel antimicrobial agents. *Expert Opinion on Therapeutic Patents, 30*(12), 949–962. https://doi.org/10.1080/13543776.2020.1853101.

22. Gul, G. C. (2025). Advances in boron compounds: Author's perspectives on their role in biotechnology from antimicrobial agents to cancer therapy. *EUCHEMBIOJ Reviews*. https://www.semanticscholar.org/paper/7ea1409d179c52f46fd65d5ad3759cdd09e76bbb (accessed on 9 May 2025).

23. Gupta, A., Jeyakumar, E., & Lawrence, R. (2021). Journey of limonene as an antimicrobial agent. *Journal of Pure and Applied Microbiology, 15*, 1094–1110. https://doi.org/10.22207/jpam.15.3.01.

24. He, Q. (2019). Antibacterial activity of traditional herbal medicine. *Access Microbiology*. https://www.semanticscholar.org/paper/1f7b0a00db553838e4691ae85c0e7fd57c30ccd0 (accessed on 9 May 2025).

25. Helal, M., & Dadachova, E. (2018). Radioimmunotherapy as a novel approach in HIV, bacterial, and fungal infectious diseases. *Cancer Biotherapy & Radiopharmaceuticals, 33*(8), 330–335. https://www.semanticscholar.org/paper/93d18f3a41318ac3b5d228b0b9eae2d75a22c9bc (accessed on 9 May 2025).

26. Hols, P., Ledesma-García, L., Gabant, P., & Mignolet, J. (2019). Mobilization of microbiota commensals and their bacteriocins for therapeutics. *Trends in Microbiology, 27*(8), 690–702. https://doi.org/10.1016/j.tim.2019.03.007.

27. Jayaseelan, V. P. (2019). *In silico* validation of the non-antibiotic drugs acetaminophen and ibuprofen as antibacterial agents against red complex pathogens. *Journal of Periodontology, 90*, 1441–1448. https://doi.org/10.1002/jper.18-0673.

28. Kim, S. M., Heo, H. R., Kim, C. S., & Shin, H. H. (2024). Genetically engineered bacteriophages as novel nanomaterials: Applications beyond antimicrobial agents. *Frontiers in Bioengineering and Biotechnology, 12*. https://www.semanticscholar.org/paper/e7239fbd5472e811d077812c41b6ba0bebc211c5 (accessed on 9 May 2025).

29. Kumari, B., Arya, N. G., Neeta, & Verma, P. (2025). Antimicrobial textiles: Innovations, challenges, and applications for health and hygiene. *Asian Journal of Research in Biochemistry*. https://www.semanticscholar.org/paper/05300d25d3a3688bb6782f362d48e00b041744b1 (accessed on 9 May 2025).

30. Langendonk, R. F., Neill, D. R., & Fothergill, J. L. (2021). The building blocks of antimicrobial resistance in *Pseudomonas aeruginosa*: Implications for current resistance-breaking therapies. *Frontiers in Cellular and Infection Microbiology, 11*, 665759. https://doi.org/10.3389/fcimb.2021.665759.

31. Li, Y., Xiao, P., Wang, Y., & Hao, Y. (2020). Mechanisms and control measures of mature biofilm resistance to antimicrobial agents in the clinical context. *ACS Omega, 5*, 22684–22690. https://doi.org/10.1021/acsomega.0c02294.

32. Matanic, A., Bayerl, C., Berg, M., Blount, B. W., Boguniewicz, M., Bourinbaiar, A. S., Bradshaw, J., et al. (2012). Antimicrobial peptides and skin: A paradigm of translational medicine. https://core.ac.uk/download/16432237.pdf (accessed on 9 May 2025).

33. Murata, M., Sugimoto, M., Mizuno, H., Kanno, T., & Satoh, K. (2020). Clarithromycin versus metronidazole in first-line *Helicobacter pylori* triple eradication therapy based on resistance to antimicrobial agents: Meta-analysis. *Journal of Clinical Medicine, 9*(2), 543. https://doi.org/10.3390/jcm9020543.

34. Pal, K., Sarkar, P., Anis, A., Wiszumirska, K., & Jarzębski, M. (2021). Polysaccharide-based nanocomposites for food packaging applications. *Materials, 14*, 5549. https://doi.org/10.3390/ma14195549.

35. Patra, J. K., Das, G., Fraceto, L. F., Campos, E. V. R., Rodríguez-Torres, M. P., Acosta-Torres, L. S., Díaz-Torres, L. A., et al. (2018). Nano based drug delivery systems: Recent developments and future prospects. *Journal of Nanobiotechnology, 16*. https://doi.org/10.1186/s12951-018-0392-8.

36. Pilatz, A., Dimitropoulos, K., Veeratterapillay, R., Yuan, Y., Omar, M. I., MacLennan, S., Cai, T., et al. (2020). Antibiotic prophylaxis for the prevention of infectious complications following prostate biopsy: A systematic review and meta-analysis. *The Journal of Urology, 204*, 224–230. https://doi.org/10.1097/ju.0000000000000814.

37. Rhodes, A., Evans, L., Alhazzani, W., Levy, M. M., Antonelli, M., Ferrer, R., Kumar, A., et al. (2017). Surviving sepsis campaign: International guidelines for management of sepsis and septic shock: 2016. *Critical Care Medicine, 45*, 486–552. https://doi.org/10.1097/ccm.0000000000002255.
38. Ribeiro, A. I., Dias, A., & Zille, A. (2022). Synergistic effects between metal nanoparticles and commercial antimicrobial agents: A review. *ACS Applied Nano Materials, 5*, 3030–3064. https://doi.org/10.1021/acsanm.1c03891.
39. Rowley, J., Vander Hoorn, S., Korenromp, E. L., Low, N., Unemo, M., Abu-Raddad, L. J., Chico, R. M., et al. (2019). Chlamydia, gonorrhoea, trichomoniasis, and syphilis: Global prevalence and incidence estimates, 2016. *Bulletin of the World Health Organization, 97*, 548–562. https://doi.org/10.2471/blt.18.228486.
40. Sabah, T. Q., & Baqer, S. R. (2024). Design, synthesis, and evaluation of some metal ion complexes of mannich base derived from 2-mercaptobenzimidazole as potential antimicrobial agents. *Iraqi Journal of Chemical and Petroleum Engineering*. https://www.semanticscholar.org/paper/4cb1dbf6feb1a13bd51491f273d35faa66defd2b (accessed on 9 May 2025).
41. Salam, M. A., Al-Amin, M. Y., Tabassoom Salam, M., Pawar, J. S., Akhter, N., Rabaan, A. A., & Alqumber, M. A. A. (2023). Antimicrobial resistance: A growing serious threat for global public health. *Healthcare, 11*(13), 1946. https://doi.org/10.3390/healthcare11131946.
42. Sherry, N., Lee, J. Y. H., Giulieri, S., Connor, C. H., Horan, K., Lacey, J. A., Lane, C., et al. (2025). Genomics for antimicrobial resistance—Progress and future directions. *Antimicrobial Agents and Chemotherapy*. https://www.semanticscholar.org/paper/7ec919db9e70fa7de46f49958443bf83819948fd (accessed on 9 May 2025).
43. Shewale, M. M., Mali, K. K., Jatte, K. P., & Marale, P. S. (2025). Silver nanoparticles as broad-spectrum antimicrobial agents: Applications, challenges, and future directions in microbial control. *International Journal of Drug Delivery Technology*. https://www.semanticscholar.org/paper/c274f1fadbd76e1fe3ab77634a519180a1a86cc1 (accessed on 9 May 2025).
44. Siburian, E., Hayun, H., & Suryadi, H. (2025). A review on Mannich base derivatives of some natural compounds: Antimicrobial activities. *Eduvest–Journal of Universal Studies*. https://www.semanticscholar.org/paper/ffc91f69f8a7c4df2cc7509e74ce3ebcfed63694 (accessed on 9 May 2025).
45. Silvan, J., Zorraquín-Peña, I., González de Llano, D., Moreno-Arribas, M., & Martinez-Rodriguez, A. (2018). Antibacterial activity of glutathione-stabilized silver nanoparticles against *Campylobacter* multidrug-resistant strains. *Frontiers in Microbiology, 9*. https://www.semanticscholar.org/paper/ee12a3aacfbc6f57fe9de352f4663952ec166dc0 (accessed on 9 May 2025).
46. Singh, J., Dutta, T., Kim, K. H., Rawat, M., Samddar, P., & Kumar, P. (2018). 'Green' synthesis of metals and their oxide nanoparticles: Applications for environmental remediation. *Journal of Nanobiotechnology, 16*. https://doi.org/10.1186/s12951-018-0408-4.
47. Solanki, S., & Bhatt, H. (2025). Emerging frontiers in antimicrobial therapy: The role of nitrogen-containing heterocyclic compounds in overcoming drug-resistant infections. *Research Review International Journal of Multidisciplinary*. https://www.semanticscholar.org/paper/fda6696dcdfe148270a4ac351d51180b5afaead2 (accessed on 9 May 2025).
48. Spirescu, V. A., Chircov, C., Grumezescu, A. M., & Andronescu, E. (2021). Polymeric nanoparticles for antimicrobial therapies: An up-to-date overview. *Polymers, 13*, 724. https://doi.org/10.3390/polym13050724.

49. Suriyaprom, S., Mosoni, P., Léroy, S., Kaewkod, T., Desvaux, M., & Tragoolpua, Y. (2022). Antioxidants of fruit extracts as antimicrobial agents against pathogenic bacteria. *Antioxidants, 11*, 602. https://doi.org/10.3390/antiox11030602.

50. Talapko, J., Meštrović, T., Juzbašić, M., Tomas, M., Erić, S., Horvat Aleksijević, L., Bekić, S., et al. (2022). Antimicrobial peptides—Mechanisms of action, antimicrobial effects, and clinical applications. *Antibiotics, 11*, 1417. https://doi.org/10.3390/antibiotics11101417.

51. Thalia, O. P. (2025). Emerging technologies in antimicrobial resistance research. *Research Invention Journal of Engineering and Physical Sciences*. https://www.semanticscholar.org/paper/736b1fd28f014e03c13f9ad920bf6ecedd42036d (accessed on 9 May 2025).

52. Vaou, N., Stavropoulou, E., Voidarou, C., Tsigalou, C., & Bezirtzoglou, E. (2021). Towards advances in medicinal plant antimicrobial activity: A review study on challenges and future perspectives. *Microorganisms, 9*(10), 2041. https://doi.org/10.3390/microorganisms9102041.

53. Veiko, A. G., Olchowik-Grabarek, E., Sękowski, S., Roszkowska, A., Лапшина, E. A., Dobrzyńska, I., Zamaraeva, M., et al. (2023). Antimicrobial activity of quercetin, naringenin, and catechin: Flavonoids inhibit *Staphylococcus aureus*-induced hemolysis and modify membranes of bacteria and erythrocytes. *Molecules, 28*, 1252. https://doi.org/10.3390/molecules28031252.

54. Vigašová, D., Nemergut, M., Lišková, B., & Damborský, J. (2021). Multi-pathogen infections and Alzheimer's disease. *Microbial Cell Factories, 20*. https://doi.org/10.1186/s12934-021-01520-7.

55. Yan, X., Li, X., Yu, P., Wang, L., & Zhao, Q. (2024). Nanozymes as antibacterial agents: New concerns in design and enhancement strategies. *Chembiochem: A European Journal of Chemical Biology*. https://www.semanticscholar.org/paper/4d3d514ea3a2028e91177466ee6073adfc5c0c77 (accessed on 9 May 2025).

56. Yang, Y., & Zhang, T. (2019). Antimicrobial activities of tea polyphenol on phytopathogens: A review. *Molecules, 24*, 816. https://doi.org/10.3390/molecules24040816.

57. Zuorro, A., Lavecchia, R., Contreras-Ropero, J. E., García Martínez, J. B., Barajas-Ferreira, C., & Barajas-Solano, A. (2024). Natural antimicrobial agents from algae: Current advances and future directions. *International Journal of Molecular Sciences, 25*. https://www.semanticscholar.org/paper/5472dabb3adafb38d30337063bc6b11a07f7d003 (accessed on 9 May 2025).

ENDOCRINE PHARMACOLOGY

10

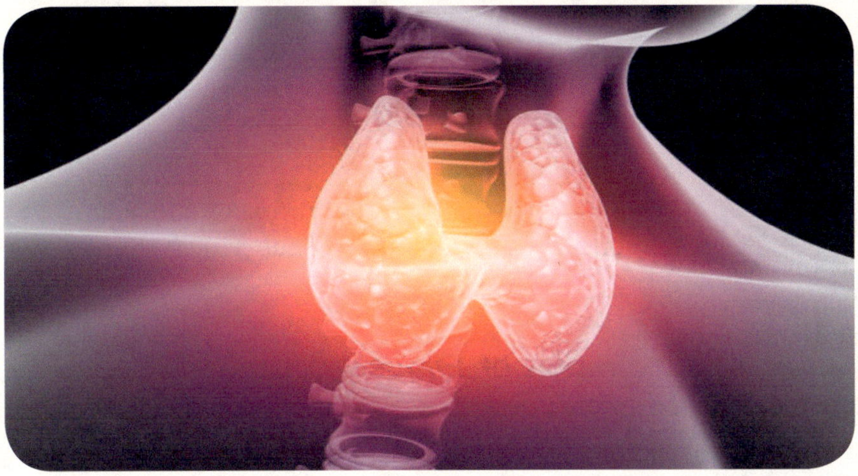

LEARNING OBJECTIVES

After studying this chapter, you will be able to:

1. Explore hormones and their mechanisms of action
2. Define major endocrine disorders
3. Know the pharmacological treatments for diabetes
4. Understand thyroid hormone replacement therapy
5. Discuss the corticosteroids and their uses
6. Explain about emerging therapies in endocrine pharmacology

Introduction

The intricate interplay of hormones in the body coordinates a vast array of physiological functions essential for homeostasis. A knowledge of these mechanisms is vital to understanding how endocrine pharmacology provides therapeutic interventions through the modification of hormonal function (Figure 10.1). Hormones are chemical messengers produced by glands and circulate in the blood to affect a particular organ, thereby controlling metabolism, growth, reproduction, and mood. The development of endocrine pharmacology enables clinicians to treat hormonal imbalances underlying such disorders as diabetes and infertility. Pharmacologic agents may either substitute for natural hormones, suppress hormone secretion, or interfere with receptor action, offering flexible means of treatment. This advanced control of endocrine messaging is a quintessential marriage of biochemistry and therapeutic science, and thus an essential branch of medicine. By understanding the principles of hormone action and drug interaction, one can realize the accuracy required in designing effective, customized endocrine therapies. Endocrine pharmacology has evolved much as a result of seeking safer and more effective hormonal pathway-targeting treatments. Conventional hormone replacement therapy or contraceptives have undesirable side effects, and hence the need to explore new drug compounds that counteract these shortcomings. For instance, ongoing research into non-hormonal male contraceptives targets the inhibition of certain enzymes and proteins essential for spermatogenesis and sperm function, including prostate-specific antigen and serine/threonine kinases, without affecting systemic endocrine homeostasis (Pereira et al., 2025). This novel approach to enzyme inhibition instead of hormone analogs hopes to minimize side effects such as mood changes and metabolic disturbances typical of hormonal regimens. These developments demonstrate the evolving nature of endocrine pharmacology, in which novel molecular targets keep redefining therapeutic concepts and enhancing patient compliance by reducing undesirable systemic side effects. Endocrine disorders frequently present with complex clinical manifestations that necessitate an integrated pharmacological strategy to correct both hormonal and metabolic derangements. Polycystic ovary syndrome (PCOS), which is a ubiquitous endocrine disease among women in reproductive age, is the ultimate example of complexity because it represents irregular menses, hyperandrogenism, and metabolic syndromes including insulin resistance (Corte et al., 2020). Successful management of PCOS with endocrine pharmacology requires regimens that recover hormonal balance while also addressing concurrently metabolic risk reduction. Pharmacotherapeutics existing currently and emerging involve both reproductive as well as systemic features and demonstrate potential improvement for long-term outcomes of health. The continuous search for new mechanisms involved in endocrine disorders continuously increases pharmacologic possibilities, with the focus being on personalized medicine in endocrine therapy. The holistic understanding validates the pivotal contribution of endocrine pharmacology in tackling varied and dynamic clinical challenges in endocrinology.

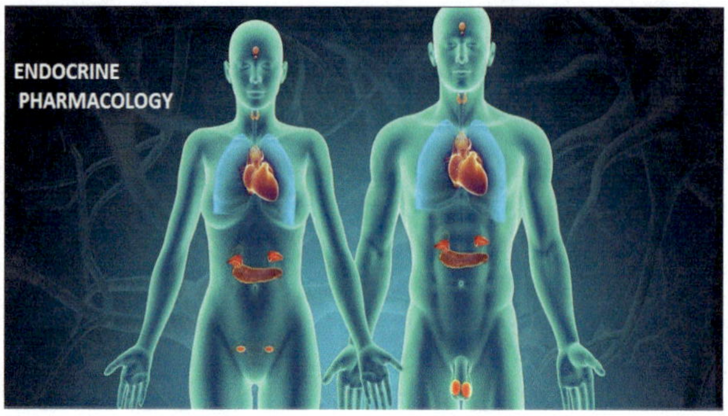

Figure 10.1. Endocrine pharmacology.

Source: Pharma Professor. (2020). *Endocrine System.* https://pharmaprofessor.com/wp-content/uploads/2020/08/EndocrineSystem1.jpg.

Definition of Endocrine Pharmacology

Chemical messenger control of body functions is a basic part of human physiology. Endocrine pharmacology, being an allied branch, deals with the study of how drugs affect the endocrine system that includes glands secreting hormones directly into the blood. The hormones control many of the biological functions like metabolism, growth, and reproduction. The field fills the gap between endocrinology and pharmacology by analyzing the processes through which synthetic or natural chemicals change hormone concentrations or receptor functions to bring about therapeutic activity. This interaction is of paramount importance because derangements in hormone function can result in varied pathological conditions. Hence, endocrine pharmacology not only investigates the processes by which drugs affect endocrine processes but also ascertains their safety and efficacy. Designing such therapeutic drugs demands a complex understanding of both chemical characteristics and physiological reactions, aiming for specific treatment with minimal side effects (Mojca et al., 2011). Endocrine pharmacology also involves a thorough assessment of drug absorption, distribution, metabolism, and excretion (ADME) processes related to hormones and hormone-like substances. These pharmacokinetic properties are crucial in defining the onset, magnitude, and duration of a drug's endocrine action. In contrast to traditional pharmacology, endocrine pharmacology has to contend with the subtlety of feedback loops and the systemic nature of hormone signaling. Thus, the pharmacodynamics of endocrine drugs require an understanding of receptor specificity, signal transduction pathways, and the possibility of receptor desensitization or downregulation. Improved computational modeling and non-animal testing techniques have improved the predictive ability of drug behavior in endocrine systems, providing insights into toxicological profiles and safety assessments. Incorporating such methods guarantees that endocrine pharmacology may develop with both scientific integrity and ethics (Mojca et al., 2011). Pharmacological therapy on the endocrine system includes a wide range of clinical uses, such as management of diabetes, thyroid diseases, and hormone replacement therapy. Endocrine pharmacology describes how these therapies produce their action by mimicking, augmenting, or blocking hormone activity. For instance, insulin analogs attempt to normalize glycemic control by mimicking the action of endogenous insulins, while anti-thyroid agents curb overproduction of thyroid hormones. The branch also researches newer agents that seek to modulate endocrine disruptors or act upon hormone receptors with increased specificity. Due to the delicate nature of the endocrine system, small changes in hormone levels have extreme systemic implications. Hence, endocrine pharmacology is characterized by a careful definition of dose-response relationships, therapeutic windows, and toxicities. This delicate balancing act with the aid of advancing experimental and computational capabilities embodies the dynamic and interdisciplinary character of the field.

Importance in Medical Treatment

Endocrine pharmacology has evolved dramatically and has changed the face of medical treatment, especially in the management of intricate hormonal disorders (Figure 10.2). The complex pathophysiology of endocrine disease frequently necessitates a judicious pharmacologic strategy to reestablish homeostasis as well as relief of symptoms. For example, PCOS, an extremely common endocrine condition, is best treated by employing therapeutic strategies that combine lifestyle intervention with pharmacotherapy to address symptoms of menstrual irregularities as well as hyperandrogenism effectively. The significance of adding vitamins and supplements, including vitamins D and E and inositol, to traditional medications reflects the extent to which endocrine pharmacology is more than mere prescriptions of drugs to include general patient care. These combined treatments enhance fertility and reduce metabolic risks but also minimize long-term consequences such as cardiovascular disease (CVD) and diabetes, which illustrates the essential role precision medicine plays in endocrine therapy (Turek et al., 2024). This multidisciplinary approach illustrates how pharmacologic management is a keystone in enhancing patient quality of life and disease outcomes. The nature of endocrine disorders often requires careful management of comorbid conditions to achieve optimal therapeutic outcomes, a paradigm that is being increasingly accepted in general medical treatment models. Endocrine modulation is crossed with cardiovascular pharmacology in conditions like heart failure with reduced ejection fraction, where neurohormonal agents must be titrated carefully to balance effectiveness with side effects such as hypotension and electrolyte imbalances. The subtlety in dose increases and handling of treatment-limiting challenges underscores the need for personal care pharmacologically in ensuring that maximum tolerated doses are reached safely. Additionally, these strategies highlight the importance of adjunctive interventions, such as rehabilitation and nutritional support, in the augmentation of the effectiveness of pharmacotherapy for endocrine-associated comorbidities. All of these considerations serve to illustrate that effective endocrine pharmacology relies not only on the choice of drug but also on integrative patient care to maximize clinical success (Bak et al., 2023).

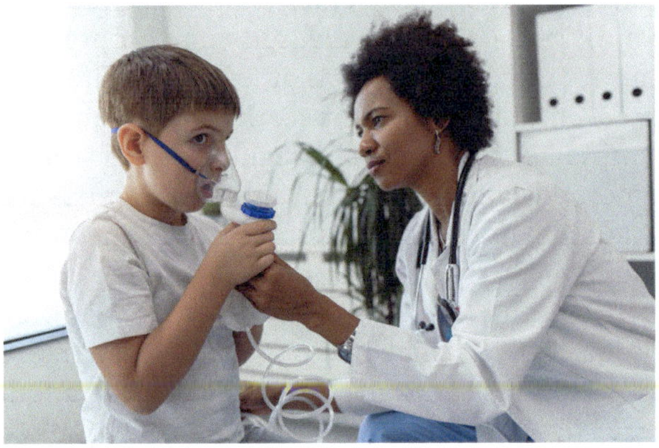

Figure 10.2. Medical treatment.

Clinical management in endocrine pharmacology is vital for the treatment of acute symptoms as well as to avoid chronic complications resulting from hormonal imbalance. Endocrine-targeted therapies have a significant effect on the course of disease, with therapy ranging from replacement hormones to inhibitors of hormone synthesis or action. Notably, the therapeutic effect is optimized when pharmacologic interventions are complemented by changes in lifestyle and diet, evidencing an integrated treatment model. This multifaceted model is crucial in diseases like diabetes, thyroid disease, and PCOS, where pharmacologic therapy controls biochemical derangements while lifestyle modification alters susceptibility and severity of the disease. The role of early treatment and personalized therapy, which endocrine pharmacology plays so crucially, demonstrates its essential role in contemporary medicine. The focus on both pharmacologic and non-pharmacologic approaches enhances clinical practice, enhancing prognoses and improving patient-centered care (Bak et al., 2023; Turek et al., 2024).

Overview of Endocrine System Functions

The body's maintenance of internal stability depends significantly on a system of signaling molecules that regulate the physiological processes over a period of time. These chemical messengers are called hormones and play their role in being secreted by specialized glands located around the body, which constitute the endocrine system. In contrast to the quick action of nerve impulses, hormones take longer to work but have longer-lasting impacts. They control a variety of vital functions like growth, metabolism, reproduction, and stress responses by interacting with specific receptors on target cells. This complex system makes sure that several organs work in concert to satisfy the dynamic demands of the organism. Knowledge of these basic mechanisms is crucial for pharmacological interventions to correct endocrine imbalances or augment hormonal activity. Of all the endocrine glands, the adrenal glands are unique in their wide-ranging function in metabolism, immunity, and coping with stress. Situated atop the kidneys, they secrete hormones such as cortisol, aldosterone, and adrenaline that regulate blood pressure, glucose metabolism, and immune function. Synthesis of these hormones relies on the steroidogenic pathway of the adrenal cortex, and any derangement of this pathway can have severe physiological effects. Endocrine-disrupting chemicals (EDCs) like flame retardants and bisphenols have been demonstrated to interfere with adrenal function and morphology, and the gland's susceptibility to environmental toxins (Li et al., 2025). Identification of the EDCs' impact emphasizes the importance of rigorous testing of such chemicals to ensure adrenal health as well as general endocrine equilibrium. Aside from the classical endocrine glands, natural products with bioactive compounds are further researched for modulating the endocrine system. An example is the areca nut, which is commonly used in Chinese medicinal practice. Alkaloids and polyphenols in the areca nut have anti-inflammatory and antioxidant activities. These bioactive compounds act on the nervous, digestive, and more importantly on the endocrine systems, presenting potential therapeutic applications in the field of endocrine pharmacology. Although the therapeutic benefits of such plant materials provide exciting leads for the development of new drugs, their mechanisms and safety profiles must be thoroughly studied. Improvements in pharmacological studies of natural compounds may therefore underpin traditional strategies for controlling endocrine diseases (Sun et al., 2024).

10.1. Hormones and Their Mechanisms of Action

Learning Outcome

1. Types of Hormones (Steroid Versus Peptide)
2. Mechanisms of Hormone Action
3. Receptor Types and Signaling Pathways

The complex communication networks in the human body are highly dependent on biochemical messengers that control physiological processes with high precision. Of these, hormones are crucial agents, converting signals into synthesized molecules that affect cellular activities in a wide range of tissues. Such substances can be categorized broadly depending on their solubility and receptor interactions, which determine their mechanisms of action. Lipid-soluble steroid hormones pass through the plasma membrane to bind with intracellular receptors, regulating gene transcription and thereby protein synthesis (Figure 10.3). Water-soluble peptides and amines, on the other hand, bind with receptors in the membrane, triggering a series of second messenger reactions that convert extracellular stimuli to proper cellular responses. This dualism of hormonal action reflects the sophistication of endocrine control, emphasizing its versatility in achieving homeostasis and reacting to environmental signals (Arnold et al., 2001). Going deeper into the molecular mechanisms, the binding affinity and receptor specificity are the determining factors of the efficacy and result of the hormone. Membrane receptors tend to employ G-protein coupled mechanisms or tyrosine kinase activities to amplify the signal so that it is rapid and under control. These pathways not only impact enzymatic functions but also affect ion channel permeability and cellular metabolism, allowing organisms to precisely modulate their physiological conditions. Alternatively, steroid hormones bind to nuclear receptors to create hormone-receptor complexes acting as transcription factors and directly impacting gene expression patterns over a longer timescale. This genomic pathway enables extended metabolic regulation and differentiation processes essential in development and adaptation. Knowledge of these mechanisms is central to pharmacology, since numerous therapeutic drugs are created to imitate or block hormone action, to provide targeted and effective interventions (Arnold et al., 2001). Aside from biochemical complexity, the role of sex hormones and gender factors adds a profound level of variability to endocrine mechanisms. Sex hormones like estrogens, progesterone, and testosterone not only dictate biological differences but also are important in modulating receptor sensitivity and downstream signaling pathways. These differences can both influence physiological responses as well as the pharmacodynamics of hormone therapies.

In addition to biological sex, gender-related behavior and environmental exposures might also be responsible for further modifying hormone interactions and clinical responses, emphasizing the need for a personalized strategy in endocrine pharmacology. Understanding these factors increases the promise of precision medicine by individualizing treatments based on a person's hormonal make-up and sociocultural environments, hence maximizing therapeutic outcomes and patient management.

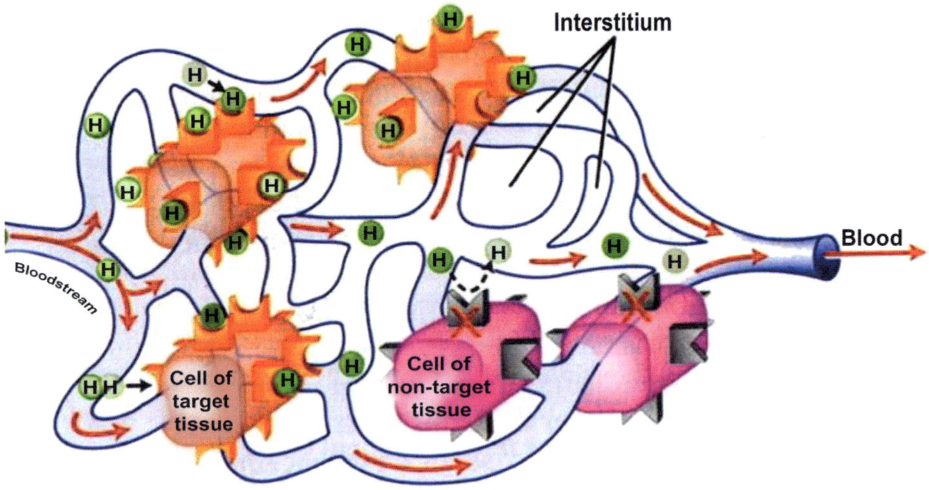

Figure 10.3. Hormones and their mechanisms of action.

Source: Slideserve. (n.d.). *Mechanism of Hormone Action.* https://image.slideserve.com/282016/mechanism-of-hormone-action1-l.jpg.

10.1.1. Types of Hormones (Steroid Versus Peptide)

Hormonal communication is the bedrock of endocrine pharmacology by facilitating a diverse range of physiological activities through chemical messengers. Of these messengers, steroid and peptide hormones are two basic categories with considerable differences in structure and action mechanism. Steroid hormones are steroid lipids derived from cholesterol that can easily diffuse across cell membranes and bind directly to intracellular receptors. When bound, such complexes generally translocate to the nucleus, having an effect on gene transcription and protein synthesis that leads to less rapid but longer cellular responses. Peptide hormones, however, are hydrophilic and can freely cross neither the lipid bilayer nor phospholipid bilayers since they bind to cell surface receptors, initiating secondary messenger cascades that rapidly modify cell function. Recognizing these differences is essential for pharmacological treatment of targeted endocrine pathways because kinetics and sites of action vary significantly among these types of hormones (Alexander et al., 2022). Mechanisms of steroid and peptide hormone synthesis and release also demonstrate important pharmacologic considerations in endocrine treatment. Steroid hormones are on-demand synthesized within endocrine tissues like the adrenal cortex or gonads due to their lipophilic character and limitations of storage. They require transport bound to carrier proteins within the bloodstream, affecting their bioavailability and half-life. Peptide hormones, on the other hand, are synthesized as larger precursor proteins and are stored in secretory vesicles so that they can be released rapidly on stimulation. These peptide hormones possess shorter half-lives in plasma as a result of enzymatic breakdown, necessitating novel approaches to drug formulation and administration. In addition, receptor sensitivity and downregulation kinetics vary, affecting drug dosing and efficacy. Such biochemical and physiological features need to be carefully considered in the development of hormone-based pharmacotherapies (Alexander et al., 2022). Pharmacodynamic profiles of steroid versus peptide hormones point toward divergent clinical implications and therapeutic challenges. Steroid hormones nuclear receptor mediation to transcriptional modulation achieves, to be beneficial in chronic diseases involving prolonged tissue remodeling, osteoporosis treatment where anabolic or antiresorptive drugs simulate steroidal actions. Yet, with prolonged action, they also produce delayed side effects, requiring close dosage control. Peptide hormones, through membrane-bound receptors and intracellular signaling mechanisms, achieve quick physiological effects, as seen with insulin analogs in the control of glycemia. However, their enzymatic vulnerability necessitates continuous dosing or altered-release products. The receptor selectivity and signal transduction mechanisms utilized by each hormone category highlight specialized approaches in drug development, with a focus on highlighting the need for a comprehensive knowledge of hormone categories to optimize endocrine pharmacologic therapy (Figure 10.4).

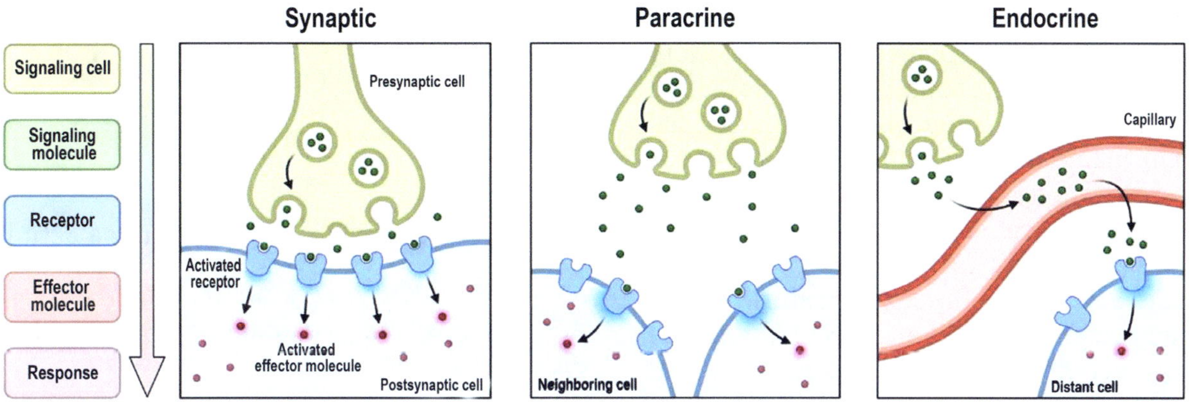

Figure 10.4. Types of hormones.

Source: EndoConsult. (n.d.). *Chemical Signaling.* https://endoconsult.b-cdn.net/wp-content/uploads/chemical-signaling.png.

10.1.2. Mechanisms of Hormone Action

The interaction of hormones with their receptors leads to a cascade of cellular events essential for the preservation of physiological equilibrium. Hormones may engage in different pathways based on their molecular characteristics and receptor specificity. For example, peptide hormones preferentially bind to membrane-bound G protein–coupled receptors (GPCRs) and activate intracellular signaling cascades through second messengers like cyclic AMP. This increase in signal makes a minimal quantity of hormone molecules bring considerable cellular response. However, steroid hormones, on the basis of being hydrophobic in nature, diffuse directly across the plasma membrane and attach themselves to intracellular receptors modulating gene transcription directly. This system is important for governing biological activity from metabolic, through growth to reproductive function. Understanding these pathways not only illuminates basic biological mechanisms but also guides drug development approaches designed to modulate hormone action for therapeutic gain in diseases such as diabetes and thyroid disease. Surprisingly, advances in structural biology over the last few years have provided further insights into how family B GPCRs transmit hormone action, involving a "two-site" ligand binding mechanism that enables effective receptor activation. The parathyroid hormone receptor type 1 (PTHR1) illustrates this paradigm, with ligands including parathyroid hormone and its related proteins activating discrete receptor domains to promote signaling. Remarkably, PTHR1 exhibits the capacity for prolonging signaling after internalization to endosomes, implying a more prolonged temporal scope to hormone action beyond the plasma membrane. Such endosomal signaling maintains such pathways as Gαs/cAMP, which regulate calcium homeostasis and bone metabolism. Such subtle insight highlights possible directions for the design of drugs that take advantage of receptor trafficking and compartmentalized signaling, providing subtle control over hormone-mediated physiological processes in endocrine therapy (Gardella et al., 2015). In the clinic, the exploitation of mechanisms of hormone action has transformed treatment modalities for hormonally mediated diseases. For instance, in hormone receptor–positive breast cancer, modifying estrogen receptor activity by endocrine therapy interrupts cancer cell growth through antagonism of hormone signaling pathways. In like manner, combination therapies of targeted agents and hormone therapies maximize therapeutic benefit by targeting multiple nodes within hormone signaling networks. These examples illustrate how molecular understanding of hormone-receptor interaction and downstream impact is translated into practical clinical maneuvers. Additionally, continuous trials focus on leveraging synergistic effects between new drugs and conventional endocrine therapy to bypass resistance and enhance patient benefits. These advances represent the changing scope of endocrine pharmacology, whereby a thorough comprehension of hormone action mechanisms directs pioneering and targeted therapy approaches (Figure 10.5) (Cao et al., 2024).

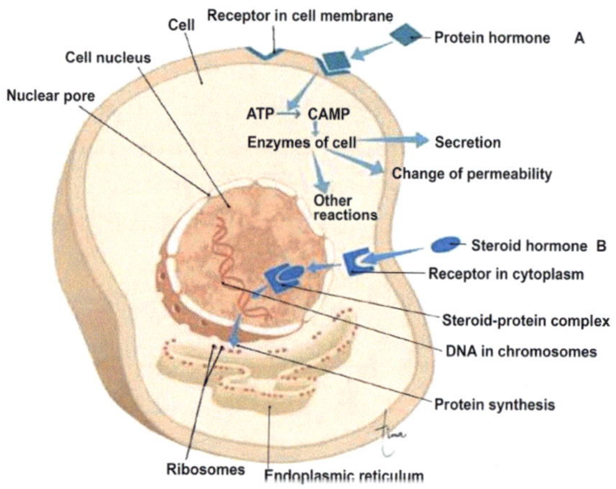

Figure 10.5. Mechanisms of hormone action.

Source: BrainKart. (n.d.). *Mechanisms of Hormone Action.* https://img.brainkart.com/imagebk19/FICIN9g.jpg.

10.1.3. Receptor Types and Signaling Pathways

The intricacy of endocrine pharmacology is deeply impacted by the heterogeneity of receptor types and their corresponding signaling pathways, which determine cellular responses to hormonal signals (Figure 10.6). Of these, nuclear receptors like estrogen receptors (ER) are central, acting as ligand-activated transcription factors that modulate gene expression and cellular growth. In breast cancer, ER signaling is pivotal to tumor growth and progression, with ESR1 gene mutations changing receptor function and making therapeutic approaches challenging. These mutations may cause ligand-independent activity, making classical endocrine therapies less effective and facilitating resistance mechanisms. The interaction between tumor cells and their microenvironment also modulates signaling dynamics, with players such as chemokines and co-receptors amplifying pro-survival and metastatic pathways. Clarifying these receptor interactions and downstream events is essential for the development of targeted therapies that can bypass resistance and enhance outcomes for patients (Lomonaco et al., 2025). Signaling pathways triggered by hormone receptors are not limited to the nuclear compartment but include intricate networks such as the PI3K/AKT/mTOR and MAPK cascades, which converge to integrate extracellular stimuli and affect cell cycle progression, metabolism, and apoptosis. Pharmacologic agents against such pathways have proven to be promising by interrupting significant nodes of cancer cell survival and growth networks. Examples include novel selective estrogen receptor degraders (SERDs) and modulators (SERMs) with increased receptor targeting and enhanced pharmacokinetic profiles, filling the gaps of previous therapies. Proteolysis-targeting chimeras (PROTACs) are also new agents that induce selective hormone receptor degradation and overcome resistance to drugs. Combination regimens involving inhibitors of CDK4/6, PI3K, or mTOR with endocrine agents are a promising approach to overcome compensatory signaling pathways and enhance antitumor activity (Abdullaeva et al., 2025). Recent studies point to the therapeutic value of targeting certain chemokine signaling axes that cross-talk with hormone receptor pathways, e.g., the CCL5-CCR5 interaction involved in endocrine resistance and metastasis. Interference with this pathway by receptor antagonists such as maraviroc has shown to reduce tumor growth and metastatic spread, proposing a promising adjunct to standard endocrine therapies. Elucidation of the interplay between receptor mutations, ligand-dependent as well as independent signaling, and the tumor microenvironment continues to be critical to the advancement of targeted therapies. Breakthroughs in defining these signaling networks offer a model for combining novel molecular targets with known endocrine pharmacology with the ultimate goal of bypassing resistance and maximizing precision medicine strategies in hormone-dependent cancers (Lomonaco et al., 2025).

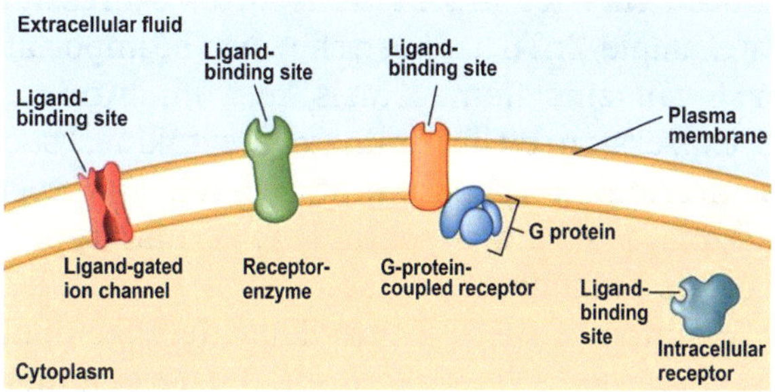

Figure 10.6. Receptor types and signaling pathways.

Source: Slideserve. (n.d.). *Types of Receptors.* https://image.slideserve.com/405011/types-of-receptors-l.jpg.

Test Your Knowledge

1. What is the mechanism of steroid hormones in gene regulation?
2. How do steroid hormones influence gene transcription?

10.2. Major Endocrine Disorders

Learning Outcome

1. Diabetes Mellitus
2. Thyroid Disorders
3. Adrenal Insufficiency

Endocrine disorders tend to result from disturbances in hormone production, secretion, or receptor action and hence give rise to systemic imbalance and a range of clinical presentations (Figure 10.7). Among the most common disorders, diabetes mellitus has a particularly widespread effect on metabolic control. This disorder is most often caused by defects in insulin production or function, and recent work has highlighted the mediation of β-cell dysfunction by cytokine-induced changes in zinc transporter expression. For example, ZnT8 has been shown to be important for β-cell zinc homeostasis, and inhibition of its expression by inflammatory cytokines such as interleukin-1β potentiates β-cell apoptosis and plays a role in both type 1 and type 2 diabetes pathogenesis (Rabinovitch et al., 2009). Recognition of these intracellular derangements has far-reaching implications in the development of therapies directed toward β-cell preservation and function, demonstrating the complex interplay of immune signaling and endocrine regulation. In addition to metabolic disorders, environmental exposures also play an important role in endocrine disruption. Chemicals like nonylphenol and octyl phenol, classified as xenoestrogens, have agonist or antagonist effects toward endogenous estrogens and disrupt estrogen receptor signaling pathways. Exposure to such agents ruins cellular redox status and mitochondrial function of liver cells, as evidenced by elevated formation of reactive oxygen species and nitric oxides accompanied by damaged mitochondrial proton gradients (Arese et al., 2018). These biochemical disturbances indicate that chronic exposure to such ECMOs would lead to a variety of disorders, including reproductive malfunction and hormone-sensitive cancers. Pharmacological management in such situations calls for careful handling, overcoming not only the receptor-level interference but also the downstream consequences of oxidative stress to reclaim endocrine homeostasis. The multifaceted nature of primary endocrine disorders carries over even to thyroid disorders, which present with hypo- or hypersecretion of thyroid hormones and have far-reaching effects on metabolism, cardiovascular health, and neurological function. Pharmacologic therapy has long centered on hormone replacement or inhibition of synthesis but increasingly reflects emerging understanding of molecular mechanisms for greater therapeutic specificity. For instance, changes in mitochondrial bioenergetics and markers of oxidative stress involved in endocrine cell damage point to adjunct measures reducing cellular injury beyond the modulation of hormones per se. This synergistic view points to the importance of interdisciplinarity in endocrine pharmacology, the integration of hormone-targeting therapies with antioxidants or mitochondrial stabilizers, and thus conceivably enhancing outcomes in those diseases where endocrine gland integrity is lost through environmental or autoimmune injury.

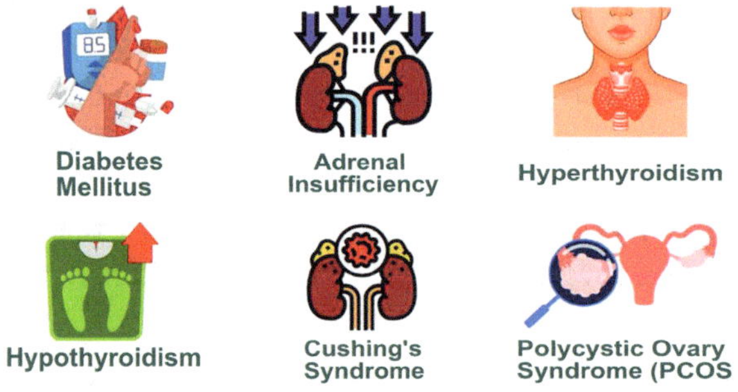

Figure 10.7. Major endocrine disorders.

Source: **Shopify.** (n.d.). *Major Endocrine Disorders.* https://cdn.shopify.com/s/files/1/0789/3781/7379/files/25.png?v=1720715274.

10.2.1. Diabetes Mellitus

The heterogeneity of endocrine disorders requires a sophisticated appreciation of both biological and sociocultural determinants that affect disease expression and response to therapy. For diabetes mellitus, sex hormones and gender differences significantly influence metabolic regulation as well as response to drug therapy. The interaction between estrogens, progesterone, and testosterone influences insulin sensitivity and glucose metabolism, which can result in differences in disease prevalence and progression between men and women. In addition, gender-specific behaviors and societal expectations can impact lifestyle factors such as diet and exercise, thus affecting diabetes control and therapeutic response. It is important to appreciate these distinctions in order to develop personalized medicine that seeks to maximize diagnostic precision and therapeutic strategies that are specific to a person's endocrine context and social setting (Appetecchia et al., 2018). This shift of paradigm calls for incorporating considerations of sex and gender into endocrine pharmacology research and clinical care. Pathophysiology of diabetes mellitus is mainly caused by a lack of insulin production or a failure in insulin action, leading to hyperglycemia. Chronic elevation of blood glucose is the basis for development of most diabetic complications that have a devastating impact on organ systems and quality of life in patients. Pharmacologic management of diabetes aims at restoration of glucose homeostasis either by insulin replacement or increasing insulin sensitivity. Aside from traditional drug medicines, ongoing studies investigate natural biomolecules with antidiabetic activity, including ones from plants such as *Smallanthus sonchifolius* (yacon). Yacon leaf has shown promise to regulate glucose metabolism and enhance insulin function, indicating they may be useful complementary drugs in diabetes prevention and treatment. Researching such plant compounds opens up the therapeutic tool kit in endocrine pharmacology to possibly provide more cost-effective and integral treatment possibilities (Genta et al., 2015). Successful management of diabetes calls for holistic approaches that involve both pharmacological ingenuity and patient-specific care. The chronic nature of diabetes mellitus (Figure 10.8) necessitates long-term compliance with drugs that correct either the insulin deficiency or resistance typical of the condition.

Endocrine pharmacology increasingly recognizes the need to tailor treatment according to patient-specific factors such as genetic susceptibility, hormonal status, and gender-related factors. Current progress underscores the combination of conventional drug treatments with adjuncts of natural origin, which potentially increases efficacy while minimizing side effects. Furthermore, knowledge of how these disparate therapies act provides clinicians with the opportunity to tailor regimens not only to control blood glucose but also to minimize the risk of complications. The continuous evolution in this area points to a shift toward increasingly personalized, effective, and inclusive management of diabetes (Appetecchia et al., 2018; Genta et al., 2015).

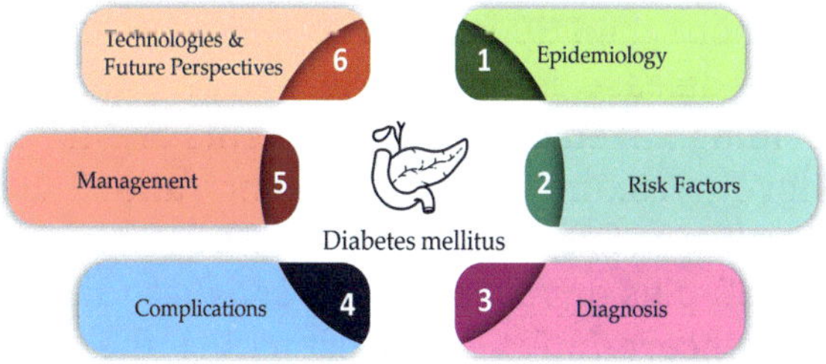

Figure 10.8. Diabetes mellitus.

Source: MDPI. (2021). *[Image showing diabetic mechanisms or pathways]. Diabetology, 2*(1). https://pub.mdpi-res.com/diabetology/diabetology-02-00004/article_deploy/html/images/diabetology-02-00004-ag.png?1618555525.

10.2.2. Thyroid Disorders

The intricacy in the treatment of endocrine diseases requires knowledge of biological sex and gender differences, which carry significant significance for thyroid pathophysiology and pharmacological treatment. Estrogen and androgen, the sex hormones, influence different physiological systems and the incidence as well as clinical presentation of thyroid diseases. For example, autoimmune thyroid diseases present an increased incidence in women as a result of estrogen's immunomodulatory effects (Figure 10.9). Identifying these sex-specific hormonal effects is important for individualizing thyroid disorder therapies and enhancing therapeutic effectiveness. Also, the difference between sex as a biological variable and gender as a sociocultural construct underscores the requirement for personalized medicine approaches in endocrine pharmacology, since gender roles and behaviors could affect disease management and patient compliance with therapy. This gender-sensitive strategy would maximize early diagnosis, risk stratification, and personalized treatment strategies in thyroid diseases (Appetecchia et al., 2018). Subclinical hypothyroidism, defined by an elevated thyroid-stimulating hormone (TSH) but normal free thyroxine levels, presents special challenges in elderly patients, especially those aged more than 80 years. The clinical relevance of this disease is still unclear, with literature providing mixed evidence of benefits and harms of levothyroxine therapy. Recent randomized controlled trials, such as the TRUST trial and IEMO 80-plus thyroid trial, have sought to address these uncertainties by investigating the effect of levothyroxine on cognitive function, quality of life, and physical symptoms in this patient group. The studies use intense methodology, placebo-controls, and dose titration to identify the therapeutic benefit as well as keep track of negative cardiovascular events like atrial fibrillation or heart failure. The collective evidence from these landmark studies holds the potential to further define clinical guidelines and guide targeted pharmacologic management of subclinical hypothyroidism in extremely old patients (Blum et al., 2018). Pharmacologic therapy in thyroid disease must also consider the wide range of disease presentations, from hypothyroidism to hyperthyroidism, each with unique therapeutic agents. Levothyroxine remains the cornerstone for hypothyroidism treatment, restoring hormone levels and alleviating systemic symptoms; however, its dosing requires careful titration to avoid overtreatment and adverse effects. Conversely, hyperthyroid states often necessitate antithyroid drugs, radioactive iodine, or surgery, depending on etiology and severity. New understanding of thyroid hormone receptor isoforms and intracellular signaling has driven the creation of new therapeutics that target specific pathways, potentially providing more targeted control of thyroid hormone action. The incorporation of pharmacogenomics and personalized medicine into endocrine pharmacology has the potential to further optimize thyroid disorder treatments, improving both safety and efficacy in diverse patient populations.

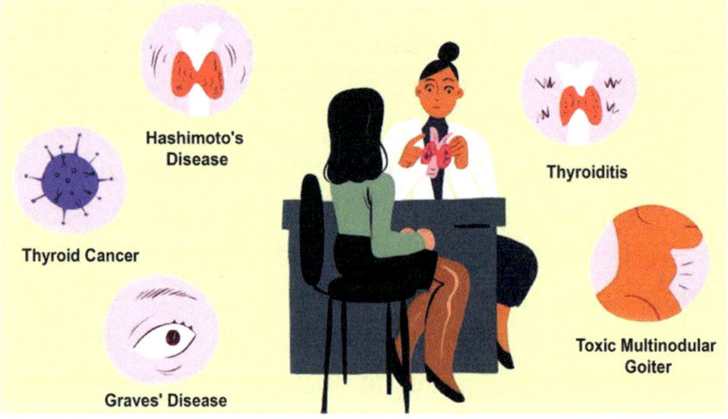

Figure 10.9. Thyroid disorders.

Source: Verywell Health. (n.d.). *Thyroid disease overview*. https://www.verywellhealth.com/thmb/EH9fRFiO_NLY0WUZ0v2zeMTdRHY=/6000x4000/filters:no_upscale():max_bytes(150000):strip_icc()/thyroid-disease-overview-4014636_final-87af4e82207a4559879610af06ea90b51-0c27c93ae9264d6fb9703fd12c918056.png.

10.2.3. Adrenal Insufficiency

The intricate interaction between the endocrine glands and their hormonal secretions achieves homeostasis and responds to physiological stress, and the adrenal cortex is a vital part of this system. Adrenal insufficiency, a state of insufficient production of glucocorticoids, mineralocorticoids, or both, results from disruption in adrenal hormone synthesis or secretion. It may result from primary damage to the adrenal glands or secondary to dysfunction of the pituitary or hypothalamus. From a drug perspective, knowing the mechanisms of hormone deficiency guides diagnosis and treatment. Glucocorticoid replacement is still the mainstay of treatment, which requires judicious dose titration to simulate physiological circadian patterns and avoid complications like iatrogenic Cushing's syndrome. In the clinic, early identification of adrenal insufficiency (Figure 10.10) and prompt pharmacologic management are key in avoiding crisis situations, emphasizing the need for endocrinological vigilance. Although adrenal insufficiency can manifest with subtle clinical characteristics early on, it carries a severe threat of adrenal crisis if untreated or triggered by stressors. Adrenal crisis is a medical emergency with hypotension, electrolyte disturbances, and shock, usually accompanied by nonspecific signs that make immediate diagnosis difficult. Successful management involves the rapid intravenous administration of glucocorticoids with fluid resuscitation. In spite of medical training placing strong emphasis on "sick day rules," resistance to dose escalation or switch to parenteral therapy can lead to morbidity and mortality in these individuals. Pharmacological protocols for the treatment of adrenal insufficiency thus need to incorporate stress dosing instructions and patient education to minimize the occurrence of adrenal crisis. The delicate balance between proper glucocorticoid supplementation and prevention of overtreatment requires both clinical judgment and pharmacologic accuracy (Bhardwaj et al., 2020). In managing adrenal insufficiency, coexistence with other endocrine dysfunctions must be taken into account because polyendocrine involvement alters treatment requirements.

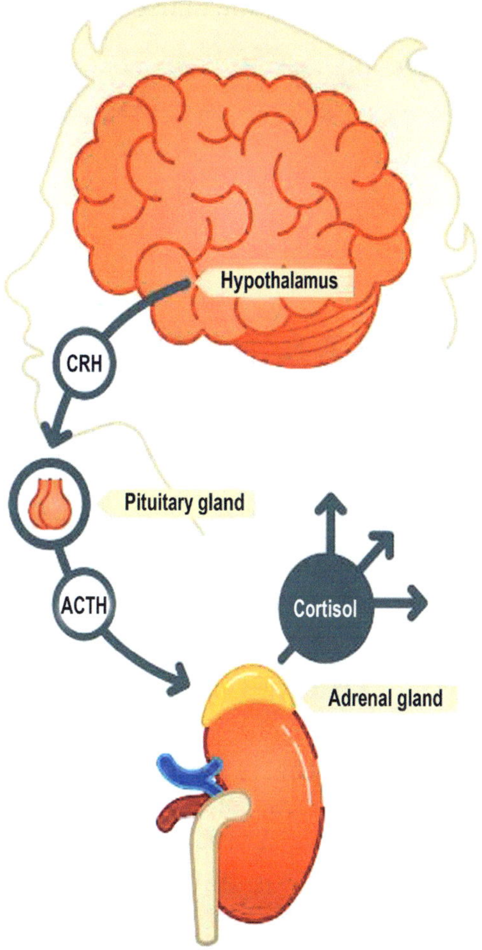

Figure 10.10. Adrenal insufficiency.

Source: National Institute of Diabetes and Digestive and Kidney Diseases. (n.d.). *Cortisol creation*. U.S. Department of Health and Human Services. https://www.niddk.nih.gov/-/media/Images/Health-Information/Endocrine-Diseases/cortisol-creation.jpg?imbypass=true.

For example, plasma protein loss in nephrotic syndrome indirectly impinges on hormone dynamics by enhancing binding globulin and hormone urinary excretion, thus making adrenal hormone bioavailability more complicated. As much as this occurrence is better understood in thyroid disease to precipitate hypothyroidism, the same tenets may extend to adrenal hormone pharmacokinetics and responsivity. Identifying such subtleties helps to maximize replacement therapy, particularly in patients with impaired endocrine reserves or comorbid nephropathies. Therefore, pharmacologic treatment must be tailored, considering associated endocrine disturbances and protein loss syndromes, to enhance outcomes and avoid overtreatment or undertreatment (Barbano et al., 2017).

Test Your Knowledge

1. What is the main cause of endocrine disorders related to hormone production?
2. Why is it important to consider biological sex in the treatment of endocrine diseases?

10.3. Pharmacological Treatments for Diabetes

Learning Outcome

1. Insulin Therapy
2. Oral Hypoglycemic Agents
36. Newer Diabetes Medications (GLP-1 Agonists, SGLT2 Inhibitors)

The treatment of diabetes mellitus has changed over time, with a focus on the restoration of normal glucose homeostasis through multiple pharmacologic interventions. Most traditional treatments often include exogenous insulin therapy in replacement of the endogenous deficiency of insulin in type 1 diabetes. Still, the challenges of insulin treatment, including risks of hypoglycemia and patient noncompliance, have driven exploration into other therapy options. Of these, natural products from medicinal plants have been of interest because of their potential for multifaceted mechanisms and low side effect profiles. For example, the bioactive constituents in *Smallanthus sonchifolius* leaves have shown promising antidiabetic activity, indicating a prophylactic as well as therapeutic role. These chemicals can act by influencing insulin sensitivity and glucose metabolism, marking the potential of plant pharmacology in the treatment of diabetes-associated metabolic derangements (Genta et al., 2015). This method widens the scope beyond traditional therapy by incorporating complementary approaches that could enhance patient outcomes. Aside from plant-originating medications, combination therapy has proven significant in increasing the efficacy of therapy in diabetes models. Experimental research using combined extracts of *Vernonia amygdalina* and *Gongronema latifolium* showed substantial enhancements in glycemic regulation and pancreatic tissue histomorphology in streptozotocin-induced diabetic rats. The combined extracts not only lowered serum glucose levels equivalently to insulin therapy but also supported the regeneration of pancreatic β-cells, as indicated by histologic exams. This β-cell regeneration implies an innate repair process, which is not tackled by orthodox insulin treatment but rather works essentially through extra-pancreatic mechanisms without eliciting islet cell regeneration. Through the augmentation of endogenous insulin secretion and beta-cell recuperation, these phytotherapeutic treatments would enhance current pharmacologic regimens and possibly reframe disease outcome in diabetes (Akpantah et al., 2011). These results highlight the need to investigate plant compounds with regenerative properties as adjunct therapy or substitutes for man-made drugs. The pharmacological management of diabetes remains to grow with the addition of both man-made and natural agents, as an increasing picture of the endocrinological complexity of the disease emerges. Management is frequently most effective through action on several pathophysiologic factors, such as insulin deficiency, insulin resistance, and pancreatic β-cell integrity. While traditional insulin and oral hypoglycemic drugs continue to be cornerstones, the advent of bioactive plant substances provides new mechanistic pathways. These treatments, particularly when used in combination with current agents, have the potential to enhance glycemic control and improve islet cell preservation or regeneration. Notably, proof that some plant extracts have regenerative activity heralds a paradigm shift towards not only symptomatic therapies but also those that target underlying cellular injury. These developments underscore the interactive dynamics of endocrine pharmacology and integrative therapeutic approaches, opening doors to novel therapy in diabetes treatment (Akpantah et al., 2011; Genta et al., 2015).

10.3.1. Insulin Therapy

Optimal treatment of chronic endocrine disorders usually depends on the delicate balance between therapeutic action and physiological control. With diabetes mellitus, wherein endogenous insulin release is defective or deficient, exogenous insulin treatment becomes a critical necessity for metabolic regulation (Figure 10.11). The pharmacologic use consists of multiple insulin preparations, customized by onset, peak, and duration, to simulate natural insulin secretion rates. Rapid-acting insulins are generally employed to manage postprandial glucose peaks, whereas longer-acting analogs deliver basal insulin levels. This regimen necessitates precise dose adjustment according to patient-specific parameters like food intake, exercise, and concurrent diseases. In addition, improvements in insulin delivery systems, such as pens, pumps, and continuous glucose monitoring integration, have improved therapeutic efficacy and patient compliance. The complexity of insulin treatment reflects the overall endocrine pharmacologic challenges, placing a high priority on individualized treatment strategies that reduce the risk of hyperglycemia without increasing the risk of hypoglycemia. The physiologic substrates for insulin treatment extend from glucose homeostasis to influencing multiple metabolic pathways essential to systemic health. The anabolic effects of insulin favor glycogen deposition, lipogenesis, and protein synthesis, underlining its key role in the storage and use of energy. Defects or insulin resistance interfere with these processes, leading to complications like diabetic ketoacidosis and long-term vascular damage. In clinical situations with PCOS, insulin sensitizers enhance the effectiveness of insulin therapy by enhancing peripheral glucose uptake and lowering hyperinsulinemia, which is commonly involved in PCOS pathogenesis. While insulin treatment of PCOS directly is not frequent, the interaction between insulin control and endocrine disorders dictates the imperative of multidisciplinary pharmacological interventions. These findings reinforce the imperative for further research into the mechanisms of insulin and therapeutic developments in endocrine pharmacology (Prudence et al., 2024). Insulin-related complications compounded by improper insulin therapy also reinforce the imperative of holistic treatment programs to manage systemic comorbidities. For example, the development of diabetic nephropathy is an immune-mediated cellular damage that is exacerbated by metabolic dysregulation, and thus requires a two-pronged approach to glycemic control and renal protection. Drugs like renin-angiotensin-aldosterone system (RAAS) inhibitors and sodium-glucose co-transporter-2 inhibitors are synergistic with insulin therapy by lowering glomerular hypertension and enhancing renal outcomes, illustrating synergy between endocrine and nephrological pharmacology. Management of non-pharmacological elements such as diet, weight control, and lifestyle changes is equally important in maximizing insulin effectiveness and avoiding complications. Therefore, insulin therapy is a cornerstone of endocrine care strategies that needs to be combined with multidisciplinary interventions to facilitate integral patient care (Anders et al., 2023).

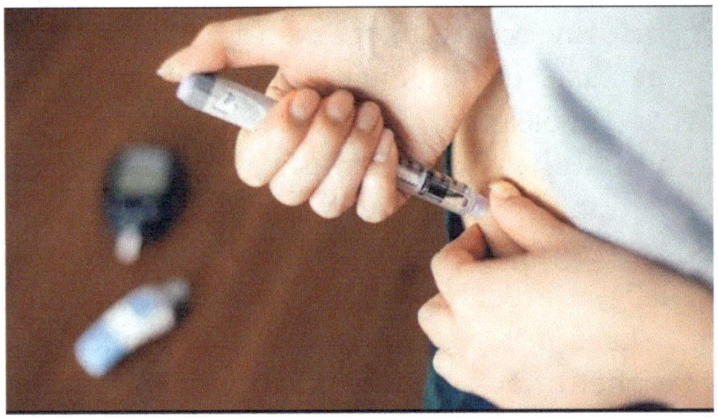

Figure 10.11. Insulin therapy.

Source: Everyday Health. (n.d.). *Habits That Sabotage Insulin Therapy.* https://images.everydayhealth.com/images/diabetes/cs-habits-that-sabotage-insulin-therapy-01-722x406.jpg.

10.3.2. Oral Hypoglycemic Agents

The treatment of diabetes mellitus (DM) has undergone changes with the advent of several pharmacologic agents acting on multiple pathophysiological mechanisms. Oral hypoglycemic agents are one of the cornerstones in the management of type 2 diabetes by enhancing glycemic control without the use of insulin injections. These agents can be classified broadly into several classes, such as sulfonylureas, biguanides, thiazolidinediones, DPP-4 inhibitors, SGLT2 inhibitors, and meglitinides, each having a distinct mechanism of action. For example, biguanides decrease hepatic glucose production and enhance insulin sensitivity, whereas sulfonylureas induce pancreatic insulin secretion. Agent selection must be a careful consideration of patient-specific characteristics, comorbidities, and possible side effects. Oral hypoglycemic agents in perioperative periods require specific vigilance owing to changed metabolic requirements and risks of hypoglycemia, highlighting the need for individualized medication management in surgical patients to ensure optimal glycemic control (Rajan et al., 2024). Pharmacodynamics and pharmacokinetics play an important role in the clinical use of oral hypoglycemic drugs. Onset, action duration, and metabolic pathways determine both efficacy and safety profiles. For instance, metformin, a commonly used biguanide, has a long half-life and inhibits mainly hepatic gluconeogenesis, hence is effective and in most patients relatively safe. But in renal-impaired or hepatic-impaired patients, its risk for lactic acidosis requires careful dosing or withdrawal. But sulfonylureas, though effective in stimulating insulin secretion, pose more risk of hypoglycemia, especially in elderly subjects or those with unpredictable oral intake. Newer classes like SGLT2 inhibitors not only reduce blood glucose through glucose excretion by the kidney but also have favorable cardiovascular effects. Merging these pharmacologic subtleties allows clinicians to fine-tune treatment regimens designed to a specific patient profile. Proper monitoring when initiating or altering treatment is key to achieve balanced glycemic control and reduce unwanted effects (Rajan et al., 2024). As much as the clinical value of oral hypoglycemic agents is considerable, some limitations remain to their use within endocrine pharmacology. Adherence to medication, affecting treatment outcomes, can be disrupted by complicated regimens and side effects like gastrointestinal (GI) intolerance or weight gain. In addition, drug interactions and comorbidities complicate pharmacologic therapy in diabetes. Growing evidence highlights the necessity for detailed guidelines on perioperative management of these drugs, considering changed drug metabolism and possible influence on surgical outcome. Recommendations emphasize individualized methods, such as temporary withholding of some agents to minimize the risk of hypoglycemia and lactic acidosis with surgical stress (Rajan et al., 2024).

Although the Endocrine Society publishes extensive recommendations for hormone therapies, the same level of rigor for standardizing oral hypoglycemic agent protocols is still a developing component of endocrinology practice. Further research must be conducted to further develop therapeutic strategies and enhance patient-centered outcomes in the pharmacologic treatment of diabetes.

10.3.3. Newer Diabetes Medications (GLP-1 Agonists, SGLT2 Inhibitors)

The advent of glucagon-like peptide-1 (GLP-1) receptor agonists and sodium–glucose cotransporter 2 (SGLT2) inhibitors represents a major paradigm shift in diabetes pharmacotherapy, illustrative of a greater appreciation of glucose homeostasis and systemic disease modulation. Unlike earlier agents that primarily affected insulin secretion or sensitivity, these novel classes utilize separate physiological mechanisms. GLP-1 agonists increase glucose-dependent insulin secretion and inhibit glucagon secretion, whereas SGLT2 inhibitors decrease renal glucose reabsorption with glucosuria promotion.

This two-mechanism intervention not only enhances glycemic control but also is associated with overall metabolic advantage, such as weight loss and cardiovascular protection. Together, the drugs provide individualized choices that capture the heterogeneity of diabetes, improving personalized medicine models and transforming clinical profiles beyond glycemic markers. Apart from glycemic control, therapeutic use by SGLT2 inhibitors and GLP-1 receptor agonists, in addition to organ protection of the kidney and nervous system, has great promise. Recent observational research and meta-analyses have shown that SGLT2 inhibitors have renoprotective properties separate from their glucose-lowering abilities. One comparative review revealed that SGLT2 inhibitor-treated patients had slower deterioration in estimated glomerular filtration rate (eGFR), with decreased chronic kidney disease (CKD) progression than GLP-1 receptor agonist users. Interestingly, these renal effects are seen even with smaller HbA1c improvements, indicating pleiotropic action, possibly mediated by hemodynamic regulation and anti-inflammatory effects. These observations reinforce the position of SGLT2 inhibitors as ideal drugs in patients with diabetes complicated by renal comorbidities, reaffirming their place in endocrine pharmacology in its fullest sense (Fadini et al., 2024).

Notably, the neuroprotective potential of these newer class III diabetes drugs is now being unraveled, with its implications extending beyond metabolic parameters. Recent network meta-analyses have investigated the prophylactic efficacy of GLP-1 receptor agonists and SGLT2 inhibitors in neurodegenerative diseases. While varying results, a single SGLT2 inhibitor, dapagliflozin, showed significant reduction in Parkinson's disease incidence, pointing towards a novel protection potentially due to its selective SGLT2 inhibition. This selectivity introduces interesting questions regarding drug-target interactions and neurobiology, making dapagliflozin a promising drug for preventive neurology interventions among at-risk populations. Though more investigation is needed, these new findings shed light on the widening therapeutic horizons of endocrine pharmacology where prevention of metabolic and neurodegenerative diseases converge (Tseng et al., 2025) (Figure 10.12).

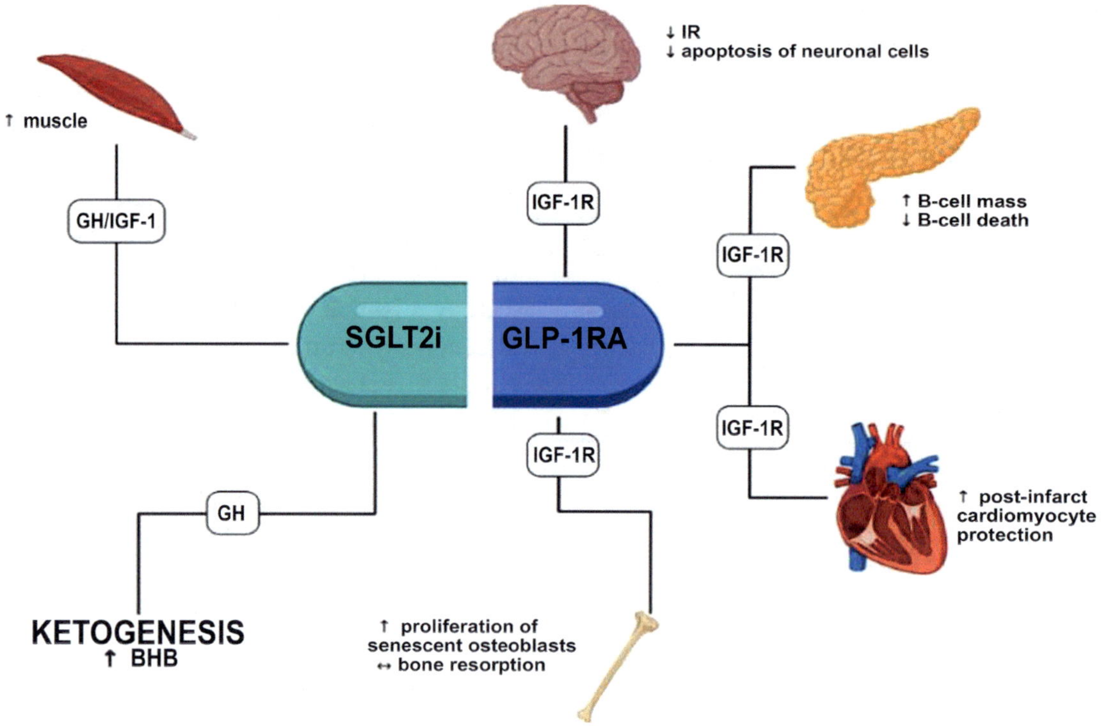

Figure 10.12. Newer diabetes medications (GLP-1 agonists, SGLT2 inhibitors).

Source: Frontiers in Endocrinology. *GLP-1 Agonists and SGLT2 Inhibitors in Diabetes Management.* Frontiers. https://www.frontiersin.org/files/Articles/846903/fendo-13-846903-HTML/image_m/fendo-13-846903-g001.jpg.

Test Your Knowledge

1. What is the primary goal in the treatment of diabetes mellitus?
2. What is the primary purpose of oral hypoglycemic agents in diabetes treatment?

10.4. Thyroid Hormone Replacement Therapy

Learning Outcome

1. Levothyroxine for Hypothyroidism
2. Antithyroid Medications for Hyperthyroidism
3. Monitoring and Adjusting Therapy

The best management of hypothyroidism is the restoration of normal levels of thyroid hormones, mainly achieved by hormone replacement therapy. Synthetic thyroxine (T4), the most commonly used medication, is still the mainstay of treatment because of its effectiveness and uniform pharmacokinetic pattern. Administration is usually oral dosing, precisely adjusted to replicate physiological hormone levels and relieve symptoms of thyroid hormone deficiency. The patient's age, weight, cardiovascular status, and comorbidities determine dosing regimens, which need to be individualized by the clinician. Importantly, there is difficulty in the more severe state of hypothyroidism, such as myxedema coma, where there is impairment of absorption from tablets. In these urgent situations, even other formulations like liquid levothyroxine have proven to be beneficial by optimizing bioavailability and facilitating more immediate action of therapy, thereby enhancing clinical efficacy in the acute environment (Bado et al., 2024). This reflects the advancing pharmacological strategies targeting optimal thyroid hormone replacement. Pregnancy places multifaceted physiological challenges on the thyroid axis, making careful monitoring and titration of thyroid hormone replacement in patients with hypothyroidism necessary. Disrupted maternal thyroid function can lead to serious unfavorable outcomes such as preeclampsia and impaired fetal growth, highlighting the need for proper levothyroxine dosing in pregnancy. Empirical evidence indicates a high incidence of hypothyroidism in pregnant women, with most needing incremental doses to achieve euthyroid status and prevent obstetric and perinatal complications (Johnson et al., 2020). Regular screening for thyroid disease in pregnancy followed by prompt initiation or dose titration of levothyroxine has been shown to prevent risks to mother and fetus effectively. These clinical observations highlight the pivotal interface between endocrine pharmacology and obstetrics to ensure maternal-fetal health. The use of thyroid hormone replacement therapy is more than mere routine management of hypothyroidism and involves issues of formulation, absorption, and patient-specific variables. Liquid formulations of levothyroxine have become useful alternatives in situations involving compromised GI absorption, as in critically ill patients or those with malabsorption syndromes. Through avoidance of some inherent limitations of tablet preparations, liquid forms allow for more uniform and more immediate delivery of active hormone, an important benefit in life-threatening circumstances such as myxedema coma (Bado et al., 2024). In addition, extensive screening programs such as neonatal TSH screening emphasize the critical necessity of early detection and intervention in thyroid disease throughout life (Johnson et al., 2020). Inasmuch as the pharmacology of thyroid hormone replacement continues to evolve, these subtle strategies for thyroid hormone replacement highlight the need for personalized therapy approaches that maximize therapeutic effectiveness while excluding adverse effects (Figure 10.13).

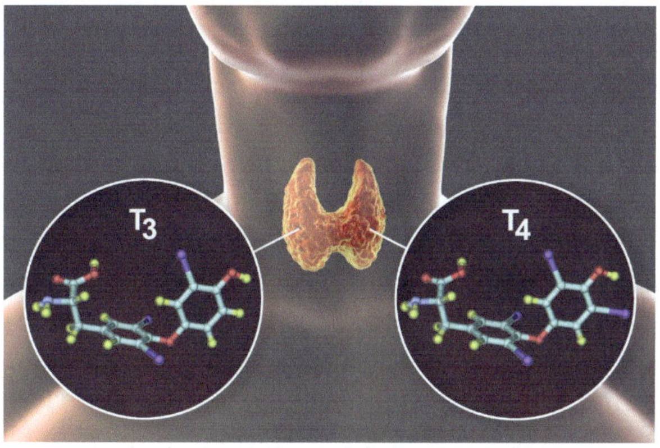

Figure 10.13. Thyroid hormone replacement therapy.

Source: Natural Bio Health. (2020). *Austin Thyroid Hormone Therapy T3 T4.* https://naturalbiohealth.com/wp-content/uploads/2020/10/Austin-Thyroid-Hormone-Therapy-T3-T4-scaled.jpeg.

10.4.1. Levothyroxine for Hypothyroidism

Successful treatment of endocrine disorders depends upon the accurate replacement of the lacking hormone, and this is especially important in hypothyroidism—a state of decreased production of thyroid hormone. Levothyroxine, a synthetic version of thyroxine (T4), is the foundation of therapy because it has the capacity to normalize levels of thyroid hormones and normalize metabolism (Figure 10.14). Its pharmacokinetics permits daily administration, with peripheral conversion at a slower rate to the more active triiodothyronine (T3) to maintain a stable and physiologic level of hormone replacement. Titration of levothyroxine dosage must be done carefully, primarily based on serum TSH levels, to maintain successful symptom control with a minimum of side effects. Individualized therapy necessitates continued clinical assessment because variables such as varied absorption and patient compliance affect treatment efficacy. Therefore, levothyroxine continues to be irreplaceable in attaining euthyroidism and alleviating the systemic effects of hypothyroidism in endocrine pharmacology. Patterns of clinical practice show significant heterogeneity in the diagnosis and management of hypothyroidism, especially regarding monitoring and utilization of levothyroxine. Although measurement of serum TSH is almost universal, other pertinent thyroid parameters like free T4 and thyroid antibody titers show variable use, perhaps indicative of differing clinical priorities or resource constraints. Additionally, treatment regimens go beyond levothyroxine monotherapy, with combination therapies or desiccated thyroid extracts used by some clinicians, even though levothyroxine has an established safety and efficacy profile. This heterogeneity highlights the importance of standardized guidelines to maximize patient outcomes and facilitate care delivery, particularly in academic endocrine centers where training informs future practice. This variability can be addressed to foster more uniform and evidence-based use of levothyroxine, enhancing symptom control and minimizing excessive testing in hypothyroid patients (Shim et al., 2019). In addition to pharmacologic factors, hypothyroidism treatment with levothyroxine also needs to consider immune-related events, especially in patients undergoing immunotherapies, where autoimmune endocrinopathies are likely to occur. Expert opinion urges caution with close monitoring and hormone replacement with a view to preventing premature cessation of life-saving oncologic treatment. In levothyroxine-dependent hypothyroidism occurring as an immune-related adverse event, therapy is usually continued in addition to corticosteroid treatment and other immunosuppressive therapies when indicated. Significantly, endocrine toxicities are unique in that the use of hormone replacement facilitates the ability to maintain immune checkpoint inhibitor therapy, representing a subtle compromise between modulating adverse effects and maintaining anticancer activity. Thus, the role of levothyroxine transcends the relief of symptoms to facilitating multidisciplinary management in complex clinical cases, underscoring its central position in endocrine pharmacology (Bryan et al., 2021).

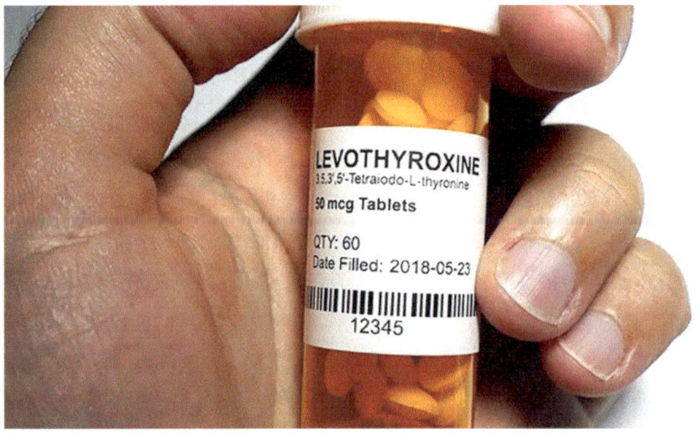

Figure 10.14. Levothyroxine for hypothyroidism.

Source: MedPage Today. (n.d.). *Levothyroxine for Hypothyroidism*. https://assets.medpagetoday.net/media/images/93xxx/93206.jpg.

10.4.2. Antithyroid Medications for Hyperthyroidism

The management of hyperthyroidism is most commonly with antithyroid drugs, which are aimed at blocking the production of thyroid hormones (Figure 10.15). Of these drugs, carbimazole and its active metabolite methimazole (MMI) have become the most widely used drugs because they are effective and have a good safety profile. Clinical practice has consistently favored carbimazole for its ability to adequately control the hypermetabolic state induced by excessive thyroid hormone production. Despite the availability of various drugs for hyperthyroidism, carbimazole remains the cornerstone of pharmacological treatment, especially in ambulatory patients, as observed in recent drug utilization studies conducted at specialty endocrinology centers. These trends reflect ongoing clinical dependence on carbimazole in the therapeutic armamentarium and indicate the changing trends in endocrine pharmacology to optimize patient care (Ramachandran et al., 2020). Although methimazole has become the preferred drug in hyperthyroidism management, especially following the fall of propylthiouracil (PTU), the safety aspects of these drugs continue to be a matter of concern in prescribing. PTU, which was highly used, has been linked to serious hepatotoxicity and has resulted in substantial morbidity and mortality, particularly among children. The risk of liver failure associated with PTU is considerably greater than that of methimazole and has led to recommendations against its use outside of the first trimester of pregnancy in children. Neither the incidence nor the timing of liver injury due to PTU is dose-dependent or predictable by time, making clinical monitoring difficult. Methimazole, on the other hand, is more likely to induce less severe hepatic side effects, primarily cholestasis, in the elderly, which has helped to make it more popular with clinicians (Malozowski et al., 2010). These differences emphasize the need for individualized treatment in endocrine pharmacology, weighing efficacy against possible toxicities. In spite of the thoroughly documented hepatotoxic potential of PTU, it continues to be used in a significant percentage of patients, continuing to raise alarm among medical practitioners. Data suggest that a notable proportion of patients continue to be treated with PTU as a first-line agent, either because of historical prescribing practices or certain clinical factors like pregnancy. The delay in regulatory responses to PTU's black box warnings reflects pharmacovigilance challenges, in part resulting from underreporting of adverse drug reactions (ADRs) and the relative rarity of severe events compared to total exposure. In addition, technological advances in data mining and increasing interactions among clinicians, academic organizations, and regulatory bodies have underscored the paramount importance of ongoing surveillance and education on antithyroid drug choice. These advances reaffirm the need for safer pharmacotherapeutic options, further supporting methimazole as the agent of choice outside of narrow exceptions (Malozowski et al., 2010).

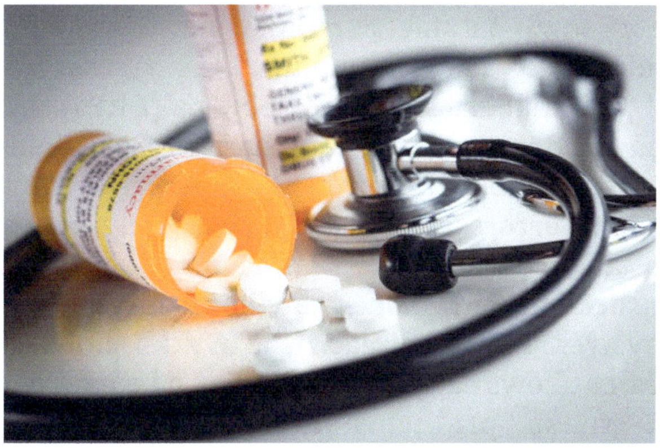

Figure 10.15. Antithyroid medications for hyperthyroidism.

Source: CTFA. (n.d.). *Antithyroid Medications for Hyperthyroidism.* https://images.ctfassets.net/yixw23k2v6vo/ew_wysiwyg_fid4968_asset/0400c9d666ed1d59ffcf19b92931cafb/69066886_M.jpg.

10.4.3. Monitoring and Adjusting Therapy

Successful management of endocrine diseases relies on careful monitoring of pharmacologic treatment to achieve therapeutic effectiveness while avoiding harmful effects (Figure 10.16). Because many treatments for endocrine disease consist of narrow therapeutic indexes, e.g., lithium therapy for bipolar disorder (BD), frequent measurement of drug levels is critical. Evidence shows that a single exposure to high lithium levels over 1.0 mmol/L can cause an abrupt deterioration of renal function as reflected by falls in estimated glomerular filtration rate within three months. This highlights the importance of having tight monitoring protocols, ideally at intervals not exceeding three months, to early detect and treat potential toxicity before permanent damage sets in. This vigilance contributes towards the maintenance of clinical equilibrium, maximizing renal safety, and individualizing therapy adjustments according to patient response, thus conforming to best practice recommendations in endocrine drug therapy (Anderson et al., 2014). In addition to laboratory parameter monitoring, therapeutic monitoring also encompasses the assessment of potential drug-related problems (DRPs) that may undermine treatment success. In diabetic patients, the incidence of DRPs—ranging from dosing errors and inappropriate drug choice to adverse effects—is significantly higher and associated with moderate clinical importance. Involvement of pharmacists in multidisciplinary teams allows early identification and correction of these problems through medication reconciliation and tailored patient interviews. Most of the clinical interventions suggested by pharmacists have been demonstrated to gain physician acceptance, supporting their contribution to optimizing endocrine therapy. This interdisciplinary practice not only encourages safety but also facilitates dynamic management of medication regimens in relation to patient-specific issues, as an illustrative aspect of endocrine disease monitoring therapy (Wong et al., 2017). Optimal management of endocrine pharmacotherapy is facilitated by a rigorous system of analyzing patient outcomes and adjusting treatment as needed. Monitoring involves clinical metrics, biochemical measurements, and patient compliance, all of which are necessary for educated therapeutic adjustment. Not accommodating therapy to changing physiological or pathological conditions may lead to reduced efficacy or enhanced risk of complications. For example, continuous monitoring of renal function and lithium levels is essential to avoid nephrotoxicity, and regular checking of dosing and drug selection avoids unnecessary harm in diabetes. Prioritizing a patient-focused, evidence-based monitoring approach guarantees that endocrine therapy remains effective and safe in the long run, highlighting the interplay between pharmacologic surveillance and personalized care (Anderson et al., 2014; Wong et al., 2017).

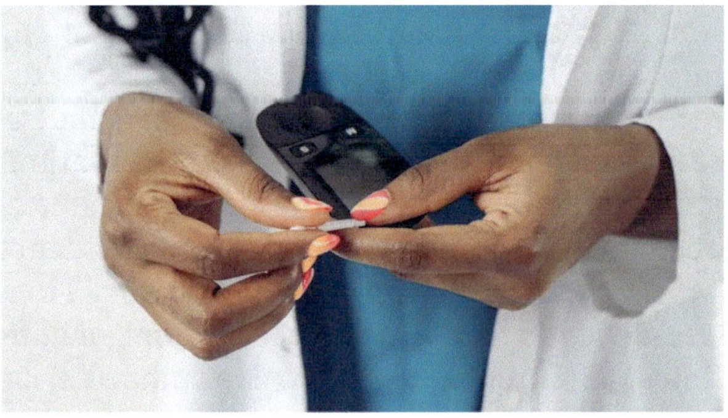

Figure 10.16. Monitoring and adjusting therapy.

Source: Feminine Health (2024). *Monitoring and Adjusting HRT. https*://femininehealth.org/wp-content/uploads/2024/09/monitoring-and-adjusting-hrt-c5fe5e9a-cover-photo.webp.

Test Your Knowledge

1. What is antithyroid medication commonly used to treat hyperthyroidism.
2. Why is monitoring therapy important in clinical practice?

10.5. Corticosteroids and Their Uses

Learning Outcome

1. Mechanism of Action of Corticosteroids
2. Indications for Corticosteroid Therapy
3. Side Effects and Management

The delicate equilibrium of hormonal control in the body frequently requires pharmacological correction to re-establish homeostasis in disease conditions. Among such treatments, corticosteroids are a well-established option on account of their multifaceted physiological action, especially in regulating inflammatory and immune responses. The synthetic glucocorticoid dexamethasone is a common choice in clinical practice on account of its strong anti-inflammatory as well as immunosuppressive actions. But their impact transcends immediate therapeutic effects; exposure at pivotal developmental windows, like the intrauterine environment, can trigger permanent changes in the function of the hypothalamic-pituitary-adrenal (HPA) axis. This modulation is proven through diminished HPA activity after prenatal glucocorticoid exposure that can normalize postpartum but continues to have blunted reactivity to stressors during early infancy. These results highlight the intricacy of corticosteroid pharmacology, in which clinical benefit has to be balanced against possible long-term endocrine consequences (1994 effect of corticosteroids for fetal maturation on perinatal outcomes et al., 2009). The application of corticosteroids in reproductive medicine is a classic example of the overlap between therapeutic need and developmental sensitivity. Administration of dexamethasone to pregnant women demonstrates a significant use, stimulating fetal lung maturation and enhancing neonatal thermoregulation in preterm infants. This therapeutic effect has resulted in extensive use of dexamethasone for maternal-fetal treatments in human and veterinary medicine. However, the safety profile of short-term use is different from issues with long-term or repeated dosing, which can negatively impact fertility and pregnancy. Animal models form a basis for these risks, although species differences complicate direct extrapolation to human physiology. Thus, judicious pharmacokinetic and clinical assessment continues to be crucial when using corticosteroids in reproductive settings in order to maximize therapeutic efficacy with minimal ill effects (Adebayo et al., 2017). Outside reproductive medicine, there is a well-established role for corticosteroids in a variety of medical specialties, with their ability to direct endocrine and immune function. They are invaluable in managing autoimmune disease, allergies, and some cancers because of their modulating actions on cytokine synthesis and immune cell function. Their efficacy clinically relies on their capacity to act like endogenous hormones, but their systemic action requires careful titration to minimize untoward consequences such as suppression of the HPA axis, metabolic derangement, and enhanced infection risk. A clear grasp of corticosteroid pharmacodynamics and pharmacokinetics is essential to the tailoring of treatment regimens, to assure successful therapy while minimizing iatrogenic complications. As further research further refines our understanding, the strategic application of corticosteroids continues to be a foundation of endocrine pharmacology.

10.5.1. Mechanism of Action of Corticosteroids

The physiological action of stress is mediated through a sophisticated interaction between the HPA axis and other neurotransmitter systems. The basis of how corticosteroids act at the molecular level is formed through this interaction. Following secretion, corticosteroids diffuse through cell membranes to bind intracellular glucocorticoid receptors (GRs) within the cytoplasm. This complex of hormone and receptor then translocates to the nucleus where it acts as a transcription factor by binding with glucocorticoid response elements of DNA. Thus, corticosteroids regulate the expression of genes, leading to upregulation or inhibition of target proteins that control inflammation, immune responses, and metabolism. These genomic processes occur within hours to days, pointing towards the role of the hormone in long-term physiological regulation compared to the instantaneous response, contributing partly to their effectiveness in controlling chronic inflammatory disease. Outside the traditional genomic pathways, corticosteroids have been found to impact many neuroendocrine functions by virtue of non-genomic processes acting even more quickly inside the cell (Figure 10.17). These include membrane-bound GR interactions that modify intracellular signal cascades like protein kinase activation and the modulation of calcium flux. An important feature of corticosteroid action includes their regulatory influence upon the serotonergic system that was demonstrated to modulate the functioning of the HPA axis and thereby affect stress-related endocrine feedback loops. Experimental data indicate serotonin receptor subtypes like 5-HT7 to be involved in overactivation of the HPA axis during chronic stress disorders and imply that corticosteroids could indirectly influence mood and behavior via these receptors. Such findings suggest an integrative endocrine system wherein corticosteroid signaling crosses pathways with neurotransmitter systems, thus adjusting both physiological and psychological adjustments to stress (José, 2014).

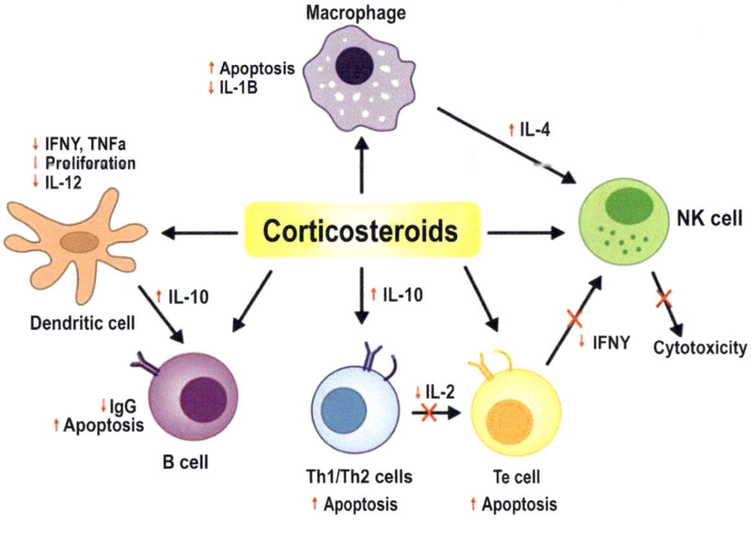

Figure 10.17. Mechanism of action of corticosteroids.

Source: Ordonez, A. A. (2014). *Mechanism of Action of Corticosteroids* [Figure 3]. In *Novel Adjunctive Therapies for the Treatment of Tuberculosis.* ResearchGate.

Although corticosteroids are invaluable in managing many endocrine and inflammatory illnesses, their extremely active mechanism of action also sets patients up for a range of adverse effects, making careful clinical use imperative. The very intense gene regulatory effects of corticosteroids do not only act on the immune response but influence metabolic pathways, bone remodeling, and CNS homeostasis. Therefore, side effects including adrenal suppression, osteoporosis, hyperglycemia, and psychiatric disturbances tend to occur with long-term or high-dose therapy. These complications highlight the fine line between therapeutic effect and toxicity inherent in corticosteroid pharmacology. Successful management aims to minimize systemic exposure yet maximize targeted anti-inflammatory effect, a consideration of the complexity of corticosteroid action and systemic penetration (Liu et al., 2013).

10.5.2. Indications for Corticosteroid Therapy

The clinical usefulness of corticosteroids ranges over a broad spectrum of illnesses, taking advantage of their powerful anti-inflammatory and immunosuppressive properties. These qualities make corticosteroids invaluable in the control of diseases that are characterized by exaggerated or dysregulated immune responses or inflammation. Such diseases include autoimmune disorders like systemic lupus erythematosus, rheumatoid arthritis, and inflammatory bowel disease, which often need to be treated with corticosteroids to dampen immune-mediated tissue injury. Outside of autoimmune causes, corticosteroids play a pivotal role in managing allergic reactions and asthma attacks, where their prompt suppression of inflammatory cascades improves symptoms and forestalls exacerbation. Corticosteroid utility also extends to transplantation medicine, where they suppress graft rejection by inhibiting immune activation. Together, these signs reveal the extensive clinical utility of corticosteroid treatment in endocrine pharmacology, highlighting its function in controlling pathologic immune and inflammatory mechanisms in a wide range of medical situations (Alexander et al., 2022). Aside from autoimmune and inflammatory diseases, corticosteroid treatment is also central to the control of endocrine diseases themselves, most notably adrenal insufficiency. Key adrenal insufficiency, like Addison's disease, requires long-term corticosteroid replacement to make up for impaired endogenous corticosteroid secretion. Supplementation with hormones eliminates potentially life-threatening manifestations of glucocorticoid deficiency, such as hypotension, weakness, and electrolyte disturbances. Corticosteroids are also used in congenital adrenal hyperplasia, where defects of enzymes necessary for cortisol production lead to the necessity of exogenous glucocorticoids to correct homeostasis and inhibit abnormal androgen secretion. Interestingly, corticosteroids play a crucial part in managing cerebral edema as a result of brain tumor or trauma, evidence of their applications beyond traditional endocrine indications. These diverse endocrine-related uses show the basic role corticosteroids play in hormone replacement and symptomatic treatment in the context of critical care and metabolics (Alexander et al., 2022). Recent global health emergencies have further underlined the relevance of corticosteroids in the management of infectious diseases, demonstrating changing indications in the era of emerging pathogens. Most strikingly, with the COVID-19 pandemic, corticosteroids like dexamethasone were found to be life-saving treatments in severe cases featuring hyperinflammatory conditions and respiratory failure. Corticosteroid administration at appropriate times in these patients decreased mortality by dampening cytokine storm phenomena and augmenting pulmonary function. Yet this use also emphasized the necessity of accurate therapeutic standards informed by strong clinical evidence and expert opinion. Quick updates in guidelines by esteemed panels also point to the dynamic character of corticosteroid indications as new information becomes available. This dynamic nature mirrors the ongoing way in which corticosteroid pharmacotherapy evolves within endocrine and infectious disease frameworks, supporting the imperative for continued investigation and evidence-based use.

10.5.3. Side Effects and Management

The complex homeostasis of endocrine function can be readily deranged by pharmacologic therapy intended to alter hormone concentrations or receptor activity. Though endocrine medication provides therapeutic benefit in hyperfunction states such as prolactinomas, hypothyroidism, and diabetes, its use is often accompanied by side effects that need to be closely monitored and managed (Figure 10.18). For example, dopamine agonists employed in the management of prolactinoma cause nausea, orthostatic hypotension, and on occasion, abnormalities in cardiac valves. Knowledge regarding these side effects is imperative for clinicians to achieve optimal therapeutic regimens and ensure patient compliance. Adjustment of dosage, gradual titration, and supportive therapy while administering these medications usually minimizes these problems. Further, routine cardiovascular assessment and patient education continue to be essential measures in the prevention of severe side effects of endocrine medicines, emphasizing the importance of an individualized and multidisciplinary care approach (Yogeeta et al., 2024). Development in endocrine pharmacology continues with new therapeutic drugs, but these advances come with complicated side effect profiles that tax traditional management models. Of special interest is increasing awareness of ocular side effects of anticancer agents with hormonal properties, which may strongly influence patients quality of life. Blepharoconjunctivitis and dry eye disease have been significantly reported with drugs such as methotrexate, anastrozole, and docetaxel. These ocular surface disorders are caused by inflammatory and cytotoxic actions, which highlight the need for early detection and treatment. Preventive strategies could involve the use of lubricating eye drops, anti-inflammatory drugs, and coordination with ophthalmologists to anticipate and treat such side effects efficiently. Management of such multifaceted toxicities maintains therapeutic efficacy without sacrificing patient health (Vitiello et al., 2024). Side effect management in endocrine pharmacology involves a multifaceted approach incorporating pharmacovigilance, patient counseling, and adjunct therapies specific to certain types of adverse effects. Endocrine medications tend to affect more than one physiological system, so side effect profiles are complex and at times unforeseeable. Routine laboratory tests, monitoring of hormonal levels, and symptomatology thus have a crucial role to play in informing dosage adjustments and therapeutic changes. Where side effects threaten treatment adherence or safety, clinicians have to balance the risk-benefit ratio carefully. Utilizing multidisciplinary teams, such as endocrinologists, pharmacists, and other experts, increases the ability to predict, identify, and prevent adverse events, maximizing therapeutic effects. In the end, successful management not only prevents toxicity but also maximizes long-term effectiveness of endocrine pharmacotherapy, confirming its essential role in chronic disease management (Vitiello et al., 2024; Yogeeta et al., 2024).

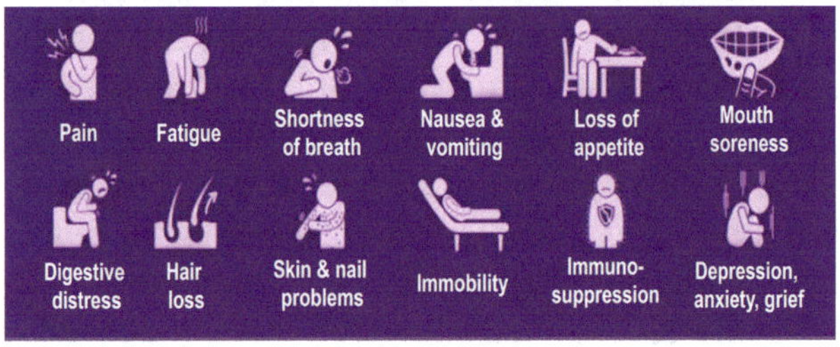

Figure 10.18. Side effects and management.

Source: Poon, D. (2023). *Common Side Effects of Cancer. https*://dyhpoon.com/wp-content/uploads/2023/02/drdonaldpoon_common-side-effects-of-cancer-768x320.jpg.

Test Your Knowledge

1. How can pharmacologic therapy disrupt endocrine homeostasis?
2. What is the primary mechanism of action of corticosteroids at the cellular level?

10.6. Emerging Therapies in Endocrine Pharmacology

Learning Outcome

1. Gene Therapy Approaches
2. Novel Drug Delivery Systems
3. Personalized Medicine in Endocrine Disorders

Molecular biology advances have offered astonishing revelations into endocrine disorder mechanisms, opening avenues for novel therapeutic avenues. An exciting potential lies in modulating the 18-kDa translocator protein (TSPO), a mitochondrial membrane protein that has been implicated in cholesterol transport and steroidogenesis. Beyond steroidogenesis, TSPO's role affects fundamental cellular functions such as apoptosis and autophagy through its interactions with proteins such as the voltage-dependent anion channel. Even with its discovery years ago, recent structural elucidations have furthered insights into TSPO's functional complexity, opening new avenues for pharmacological interventions geared towards the restoration of endocrine homeostasis. Targeted TSPO ligands have the potential not only to regulate steroidogenesis but also to modulate mitochondrial quality control processes, which may counteract endocrine dysfunction resulting from cell stress or inflammation. Such new therapies represent a movement away from symptom management and toward the correction of underlying molecular dysfunctions integral to endocrine disorders (Aghazadeh et al., 2016). Metabolic disorders marked by deranged glucose homeostasis constitute a substantial and rising public health problem, with increased motivation to improve on therapeutic possibilities. Diabetes mellitus, especially types 1 and 2, represents this issue with rising incidence attributed to population dynamics as well as lifestyle across the globe. Emerging pharmacological strategies focus on enhancing insulin secretion, improving insulin sensitivity, and mitigating complications associated with chronic hyperglycemia. Beyond traditional therapies, novel agents targeting pathways involved in beta-cell preservation and inflammatory modulation are under investigation. These approaches aim to address the heterogeneous etiology of diabetes, tailoring treatment regimens to patient-specific pathophysiology. The growing knowledge base of diabetes pathogenesis allows for more targeted pharmacological interventions, better glycemic control, and decreased disease burden (Amir et al., 2023). New endocrine therapies also include a paradigm of personalized medicine, leveraging genetic and molecular profiling to maximize drug effectiveness and reduce side effects. Receptor biology and signal transduction advances have led to the discovery of new classes of selective modulators that can fine-tune hormonal responses. For example, thyroid hormone receptor agonists and antagonists have pinpointed control of metabolic rate and cardiovascular performance, yet no sweeping systemic consequences occur. Additionally, peptide therapeutics targeting pathways in gut hormones like GLP-1 receptor agonists exhibit wide promise for treatment of diabetes and obesity through utilizations of endogenous regulatory mechanisms. These advances, bolstered by innovative delivery systems and biomarker-guided dosing, mark a new age of endocrine pharmacology in which treatment regimens are optimized to the individual patient to promote better clinical outcomes and quality of life. Harmonization of molecular information with clinical use is a hallmark of the future of endocrine therapeutics in the 21st century.

10.6.1. Gene Therapy Approaches

Advances in molecular biology have transformed the treatment of endocrine disease, and gene therapy now offers a novel solution to mend underlying genetic defects. In contrast to traditional pharmacological interventions that affect symptoms or hormonal levels, gene therapy seeks to correct or modify defective gene expression leading to endocrine dysfunction. This method comprises the introduction, modification, or suppression of precise genes in target cells, using viral vectors or new delivery mechanisms to provide persistent therapeutic effects. In endocrine pharmacology, gene therapy presents the possibility for accurate modulation of hormone secretion and receptor activity to enhance disease states and reduce systemic side effects common in conventional hormone replacement therapies. These innovations require a strong grasp of gene regulation, cellular uptake processes, and immune reactions to provide efficacy and safety in clinical use. One of the challenges in creating gene therapies for endocrine disorders is finding the best molecular targets and delivery systems to provide specificity and avoid off-target effects. This involves thorough knowledge of the genetic and epigenetic determinants affecting hormone signaling pathways and receptor sensitivity. For instance, some subtypes of breast cancer—based on hormone receptor status—represent the complexity of molecular targets that may be amenable to gene-directed interventions. Blending multi-target network approaches enables scientists to determine synergistic interactions between compounds and potential gene targets and to move forward with personalized therapeutic approaches suitable for particular endocrine cancers (Yang et al., 2018). These strategies emphasize the need for the integration of classical pharmacology with advanced gene therapy methods in order to maximize results in endocrine-related cancers and metabolic syndromes. In addition, the use of epigenetic modifiers like histone deacetylase inhibitors has been particularly encouraging in increasing the efficacy of gene therapy in endocrine oncology. These drugs have the ability to change chromatin conformation, hence controlling gene expression and enhancing responsiveness to gene transfer as well as subsequent therapies. For example, the agents such as ethnostate have shown the ability to enhance immune responses and reverse endocrine resistance mechanisms in hormone-positive breast cancer. Such synergistic potential indicates the function of epigenetic regulation in improving gene therapy strategies, especially in evading endocrine resistance and increasing therapeutic longevity (Trapani et al., 2017). The future of endocrine pharmacology is in combining gene therapy with epigenetic and immunomodulatory approaches, setting the stage for more effective and tailored treatments (Figure 10.19).

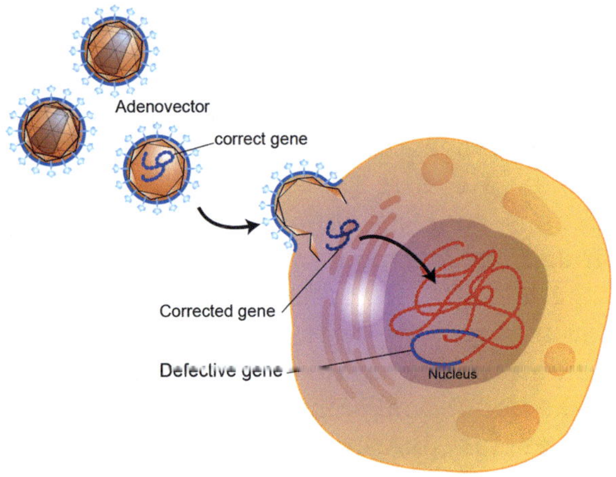

Figure 10.19. Gene therapy approaches.

Source: National Human Genome Research Institute. (n.d.). *Gene Therapy*. U.S. Department of Health and Human Services. https://www.genome.gov/sites/default/files/tg/en/illustration/gene_therapy.jpg.

10.6.2. Novel Drug Delivery Systems

Progresses in drug delivery science have radically changed the dynamics of endocrine pharmacology through improved therapeutic effectiveness and reduced systemic side effects. Conventional routes of administration create fluctuating hormone concentrations, degrading treatment efficacy and worsening side effects. New drug delivery systems overcome such obstacles by facilitating controlled and targeted delivery of endocrine drugs. For example, peptide hormones with low half-lives, including vasoactive intestinal peptide, are advantageously encapsulated within nanocarriers that shield them from enzymatic hydrolysis and enhance bioavailability. Such systems provide sustained plasma levels that simulate physiological secretion rates, thus maximizing hormonal signaling and minimizing dosing frequency. These new strategies not only enhance compliance in patients but also provide new doors to treating complex endocrine diseases by modulating cellular mechanisms more specifically (Akiba et al., 2019). The inclusion of antibody-drug conjugates (ADCs) in endocrine drugology best explains the capability of new delivery platforms to promote specificity with reduced adverse effects. An important example is trastuzumab emtansine (T-DM1), a drug-antibody conjugate that specifically targets HER2-positive breast cancer, a disease modulated by endocrine pathway signaling. T-DM1 is a monoclonal antibody conjugated to a cytotoxic agent, and it selectively delivers the cytotoxin to tumor cells expressing the HER2 receptor. This targeting significantly enhances antitumor activity and tolerability over traditional chemotherapy. In addition, continuous clinical trials explore its activity in earlier therapy contexts, highlighting the promise of new drug delivery systems to redefine endocrine-type cancer treatment modalities by achieving resistance reversal and reducing systemic toxicity (Hurvitz et al., 2014). Novel drug delivery methods in endocrine pharmacology also focus on individualized medicine using ligand-receptor targeting and responsive release mechanisms. These devices are designed to discharge hormonal agents in response to certain physiological cues, thus delivering site-specific therapeutic action. For instance, glucose-sensitive insulin delivery platforms ensure dynamic release of hormone, real-time adjustment with blood glucose levels, and consequently improved glycemic control and protection against hypoglycemia. Moreover, receptor-targeted nanoparticles are capable of targeting endocrine glands or hormone-responsive tissues and can allow the localized drug delivery with excellent precision. Such specificity not only optimizes therapeutic effects but also minimizes unwanted interactions in peripheral tissues, which underscores the central importance of innovative drug delivery systems (Figure 10.20) in optimizing endocrine therapy across a variety of clinical settings (Akiba et al., 2019; Hurvitz et al., 2014).

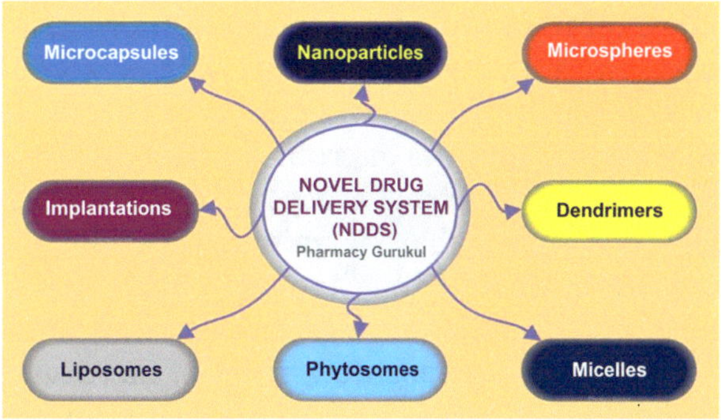

Figure 10.20. Novel drug delivery systems.

Source: Natural Bio Health. (2020). *Austin Thyroid Hormone Therapy T3 T4.* https://i.ytimg.com/vi/fhvi8accAjI/maxresdefault.jpg.

10.6.3. Personalized Medicine in Endocrine Disorders

New advances in the fields of molecular biology and genomic sciences have redynamically shifted the paradigms in the management of multifactorial diseases, including endocrine disorders. Traditional endocrine pharmacology adopts a one-size-fits-all principle, and therefore it may lead to ineffective therapy due to variability among patients. Personalized medicine, however, makes therapy person-specific based on genetic, environmental, and lifestyle determinants, thereby increasing drug efficacy with decreased side effects. For instance, genetic variation in sensitivity or metabolism of hormone receptors is a prime determinant of drug response to diseases like diabetes mellitus and thyroid disorders. Incorporation of pharmacogenomics in the clinical context allows for proper titration of doses as well as application of the most appropriate pharmacological therapeutics. Personalized care also allows for early detection of patients susceptible to drug toxicity or resistance, improving disease management in general. Therefore, the integration of personalized medicine into endocrine pharmacology is a significant step towards better and safer treatment protocols (Alexander et al., 2022). Endocrine disorders are generally marked by complex interactions between hormonal pathways and systemic physiological processes, which are further added to by the effect of the microbiota. New evidence suggests that microbial ecosystems, particularly in the gut, are capable of manipulating endocrine function by modulating immune response and systemic inflammation. Dysbiosis, or imbalance in microbiota composition, may be implicated in the pathogenesis and onset of endocrine disorders such as obesity, diabetes, and thyroid conditions. Understanding such interactions between microbiota and endocrinology holds new avenues for personalized therapeutic interventions. The treatment of the host not only based on their genetic profile but also based on their structure of the microbiota will likely make drugs more effective and diminish disease progression. Such integrative methods, including microbiota modulation, highlight the utility of personalized medicine in enhancing endocrine pharmacology and facilitating new treatment strategies aimed at re-balancing such cross-talking systems (Hou et al., 2022). Although maintaining extremely promising promise, utilization of personalized medicine in endocrine pharmacology is beset by numerous challenges. Variability in genetic testing with respect to accessibility and ease of interpretation of multi-omic data are significant barriers to clinical applicability. Additionally, the dynamic nature of variability of endocrine disease, which can shift over time of life, environmental exposure, and lifestyle, necessitates real-time tracking and adaptive treatment regimens. Ethical concerns like confidentiality of the patient and equal access to customized therapies must also be addressed. However, ongoing advances in bioinformatics tools, artificial intelligence, and wearable monitors are progressively overcoming these constraints, allowing real-time patient-specific management. With studies increasingly elucidating the molecular and microbiota-related origin of endocrine diseases, personalized medicine is at the threshold of revolutionizing endocrine pharmacology since it is capable of rendering extremely individualized and responsive therapy (Alexander et al., 2022; Hou et al., 2022).

Test Your Knowledge

1. What is meant by emerging therapies in endocrine pharmacology?
2. Which of Personalized Medicine in Endocrine Disorders?

SUMMARY

Endocrine pharmacology advances have meaningfully progressed our comprehension of hormone-related ailment as well as their therapeutic measures. This advancement is best illustrated by current studies investigating the complex functions of vitamin D in the treatment of thyroid cancer, where network pharmacology and molecular docking methods have identified key target genes and signaling pathways involved in disease regulation. Of particular interest, vitamin Ds inhibition of thyroid cancer cell growth and repression of ESR1 expression shed light on the intricate biological processes at play, underscoring the potential for using endogenous compounds to attain targeted therapeutic effects. These integrative strategies highlight the importance of probing several molecular targets and pathways towards creating effective endocrine treatments in highlighting the requirement of an exhaustive outlook in navigating the complexity of endocrine cancer (Liu et al., 2024). Endocrine disorders are highly complex, moving beyond oncology to include disorders in children, such as in childhood precocious puberty, whereby conventional drugs introduce new pharmacologic perspectives. By applying the use of sophisticated analytical tools in conjunction with network pharmacology, the multicomponent nature of such herbal drugs as Zhibai Dihuang pill has been explained and elucidated, disclosing active constituents and their interaction with major endocrine targets PIK3CA and CYP19A1. This polypharmacological profiling supports the worth of combining conventional medicinal knowledge with modern scientific methodologies to disclose the therapeutic efficacy mechanisms. Additionally, delineation of critical signaling pathways, including cAMP and neuroactive ligand-receptor interactions, offers underlying justification for the creation of novel therapeutics that are holistic and mechanism-based (Zhang et al., 2024). In conclusion, the changing landscape of endocrine pharmacology highlights the need for interdisciplinary research approaches incorporating molecular, cellular, and systemic analyses to refine treatment modalities. The integration of network pharmacology, molecular docking, and experimental confirmation provides a robust platform to traverse the intricate signaling networks that define endocrine disorders. This holistic approach not only streamlines drug discovery but also facilitates precision medicine by delineating actionable targets and clarifying drug mechanisms. Multidisciplinary efforts are necessary to take these findings to clinical bedside, ultimately leading to better patient outcomes in various endocrine pathologies. Therefore, continued research in this area holds the promise of improving therapeutic interventions and driving personalized medicine to address endocrine system complexities (Liu et al., 2024; Zhang et al., 2024).

Summary of Key Points

Endocrine pharmacology involves the investigation and use of drugs that affect the body's hormonal systems to correct imbalances or regulate physiological processes. A critical insight is gained by analyzing how drugs engage with particular hormone receptors and signaling pathways to manage endocrine diseases effectively. For example, treatment approaches for PCOS utilize intricate formulations that act on multiple molecular targets, reflecting the multidimensional aspect of endocrine modulation. Through the use of network pharmacology and molecular docking methods, scientists have established core targets and bioactive compounds which offer a mechanistic rationale for enhanced therapeutic effectiveness in PCOS treatment. Such holistic methodology points towards the leap from one-target therapy to more integrated modalities that value the polygenic and multifactorial nature of endocrine disorders (Ouyang et al., 2024). These findings emphasize the revolutionary value of pharmacology in individualizing effective endocrine therapies.

Current advances in endocrine pharmacology also attest to the need for quantitative integration to overcome challenges inherent in drug development, especially for rare endocrine-related diseases. The discipline is beset by huge challenges such as poor understanding of disease natural histories, heterogeneity in patient responses, and recruitment issues in clinical trials. Focusing on biomarker usage innovations, statistical approaches, and model-based drug development, today's research emphasizes a data-centric paradigm to facilitate therapeutic optimization and regulatory approval workflows. Cooperative platforms, such as public-private collaborations, have now become crucial to improving clinical trial efficiency and enabling knowledge sharing. These developments enable faster development of safe and efficacious endocrine medicines addressing both prevalent and uncommon disorders, promoting systemic alignment of multi-disciplinary knowledge to prevail over drug discovery and patient treatment barriers (Krishna et al., 2024). Such strategies hold the potential to streamline and accelerate endocrine pharmacotherapy. Overall, endocrine pharmacology is being transformed through integrative and quantitative approaches that enhance our knowledge of hormone regulation and its pharmacologic manipulation. The discovery of new drug targets and bioactive molecules with the help of advanced analysis tools is a critical step towards the treatment of multifaceted endocrine disorders such as PCOS. In parallel, the inclusion of groundbreaking regulatory science and cooperative efforts provides emerging drugs more precision and effectiveness, especially for uncommon endocrine disorders with few therapeutic alternatives. Collectively, these major advances represent a dynamic discipline that combines molecular understanding with clinical pragmatism to facilitate personalized and adaptive endocrine therapies. As the field evolves, ongoing focus on integrated data analysis and cross-disciplinary collaboration will be critical to fully unlock the therapeutic potential of endocrine pharmacology (Krishna et al., 2024; Ouyang et al., 2024).

KEY TERMS FROM THIS CHAPTER

Hormone replacement
Mechanisms of action
Endocrine pharmacology
Medical treatment
Endocrine-disrupting chemicals (edcs)
Pharmacology
Pharmacologic
Pharmacological treatment
Endocrine pharmacology
Polycystic ovary syndrome (pcos)
Endocrine pharmacology
Clinical management
Hormone action
Selective estrogen receptor degraders (serds)
Clinical care
Hyperglycemia

CRITICAL THINKING QUESTIONS

1. **Which of the following drugs is used in the treatment of hyperthyroidism?**
   a. Levothyroxine
   b. Methimazole
   c. Liothyronine
   d. Iodide 131
2. **Which of the following is a DPP-4 inhibitor used in the management of type 2 diabetes?**
   a. Metformin
   b. Sitagliptin
   c. Acarbose
   d. Glipizide
3. **The mechanism of action of propylthiouracil includes?**
   a. Stimulating thyroid hormone release
   b. Blocking thyroid peroxidase and conversion of T4 to T3
   c. Mimicking TSH
   d. Inhibiting thyroid-stimulating immunoglobulins
4. **Insulin glargine is best classified as?**
   a. Rapid-acting insulin
   b. Short-acting insulin
   c. Intermediate-acting insulin
   d. Long-acting insulin
5. **Which of the following is a side effect commonly associated with glucocorticoids?**
   a. Hypoglycemia
   b. Osteoporosis
   c. Bradycardia
   d. Weight loss

Short Answer Questions

1. Difference between peptide, steroid, and amino acid-derived hormones in terms of their mechanisms of action?
2. Discuss the differences between Type 1 and Type 2 diabetes in terms of pathophysiology and pharmacological treatment strategies?
3. What is the mechanism of action thyroid hormone replacement therapy?
4. List the primary clinical indications for corticosteroid therapy?
5. What is emerging therapies in endocrine pharmacology?

Answer to Critical Thinking Questions

1. (b) 2 (b) 3. (b) 4. (d) 5. (b)

REFERENCES

1. Abdullaeva, S., Abdullaeva, P., Gabdrahimova, R., Nazmieva, K., Neganova, M., Liu, J., Samsonov, M., et al. (2025). Analysis of the main directions in the development of mono and combination pharmacotherapy acting on hormonal signaling pathways of breast cancer according to the FDA databases and ClinicalTrials.gov. *Current Medicinal Chemistry.* https://www.semanticscholar.org/paper/43f0998a087cb1e4cbd2fb11d16aab6c1b4be953 (accessed on 9 May 2025).
2. Adebayo, A., Mshelia, G. D., Ojo, N. A., Uchendu, C., et al. (2017). The use of dexamethasone in animals: Implication for fertility, pregnancy and extrapolation of the animal data to humans. https://core.ac.uk/download/478279699.pdf (accessed on 9 May 2025).
3. Aghazadeh, M., Aghazadeh, T., Alho, H., Amitani, M., Anholt, R. R. H., et al. (2016). TSPO: Kaleidoscopic 18-kDa amid biochemical pharmacology, control and targeting of mitochondria. https://core.ac.uk/download/36779164.pdf (accessed on 9 May 2025).
4. Akiba, Y., Iwasaki, M., & Kaunitz, J. D. (2019). Recent advances in vasoactive intestinal peptide physiology and pathophysiology: Focus on the gastrointestinal system. https://core.ac.uk/download/286729137.pdf.
5. Akpantah, A., Amabe, M., Akpaso, M. I., Atangwho, I. J., Ebong, P. E., et al. (2011). Effect of combined leaf extracts of *Vernonia amygdalina* (bitter leaf) and *Gongronema latifolium* (utazi) on the pancreatic beta-cells of streptozotocin-induced diabetic rats. https://core.ac.uk/download/30437207.pdf (accessed on 9 May 2025).
6. Alkalay, A., Anderson, J., Andrews, K., Arlt, W., Arnold, R., Asa, S., et al. (2009). Effects of intrauterine exposure to synthetic glucocorticoids on fetal, newborn, and infant hypothalamic-pituitary-adrenal axis function in humans: A systematic review. *Unpublished manuscript.* https://core.ac.uk/download/18242225.pdf (accessed on 9 May 2025).
7. Amir, M., Asif, M., Hussain, A., Jamil, S., et al. (2023). An updated review on anti-diabetic agents and their functions: A comparative study. https://core.ac.uk/download/590905601.pdf (accessed on 9 May 2025).
8. Anders, H. J., Fernández-Juárez, G., Vaglio, A., Romagnani, P., & Floege, J. (2023). CKD therapy to improve outcomes of immune-mediated glomerular diseases. *Nephrology, Dialysis, Transplantation.* https://www.semanticscholar.org/paper/47e9fb8b19765676d2dc40010ab473813eb996a1 (accessed on 9 May 2025).
9. Anderson, T., Bazire, S., Desborough, J., Kirkham, D., et al. (2014). One lithium level >1.0 mmol/L causes an acute decline in eGFR: Findings from a retrospective analysis of a monitoring database. https://core.ac.uk/download/29109947.pdf (accessed on 9 May 2025).
10. Appetecchia, M., Lauretta, R., Romanelli, F., & Sansone, A. (2018). Gender in endocrine diseases: Role of sex gonadal hormones. https://core.ac.uk/download/188826984.pdf (accessed on 9 May 2025).
11. Arese, M., Magnifico, M. C., Popov, M., Sarti, P., et al. (2018). Nonylphenol and octylphenol differently affect cell redox balance by modulating the nitric oxide signaling. https://core.ac.uk/download/158822283.pdf (accessed on 9 May 2025).
12. Arnold, B. S., Gross, T. S., McDonald, K., & Spulveda, M. S. (2001). Relations of environmental contaminants, algal toxins, and diet with the reproductive success of American alligators on Florida lakes. https://core.ac.uk/download/11016994.pdf (accessed on 9 May 2025).

13. Bado, M., Bednarczyk, P., Bilecki, K., Duda, M., et al. (2024). Liquid levothyroxine: Efficacy and application in the treatment of myxoedema coma–A narrative review. https://core.ac.uk/download/620863142.pdf (accessed on 9 May 2025).

14. Bak, M., & Choi, J. O. (2023). Optimization of guideline-directed medical treatment for heart failure patients with reduced ejection fraction. *The Korean Journal of Internal Medicine, 38*, 595–606. https://www.semanticscholar.org/paper/7adac25c580a6760de5aa87e1f6af804f013815b (accessed on 9 May 2025).

15. Barbano, B., Cianci, R., Di Mario, F., Gigante, A., et al. (2017). Hypothyroidism and nephrotic syndrome: Why, when and how to treat. https://core.ac.uk/download/132156565.pdf (accessed on 9 May 2025).

16. Bhardwaj, A., Kapoor, K., Kem, A., Singh, A., et al. (2020). Adrenal crisis: A rare endocrine emergency with challenging diagnosis. https://core.ac.uk/download/543133776.pdf (accessed on 9 May 2025).

17. Bhasin, S., Brito, J. P., Cunningham, G. R., Hayes, F. J., Hodis, H. N., Matsumoto, A. M., Snyder, P. J., et al. (2018). Testosterone therapy in men with hypogonadism: An Endocrine Society* clinical practice guideline. *The Journal of Clinical Endocrinology & Metabolism, 103*(5), 1715–1744. https://doi.org/10.1210/jc.2018-00229 (accessed on 9 May 2025).

18. Bhimraj, A., Morgan, R. L., Shumaker, A. H., Lavergne, V., Baden, L. R., Cheng, V. C. C., Edwards, K. M., et al. (2020). Infectious Diseases Society of America guidelines on the treatment and management of patients with COVID-19 (April 2020). *Clinical Infectious Diseases, 78*(e83–e102). https://doi.org/10.1093/cid/ciaa478.

19. Blum, M. R., Dekkers, O. M., Den Elzen, W. P. J., Du Puy, R. S., et al. (2018). Study protocol: A randomized controlled trial on the clinical effects of levothyroxine treatment for subclinical hypothyroidism in people aged 80 years and over. https://core.ac.uk/download/161514514.pdf (accessed on 9 May 2025).

20. Bremer, S., Burton, J., Casati, S., Coecke, S., Corvi, R., Desprez, B., Dumont, C., et al. (2014). Alternative methods for regulatory toxicology–A state-of-the-art review. https://core.ac.uk/download/38628483.pdf (accessed on 9 May 2025).

21. Cao, L. Q., Sun, H., Xie, Y., Patel, H., Bo, L., Lin, H., & Chen, Z. S. (2024). Therapeutic evolution in HR+/HER2- breast cancer: From targeted therapy to endocrine therapy. *Frontiers in Pharmacology, 15*. https://www.semanticscholar.org/paper/a80cf754333fa4c5d542dfc5fc64934b8f597f72 (accessed on 9 May 2025).

22. De Medeiros Pereira, L., Santos, T., Silva, E., Costa, I., & Silva, W. (2025). Non-hormonal male contraceptives: A promising pharmacological alternative. *Revita de Pathologic do Tocantins.* https://www.semanticscholar.org/paper/12e847d9c37e4f6bc15378aca25552b8acfaab75 (accessed on 9 May 2025).

23. Della Corte, L., Foreste, V., Barra, F., Gustavino, C., Alessandri, F., Centurioni, M., Ferrero, S., et al. (2020). Current and experimental drug therapy for the treatment of polycystic ovarian syndrome. *Expert Opinion on Investigational Drugs, 29*, 819–830. https://www.semanticscholar.org/paper/c4968ae090642a00990d2b4dec7f160758321ab8 (accessed on 9 May 2025).

24. Fadini, G. P., Longato, E., Morieri, M., Bonora, E., Consoli, A., Fattor, B., Rigato, M., et al. (2024). Comparative renal outcomes of matched cohorts of patients with type 2 diabetes receiving SGLT2 inhibitors or GLP-1 receptor agonists under routine care. *Diabetology, 67*, 2585–2597.

https://www.semanticscholar.org/paper/cb4457888508938e4a38db868053514484acdd7e (accessed on 9 May 2025).

25. Gardella, T., & Vilardaga, J. (2015). International Union of Basic and Clinical Pharmacology. XCIII. The parathyroid hormone receptors—Family B G protein–coupled receptors. *Pharmacological Reviews, 67*(2), 310–337. https://www.semanticscholar.org/paper/e50c8d7205fbabf10c2aca2b88edf22ad515b731 (accessed on 9 May 2025).

26. Gatnik, M. F., Lapenna, S., Lo Piparo, E., Mostrag-Szlichtyng, A., Serafimova, R., & Worth, A. (2011). The use of computational methods in the toxicological assessment of chemicals in food: Current status and future prospects. https://core.ac.uk/download/38621283.pdf (accessed on 9 May 2025).

27. Genta, S. B. de F., Honore, S. M., & Sanchez, S. S. del V. (2015). *Smallanthus sonchifolius* (Yacon) leaves: An emerging source of compounds for diabetes management. https://core.ac.uk/download/159286606.pdf (accessed on 9 May 2025).

28. Hou, K., Wu, Z. X., Chen, X. Y., Wang, J. Q., Zhang, D., Xiao, C., Zhu, D., et al. (2022). Microbiota in health and diseases. *Signal Transduction and Targeted Therapy, 7*, Article 135. https://doi.org/10.1038/s41392-022-00974-4.

29. Hurvitz, S. A., Olevsky, O., & Sadeghi, S. (2014). Profiling and targeting HER2-positive breast cancer using trastuzumab emtansine. https://core.ac.uk/download/323079599.pdf.

30. Johnson, M. S., & Justin, S. A. (2020). A prospective study on evaluation of maternal and foetal outcomes of hypothyroidism with levothyroxine and prevalence of hypothyroidism in pregnancy in a tertiary care teaching hospital in Kerala. https://core.ac.uk/download/539896378.pdf (accessed on 9 May 2025).

31. Krishna, R., Sebastien, B., Corriol-Rohou, S., Cheung, S. Y. A., Liu, J., & Suryawanshi, S. (2024). Pediatric rare diseases development in the pharmaceutical industry: An international consortium for innovation and quality in pharmaceutical development, Clinical Pharmacology Leadership Group–Pediatrics Working Group, Rare Diseases Subteam whitepaper examining the current landscape and recommendation. *Clinical Pharmacology and Therapeutics.* https://www.semanticscholar.org/paper/9311217e05e626b49345b81d37f3e11a2db2ffce (accessed on 9 May 2025).

32. LeBoff, M. S., Greenspan, S. L., Insogna, K., Lewiecki, E. M., Saag, K. G., Singer, A., & Siris, E. S. (2022). The clinician's guide to prevention and treatment of osteoporosis. *Osteoporosis International, 33*, 2049–2102. https://doi.org/10.1007/s00198-021-05900-y.

33. Li, Z., & Robaire, B. (2025). Effects of endocrine-disrupting chemicals on adrenal function. *Endocrinology, 166*. https://www.semanticscholar.org/paper/b6d42a0487f515be3698aa7b6eb21c7542778c44 (accessed on 9 May 2025).

34. Liu, B., Hou, B., Zhao, Y., Gao, F., Dong, X., & He, J. (2024). Investigating potential mechanisms of vitamin D against thyroid cancer via network pharmacology and experimental validation. *Chemical Biology & Drug Design, 104*(1), e14586. https://www.semanticscholar.org/paper/9a60343fb05348d2e057cbb874c6c38b3965b53f (accessed on 9 May 2025).

35. Liu, D., Ahmet, A., Ward, L. M., Krishnamoorthy, P., Mandelcorn, E. D., Leigh, R., Brown, J. P., et al. (2013). A practical guide to the monitoring and management of the complications of systemic corticosteroid therapy. *Allergy, Asthma & Clinical Immunology, 9*, 30. https://doi.org/10.1186/1710-1492-9-30.

36. Lomonaco, D., & Jin, K. (2025). Abstract 4414: Targeting CCL5 signaling pathway in endocrine resistant breast cancer therapy. *Cancer Research*. https://www.semanticscholar.org/paper/a51a15ed8bed99b432ae35353099159e5586b083 (accessed on 9 May 2025).

37. Lyon, A. R., López-Fernández, T., Couch, L. S., Asteggiano, R., Aznar, M. C., Bergler-Klein, J., Boriani, G., et al. (2022). 2022 ESC guidelines on cardio-oncology developed in collaboration with the European Hematology Association (EHA), the European Society for Therapeutic Radiology and Oncology (ESTRO), and the International Cardio-Oncology Society (IC-OS). *European Heart Journal, 43*, 4229–4361. https://doi.org/10.1093/eurheartj/ehac244.

38. Malozowski, S., & Chiesa, A. (2010). Propylthiouracil-induced hepatotoxicity and death. Hopefully, never more. *The Journal of Clinical Endocrinology & Metabolism, 95*(7), 3161–3163. https://www.semanticscholar.org/paper/41ac55d3666c01531814678436fc65d1a2a1be49 (accessed on 9 May 2025).

39. Ouyang, T., Chen, Y., Wang, Y., Xie, Y., Li, H., & Zhao, M. (2024). Exploring the mechanism of adjustment formula related to Siwu Decoction in the treatment of polycystic ovary syndrome based on network pharmacology. *2024 IEEE International Conference on Big Data (BigData)*. https://www.semanticscholar.org/paper/55963182f60ca0554baead671cd47a91338bfc41 (accessed on 9 May 2025).

40. Rabinovitch, A., Chausmer, A. B., Ertman Karlsen, A., Roussel, A. M., Petersen, A. B., Kutlu, B., Kim, B. J., et al. (2009). Zinc transporter gene expression is regulated by pro-inflammatory cytokines: A potential role for zinc transporters in beta-cell apoptosis? https://core.ac.uk/download/pdf/8265885.pdf.

41. Rajan, N., Duggan, E. W., Abdelmalak, B., Butz, S., Rodriguez, L. V., Vann, M. A., & Joshi, G. P. (2024). Society for Ambulatory Anesthesia updated consensus statement on perioperative blood glucose management in adult patients with diabetes mellitus undergoing ambulatory surgery. *Anesthesia & Analgesia, 139*, 459–477. https://doi.org/10.1213/ane.0000000000006791.

42. Ramachandran, S., Swethanjali, D., Himabindu, M., Devaki, K., Sripada, R., DeepakSrinivas, E., Chakravarthy, M., et al. (2020). Drug utilization evaluation on antidiabetic, thyroid and antithyroid drugs. *Biomedical and Pharmacology Journal*. https://www.semanticscholar.org/paper/e5b2c9415c2e6ebe4cba415bb7758101596d7309 (accessed on 9 May 2025).

43. Rodrigues, P. A., Madhusri, M., & Anjali, M. (2024). A narrative review of polycystic ovarian syndrome. *The Thai Journal of Pharmaceutical Sciences*. https://www.semanticscholar.org/paper/07dc592846e5c86e99d48cf1e6e423c2e2d5bfc2 (accessed on 9 May 2025).

44. Schneider, B. J., Naidoo, J., Santomasso, B., Lacchetti, C., Adkins, S., Anadkat, M. J., Atkins, M. B., et al. (2021). Management of immune-related adverse events in patients treated with immune checkpoint inhibitor therapy: ASCO guideline update. *Journal of Clinical Oncology, 39*, 4073–4126. https://doi.org/10.1200/jco.21.01440.

45. Shim, J., Lin, T., Dashiell-Earp, C., Nechrebecki, M., & Leung, A. M. (2019). Endocrinology practice patterns of hypothyroidism and osteoporosis management in a U.S. tertiary academic medical center. *Clinical Diabetes and Endocrinology, 5*, 8. https://doi.org/10.1186/s40842-019-0085-8.

46. Sun, H., Yu, W., Li, H., Hu, X., & Wang, X. (2024). Bioactive components of Areca nut: An overview of their positive impacts targeting different organs. *Nutrients, 16*. https://www.

semanticscholar.org/paper/65cd664f250ad2b6ee485e34e61b3fc9666db112 (accessed on 9 May 2025).

47. Terrón, J. A. (2014). Novel insights into the potential involvement of 5-HT7 receptors in endocrine dysregulation in stress-related disorders. *Reviews in the Neurosciences, 25*, 439–449. https://doi.org/10.1515/revneuro-2014-0017.

48. Trapani, D., Espósito, A., Criscitiello, C., Mazzarella, L., Locatelli, M., Minchella, I., Minucci, S., et al. (2017). Entinostat for the treatment of breast cancer. *Expert Opinion on Investigational Drugs, 26*, 965–971. https://doi.org/10.1080/13543784.2017.1353077.

49. Tseng, P., Zeng, B. Y., Hsu, C. W., Hung, C. M., Carvalho, A. F., Stubbs, B., Chen, Y. W., et al. (2025). The pharmacodynamics-based prophylactic benefits of GLP-1 receptor agonists and SGLT2 inhibitors on neurodegenerative diseases: Evidence from a network meta-analysis. *BMC Medicine, 23.* https://www.semanticscholar.org/paper/39cf546917eaa806b3f6581b65c5b7f170a39fef (accessed on 9 May 2025).

50. Turek, M., Wojciechowska, K., Jaroń, A., Jastrzębska, K., Wiklińska, A., Witkowska, M., Skotnicka, J., et al. (2024). PCOS–The importance of diet, physical activity, and other non-pharmacological methods in treatment. *Quality in Sport.* https://www.semanticscholar.org/paper/d90015d86d66065a17dcdbf95a03fc1ae96ec57b (accessed on 9 May 2025).

51. Vitiello, L., Lixi, F., Coco, G., & Giannaccare, G. (2024). Ocular surface side effects of novel anticancer drugs. *Cancers, 16.* https://www.semanticscholar.org/paper/e72f0392f0fe05d5804f3ccf054412eb48fc4ec7 (accessed on 9 May 2025).

52. Wong, I. C. K. (2017). *Improving Medication Safety and Diabetes Management In Hong Kong–A Multi-Disciplinary Approach.* https://core.ac.uk/download/79557356.pdf (accessed on 9 May 2025).

53. Yang, K., Zeng, L., & Ge, J. (2018). Exploring the pharmacological mechanism of Danzhi Xiaoyao Powder on ER-positive breast cancer by a network pharmacology approach. *Evidence-Based Complementary and Alternative Medicine, 2018*, Article 5059743. https://doi.org/10.1155/2018/5059743.

54. Yogeeta, F., Rauf, S. A., Devi, M., Imran, K., Ahmed, R., Aruwani, P. K., Saad, M., et al. (2024). Prolactinoma: Navigating the dual challenge of side effects and treatment strategies–A comprehensive review. *Annals of Medicine and Surgery, 86*, 4613–4623. https://www.semanticscholar.org/paper/a4af64e41b4cfd567f4b0ea91bab24f12ecc00d1 (accessed on 9 May 2025).

55. Zhang, J., Yang, Q., Wulu, J., & Zhang, Z. (2024). Integrated multicomponent analysis based on ultra-high-performance liquid chromatography coupled with quadrupole-Exactive Orbitrap mass spectrometry and network pharmacology to elucidate the effective constituents and potential mechanism of Zhibai Dihuang pill in treating childhood precocious puberty. *Rapid Communications in Mass Spectrometry, 38*(16), e9831. https://www.semanticscholar.org/paper/7cc03e77c4ec9d9bb4207d74561a0f7078d9e182 (accessed on 9 May 2025).

DRUGS USED IN CANCER CHEMOTHERAPY

11

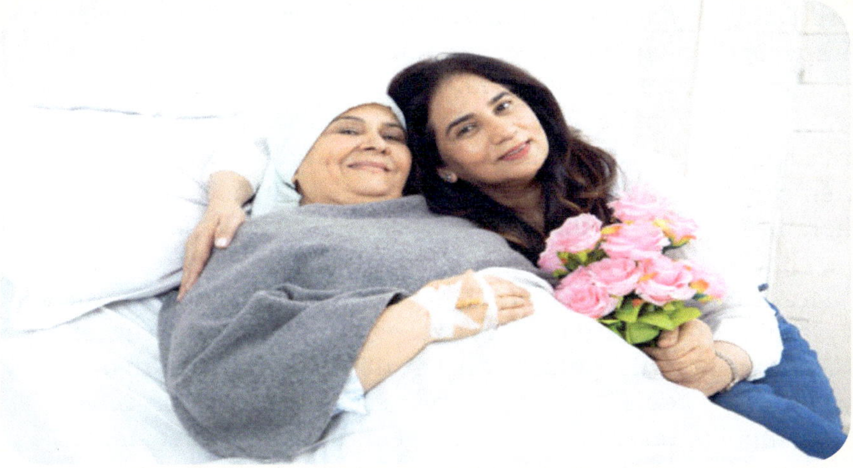

LEARNING OBJECTIVES

After studying this chapter, you will be able to:

1. Explain types of chemotherapy drugs
2. List the mechanisms of action
3. Describe of commonly used chemotherapy drugs
4. Discuss the side effects of chemotherapy
5. Explore targeted therapy versus traditional chemotherapy
6. Define advances in chemotherapy

Introduction

The complexity of the disease of cancer requires multidirectional methods of effective treatment, and chemotherapy occupies a leading place. Chemotherapy uses a range of drugs intended to suppress the growth of actively dividing cells that is typical of cancer. Drugs vary in their chemical composition, activity mechanism, and selectivity, acting upon the heterogeneity of the biological behavior of tumor cells. In spite of tremendous progress in the area, limitations like drug resistance, side effects, and inconsistent patient responses still limit the therapeutic efficacy of chemotherapy. It is critical to understand these factors in order to maximize treatment regimens and enhance patient outcomes through precision medicine and novel drug development. This introduction provides the background context for discussing the types and roles of drugs employed in cancer chemotherapy. One of the critical components of modern cancer chemotherapy is the targeting of the tumor microenvironment to bypass hypoxia-imposed limitations, a state of reduced oxygen tension in solid tumors. Tumor hypoxia is responsible for aggressive cancer growth and resistance to traditional treatments, such as chemotherapy. Hypoxia-inducible factors (HIFs), transcription factors that respond to low oxygen levels, induce tumor survival and metastasis. Attempts to block HIF activity have become a potential strategy in cancer therapy to make tumors more sensitive to chemotherapy and minimize metastasis. The creation of HIF-1/2 inhibitors represents a milestone, as demonstrated in recent research on their structural characteristics and anticancer activity. The inhibitors hold the promise of enhancing chemotherapy by interfering with hypoxia-mediated tumor adaptation (Mustafa et al., 2024). Another key innovation in chemotherapy is to improve drug delivery systems to ensure maximum efficacy with minimal toxicity. Platinum-based therapies, including cisplatin and carboplatin, have been mainstays of chemotherapy for decades but are frequently hampered by systemic toxicities due to free circulating drug. The use of these drugs in combination with hydrogel-based delivery systems has been promising to overcome these shortcomings. Hydrogels based on biocompatible materials such as polysaccharides and polypeptides facilitate controlled and localized drug release, enhancing tumor targeting and minimizing toxic systemic exposure. This combination system not only maximizes therapeutic effectiveness through continuous drug availability but also minimizes side effects through slow degradation of the carrier inside the body. Such inventions mark a seminal advancement toward safer and more effective chemotherapy regimens (Yao et al., 2023).

Definition of Chemotherapy

The management of cancer has changed dramatically over the last hundred years, with a variety of therapeutic options now at hand to fight cancer cells. Amongst them, chemotherapy continues to be a cornerstone in the management of systemic cancers that are not accessible to localized treatments alone like surgery or radiation. Chemotherapy is the application of cytotoxic agents that are meant to disrupt rapidly growing cancer cells by targeting several cell mechanisms critical to proliferation and survival (Figure 11.1). These drugs target cells at different phases of the cell cycle, interfering with DNA synthesis, the formation of the mitotic spindle, or protein synthesis, leading to eventual destruction of the cancer cell. The accuracy and sophistication of chemotherapy have been enhanced by advances that now make it possible to administer intraperitoneally in conjunction with hyperthermia, a method that has been proven to enhance disease-free survival in some cancers like advanced ovarian cancer (Llueca et al., 2023). The biochemical basis of chemotherapy is dependent on its capability to take advantage of the weakness of cancer cells while avoiding damage to normal tissues as much as possible. This selectivity is because cancer cells typically display dysregulated growth and defective repair processes that render them more vulnerable to agents inducing DNA damage or proteotoxic stress. Molecular processes like the unfolded protein response and endoplasmic reticulum-associated degradation are pivotal for cellular homeostasis and have been targeted for new chemotherapy strategies. For example, the valosin-containing protein (VCP), involved in protein degradation and stress response, has been found to exhibit variable expression in cancers including acute myeloid leukemia and correlated with prognosis and therapeutic outcome. Inhibiting proteins like VCP would be expected to augment chemotherapy activity by interfering with mechanisms of cancer cell survival (Hoff et al., 2021). Theoretically, chemotherapy is not a one-size-fits-all treatment but rather a set of agents whose efficacy is achieved through a wide variety of molecular targets and pharmacokinetics. This diversity facilitates combination regimens that will be able to overcome resistance and reduce adverse effects. The ultimate goal remains the same: to eliminate cancer cells with the least harm to patient quality of life. Additionally, changes in delivery of chemotherapy, as in heated intraperitoneal chemotherapy after surgery, illustrate the continued pursuit to maximize therapeutic outcomes and reduce toxicities. These developments reinforce the need to view chemotherapy not merely as a drug class but as a reactive therapeutic modality that is being evolved continuously based on clinical studies and molecular findings (Llueca et al., 2023).

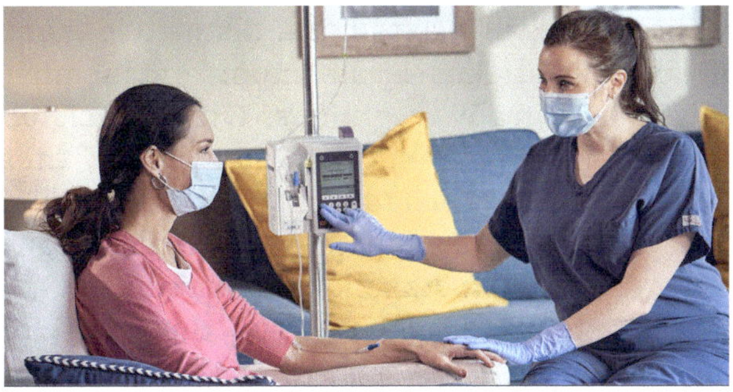

Figure 11.1. Chemotherapy treatment of cancer.

Source: City of Hope. (2021). *Chemotherapy. https*://cdn.cancercenter.com/-/media/ctca/images/others/blogs/2021/03-march/blog-chemotherapy-l.jpg.

Importance of Chemotherapy in Cancer Treatment

The multi-cellular nature of cancer requires a multi-modal approach to treatment, with chemotherapy serving as the central intervention. Cancer cells, having originated from one or more tissues, have an accelerated and unchecked growth pattern, rendering them excellent targets for cell division-inhibiting cytotoxic agents that cause apoptosis. Chemotherapy provides a systemic treatment able to access metastatic cells at distant sites beyond the original tumor location, hence targeting the disease's disseminated nature. But administration of chemotherapeutic agents is not problem-free; adverse drug reactions (ADRs) often complicate the course of treatment. Research underscores the need to conscientiously monitor and maintain control over these ADRs, including nausea, anemia, and gastrointestinal (GI) upset, in order to maximize efficacy while maintaining patient quality of life. The judicious evaluation and attenuation of such effects are essential for ensuring maximal therapeutic gain at minimal risk, highlighting the value of chemotherapy as an effective and delicate component of cancer therapy (Gupta et al., 2019). Its role is not limited to direct cytotoxicity against cancer cells, as increasing evidence points to extensive interactions with the host immune system. The immunomodulation of immune cells, both innate and adaptive, by treatment can affect therapeutic outcomes, either promoting or impairing cancer eradication. Cytotoxic chemotherapy has been found to modulate immune cell phenotypes and functions, thus influencing tumor microenvironments and systemic immunity. Harnessing these immunomodulatory effects offers a promising strategy to enhance treatment efficacy, especially in advanced metastatic cancers where conventional strategies are often ineffective. This twofold effect—coinciding direct killing of tumor cells with activation of the immune system—accentuates chemotherapy's changing role as a multifunctional agent, not just for reduction of tumors but also for modulation of the immune system to achieve improved long-term management of cancer growth (Acharyya et al., 2015). Even though it plays an irreplaceable part in oncologic therapy, chemotherapy's value is ultimately linked to its integration with other therapeutic modalities and patient-specific management approaches. The strategic integration of chemotherapy with surgery, radiation, and specific targeting can maximize tumor control and survival. Also critical is ongoing scrutiny of therapeutic regimens to reduce toxicity and improve patient compliance. Spotlighting early detection of adverse effects and individualized dose tailoring illustrates how contemporary oncology attempts to increase chemotherapy's benefit-to-risk ratio. Finally, chemotherapy is still a mainstay of cancer therapy because of its flexibility in various types and stages of cancer, its capacity to be systemic against micro-metastases, and its compatibility with immunotherapeutic innovations, representing an essential element in the holistic battle against cancer (Acharyya et al., 2015; Gupta et al., 2019).

11.1. Types of Chemotherapy Drugs

Learning Outcome

1. Alkylating Agents
2. Antimetabolites
3. Plant Alkaloids

The face of oncology has changed considerably with the introduction and establishment of a number of classes of chemotherapy drugs that have been engineered to target cancer cells at different phases of their life cycle (Figure 11.2). Among these, alkylating agents work by directly harming DNA, blocking replication and transcription, and hence causing death to cancer cells. Antimetabolites, another very important category, structurally resemble the normal substances found in a cell and affect DNA and RNA synthesis, thus hindering cell division. Plant alkaloids and natural products also interfere with the mitotic spindle machinery or act by inhibiting topoisomerase enzymes, which are necessary for cell division and DNA replication. Every class has a distinctive mode of action and thus is an important member of chemotherapy regimens with precision for specific types and stages of cancer, thus contributing to targeted treatment approaches. One promising development in chemotherapy is the use of the metabolic weaknesses that are cancer cell-specific, more notably their need for specific amino acids such as methionine. This dependence, referred to as the Hoffman effect, characterizes cancer cells from normal cells because they need to consume much higher amounts of methionine for growth and survival.

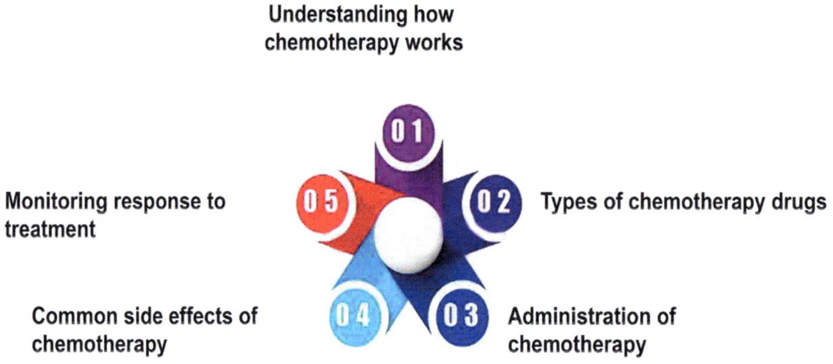

Figure 11.2. Types of chemotherapy drugs.

Source: Google Images. (n.d.). *Types of Chemotherapy Drugs. https*://encrypted-tbn0.gstatic.com/images?q=tbn:ANd9GcQ15YwOs7GzSCybeo49KbqF8E0zRcCbmSrPxw&s.

Novel treatments that involve methionine restriction or the intravenous injection of recombinant methioninase (rMETase) have shown the promise to stop cancer cells in key stages of the cell cycle, increasing the effectiveness of concurrent cytotoxic agents. Such combination therapies take advantage of this selective sensitivity by synergistically enhancing the sensitivity of cancer cells to chemotherapy drugs while leaving normal cells unaffected, potentially lowering side effects and enhancing outcomes in a wide range of malignancies (Kubota et al., 2023). Combination chemotherapy is another important modality in cancer therapy, where two or more drugs with different mechanisms are given together to enhance therapeutic effectiveness and counteract drug resistance. This approach is particularly effective when the drugs target different signaling pathways or cellular processes, minimizing the likelihood of cancer cell survival. For example, 5-fluorouracil (5-FU), a widely utilized antimetabolite, is often paired with complementary agents like melatonin, which has been shown to inhibit tumor growth and induce apoptosis. The synergistic interaction between such compounds can enhance tumor suppression beyond the effects of monotherapy, leading to better patient prognoses. Studies investigating these blended regimens also continue to refine the therapeutic interventions available, enhancing both efficacy and tolerability in cancer patients (Mafi et al., 2023).

11.1.1. Alkylating Agents

The cancer treatment landscape has changed with a focus on therapeutic agents that directly act on tumor cell growth. Of these, alkylating agents occupy a pivotal role because they have the capacity to interfere with the very fabric of cancer cell DNA (Figure 11.3). These agents act by alkylating DNA, primarily at the N7 position of guanine bases, resulting in the formation of DNA adducts that inhibit replication and transcription. Such interference eventually causes apoptosis in the rapidly dividing cancer cells, a mechanism that supports their clinical value. Although effective, the complexity of adduct formation within DNA and subsequent cellular responses remains to be fully defined, particularly as these molecular interactions impact treatment response and drug resistance profiles. More research has aimed to define the individual adducts that are formed and their implication as potential biomarkers for therapeutic response prediction, optimizing the individualized application of alkylating drugs in personalized cancer care (Li, 2024). The clinical use of alkylating agents is widespread among many malignancies and thus forms the backbone of chemotherapy regimens. Their therapeutic utility, though, is frequently foiled by the creation of multidrug resistance (MDR), a process that considerably impairs treatment success. MDR in cancer cells can originate from multiple mechanisms, such as improved DNA repair functions that mend damage caused by alkylation before apoptosis is triggered. In addition, resistance can be mediated by heightened efflux of active ingredients from cells and drug metabolism changes that lower intracellular availability of drugs. The interactive dynamics of these factors result in treatment failure and underscore the need for new approaches to overcome resistance. Research continues to examine the biochemical mechanisms of MDR, aiming to develop alkylating derivatives or adjunct therapies with the potential to overcome such barriers in cancer chemotherapy (Bukowski et al., 2020). Advances have also aimed at the incorporation of alkylating agents into new molecular and targeted therapies for enhanced clinical results. By combining conventional DNA-altering drugs with drugs that alter signaling pathways or epigenetic status, scientists hope to maximize cytotoxicity while reducing systemic toxicity. The use of DNA adducts as biomarkers has become increasingly important in this regard, providing a predictive assessment of patient responsiveness and informing dose optimization. Further, knowledge of the metabolic activation needed for some alkylating agents provides insight into interpatient variability and informs individualized treatment modifications. Continuous clinical trials and preclinical research are central to the development of refining the use of alkylating agents so that they remain relevant through innovations that overcome resistance mechanisms and enhance specificity (Bukowski et al., 2020; Li, 2024).

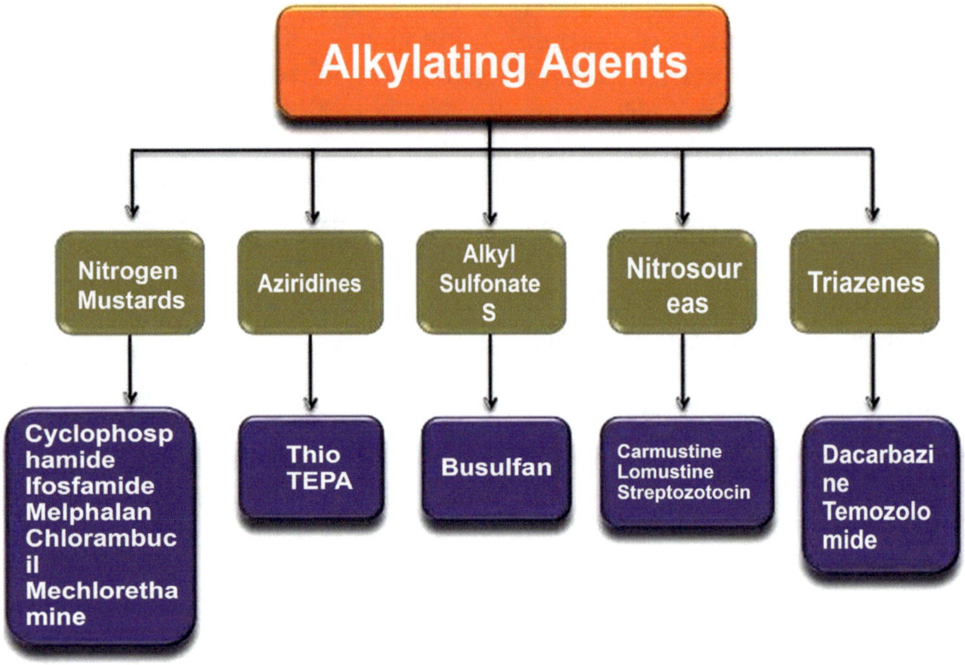

Figure 11.3. Alkylating agents.

Source: **Thomas, N.** (2016). *Alkylating Agents* [Slide 3]. In *Alkylating agents by Dr. Neenu Thomas.* SlideShare. https://image.slidesharecdn.com/alkylatingagents-160107015119/95/alkylating-agents-by-drneenu-thomas-3-638.jpg?cb=1452131548.

11.1.2. Antimetabolites

The subtle interference with cellular metabolism is a promising direction for cancer chemotherapy, especially by exploiting antimetabolites. Antimetabolites interfere by emulating normal substrates in essential biochemical pathways, and this interruption of DNA and RNA synthesis is critical to the rapidly growing cancer cells. In contrast to conventional cytotoxic agents that non-selectively damage proliferating tissue, antimetabolites are specific in that they block nucleotide synthesis or insert false nucleotides into nucleic acids, causing fatal errors during replication. This disruption disproportionately impacts tumor cells because of their high metabolic rates. Nevertheless, clinical use of antimetabolites must be carefully planned with regard to dosage and administration schedules to achieve optimal therapeutic benefit while avoiding side effects like myelosuppression and mucositis. Recent developments in molecular profiling have enriched our knowledge of how antimetabolites engage with cancer-restricted genetic landscapes. The discovery of gene expression signatures, especially those of thymidylate synthase pathways, highlights the promise of individualized chemotherapy treatments. This sensitivity profile guides the application of fluoropyrimidines, a subset of thymidylate synthase-targeting antimetabolites, helping oncologists personalize treatment regimens for ovarian serous adenocarcinoma and other cancers. By incorporating bioinformatic tools analyzing gene signatures and molecular pathways, clinicians are able to forecast drug sensitivity and resistance, making chemotherapeutic interventions more precise. These advances represent the direction towards the rationalization of antimetabolite use by bridging genetic information with pharmacological characteristics (Lockwood et al., 2015). Though effective, antimetabolites tend to induce difficult side effects, such as chemotherapy-induced alopecia, which continues to be alarming for patients and is underappreciated in clinical practice.

The influence of hair loss depends upon drug dose, administration regimen, and patient characteristics and necessitates the use of a multidisciplinary approach to counteract this side effect. The latest research promotes the creation of standardized criteria to evaluate alopecia risk prior to, during, and after antimetabolite therapy to improve patient quality of life. Minimizing these toxicities through anticipatory measures represents a holistic approach to cancer chemotherapy, aligning cytotoxic efficacy with patient-focused attention (Carlesimo et al., 2017).

11.1.3. Plant Alkaloids

The quest for fruitful cancer therapies has shifted more and more towards naturally occurring compounds, especially those derived from plants. Of these, the plant alkaloids (Figure 11.4) have been key contributors to chemotherapy as a result of their strong cytotoxic activity and capacity to disrupt cancer cell proliferation. Traditionally, drugs such as vincristine and vinblastine, which are derived from *Catharanthus roseus*, have become staples in cancer therapy protocols, interfering with microtubule dynamics and thereby arresting mitosis. Likewise, paclitaxel, which is derived from the plant *Taxus baccata*, stabilizes microtubules to prevent cell division. The action of these alkaloids tends to often involve apoptosis induction or cell cycle arrest, which tends to effectively reduce malignant proliferation. Recent studies continue to examine novel plant alkaloids for their prospects in improving cancer selectivity as well as diminishing side effects, highlighting the significance of plant botanical origins in contemporary chemotherapy (Karagil et al., 2025). Resistance to chemotherapeutic agents continues to be an immediate problem in cancer therapy, especially due to MDR phenomena. Tumor cells often acquire MDR through overexpression of ATP-binding cassette (ABC) transporters like P-glycoprotein and multidrug resistance-associated proteins, which actively efflux chemotherapeutic drugs and lower their intracellular levels. Promisingly, certain plant alkaloids have shown potential not just as anticancer agents but also as modulators of MDR processes. The natural agents can be a hindrance to transporter action, and thereby restore the activity of chemotherapeutics in drug-resistant tumors.

By making cancer cells sensitive to known drugs, plant alkaloids have a potential adjunctive therapy, possibly enhancing the clinical outcome of cancers with a high incidence of MDR, e.g., GI cancers (Perazzoli et al., 2025). Though on the horizon of biological activity of plant alkaloids is encouraging, there are a number of challenges awaiting them before they could find universal application in clinical oncology. Most of the early reports of pro-apoptotic and anti-proliferative activities are restricted to *in vitro* studies, which fail to accurately mimic the complexity of the tumor microenvironment and are not subjected to pharmacokinetics like bioavailability. Furthermore, selectivity issues remain, as strong alkaloids can be cytotoxic against normal cells as well, highlighting the demands of accurate dosing and delivery procedures. To translate bench to bedside, strict clinical trials are necessary to delineate safe and effective concentrations and to monitor long-term therapeutic effects. Clarification of the molecular mechanisms involved in plant alkaloid-targeted pathways, such as those that involve caspases and cell cycle regulators, provides a robust basis for translational research in the future (Karagil et al., 2025).

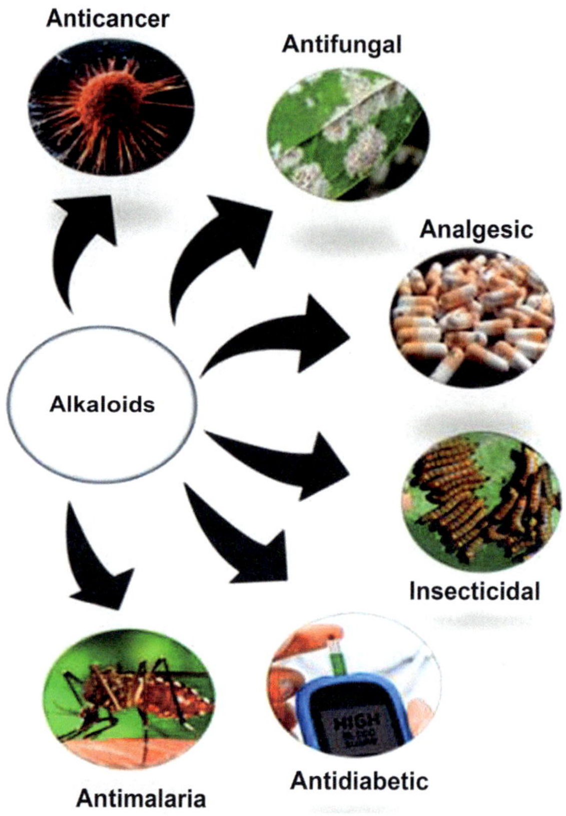

Figure 11.4. Plant alkaloids.

Source: MDPI. (2023). *Illustration of Molecular Interactions. Molecules, 28*(5578). https://www.mdpi.com/molecules/molecules-28-05578/article_deploy/html/images/molecules-28-05578-g001-550.jpg.

Test Your Knowledge

1. Which of the Types of Chemotherapy Drugs?
2. What is antimetabolite in chemotherapy?

11.2. Mechanisms of Action

Learning Outcome

1. DNA Damage and Repair Inhibition
2. Disruption of Cell Division
3. Induction of Apoptosis

The intricate interaction between chemotherapeutic agents and tumor cells is at the center of successful cancer therapy. Most anticancer drugs work by binding to rapidly proliferating cells, a characteristic of tumor tissue, and thus interfering with vital cellular functions like DNA replication and mitosis. Drugs such as doxorubicin insert themselves between DNA strands, hindering the replication machinery, whereas compounds such as paclitaxel stabilize microtubules, blocking their disassembly required for cell division. Yet, beyond these traditional mechanisms, new data indicate that the use of natural compounds such as curcumin together with chemotherapy may increase efficacy and decrease toxicity. Curcumin has been demonstrated to regulate several molecular pathways implicated in cell growth and apoptosis, offering a synergistic possibility with conventional cytotoxic drugs to induce tumor cell death by means of cooperative mechanisms of action (Bee et al., 2019). This multi-target strategy could provide a promising route for drug resistance avoidance and improvement in therapeutic selectivity in cancer chemotherapy. Elucidation of the basis of chemotherapeutic mechanisms includes the control of related adverse effects, which frequently occur due to these drugs' lack of absolute specificity for cancer cells. Alopecia caused by chemotherapy, for example, is a distressing and common side effect indicating destruction of rapidly proliferating hair follicle cells. The degree of hair loss varies with several factors, such as drug type, dose, dosing schedule, and patient-related factors. The molecular basis is through cytotoxicity on the anagen cycle of hair follicles, which are extremely sensitive to DNA damage and mitotic interference induced by chemotherapy (Carlesimo et al., 2017). Understanding these pathways not only illuminates alopecia's pathophysiology but also underscores the need to bring mechanism-based approaches for minimizing undesirable toxicity with maintenance of antitumor activity. Recent advances in mechanism of drug action understanding have also given rise to new formulations and combination treatments for enhancing therapeutic efficacy. Nanoformulations of chemotherapeutic agents in association with biologically active natural products have been an important advancement. This strategy improves drug delivery and cellular uptake, and may modulate molecular targets for cancer cell survival and drug resistance (Bee et al., 2019). Through the use of mechanisms such as enhanced permeability and retention effect, combined therapies provide increased intratumoral drug concentration, thus ensuring maximal cytotoxicity on cancer cells and reduced systemic toxicity. This changing paradigm illustrates the significance of mechanism-based research in the improvement of cancer chemotherapy, emphasizing a trend toward personalized, targeted, and multifaceted treatment modalities that take into account both tumor biology and host response in an integrated manner.

11.2.1. DNA Damage and Repair Inhibition

The delicate balance between damage to and repair of DNA is an essential regulator of cell fate, particularly in cancer cells whose genomic stability tends to be lost (Figure 11.5). Chemotherapeutic drugs take advantage of this weakness by causing DNA damage in excess of the malignant cells' ability to repair, hence triggering apoptosis or senescence. Some drugs further increase this effect by inhibiting simultaneously the pathways for DNA repair, making genomic instability even worse and de facto sensitizing cancer cells to treatment. For instance, natural products like β-caryophyllene have been able to modulate the DNA damage response as well as increase the cytotoxicity of anticancer drugs such as doxorubicin. They cause cancer cells to arrest in certain phases of the cell cycle and decrease repair markers like γH2AX, thus enhancing DNA damage and apoptotic signaling. Simultaneously, these drugs have the potential to display protective actions against nonmalignant cells, demonstrating a complex dual function in chemotherapy that optimizes tumor cell killing and reduces bystander toxicity (Giacomo et al., 2020). Breakthroughs in molecular oncology have ushered in the era of precision targeting of specific DNA repair deficiencies that are typical of most malignancies. Tumors with mutations in homologous recombination repair gene homologs, such as BRCA1 and BRCA2, are more sensitive to inhibitors of alternative repair proteins like poly ADP ribose polymerase (PARP). PARP inhibitors, such as Olaparib, inhibit single-strand break repair, resulting in the accumulation of DNA damage and eventually overwhelming the defective repair machinery in cancer cells. This synthetic lethality strategy has shown encouraging efficacy, particularly in cancers with inherent BRCA mutations, through the transformation of a genetic defect into a therapeutic weakness. Prostate cancer clinical trials reflect Olaparib's ability to take advantage of DNA repair deficiency, achieving better outcomes and tolerability compared to standard chemotherapy, thus being a paradigm shift in precision oncology (Felice et al., 2017).

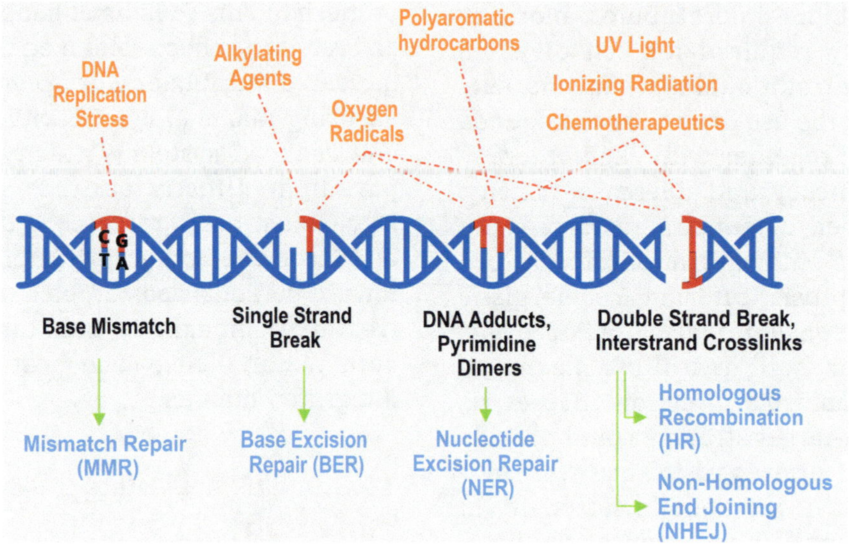

Figure 11.5. DNA damage and repair inhibition.

Source: BPS Bioscience. (n.d.). *DNA Replication and Repair Diagram.* https://bpsbioscience.com/media/wysiwyg/Landing_Pages/DNA_Replication_and_Repair_diagram.png.

Targeting DNA repair mechanisms provides a strategic benefit by taking advantage of the inherent genetic instability of cancer cells to create selective cytotoxicity. DNA-damaging chemotherapy drugs, when used with repair inhibitors, increase therapeutic activity by blocking malignant cells from fixing lethal lesions. Yet this combination must be accurately modulated to prevent undue toxicity to normal tissues. The differential impacts reported in cancer versus nonmalignant cells by combination therapies highlight the intricacy of DNA repair modulation within treatment regimens.

For example, reduction of oxidative stress and differential modulation of signaling pathways such as STAT3 can synergistically enhance DNA damage-induced apoptosis in cancer cells without harming healthy cells, implicating a subtle balance between cellular signaling, DNA damage response, and repair inhibition. These results point towards the possibility of realizing enhanced therapeutic indices via the targeted inhibition of DNA repair pathways (Giacomo et al., 2020).

11.2.2. Disruption of Cell Division

The effectiveness of most cancer chemotherapy agents comes from their ability to disrupt the very process of cell division, which is highly aberrant in cancer cells. Disruption of the mitotic machinery halts the brisk proliferation of tumors, thus inhibiting tumor growth. Chemotherapeutic drugs do so by disrupting different phases of the cell cycle, largely mitosis, where segregation of chromosomes takes place. This interference typically involves the destabilization or stabilization of microtubules, structures crucial for chromosome movement. Through disturbance in these microtubules, drugs inhibit normal spindle formation, resulting in mitotic arrest and eventual induction of apoptosis in cancer cells. This method also has an effect on dividing normal cells, producing the usual toxic side effects characteristic of chemotherapy. Comprehension of these dynamics has spurred the creation of agents more selectively targeting cancer cell weaknesses at the time of division with the goal of enhancing therapeutic benefit and diminishing systemic toxicity (Acharyya et al., 2015). Within the myriad classes of chemotherapeutic drugs, tubulin antagonists are a particular class that focuses on the microtubules central to cell division. These drugs either induce microtubule depolymerization or hyper stabilization, preventing dynamic remodeling, which is needed for mitotic spindle assembly. This results in the failure of cells to complete mitosis, activating cell death machinery. More recent work has shown the disruption caused by these drugs to be more far-reaching than mitotic arrest. For instance, Spong statin 1, an extremely potent experimental drug, not only inhibits mitotic activities but also exerts effects on angiogenesis via mechanisms that are nonmitotic. This two-way action intensifies its antitumor activity by inhibiting tumor vascularization as well as arresting cell proliferation. The study on the mechanism of Spong statin 1 proved its protein kinase Cα inhibition, an important controller in angiogenesis, and opened new avenues for tubulin-targeting drugs (Bruns et al., 2009). Aside from directly inhibiting mitosis, cell division disruption caused by chemotherapy agents initiates a multifaceted interplay with the immune system of the host, impacting therapeutic effects. Cytotoxic drugs induce not only cell killing but also affect immune cells composition, phenotype, and function within the tumor microenvironment. Immunomodulation has the potential to increase antitumor immune responses or, in opposition, facilitate immune evasion, making the treatment more difficult. Thus, the efficacy of chemotherapy goes beyond its cytotoxic effect on proliferating cells to encompass its ability to redefine immune landscape towards tumor clearance. The interplay between cell division disruption and immune activation presents possibilities for combining cytotoxic drugs with immunotherapies, with the goal of synergistically enhancing cancer treatment effectiveness and overcoming resistance mechanisms inherent in both tumor and host factors (Acharyya et al., 2015).

11.2.3. Induction of Apoptosis

Their tendency to escape programmed cell death, a natural mechanism called apoptosis, is the high degree of cancer cell complexity. More chemotherapy agents have been designed to reverse this escaping by actively triggering apoptosis in cancer cells (Figure 11.6). This thoughtful induction cuts across the cancer cell survival pathways, resulting in orchestrated cell disassembly and death, which brings a stop to tumor growth. Such drugs target intracellular signals that are in charge of cell cycle control and induction of apoptosis selectively, which is essential in reducing harm to normal cells. Advances have located molecules such as bacteriocins, which are cationic and amphiphilic with the ability to bind to cancer cell membranes specifically while leaving healthy tissue untouched. This specificity aids them in the triggering of apoptosis intracellularly and is a determining factor when bridging the loopholes posed by conventional chemotherapy, including resistance and toxicity (Wang et al., 2024). Such advancements demote the process of apoptosis induction to a point of being fundamental to novel anticancer approaches. One of the main challenges in cancer chemotherapy is overcoming multidrug resistance, a process where tumor cells resist the cytotoxic action of multiple agents by active efflux of drugs. New compounds like androstano-arylpyrimidines have shown to modulate this resistance by promoting apoptosis induction in drug-resistant tumor cells.

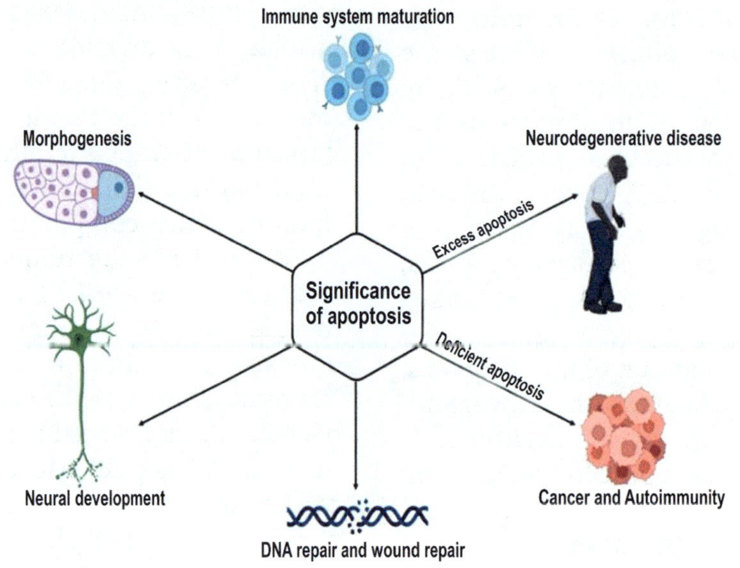

Figure 11.6. Induction of apoptosis.

Source: MDPI. (2023). *Biological Mechanism Illustration. Biomolecules, 13*(194). https://pub.mdpires.com/biomolecules/biomolecules-13-00194/article_deploy/html/images/biomolecules-13-00194-g002.png?1675052485.

By attenuating membrane efflux pumps through mechanisms involving endoplasmic reticulum stress, these compounds sensitize cancer cells to chemotherapeutic agents like Doxorubicin, resulting in increased apoptotic cell death. Notably, their efficacy surpasses that of traditional efflux inhibitors, indicating a dual function in both suppressing drug resistance and triggering apoptosis. This method shows a very promising therapeutic pathway by concurrently inhibiting the defense mechanisms of cancer cells and inducing programmed cell death, thus enhancing the overall efficacy of chemotherapy protocols (Nagy et al., 2023). Incorporation of such apoptosis-provoking agents is a landmark step toward combating resistant cancers. Knowledge about the pathways and mechanisms of apoptosis induction is prerequisite to developing more effective cancer chemotherapy drugs. Apoptosis may be triggered through intrinsic mitochondrial or extrinsic death receptor pathways, both integrating on caspase activation and causing cellular destruction. Therapies that enhance these pathways take advantage of the susceptibility of cancer cells' dysregulated signaling networks. In addition, targeting apoptosis avoids problems with nonspecific cytotoxicity by directing therapy on intrinsic cell death programs instead of killing all rapidly dividing cells indiscriminately. The definition of apoptosis-inducing molecules underscores their therapeutic potential, as in bacteriocins and steroid derivatives that exploit membrane interaction and intracellular stress response to enhance apoptosis without triggering major side effects (Wang et al., 2024). All these open the door for second-generation chemotherapeutics that do not only kill cells but also inhibit collateral damage to healthy tissue, thus enhancing patient tolerability and treatment efficacy.

Test Your Knowledge

1. How do certain chemotherapy drugs induce DNA damage?
2. How do chemotherapy drugs induce apoptotic pathways in cancer cells?

11.3. Commonly Used Chemotherapy Drugs

Learning Outcome

1. Cisplatin
2. Doxorubicin
3. Methotrexate

Among the many methods used in cancer chemotherapy, the use of certain classes of drugs continues to form the basis of treatment protocols (Figure 11.7). Alkylating agents, antimetabolites, and plant alkaloids are some of the most commonly used classes, each with a different mechanism of action against cancer cells. Alkylating agents interfere with DNA replication by covalently interacting with strands of DNA, causing cross-linking and strand breaks, thereby inhibiting cell division. Antimetabolites are structurally similar to normal substrates used in DNA and RNA synthesis, competitively binding enzymes necessary for nucleotide generation. Plant alkaloids, e.g., taxanes and vinca alkaloids, affect mitosis-critical microtubule dynamics. Drug selection based on tumor histology, stage, and molecular profile underscores the need for targeted treatment regimens that maximize therapeutic benefit with least toxicity. Progress in molecular biology has dramatically impacted chemotherapy agent development and use. By comparing gene expression profiles that are typical for a wide range of tumors, doctors are able to predict drug sensitivity, improving the choice of treatment. For instance, discovery of genes associated with angiogenesis and drug resistance, e.g., thymidylate synthase and HSP90AA1, dictates the use of targeted drugs such as tanespimycin in the treatment of ovarian cancer. These genetic signatures improve the predictive value of tumor responsiveness, with potential to better than conventional pathological grading, and represent the trend towards precision medicine. Incorporation of these molecular learnings into chemotherapy drug prescription reflects a trend away from empirical treatment towards biomarker-guided regimens, with the ultimate goal of enhancing patient outcomes (Lockwood et al., 2015).

While encouraging progress has been made, translation of molecular data into therapeutic chemotherapy regimens proves difficult. Although cell-based assays and genotyping technologies have enhanced the knowledge of drug sensitivity and resistance, inconsistencies between *in vitro* models and true tumor behavior frequently complicate therapeutic development. The poor predictive value of traditional cell lines requires the utilization of primary cultures and xenografts to more accurately reflect tumor biology. In addition, the success of EGFR-inhibiting agents highlights the importance of taking genetic mutation into account in lieu of protein overexpression in making treatment decisions. These considerations highlight the need for synthesizing molecular characterization and strong functional assays in informing chemotherapy drug selection in order to minimize reliance on empiric approaches and maximize the accuracy of cancer therapy (Andreotti et al., 2013).

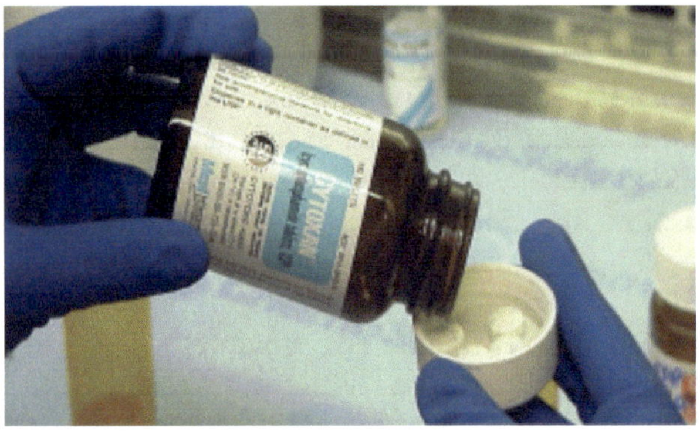

Figure 11.7. Commonly used chemotherapy drugs.

Source: Oncology Nursing Society. (n.d.). *Chemotherapy Drugs. https*://images.ctfassets.net/4dmg3l1sxd6g/77abdG9qQh0mLkOIWFKWL5/5325905d842257315a66f2c78e0420a8/chemo-drugs-4514-article.png_-_en.

11.3.1. Cisplatin

The discovery of successful chemotherapeutic agents has transformed the management of cancer, and cisplatin has been a landmark drug since its initial discovery. Cisplatin achieves its anti-cancer activity via the generation of DNA cross-links, which interfere with DNA replication and transcription, leading to apoptosis of the actively proliferating tumor cells. Although having excellent efficacy against several solid tumors, such as testicular, ovarian, and bladder carcinoma, cisplatin's administration is frequently hampered by severe side effects. Of these, nephrotoxicity, ototoxicity, and emetic nausea and vomiting are of particular concern. Mechanisms underlying these toxicities have stimulated research for optimization of cisplatin treatment, either by dose reduction or addition of antiemetic drugs, improving patient tolerance without diminishing therapeutic efficacy. Nausea and vomiting are considerably disruptive cisplatin chemotherapy side effects, considerably reducing quality of life and compliance in patients. Studies with animal models have helped identify the emetogenic action of cisplatin, allowing for studies on the efficacy of antiemetic drugs. A study with a model involving a low dose of cisplatin in dogs compared the relative efficacy of three groups of antiemetics—5-HT3 antagonists, NK1 antagonists, and D2 antagonists—showing disparate abilities in the inhibition of nausea and vomiting. In addition to behavioral ratings, this study utilized biomarkers like arginine vasopressin and cortisol for the objective evaluation of nausea severity, indicating the intricacies of its measurement and management within clinical practice (Freeman et al., 2017). The results emphasize the need for accurate antiemetic regimens in preventing the adverse effects of cisplatin. The realization of the complex nature of cisplatin-induced nausea continues to be essential for the optimization of supportive care during chemotherapy. The experience of nausea is also subjective and associated with unexplained neural pathways, making both its assessment and treatment challenging. Present knowledge calls for the employment of synergistic antiemetic regimens directed at divergent receptor pathways to more efficiently avoid nausea and vomiting caused by cisplatin. Consensus reviews continue to emphasize the necessity for better animal models and biomarkers to quantitatively measure nausea objectively and to better tailor treatment. Expansion of this knowledge would meaningfully improve cisplatin's side effect management, thus elevating patient compliance and the success of treatment overall (Aapro et al., 2015). Such a comprehensive approach to chemotherapy-induced nausea is central to ongoing advancements in cancer therapy regimens.

11.3.2. Doxorubicin

The intricacy of cancer therapy is not only in the targeting of cancer cells but also in controlling the side effects accumulated by chemotherapeutic agents. One of these agents, doxorubicin, is a part of most chemotherapy protocols because of its strong anti-cancer activity, especially against breast cancer (Figure 11.8). Yet, its therapeutic use is undermined by high toxicities, specifically cardiotoxicity, which can jeopardize patient survival. Current studies highlight the significance of genetic variations in drug metabolism as a predictor of efficacy and safety in doxorubicin treatment. Genetic polymorphisms in genes that code for cytochrome P450 enzymes and p-glycoproteins determine the pharmacokinetics of doxorubicin, which in turn determines individual responses to treatment. Knowledge of these genetic variations can facilitate personalized chemotherapy regimens that reduce side effects while maximizing therapeutic response, thereby promoting precision medicine in oncology (Alina et al., 2022). Drug delivery system advances have also appeared as key approaches to maximize the therapeutic index of doxorubicin. Conventional administration routes expose normal tissue to toxic drug action, restricting dosing increases and conferring decreasing efficacy on treatment. Novel nanocarrier-based delivery, including exosome-encapsulated doxorubicin targeted with targeting ligands such as the AS1411 aptamer, shows encouraging gains in drug specificity and safety.

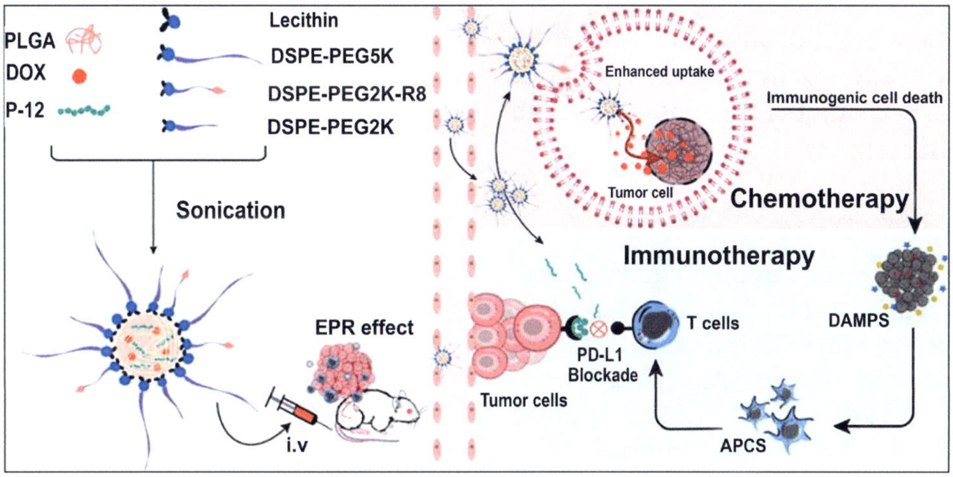

Figure 11.8. Doxorubicin.

Source: American Chemical Society (2022). *Molecular Pharmacology Illustration. Molecular Pharmaceutics*. https://pubs.acs.org/cms/10.1021/acs.molpharmaceut.2c00611/asset/images/acs.molpharmaceut.2c00611.social.jpeg_v03.

These synthetic exosomes take advantage of receptor-mediated endocytosis in nucleolin-overexpressing cancer cells to provide increased internalization and retention of doxorubicin in colorectal cancer models. Targeted delivery systems such as these promise to decrease systemic toxicity, especially cardiotoxicity, with a corresponding increase in the cytotoxic effect on cancer cells, demonstrated by both *in vitro* and *in vivo* studies (Hosseini et al., 2022).

Aside from targeted delivery and the issues of genetics, clinical efficacy of doxorubicin is also a function of achieving potent tumor suppression while minimizing its side effects. Approaches combining pharmacogenomics and new delivery platforms are being developed to overcome this problem, underscoring a shift in paradigm toward greater patient individualization. By individually adjusting dosage with respect to genetic background and the use of advanced drug carriers able to accumulate at specific sites, doxorubicin's therapeutic window can be greatly expanded. Such a multi-level approach offers potential benefits in enhancing cancer chemotherapy outcomes, overcoming the drawbacks commonly linked to anthracycline-based therapies, and maximizing the quality of life for long-term chemotherapy patients (Alina et al., 2022; Hosseini et al., 2022).

11.3.3. Methotrexate

The intricacies of cancer therapy require agents that have the ability to selectively interfere with malignant cell growth without causing excess damage to normal tissues. Antimetabolites, one of the groups of chemotherapeutic agents, do exactly this by imitating naturally occurring molecules essential for DNA and RNA formation. Of these, Methotrexate is a highly recognized folate antagonist that competes with the enzyme dihydrofolate reductase (DHFR), thereby inhibiting the formation of tetrahydrofolate, an essential cofactor in purine and thymidylate formation. This inhibition stops nucleotide biosynthesis, leading to the interference of DNA replication and repair processes crucial for highly proliferating cancer cells. Its molecular architecture, which is based on heterocyclic pteridine frameworks, reflects the significance of chemical moieties in drug activity. The significance of Methotrexate goes beyond its historical clinical application; it is still a cornerstone therapy in many neoplasms, underscoring the importance of targeted folate antagonism in the broader category of antimetabolites (Ramakrishna et al., 2025).

The clinical use of Methotrexate is complicated by its pharmacokinetics and toxicity profile, which require precise dosing and monitoring. Although its ability to cause apoptosis through nucleotide depletion is useful, the nonspecific effect on normal proliferative tissues, including bone marrow and GI mucosa, is a major source of side effects that complicate patient care. Improvements in cancer pharmacology have endeavored to maximize Methotrexate's effectiveness by altering methods of drug delivery and devising resistance countermeasures, including leucovorin rescue to salvage normal cells. In spite of its limitations, Methotrexate is highly versatile, being effective against leukemias, lymphomas, and solid tumors. Its use in multidrug regimens is the paradigm of chemotherapy, depending on synergistic drug interactions to increase anticancer efficacy while reducing toxicity (Ramakrishna et al., 2025). The field of cancer chemotherapy continues to advance with novel strategies such as drug repurposing, which explores current molecules for new anticancer uses. While Methotrexate's place is firmly established in the traditional world of chemotherapy, elucidation of its mechanism of action draws out the increasing interest in metabolic control as a therapeutic target. An analogy can be made with antidiabetic therapy, such as metformin, which also regulates cellular metabolism and has promise for being used synergistically with traditional agents like Methotrexate. This convergence of metabolic and folate pathway inhibition may have implications for future strategies that increase drug sensitivity and overcome drug resistance in cancer cells. Ongoing research is necessary to define these combined metabolic effects and maximize the clinical efficacy of drugs such as Methotrexate in combination regimens.

Test Your Knowledge

1. What is cisplatin and its primary use in cancer therapy?
2. How does doxorubicin intercalate into DNA?

11.4. Side Effects of Chemotherapy

Learning Outcome

1. Nausea and Vomiting
2. Hair Loss
3. Immunosuppression

The administration of chemotherapy, while pivotal in cancer treatment, introduces a range of adverse effects stemming from its impact on both cancerous and healthy cells (Figure 11.9). Chemotherapeutic agents typically target rapidly dividing cells, which, beyond malignancies, include essential normal cells such as those in the bone marrow, GI tract, and hair follicles. As a result, patients tend to develop such symptoms as fatigue, nausea, hair loss, and infection susceptibility because of the suppression of bone marrow. These non-specific toxicities threaten treatment tolerability and patient quality of life, and on occasion, require dosage adjustments or treatment delays. Progress in drug delivery systems, including nanomaterials, aims to alleviate these side effects through increasing selectivity for cancer cells and sparing normal tissue while decreasing systemic toxicity. Nanotechnology-based strategies hold the potential to enhance therapeutic indices and reduce collateral cytotoxicity, though more research is needed for clinical application and common use (Kumar et al., 2023). In addition to conventional chemotherapeutic agents, development of targeted therapies and immunomodulatory drugs has opened up alternative patterns of toxicity. Immune checkpoint inhibitors, as an example, revolutionize cancer care by restoring host immunity against cancer. These drugs selectively inhibit immune checkpoints such as CTLA-4 and PD-1, breaking tumor-induced immunosuppression. While overall less toxic than standard chemotherapy, immune checkpoint inhibitors can cause immune-related adverse events. These may be as mild as rash and fatigue or as severe as inflammatory syndromes involving organs such as the lung and intestine. Grasping such specific toxicities is important to effective management and is part of current efforts to individualize cancer treatment regimens to optimize efficacy while limiting side effects (Norah, 2023). The complex nature of chemotherapy side effects requires an interdisciplinary approach to the management of patients. Supportive care interventions such as antiemetics, growth factor support, and nutritional interventions are important in preventing chemotherapy-related complications. Additionally, new technologies such as nanomaterial-based drug delivery aim not only to enhance the specificity of chemotherapeutic targeting but also to increase bioavailability and diminish multidrug resistance, which is frequently responsible for treatment failure as well as further toxicity. Combining these new approaches could have the potential to transform cancer chemotherapy by equalizing high anti-cancer efficacy with a better side effect profile. Ongoing multi-disciplinary investigations and clinical authentication continue to be critical to be able to fulfill the complete capacity of these discoveries to minimize chemotherapy-induced side effect burden (Kumar et al., 2023).

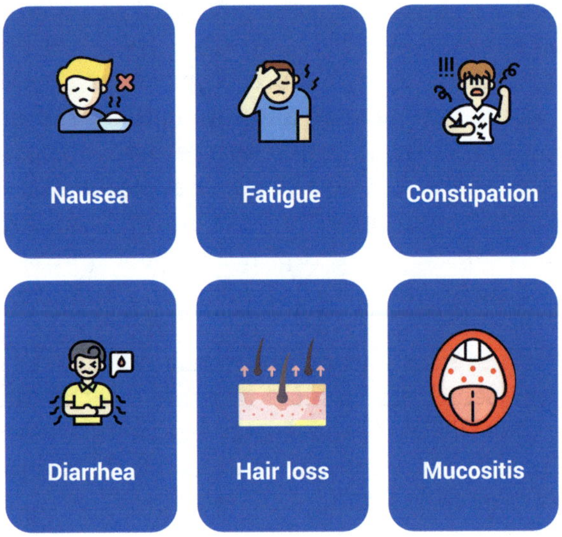

Figure 11.9. Side effects of chemotherapy.

ACTC Health (2016). *6 Ways to Deal with Chemotherapy Side Effects.*

Source: https://actchealth.com/images/way-to-deal/6-Ways-to-Deal-with-Chemotherapy-Side-effects-02.png.

11.4.1. Nausea and Vomiting

The delivery of chemotherapy, although critical to cancer therapy, tends to introduce considerable issues regarding patient comfort and compliance because of its side effects. Of these, nausea and vomiting are the most uncomfortable and frequent adverse effects (Figure 11.10). These are not only unpleasant but can have a serious impact on a patient's capacity to sustain nutrition and hydration, thereby compromising overall treatment success. The mechanisms are multi-faceted neurochemical pathways caused by anticancer agent's emetogenic activity, with much variation based on the drug and individual factors. Knowledge of chemotherapy-induced nausea and vomiting (CINV) pathophysiology has facilitated the division into acute, delayed, and anticipatory phases. These divisions assist in pharmacological management tailored to individual needs, lowering morbidity from cancer chemotherapy (Nandeesh et al., 2017). Proper management is essential in order to improve quality of life and prevent the interruption of therapy. Due to the multi-modal nature of CINV, combination regimens of drugs acting on multiple pathways have been pivotal in its control. Serotonin (5-HT3) receptor antagonists, corticosteroids, and neurokinin-1 (NK-1) receptor antagonists are the basis for prophylaxis against both acute and delayed emesis. These drugs work by disrupting the transmission of emetic messages in the central nervous system (CNS) and GI tract, thereby inhibiting the onset and spread of nausea and vomiting attacks. Although certain older agents, including dopamine antagonists and benzodiazepines, have uses in certain situations, their reduced therapeutic windows and side effect profiles restrict general use. Compliance with published clinical guidelines on antiemetic treatment not only enhances patient tolerability to intensive chemotherapy regimens but also decreases hospitalizations and healthcare expenditure, highlighting the economic and human benefit of maximizing CINV control (Nandeesh et al., 2017). Beyond the realm of pharmacology, patient-centered strategies augment the effectiveness of nausea and vomiting management during chemotherapy. Specialist cancer nursing teams have identified the importance of well-informed patient participation in efficient control of CINV. The creation of educational resources, including Patient Charters, enables patients to take an active role in care through comprehension of the rationale for antiemetic treatment and promotion of best symptom relief. These measures assist in reconciling therapeutic approaches with the needs and wishes of patients and enhance communication between healthcare professionals and patients. Integration of patient education in addition to pharmacologic measures recognizes the psychosocial aspects of CINV and encourages a more complete approach to care that maximizes compliance and psychologic well-being.

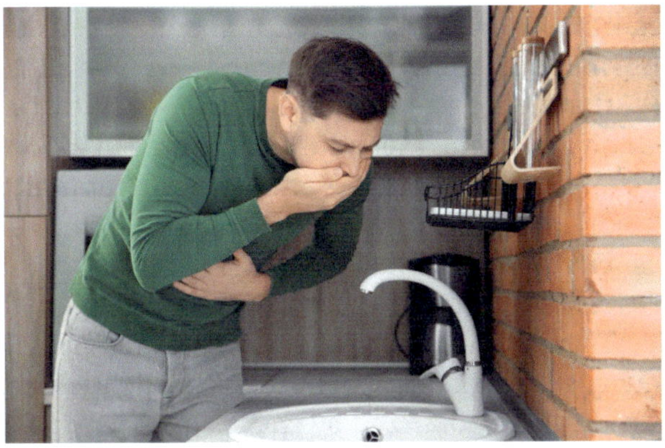

Figure 11.10. Nausea and vomiting.

Source: Apollo Hospitals (2021). *Nausea and Vomiting*. https://cdn.apollohospitals.com/health-library-prod/2021/05/Nausea-and-Vomiting-scaled.jpg.

11.4.2. Hair Loss

The side effects of cancer chemotherapy go beyond attacking malignant cells and tend to affect rapidly dividing normal tissues. Among them, the hair follicle is particularly vulnerable because of its intense mitotic activity during the anagen phase of hair growth. Chemotherapeutic drugs, particularly antimitotic drugs, cause damage that presents as chemotherapy-induced alopecia (CIA), a disconcerting condition occurring in about 65% of patients being treated. Pathophysiology comprises the disruption of mitosis in hair matrix keratinocytes, followed by mitotic arrest, apoptosis, and trachele d premature regression of hair follicles (Figure 11.11). This mechanistic understanding is best demonstrated with taxane-class drugs, which cause stabilization of microtubules and interference with segregation of chromosomes, leading to mitotic catastrophe and eventual cell death of the follicles. The clinical impact of chemotherapy-induced alopecia goes beyond appearance to adversely affect patients' psychological status and drug compliance, emphasizing the urgent need for valid preventive and therapeutic interventions (Tongyu et al., 2023). More recent work has refined the cellular and molecular pathways behind taxane-induced alopecia, showing that these drugs cause injury not only to cycling hair matrix keratinocytes but also to the relatively quiescent stem/progenitor cell populations in the outer root sheath of the hair follicle. Damage to the stem cells is of particular importance since it most likely explains why hair loss after taxane chemotherapy so frequently is permanent. Studies employing ex vivo human hair follicle cultures have shown impressive elevations in mitotic defects, micronucleation, and markers of DNA damage within keratin 15-positive stem/progenitor niches, alongside apoptosis induction. Dysfunction of these regenerative compartments undercuts the hair follicles capacity to re-enter normal cycling following treatment, resulting in persistent alopecia. These observations suggest that the design of chemotherapy regimens and the adjunctive protective therapy must include consideration of preserving stem cells in order to abrogate the enduring sequelae of anticancer therapies (Talveen et al., 2019). To meet the critical effects of chemotherapy-induced hair loss requires, in addition to its pathogenesis, devising specific interventions. At present, scalp cooling is the only FDA-approved prophylactic treatment for CIA, although its effectiveness is heterogeneous and circumscribed by practical and economic limitations. Motivated by the mechanism of taxane cytotoxicity, preclinical research has investigated pharmacological cell cycle arrest as a protective modality, using agents such as CDK4/6 inhibitors to temporarily pause cell division in hair follicle cells. This strategy seeks to make hair follicle keratinocytes and stem/progenitor cells less susceptible to disruption of mitosis by chemotherapeutics. Proofs from ex vivo assays indicate that inhibition of CDK4/6 can salvage these cells from taxane-triggered apoptosis without causing premature catagen, providing a promising route for maintaining hair follicle integrity during chemotherapy. Such new therapeutic approaches may dramatically enhance the quality of life and treatment adherence of patients by reversing one of the most psychologically distressing side effects of cancer chemotherapy (Talveen et al., 2019; Tongyu et al., 2023).

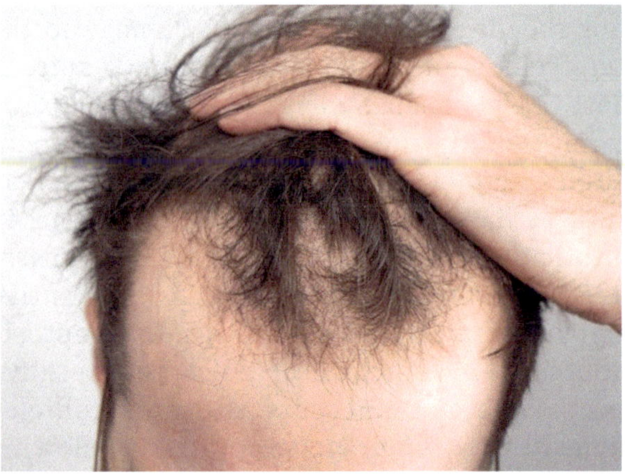

Figure 11.11. Hair loss.

Source: Hair Loss Causes. (n.d.). *Hair Loss Causes Diagram*. https://cdn.prod.website-files.com/63088c0ccad86b7cdf197d7a/65cf3278a9f36e303311239b_Hair%20Loss%20Causes.jpg.

11.4.3. Immunosuppression

The intricate interactions in the tumor microenvironment (TME) play a major role in the immunosuppressive condition seen in most cancer patients treated with chemotherapy (Figure 11.12). Cancer cells use nearby immune and stromal cells, such as T regulatory cells and monocytes, to produce a local milieu conducive to tumor survival by suppressing efficient immune responses. This immunosuppressive environment is sustained by pro-inflammatory cytokines like interleukin 6 and macrophage migration inhibitory factor, which not only enhance oncogenic signaling but also enhance immune escape mechanisms. Chemotherapy, although effective against the rapidly proliferating tumor cells, may inadvertently worsen this suppression by affecting immune cell function, eroding the host's natural antitumor immune response. The resulting immune dysfunctional state poses an enormous challenge in cancer therapy, calling for the generation of therapies that target tumor cells and the immunosuppressive TME to renew immune surveillance and enhance clinical outcomes (Wen et al., 2022). Tumor-associated macrophages (TAMs) are central as critical regulators of immunosuppression in the TME, having an impact on tumor growth and chemoresistance. These macrophages are attracted and polarized by chemokines produced by tumor cells, including CCL2 and CXCL12, which direct their invasion and regulatory activities. TAMs enhance tumor development through the release of factors that repress productive anti-tumor immune responses and facilitate angiogenesis and maintain an immunologically tolerant microenvironment. The crosstalk between TAMs and cancer cells highlights potential therapeutic targets; specifically, chemokine receptor antagonists have emerged as promising agents to disrupt this pathological communication. By modulating TAM recruitment and activity, combining these antagonists with chemotherapy or immune checkpoint inhibitors could mitigate immunosuppression and potentiate anti-cancer immunity (Qin et al., 2022). Clinical treatment of cancer more and more appreciates the need to counteract immunosuppression that is elicited by both TME and chemotherapy treatments. Standard care with chemotherapy and radiotherapy usually meets its limits in terms of tumor-mediated immune tolerance, which dampens the effectiveness of the therapy and contributes to resistance. Immune checkpoint therapy holds promise by restoring silenced cytotoxic T cells, yet its efficacy is often thwarted by the chronic immunosuppressive milieu orchestrated by the diverse cellular and molecular elements in the TME. Effective strategies that integrate cytotoxic therapies with immunomodulatory agents targeting suppressive TME constituents are pivotal in inducing long-lasting responses. This holistic view highlights the need to grasp immune evasion strategies in chemotherapy treatments with a focus on maximizing therapeutic benefit through reconstitution of strong anti-tumor immunity (Qin et al., 2022; Wen et al., 2022).

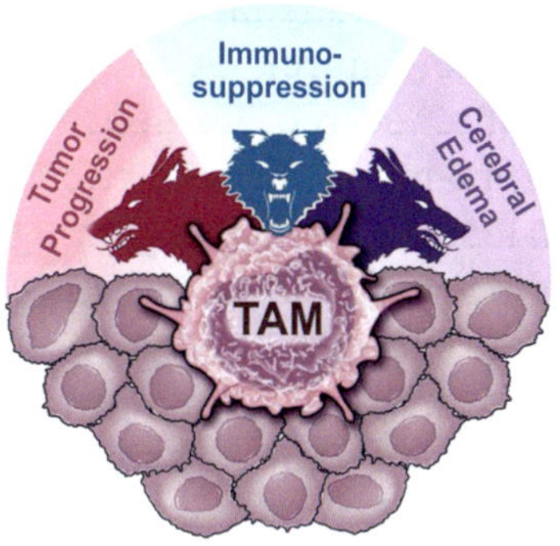

Figure 11.12. Immunosuppression tumor-associated macrophages (TAMs).

Source: Sulieman, A. M. (2021). *Tumor-Associated Macrophages (TAMs): The Cerberus of Glioblastoma (GBM).* https://www.researchgate.net/publication/350384801/figure/fig5/AS:11431281115905568@1675137562466/Tumor-associated-macrophages-TAMs-The-Cerberus-of-glioblastoma-GBM-Representation.png.

Test Your Knowledge

1. Why is it a concern during chemotherapy?
2. What is tumor microenvironment (TME)?

11.5. Targeted Therapy Versus Traditional Chemotherapy

Learning Outcome

1. Definition of Targeted Therapy
2. Comparison of Effectiveness
3. Differences in Side Effects

The history of cancer therapy has witnessed a critical transition away from general-purpose chemical toxins towards more advanced drug delivery systems. Conventional chemotherapy, based mostly on cytotoxic chemicals that indiscriminately attack dividing cells, tends to produce harmful side effects because it is not very specific, striking both normal and malignant cells. This nonspecific method, though successful in decreasing tumor burden, does so at the expense of patient quality of life by destroying tissues like the bone marrow, GI tract, and hair follicles. The emergence of targeted therapies with protein-based nanocarriers represents a major advancement in cancer pharmacology. These nanocarriers, designed to identify and bind to certain surface receptors on cancer cells, improve drug concentration in malignant tissue and spare healthy cells, thus minimizing systemic toxicity. Their biocompatibility and biodegradability also ensure less concern about safety owing to the use of synthetic delivery agents. Targeted delivery not only improves therapeutic outcomes but also opens avenues for extremely individualized cancer treatment modalities (Theivendren et al., 2025). In the wake of heightened requirements in targeting accuracy, lipid-based nanoparticles (LBNPs) have been a leading vehicle in gaining enhanced therapeutic effects in oncology. In contrast to conventional chemotherapeutic drugs that usually face barriers such as limited solubility and systemic toxicity, LBNPs bring about several specific benefits such as enhanced stability of the drug, controlled delivery, and selective tumor targeting by active and passive means. Liposomes, solid lipid nanoparticles, and hybrid lipid-polymer nanoparticles represent diverse forms of LBNPs, each tailored to optimize drug delivery and minimize off-target effects. These nanoparticles exploit enhanced permeability and retention effects within tumor microenvironments, facilitating preferential drug accumulation. Furthermore, advances in production techniques such as microfluidics enable precise control over size and surface properties, thus enhancing targeting capabilities. The combination of responsive delivery systems enables on-demand drug release, enhancing dose efficiency and patient tolerability. These advances in lipid-based delivery highlight the revolutionary potential of nanotechnology in transcending the limitations inherent in conventional chemotherapy (Chauhan et al., 2025). Even with the promising features of targeted therapies and nanocarrier systems, there are still challenges in fully substituting conventional chemotherapy. Challenges such as immunogenicity, bulk production, and stringent quality control pose barriers to clinical translation and universal adoption. Conventional chemotherapy, although less specific, enjoys decades of clinical history and established protocols, which render it universally accessible and standardly effective against a wide variety of cancer types. The success of targeted therapy is extremely dependent on the identification of suitable biomarkers and patient-specific molecular targets, rendering it more personalized but also more complicated. Moreover, drug resistance mechanisms will evolve against such targeted agents as well, forcing combination regimens that at times include traditional chemotherapy. Thus, an integrated regimen combining both therapies, taking the specificity of target therapy and broad effectiveness of chemotherapy, is envisioned to be most effective. Protein engineering and nanotechnology advancements will probably further develop this integrated model so that upcoming therapies are more efficient and less harmful to cancer patients (Chauhan et al., 2025; Theivendren et al., 2025).

11.5.1. Definition of Targeted Therapy

Cancer therapies have progressively changed their emphasis from traditional chemotherapeutic agents towards more targeted interventions that will eliminate as much damage to healthy cells as possible. Conventional chemotherapy, though good at destroying dividing cells, tends to have widespread toxicity as it is not very specific. As a response, a more sophisticated strategy called targeted therapy has been developed, aimed at disrupting certain molecular pathways implicated in tumor development and growth (Figure 11.13).

Contrary to conventional drugs that indiscriminately target dividing cells, targeted therapies are designed to identify specific biomarkers or genetic mutations specific to cancer cells. This specificity enables the creation of agents that inhibit essential signals or enzymes required for tumor survival, thus minimizing collateral damage and enhancing patient outcomes. Targeted therapy is a paradigm shift focusing on individualized treatment approaches and customized pharmacological interventions that form the basis of contemporary oncology (Alamir et al., 2015). The rationale for targeted therapy is based on the molecular diversity of cancer, being a heterogeneous array of genetic and epigenetic changes that propel the malignancy. By targeting individual-specific targets like tyrosine kinases, growth factor receptors, or mutated oncogenes, the treatments interfere with the cancer-specific mechanisms like cell proliferation, angiogenesis, and resistance to apoptosis. For example, tyrosine kinase inhibitors (TKIs) are examples of targeted agents that suppress enzymes involved in signal transduction pathways that are essential for the survival of cancer cells. This mode of treatment has been a specific success with some leukemias, such as Philadelphia chromosome-positive acute lymphoblastic leukemia (ALL), where treatment response and survival have improved dramatically with the application of TKIs. This kind of success demonstrates the ability of targeted therapy to take advantage of weaknesses inherent in the biology of the cancer instead of depending on diffuse cytotoxicity (Chiaretti et al., 2018). The establishment and delivery of targeted therapy entail extensive molecular characterization and knowledge of tumor biology per patient. Due to the potential for resistance or extreme variability between patients, treatments tend to be supplemented by targeting agents with chemotherapy or immunotherapy to maximize outcome. The intricacy of developing such treatments lies in probabilistic models that control uncertainties present in tumor behavior and patient response, making therapies both safe and effective. Such models inform scheduling and dosing to optimize tumor contraction while maintaining immune function, demonstrating a highly advanced approach to personalized medicine. Such therapeutic innovations in targeted therapy not only enhance prognostic estimates but also provide a more logical and flexible paradigm for the treatment of cancer with potential for lower toxicity and improved therapeutic specificity (Alamir et al., 2015).

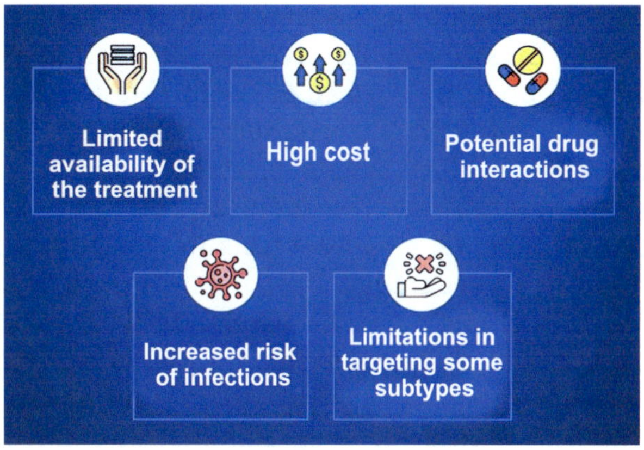

Figure 11.13. Definition of targeted therapy.

Source: ACTC. (n.d.). *Fight Breast Cancer with the Power of Targeted Therapy.* https://actchealth.com/images/fight-breast-cancer-with-the-power-of-targeted-therapy/03.webp.

11.5.2. Comparison of Effectiveness

Cancer therapy involves a multifaceted analysis of the different chemotherapeutic options due to differences in their efficacy based on tumor type as well as patient-related factors (Figure 11.14). For example, gemcitabine, which is frequently employed in pancreatic ductal adenocarcinoma, has shown restricted efficacy because the tumor microenvironments have the capacity to stimulate chemoresistance. Studies have shown that cancer-associated fibroblasts, when treated with gemcitabine, secrete exosomes that harbor microRNAs that inhibit major tumor suppressor genes like PTEN. This process reduces the efficacy of the drug's cytotoxic effect, resulting in worse prognosis despite rigorous treatment regimens. Knowledge of this interaction brings to the forefront the importance of targeting cancer cells as well as the supportive stromal microenvironment to increase chemotherapy efficacy, implying that the addition of adjunctive compounds like exosome inhibitors can better the prognosis in patients (Katherine et al., 2022). Another important consideration in evaluating the efficacy of chemotherapy medications is in the accurate dosing, which has a direct effect on the outcome of the treatment and toxicity levels. Classic dosing techniques commonly depend on body surface area (BSA) estimates using both height and weight measurements. In pediatric oncology, though, precise measurement difficulties require different measures. Research has confirmed a more straightforward BSA calculation technique based only on patient weight, yielding estimates within a 10% variation from standard methods. This simplified method ensures more consistent dosing reliability, which is critical for drug administration with narrow therapeutic windows. Although this strategy may improve chemotherapy accuracy and, subsequently, drug efficacy, care is needed in unique populations such as infants and cachectic individuals to prevent under- or overdosing (Sharkey et al., 2001). Comparing the efficacy of chemotherapeutic agents should take into consideration not only inherent drug characteristics but also aspects of drug resistance pathways and dosing precision. Chemoresistance, which is tumor microenvironment interaction and genetically mediated, can critically restrict the efficacy of otherwise effective agents such as gemcitabine. Standardized and precise dosing regimens are also necessary to optimize therapeutic benefit with minimal adverse effects, especially in susceptible populations such as pediatric patients. An integrative analysis of drug efficacy, thus, requires integration of molecular information and pharmacokinetic accuracy. In the future, cancer chemotherapy optimization will most probably rely on individualized strategies that target both resistance mechanisms and dosing schedules adjusted to patient-specific characteristics (Katherine et al., 2022; Sharkey et al., 2001).

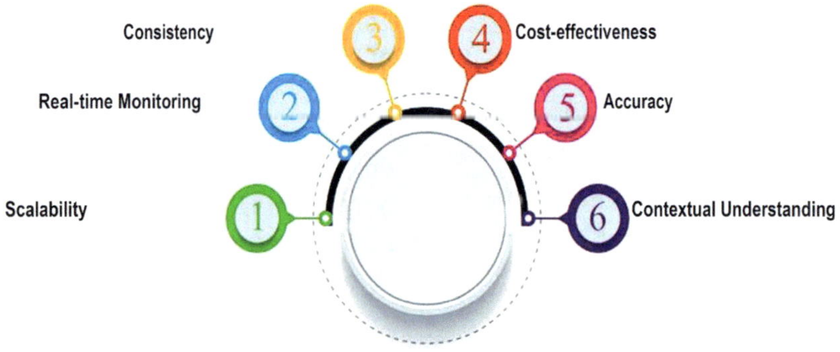

Figure 11.14. Comparison of effectiveness.

Source: https://encrypted-tbn0.gstatic.com/images?q=tbn:ANd9GcRcGJmcOrKQHKZ0DT70aOd0c97cBIZfiHf7rA&s.

11.5.3. Differences in Side Effects

The application of traditional chemotherapy agents for cancer treatment is usually followed by a wide range of side effects, mainly caused by the nonspecific mode of action of these drugs. The traditional chemotherapeutic agents act on the rapidly proliferating cells, which are not only the cancerous cells but also the normal cells like the cells present in the bone marrow, GI tract, and hair follicles. This non-selectivity causes typical side effects such as myelosuppression, mucositis, and alopecia that importantly affect patient quality of life. Additionally, severity and intensity of side effects are specific to the mechanism of action of each individual drug and its dosage regimen. For example, alkylating agents can induce long-term adverse effects like secondary malignancies, while antimetabolites are more commonly linked with GI toxicity. Such discrepancies highlight the problem of balancing therapeutic effectiveness with acceptable toxicity, spurring research for more targeted drug delivery systems in order to avoid damage to non-target tissue (Kumar et al., 2023). Recent nanotechnology has brought with it a new perspective to chemotherapy in cancer treatment by potentially overcoming the side effects normally associated with conventional therapy. Nanoparticles facilitate targeted delivery of chemotherapeutic agents exclusively to the tumor sites, minimizing systemic exposure and toxicity to the healthy tissues. The targeted delivery leads to a significantly altered side effect profile relative to traditional chemotherapy. For instance, polymeric nanoparticles have the ability to enhance drug bioavailability and stability, facilitating the release of the drug over time and lowering the peak plasma concentrations that tend to cause severe adverse effects. Moreover, surface modification of nanoparticles with targeted ligands allows for preferential tumor microenvironment accumulation, thus minimizing off-target effects like nephrotoxicity and cardiotoxicity. Even though nanoparticle-based treatments are not side effect-free, their decreased systemic effect is a huge leap in the field, which indicates a transition towards precision medicine in chemotherapy (Rizi et al., 2022). In addition to the promise of nanoparticle technologies, however, the variation in side effects also results from the distinct properties of the nanomaterials themselves, such as size, shape, and composition. Metal-based nanomaterials, for example, have shown both therapeutic effects and possible cytotoxicity based on their physicochemical properties. Smaller nanoparticles are more effective at penetrating tissues but can also cause oxidative stress and inflammation and result in unwanted toxicities. On the other hand, larger or specially shaped nanomaterials may avoid rapid immune system clearance, extending circulation time for drugs but also causing concerns regarding bioaccumulation and chronic toxicity. These subtle variations in side effects emphasize the need for rigorous preclinical screening to maximize nanomaterial design for optimal efficacy with fewer adverse consequences. Therefore, the understanding and management of the varied side effect profiles of both traditional and new chemotherapeutic agents are still critical to better cancer treatment outcomes (Kumar et al., 2023; Rizi et al., 2022).

Test Your Knowledge

1. What side effect is commonly caused by platinum-based chemotherapy agents like cisplatin?
2. What is targeted therapy in cancer treatment?

11.6. Advances in Chemotherapy

Learning Outcome

1. Development of New Drug Formulations
2. Personalized Medicine Approaches
3. Clinical Trials and Research

There has been tremendous advancement in cancer chemotherapy that has been facilitated through incorporation of nanotechnology, which has provided more accuracy in drug delivery and less systemic toxicity (Figure 11.15). Conventional chemotherapy tends to be faced with poor temporal as well as spatial control, leading to toxic side effects because of the non-specific targeting of healthy cells. Recent developments in nanomedicine using photons have brought forward innovative therapeutic strategies, such as photothermal therapy, photodynamic therapy, and photo responsive drug delivery systems, which utilize light-induced mechanisms to specifically target cancer cells. These strategies not only enhance localization of the drug but also utilize mechanisms such as hyperthermia and oxidative stress to amplify cytotoxic effects against tumors. Invention of novel nanomaterials with specific therapeutic applications further maximizes therapeutic efficacy and safety. Consequently, such novel therapies prove encouraging in preclinical studies with the potential for more powerful and less toxic chemotherapy in the near future (Baino et al., 2021). The increasing cost implications of advances in chemotherapy point to the nuanced interplay of medical innovation and resource allocation. For instance, in Australia, spending on advanced chemotherapy drugs has risen tremendously, a factor of increased demand for advanced treatments for fighting advanced cancers. Such programs that aim to enable access to these expensive drugs, like the Efficient Funding of Chemotherapy program, have witnessed high growth rates, highlighting the rising dependence on novel therapies as well as the significant economic costs they entail.

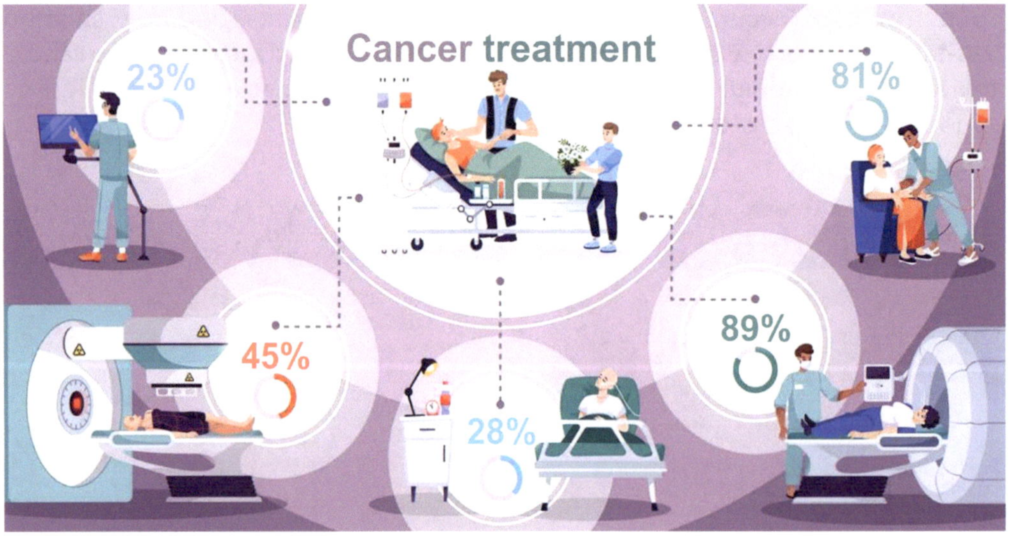

Figure 11.15. Advances in cancer chemotherapy.

Source: Sri Ramakrishna Hospital. (2021). *Latest Advancements in Cancer Treatment.* https://www.sriramakrishnahospital.com/wp-content/uploads/2021/06/Latest-Advancements-in-Cancer-Treatment.jpg.

Though such programs aim to provide even access to life-saving drugs, they also create challenges in addressing sustainability and cost-effectiveness within national healthcare systems. As cancer incidence increases around the world, ongoing growth of such funding arrangements will be necessary to support continued patient access in a timely manner without sacrificing the affordability of healthcare systems. New chemotherapy regimens are also facilitated by advancements in drug delivery and formulation, which seek to bypass resistance mechanisms and enhance patient benefits. Improved pharmacokinetic profiles obtained by the use of nanoparticle carriers or photo responsive systems provide controlled release and targeted localization in tumor tissue, overcoming the shortcomings of traditional cytotoxic drugs. In addition, these methods permit combination treatments that combine chemotherapy with adjunct therapies such as phototherapy, providing synergistic actions against drug resistant cancer cells. This intersection of technologies represents a paradigm shift away from a one-size-fits-all strategy towards personalized treatment regimens based on molecular understanding and material science. While clinical uptake is still in its infancy, these multidisciplinary advances hold the promise of optimizing the therapeutic index of chemotherapy agents, enhancing efficacy while reducing collateral damage to healthy cells (Baino et al., 2021).

11.6.1. Development of New Drug Formulations

The problem of selectively killing cancer cells with minimal damage to normal tissues continues to be a major impediment in cancer chemotherapy. Classical cytotoxic drugs, although highly effective, are generally nonselective and, therefore, produce extensive systemic toxicity. This constraint has prompted intensive efforts toward the creation of new drug delivery systems aimed at enhancing the therapeutic ratio of anticancer drugs. One of the more promising strategies is engineered carriers with site-specific localization and controlled release. For example, a new erythrocyte-based system includes magnetic targeting and viral fusion proteins to enable targeted delivery to cancer cells. These technologies not only increase malignant cell uptake of drugs but also lower the necessary dosage, thus decreasing side effects. This paradigm change in formulation development leads the charge toward more sophisticated, patient-specific chemotherapy regimens with enhanced safety and efficacy profiles (Cinti et al., 2011). In combination with cellular carriers, locoregional drug delivery has transformed delivery of chemotherapeutic drugs into inaccessible tumor sites. Systemic chemotherapy is generally ineffective in reaching peritoneal metastases because of physiological barriers and drug elimination. Recent advances such as Pressurized Intraperitoneal Aerosol Chemotherapy (PIPAC) overcome these challenges by aerosolizing medications under pressure directly into the peritoneal space. This approach improves medication distribution and allows deeper penetration into tumor nodules, with a potential for better clinical outcomes in peritoneal carcinomatosis. Moreover, PIPAC demonstrates the potential for harnessing physical and mechanical principles for drug optimization in delivering drugs, providing a solution to systemic toxicity that usually follows traditional regimens (Ceelen et al., 2019). The locoregional advancements broaden the arsenal against advanced cancers where traditional chemotherapy is still lacking. Nanotechnology is a revolutionary frontier to the development of innovative drug formulation in cancer chemotherapy. Nanomaterials facilitate the development of platforms with extended retention times and sustained release properties, overcoming the shortcomings of rapid clearance and less-than-optimal drug levels at tumor sites. Coupling nanocarriers with locoregional methods such as PIPAC maximizes the therapeutic impact by integrating targeted delivery with controlled pharmacokinetics. This intersection of nanotechnology and novel administration routes presents promising directions for the circumvention of multidrug resistance and bioavailability enhancement. In spite of significant advances, issues related to biocompatibility, toxicity, and manufacturing scalability remain, calling for ongoing interdisciplinary research. Nevertheless, the dynamic development of nanotherapeutics highlights the pivotal role of formulation science in leading cancer chemotherapy towards more efficient, personalized therapies (Ceelen et al., 2019).

11.6.2. Personalized Medicine Approaches

The intricacy of cancer treatment has long pushed against the uniform use of chemotherapy agents, with a move towards more personalized treatment approaches. Breakthroughs in cancer research today focus on the tumor microenvironments' influence on treatment outcomes, requiring patient-derived models that perfectly mimic this environment. These models, such as co-cultures of cancer cells with immune and stromal components, enable more accurate drug screening than standard cell lines. By applying such patient-specific models, scientists will be able to test the activity of many different compounds against a patients individual tumor molecular and cellular characteristics. By doing this, they have the potential to better treat disease while minimizing toxicity and resistance. Breast cancer research has already attested to the value of this approach by discovering naturally occurring compounds with targeted activity that also improve immune cell function in the tumor environment (Li et al., 2025). New technologies further enhance personalized chemotherapy by adding computational strategies to maximize the dosing schedule on the basis of multi-dimensional patient data. Conventional chemotherapy dosimetry tends to disregard the important physiological markers outside of tumor response, with a risk of side effects compromising patient health as a whole. To counteract this, novel frameworks using multi-objective decision-making and deep reinforcement learning are being created. These frameworks simulate tumor behavior in conjunction with biochemical markers to formulate treatment protocols balancing tumor annihilation with the preservation of normal physiological processes.

Through the simulation of multiple treatment regimens on patient-specific data, such algorithms can decrease treatment time and minimize side effects better than existing methodologies. This incorporation of artificial intelligence into chemotherapy design is a major step toward the realization of truly personalized medicine, moving away from one-size-fits-all regimens towards customized, adaptive treatment plans (Huo et al., 2022). The union of patient-derived experimental models and computational optimization methods represents the future of personalized oncology therapeutics. By leveraging precise biological information from patient tissue samples and pairing it with advanced algorithmic decision-making, clinicians are able to more accurately predict individual response to chemotherapeutic agents. This synergy not only increases drug efficacy by targeting pathways unique to the tumor microenvironment but also reduces systemic toxicity, enhancing quality of life during treatment. In addition, the incorporation of immune components into these models enables the investigation of the immunomodulatory actions of chemotherapy, an essential aspect in current cancer treatment. Personalized practices that draw on both biological and computing advances are a revolution in chemotherapy, ultimately leading to treatments tailored to each individual's particular cancer biology and physiological condition (Figure 11.16) (Huo et al., 2022; Li et al., 2025).

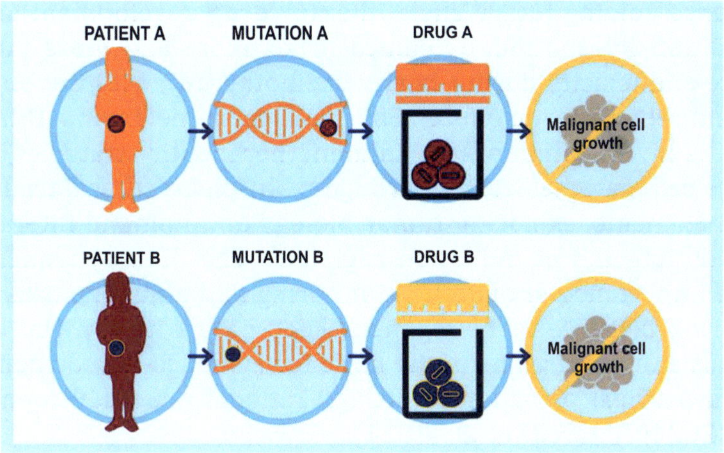

Figure 11.16. Personalized medicine approaches.

Source: Labroots. (n.d.). *Personalized Medicine Approaches.* https://d3bkbkx82g74b8.cloudfront.net/eyJidWNrZXQiOiJsYWJyb290cy1hc3NldHMiLCJrZXkiOiJfcHVibGljXC9fZmlsZXNcL3N5c3RlbVwvY2tcL3RyZW5kaW5nXC9GUCAtIFByZWNpc2lvbiBNZWQgUGFydCBJXzUzNz M0YWY3ZTkz ZTM3YzU1YTZiNTg3MzAzYTI3YWVhLnBuZyIsIm VkaXRzIjp7InJlc2l6ZSI6ey J3aWR0aCI 6MTQw MCwiZm l0Ijoi Y292ZXIifX19.

11.6.3. Clinical Trials and Research

The establishment of useful cancer chemotherapy medicines is largely based on the strict procedure of clinical trials and studies, which need to examine systematically the safety and effectiveness of the new drugs before they reach general marketability (Figure 11.17). Early-phase clinical trials are used to define the best doses and to find out about adverse effects, whereas later phases examine therapeutic effectiveness in increasing numbers of patients. This formal process guarantees that drugs showing significant clinical advantages with feasible toxicities will only advance to routine care. An example in the setting of advanced malignant melanoma is that adding systemic chemotherapy to innovative immunotherapies and targeted agents has been investigated through well-delineated clinical trials to be able to overcome resistance and provide better outcomes. The incorporation of molecular markers and genetic profiling in these trials enables more individualized treatment approaches that can maximize efficacy while reducing harm. Such adaptive research studies are essential to the development of chemotherapy regimens and enhancing survival rates in cancer patients (Natarelli et al., 2024). Meta-analyses combining evidence from several randomized controlled trials (RCTs) offer important insights into the effectiveness of combination therapies in oncology research. A case in point is the comparison of anti-angiogenic therapies in combination with chemotherapy for ovarian cancer, which showed promising improvements in progression-free survival (PFS) and objective response rates (ORR) over chemotherapy alone. Yet, these advantages tend to be associated with higher rates of severe adverse effects, indicating the need for a fine balance between therapeutic gain and toxicity. Trial sequential analysis and robust statistical designs enhance the reliability of these outcomes by limiting likely biases and verifying adequate sample sizes. Such holistic research methodologies not only inform clinical decision-making but also recognize specific areas in which new therapeutic compounds or better supportive care are necessary, hence guiding future chemotherapy drug development and clinical guidelines (He et al., 2024). Additionally, continuous clinical trials more and more target the mechanisms behind drug resistance and toxicity during cancer chemotherapy, with the objective of maximizing treatment regimens and reducing side effects. For instance, in melanoma, BRAF and MEK inhibitor resistance has led to the investigation of new immunotherapeutic strategies, including checkpoint inhibitors and adoptive cell therapies, tested through multi-phase clinical trials. These trials involve translational research elements, exploring tumor biology and immune interactions in an effort to optimize therapeutic targets and combination regimens. The fluid dynamics of clinical oncology research highlight the importance of ongoing monitoring and adjustment as new drugs enter the clinical pipeline, assuring that treatment regimens keep pace with growing scientific knowledge. Ultimately, clinical trials and research form the basis for evidence-based chemotherapy, improving the quality of life and survival of patients through rational drug development and therapeutic innovation (He et al., 2024; Natarelli et al., 2024).

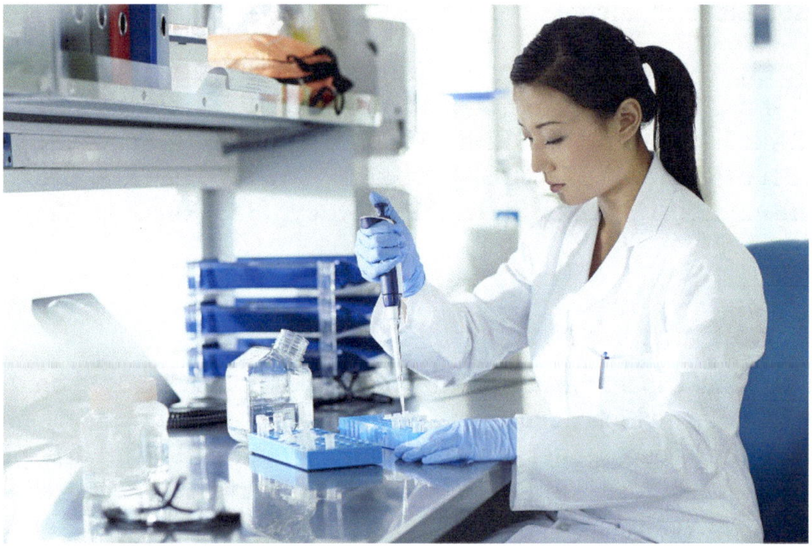

Figure 11.17. Clinical trials and research.

Source: Morsa Images (2014). *Scientist Pipetting Samples Into Eppendorf Tubes in Research Laboratory*. GettyImages. https://www.verywellhealth.com/thmb/f9422YJMZGTQa4QEiFELO_XfwPk=/1500x0/filters:no_upscale():max_bytes(150000):strip_icc()/GettyImages-487041745-5a5621df89eacc003785712e.jpg.

Test Your Knowledge

1. What is a clinical trial?
2. How does personalized medicine differ from traditional medicine?

SUMMARY

Development in cancer chemotherapy has profoundly influenced treatment outcomes, mirroring a multifaceted interrelationship among drug choice, genetics, and clinical practices. The careful manipulation and preparation of cytostatic drugs are essential for optimal efficacy and patient safety, highlighting the need for conformity to strict standards of preparation and administration. Adequate management protocols, such as aseptic procedures and control of toxicities, help with maximized therapeutic effects while limiting harm to patients and healthcare workers. However, challenges continue to exist in achieving proper dosing, especially considering differences in individual patient reactions and types of cancer. The noted inconsistencies in dose precision and labeling further underscore the necessity of sustained vigilance and precision in chemotherapy administration to enhance overall treatment efficacy and minimize adverse outcomes (Amelia et al., 2024). In addition, genetic tumor heterogeneity has become a critical determinant in chemotherapy responsiveness, informing individualized treatment strategies. Tumour mutations in oncogenes like BRAF and NRAS in melanoma are a demonstration of how molecular analysis will guide drug choice and foretell therapeutic success. In particular, the variable sensitivity of BRAF and NRAS mutant cells to a given array of chemotherapeutic drugs supports the need to incorporate genetic data into clinical decision-making. Accommodating these molecular foundations enables clinicians to individualize treatments, with the potential to strengthen effects by taking advantage of genotype-specific vulnerabilities, for instance, targeting nucleotide synthesis pathways in RAS mutant melanomas (Arozarena et al., 2014). Ultimately, the future of cancer chemotherapy resides at the convergence of deliberate pharmaceutical manipulation and molecularly guided therapeutic approaches. Ensuring strict compliance with handling protocols is vital for maintaining drug integrity and patient safety, while advancements in genetic characterization are transforming treatment paradigms into more targeted and effective regimens. Together, these elements advocate for a multidisciplinary approach, where meticulous preparation complements personalized medicine to maximize efficacy and minimize toxicity. Through the encouragement of ongoing research and incorporation of genetic findings, oncology can move towards safer and much more effective chemotherapy approaches, promising hope for better survival and quality of life for cancer patients (Amelia et al., 2024; Arozarena et al., 2014).

Summary of Key Points

The onset of chemoresistance is a major hurdle in the efficacy of cancer chemotherapy, especially in ovarian and breast cancers. The latest studies have emphasized important molecular mechanisms responsible for resistance to traditionally used agents like paclitaxel. For example, in paclitaxel-resistant ovarian cancer cells, the co-administration of deguelin with paclitaxel has been shown with promising outcomes. Deguelin resensitizes drug-resistant cells by inhibiting and reducing the expression of EGFR and its downstream signaling molecules, such as AKT, ERK, and STAT3. It also modulates pro-survival proteins of the BCL-2 family, including ultimately enhancing apoptotic processes and enhancing chemotherapy sensitivity. These observations stress targeted molecular therapy in the reversal of drug resistance, providing one potential route for the enhancement of currently available chemotherapeutic treatment (Bae et al., 2024). This strategy is essential for creating drugs that can effectively treat resistant tumors and enhance patient outcomes. Analysis of heterogeneity in cancer cell populations also helps to better define resistance mechanisms and inform therapeutic strategies. Single-cell RNA sequencing of paclitaxel-treated triple-negative breast cancer has recognized specific subsets of cells responsible for drug resistance. Of these subsets, those with AKR1C3, IDO1, and HEY1 signatures rise in incidence with extended exposure to drugs and correlate with increased inflammatory and interferon responses. Transcriptional regulators like STAT1, CEBPB, and IRF7 become essential transcription factors for developing resistance. Knowing these molecular actors offers a blueprint for combinatorial targeted therapies that can slow the progression of chemotherapy resistance. The understanding obtained through these cellular and molecular descriptions suggests direction towards custom treatment regimens designed to evade resistance mechanisms (Gao et al., 2024). In the process of synthesizing these results, it becomes apparent that successful cancer chemotherapy not only depends on drugs' cytotoxicity but also on circumventing adaptive resistance processes at the cell level. Combination strategies involving standard agents such as paclitaxel along with inhibitors of resistance-related pathways, including EGFR activation or transcription factor function, show a hopeful direction for clinical and research studies. The application of molecular biology methods together with pharmacology allows identification of new agents capable of re-establishing chemosensitivity. Finally, all of these advances highlight the need for personalized medicine strategies in oncology, where tumor biology and treatment response guide intelligent drug design and combination therapy to achieve better survival rates and quality of life for cancer patients.

KEY TERMS FROM THIS CHAPTER

- Chemotherapy
- Adverse drug reactions (ADRs)
- Modulate immune
- Cancer Chemotherapy
- Repair Inhibition
- Mechanism
- Antiemetic
- Central nervous system (CNS)
- Cancer Treatment
- Gastrointestinal (GI)
- Nevertheless
- Plant Alkaloids
- Chemotherapeutic drugs
- Tumor microenvironment (TME)
- Pharmacokinetics
- Targeted Therapy

CRITICAL THINKING QUESTIONS

1. **Which of the following is an antimetabolite used in cancer chemotherapy?**
   a. Vincristine
   b. Doxorubicin
   c. Methotrexate
   d. Cyclophosphamide
2. **Alkylating agents exert their effect by:**
   a. Inhibiting mitosis
   b. Interfering with RNA transcription
   c. Binding to tubulin
   d. Forming cross-links in DNA
3. **Which of the following is a natural plant alkaloid used in cancer therapy?**
   a. Cisplatin
   b. Vinblastine
   c. Methotrexate
   d. Imatinib
4. **Which drug is a monoclonal antibody used in HER2-positive breast cancer?**
   a. Bevacizumab
   b. Rituximab
   c. Trastuzumab
   d. Cetuximab
5. **What is the major dose-limiting toxicity of cisplatin?**
   a. Cardiotoxicity
   b. Nephrotoxicity
   c. Neurotoxicity
   d. Pulmonary fibrosis

Short Answer Questions

1. Explain the different types of chemotherapy drugs based on their mechanism of action and provide examples of each?
2. Explain the mechanisms of action of various classes of chemotherapy drugs?
3. Discuss the pharmacological profile of five commonly used chemotherapy drugs?
4. Discuss the common systemic and organ-specific side effects of chemotherapy?
5. Compare and contrast targeted therapy and traditional chemotherapy?
6. What is the advantage of using liposomal drug formulations in chemotherapy?

Answer to Critical Thinking Questions

1. (c) 2 (d) 3. (b) 4. (c) 5. (b)

REFERENCES

1. Aapro, M., Alphin, R., Andrews, P. L. R., Andrews, W., Andrews, D., André, T., Beleslin, D., et al. (2015). Nausea: Current knowledge of mechanisms, measurement and clinical impact. https://core.ac.uk/download/36778224.pdf (accessed on 9 May 2025).
2. Acharyya, S., Affara, N. I., Ahn, J., Ahn, J., Albanesi, J. P., Alizadeh, A. A., Anders, R. A., et al. (2015). Immune-mediated mechanisms influencing the efficacy of anticancer therapies. https://core.ac.uk/download/46558916.pdf.
3. Alamir, M. (2015). On probabilistic certification of combined cancer therapies using strongly uncertain models. *arXiv preprint.* http://arxiv.org/abs/1502.06218 (accessed on 9 May 2025).
4. Alturki, N. A. (2023). Review of the immune checkpoint inhibitors in the context of cancer treatment. *Journal of Clinical Medicine, 12.* https://www.semanticscholar.org/paper/82c09491941ef812154b810393945e74e08d422f (accessed on 9 May 2025).
5. Amelia, K., Emilda, K., & Tri, A. (2024). Observation of the reconstitution process and factors that influence the final condition of chemotherapy patients in private hospitals. https://core.ac.uk/download/622347478.pdf (accessed on 9 May 2025).
6. Andreotti, A. M., Batchelor, T., Corrie, P., Coxon, F., Cree, I. A., et al. (2013). Designing personalized cancer treatments. https://core.ac.uk/download/19444179.pdf (accessed on 9 May 2025).
7. Arozarena, I., Erice, O., Ferguson, J., & Goicoechea, L., et al. (2014). Differential chemosensitivity to antifolate drugs between RAS and BRAF melanoma cells. https://core.ac.uk/download/30731402.pdf (accessed on 9 May 2025).
8. Bae, S., Bae, S., Kim, H. S., Lim, Y. J., Kim, G., Park, I. C., So, K., et al. (2024). Deguelin restores paclitaxel sensitivity in paclitaxel-resistant ovarian cancer cells via inhibition of the EGFR signaling pathway. *Cancer Management and Research, 16*, 507–525. https://www.semanticscholar.org/paper/5c1a700d1f682bee15497bec759f9c192ae4fc4e (accessed on 9 May 2025).
9. Bagdasaryan, A. A., Chubarev, V. N., Smolyarchuk, E. A., Drozdov, V. N., Krasnyuk, I. I., Liu, J., Fan, R., et al. (2022). Pharmacogenetics of drug metabolism: The role of gene polymorphism in the regulation of doxorubicin safety and efficacy. *Cancers, 14*, 5436. https://doi.org/10.3390/cancers14215436.
10. Baino, F., Borges, R., de Oliveira, S. A., de Souza, A. C. S., Marchi, J., Rosa, D. S., & Seabra, A. B. (2021). Strategies for cancer treatment based on photonic nanomedicine. https://core.ac.uk/download/524608996.pdf (accessed on 9 May 2025).
11. Bruns, C. J., Fürst, R., Garczarczyk, D., & Ischenko, I., et al. (2009). Investigation of the marine compound spongistatin 1 links the inhibition of PKCα translocation to nonmitotic effects of tubulin antagonism in angiogenesis. https://core.ac.uk/download/12174630.pdf.
12. Bukowski, K., Kciuk, M., & Kontek, R. (2020). Mechanisms of multidrug resistance in cancer chemotherapy. *International Journal of Molecular Sciences, 21.* https://www.semanticscholar.org/paper/371e44b8d72cb32e2df0b54ea36c144300ec1c82 (accessed on 9 May 2025).
13. Carlesimo, M., Caro, G., Fortuna, M. C., & Garelli, M., et al. (2017). Chemotherapy-induced alopecia management: Clinical experience and practical advice. https://core.ac.uk/download/98339039.pdf (accessed on 9 May 2025).

14. Ceelen, W., De Smedt, S., Remaut, K., & Shariati, M., et al. (2019). Aerosolization of nanotherapeutics as a newly emerging treatment regimen for peritoneal carcinomatosis.

15. Chauhan, A. S., Chand, P., & Parashar, T. (2025). Lipid-based nanoparticles: Strategy for targeted cancer therapy. *BIO Integration*. https://www.semanticscholar.org/paper/88d0e48807a6bb280061855698bdf6e9db2607c1 (accessed on 9 May 2025).

16. Chiaretti, S., Hoelzer, D., & Jabbour, E. (2018). "Society of Hematologic Oncology (SOHO) State of the Art Updates and Next Questions"—Treatment of ALL. https://core.ac.uk/download/159268471.pdf (accessed on 9 May 2025).

17. Cinti, C., Grimaldi, S., Naldi, I., Taranta, M., et al. (2011). Newly engineered magnetic erythrocytes for sustained and targeted delivery of anti-cancer therapeutic compounds. https://core.ac.uk/download/pdf/8530727.pdf.

18. De Boer, R., & Harvey, R. (2025). *Growth in Expenditure on High-Cost Drugs in Australia*. https://core.ac.uk/download/pdf/30672977.pdf (accessed on 9 May 2025).

19. De Felice, F., Marampon, F., Marchetti, C., Musella, A., et al. (2017). Defective DNA repair mechanisms in prostate cancer: Impact of olaparib. https://core.ac.uk/download/141694834.pdf (accessed on 9 May 2025).

20. Dhas, Y., Biswas, N., Divyalakshmi, M. R., Jones, L. D., & Ashili, S. (2024). Repurposing metabolic regulators: Antidiabetic drugs as anticancer agents. *Molecular Biomedicine, 5*. https://www.semanticscholar.org/paper/306e67ca3167c15fc9b697f537b4194826db78d7 (accessed on 9 May 2025).

21. Di Giacomo, S., Di Sotto, A., Eufemi, M., Gulli, M., et al. (2020). Modulation of STAT3 signaling, cell redox defenses and cell cycle checkpoints by β-caryophyllene in cholangiocarcinoma cells: Possible mechanisms accounting for doxorubicin chemo sensitization and chemoprevention. https://core.ac.uk/download/323192192.pdf (accessed on 9 May 2025).

22. Dielenseger, P., Fernandez Ortega, P., Fernandez Perez, D., Jones, A., et al. (2013). Helping patients discuss CINV management: Development of a patient charter. https://core.ac.uk/download/16662894.pdf (accessed on 9 May 2025).

23. Freeman, A., Tidholm, A., Holmes, A. M., Otto, B., Pirri, C., Rojas, C., Horn, C. C., et al. (2017). Anti-nausea effects and pharmacokinetics of ondansetron, maropitant and metoclopramide in a low-dose cisplatin model of nausea and vomiting in the dog: A blinded crossover study. *BMC Veterinary Research, 12*(244), 1–12. https://core.ac.uk/download/96600362.pdf (accessed on 9 May 2025).

24. Gao, W., Sun, L., Gai, J., Cao, Y., & Zhang, S. (2024). Exploring the resistance mechanism of triple-negative breast cancer to paclitaxel through the scRNA-seq analysis. *PLOS ONE, 19*. https://www.semanticscholar.org/paper/9e6334868839ed36a233b06faa3039585fdd4844 (accessed on 9 May 2025).

25. Gupta, L., Raghavendra, L., Basavanna, S. P., & Sowmya, M. (2019). Adverse drug reactions due to cancer chemotherapy in a tertiary care hospital in south Karnataka: A prospective observational study. https://core.ac.uk/download/551597375.pdf (accessed on 9 May 2025).

26. He, H., & Zhou, F. (2024). Efficacy and safety of anti-angiogenic drugs combined with chemotherapy in the treatment of platinum-sensitive/resistant ovarian cancer: A meta-analysis with trial sequential analysis of randomized controlled trials. *Frontiers in Pharmacology, 15*.

https://www.semanticscholar.org/paper/0ba765111e3361bd85bf44156438d9bf54eb08ad (accessed on 9 May 2025).

27. Hoff, F., Qiu, Y., Brown, B., Gerbing, R., Gamis, A., Aplenc, R., Kolb, E., et al. (2021). Valosin-containing protein (VCP/p97) is prognostically unfavorable in subtypes of acute leukemia, and negatively correlates with UPR-proteins IRE1 and GRP78. *Blood*. https://www.semanticscholar.org/paper/2752de5f17ba9a47afc8e730db1b5811c9fe5851 (accessed on 9 May 2025).

28. Hosseini, N. F., Amini, R., Ramezani, M., Saidijam, M., Hashemi, S. M., & Najafi, R. (2022). AS1411 aptamer-functionalized exosomes in the targeted delivery of doxorubicin in fighting colorectal cancer. *Biomedicine & Pharmacotherapy, 155*, 113690. https://doi.org/10.1016/j.biopha.2022.113690.

29. Huo, L., & Tang, Y. (2022). Multi-objective deep reinforcement learning for personalized dose optimization based on multi-indicator experience replay. *Applied Sciences*. https://www.semanticscholar.org/paper/f31e21aec5a80f602755dff3bc307682b5faf244 (accessed on 9 May 2025).

30. Karagil, S., Szczesnowska, A., Haddad, N., Gamaethige, S. M., Coakley, E., Dawood, N., Rama, V. J., et al. (2025). How natural therapies can combat neoplastic disease by targeting key survival mechanisms and signaling pathways. *Therapeutics*. https://www.semanticscholar.org/paper/4f9e11e53957f38647975ae6655368fe3a7075e3 (accessed on 9 May 2025).

31. Kubota, Y., Han, Q., Aoki, Y., Masaki, N., Obara, K., Hamada, K., Hozumi, C., et al. (2023). Synergy of combining methionine restriction and chemotherapy: The disruptive next generation of cancer treatment. *Cancer Diagnosis & Prognosis, 3*(3), 272–281. https://www.semanticscholar.org/paper/155414b6e44e39116d568830959769db68e7bba8 (accessed on 9 May 2025).

32. Kumar, S., Shukla, M., Sharma, A., Jayaprakash, G., Tonk, R., Chellappan, D., Singh, S. K., et al. (2023). Metal-based nanomaterials and nanocomposites as promising frontier in cancer chemotherapy. *MedComm, 4*. https://www.semanticscholar.org/paper/e6d91ba8daf642587d3a8716246ebcbe44072619 (accessed on 9 May 2025).

33. Li, R., Hu, X., Ge, N., Kerin, M., & Barkley, L. (2025). Abstract 3142: Patient-derived models of breast cancer for drug screening and precision medicine approaches. *Cancer Research*. https://www.semanticscholar.org/paper/ac15043b149065de697ed61c511eff28426febc5 (accessed on 9 May 2025).

34. Li, Y. (2024). DNA adducts in cancer chemotherapy. *Journal of Medicinal Chemistry*. https://www.semanticscholar.org/paper/24cd3aa1f419038ad09ab41a200dca49e309de7e (accessed on 9 May 2025).

35. Llueca, A., Ibañez, M., Cascales, P., Gil-Moreno, A., Bebia, V., Ponce, J., Fernandez, S., et al. (2023). Neoadjuvant chemotherapy plus interval cytoreductive surgery with or without hyperthermic intraperitoneal chemotherapy (NIHIPEC) in the treatment of advanced ovarian cancer: A multicentric propensity score study. *Cancers, 15*. https://www.semanticscholar.org/paper/5c07680816e6000a65203649de919187f000fd6a (accessed on 9 May 2025).

36. Lockwood, L. A. R. (2015). Bioinformatic analysis for the validation of novel biomarkers for cancer diagnosis and drug sensitivity. https://core.ac.uk/download/30731160.pdf.

37. Mafi, A., Rezaee, M., Hedayati, N., Hogan, S. D., Reiter, R., Aarabi, M., & Asemi, Z. (2023). Melatonin and 5-fluorouracil combination chemotherapy: Opportunities and efficacy in cancer therapy. *Cell Communication and Signaling, 21*. https://www.semanticscholar.org/paper/32cc3f2af2c37da416a498e396bb486a38e33768 (accessed on 9 May 2025).

38. Muhamad, M., Rashed, M., & Winum, J. (2024). Novel anticancer drug discovery strategies targeting hypoxia-inducible factors. *Expert Opinion on Drug Discovery*. https://www.semanticscholar.org/paper/dd5c23e3cf49057da63aed83f1a1a613660e9344 (accessed on 9 May 2025).

39. Nagy, F., Adamecz, D., Baji, Á., Kiricsi, Á., Huliák, I., Rónavári, A., Kónya, Z., et al. (2023). Semi-synthetic dihydrotestosterone derivatives modulate inherent multidrug resistance and sensitize colon cancer cells to chemotherapy. *Pharmaceutics, 15*. https://www.semanticscholar.org/paper/3ed84ee7f0dee6f8f3e5e431e317fc0607ad2508 (accessed on 9 May 2025).

40. Nandeesh, B. R., & Reddy, T. M. (2017). Chemotherapy induced nausea & vomiting (CINV). https://core.ac.uk/download/544390131.pdf (accessed on 9 May 2025).

41. Natarelli, N., Aleman, S. J., Mark, I., Tran, J. T., Kwak, S., Botto, E., Aflatooni, S., et al. (2024). A review of current and pipeline drugs for treatment of melanoma. *Pharmaceuticals, 17*. https://www.semanticscholar.org/paper/f056d8d21944f7a72e3d78eca5372f4804444c96 (accessed on 9 May 2025).

42. Perazzoli, G., Mesas, C., Quiñonero, F., Doello, K., Peña, M., Cepero, A., Rodríguez-Criado, J., et al. (2025). Plant-derived molecules modulate multidrug resistance in gastrointestinal cancers: A comprehensive review. *Applied Sciences*. https://www.semanticscholar.org/paper/f88ebebfc3bb17d928f4c5d4fbf263a545d77758 (accessed on 9 May 2025).

43. Purba, T. S., Ng'andu, K., Brunken, L., Smart, E., Mitchell, E. S., Nik Hassan, N. M. K., O'Brien, A., et al. (2019). CDK4/6 inhibition mitigates stem cell damage in a novel model for taxane-induced alopecia. *EMBO Molecular Medicine, 11*. https://doi.org/10.15252/emmm.201911031.

44. Qin, R., Ren, W., Ya, G., Wang, B., He, J., Ren, S., Jiang, L., et al. (2022). Role of chemokines in the crosstalk between tumor and tumor-associated macrophages. *Clinical and Experimental Medicine, 23*, 1359–1373. https://doi.org/10.1007/s10238-022-00888-z.

45. Ramakrishna, J. K., Kotebetta Ramakrishne Gowda, P. S., Rahamanulla, A., Karadigere Nagaraju, P., Ramesh, B., & Chandramouli, M. (2025). The impact of novel purine, pyrimidine and folate analogues on cancer treatment: A review. *Journal of Young Pharmacists*. https://www.semanticscholar.org/paper/ce0cc65d37d70e5afeb567dd59259e6c44d66a54 (accessed on 9 May 2025).

46. Richards, K. E., Xiao, W., Hill, R., & USC Pancreas Research Team. (2022). Cancer-associated fibroblasts confer gemcitabine resistance to pancreatic cancer cells through PTEN-targeting miRNAs in exosomes. *Cancers, 14*. https://www.semanticscholar.org/paper/5df9c47c901b70e0127c77c2b6e41e62a7011bbb (accessed on 9 May 2025).

47. Sharkey, I., Boddy, A., Wallace, H., Mycroft, J., Hollis, R., Picton, S., & Chemotherapy Standardization Group (2001). Body surface area estimation in children using weight alone: Application in pediatric oncology. *British Journal of Cancer, 85*, 23–28. https://www.semanticscholar.org/paper/d07baa39dc0930e5bbdf927d69261992ec483737 (accessed on 9 May 2025).

48. Tan, B. L., & Norhaizan, M. E. (2019). Curcumin combination therapy: The implication and efficacy in cancer. https://core.ac.uk/download/333874177.pdf (accessed on 9 May 2025).

49. Theivendren, P., Pavadai, P., Veerachamy, S., Palanisamy, P., & Kunjiappan, S. (2025). Surface receptor-targeted protein-based nanocarriers for drug delivery: Advances in cancer therapy. *Nanotechnology*. https://www.semanticscholar.org/paper/8f5e514cd819a816da4b11506cc53d60abd9def7 (accessed on 9 May 2025).

50. Wang, Y., Wang, Y., Sun, T., & Xu, J. (2024). Bacteriocins in cancer treatment: Mechanisms and clinical potentials. *Biomolecules, 14*. https://www.semanticscholar.org/paper/0843a7e05a2a944facc43dfbe39317f4de64e071 (accessed on 9 May 2025).

51. Wen, Y., Zhu, Y. J., Zhang, C., Yang, X., Gao, Y., Li, M., Yang, H., et al. (2022). Chronic inflammation, cancer development and immunotherapy. *Frontiers in Pharmacology, 13*. https://doi.org/10.3389/fphar.2022.1040163.

52. Wikramanayake, T. C., Haberland, N., Akhundlu, A., Laboy Nieves, A., & Miteva, M. (2023). Prevention and treatment of chemotherapy-induced alopecia: What is available and what is coming? *Current Oncology, 30*, 3609–3626. https://doi.org/10.3390/curroncol30040275.

53. Yao, J., Song, S., Zhao, H., & Yuan, Y. (2023). Platinum-based drugs and hydrogel: A promising anti-tumor combination. *Drug Delivery, 30*. https://www.semanticscholar.org/paper/c077084b757088249ae2211dce6b8175cdf4b872 (accessed on 9 May 2025).

54. Yousefi Rizi, H. A., Shin, D. H., & Yousefi Rizi, S. (2022). Polymeric nanoparticles in cancer chemotherapy: A narrative review. *Iranian Journal of Public Health, 51*, 226–239. https://www.semanticscholar.org/paper/83f2d808576a3c16ec031b24efb6e5616c9e4776 (accessed on 9 May 2025).

TOXICOLOGY AND DRUG OVERDOSE

12

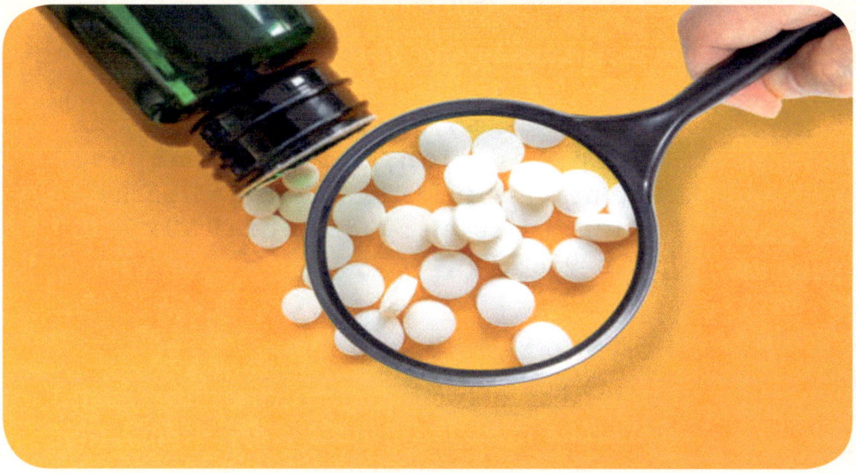

LEARNING OBJECTIVES

After studying this chapter, you will be able to:

1. List the types of drugs involved in overdoses
2. Identify the mechanisms of drug action
3. Explore signs and symptoms of drug overdose
4. Define of risk factors for drug overdose
5. Explain diagnosis of drug overdose
6. Discuss the treatment and management of overdose

Introduction

Toxicology is founded on learning about the interactions of substances with the body to result in adverse effects. Toxicology is a science that investigates the mechanisms governing the absorption, distribution, metabolism, and excretion (ADME) of toxic substances. Through studying these processes, toxicologists can determine the mechanism by which substances result in damage at cellular and systemic levels. In cases of drug overdose, toxicology becomes particularly important as it guides clinical strategies to limit injury and maximize patient outcomes. A classic case that has been extensively investigated is acetaminophen toxicity, with treatment options like acetylcysteine being refined for increased safety and efficacy. Current studies comparing streamlined dosing protocols to conventional strategies illustrate how toxicological knowledge fuels better management of drug-caused injury (Nakatsu et al., 2025). Therefore, toxicology offers the core understanding necessary for the diagnosis, treatment, and prevention of overdose-related adverse effects.

In drug overdose, toxicology also evaluates the challenges posed by polypharmacy and drug interactions. Overdoses often consist of more than one substance, which makes management clinical in nature due to synergistic toxic effects potential. For example, psychotropic drug families such as benzodiazepines, antiepileptics, and antidepressants have risks for respiratory aspiration if used collectively. Toxicological assessment usually takes such interaction effects into account, since co-administration may potentiate toxicity and enhance risk of death. Extensive worldwide evidence from pharmacovigilance programs emphasizes the importance of such multi-drug effects on adverse outcomes, especially in susceptible subgroups such as the elderly. Such enhanced sensitivity underlies safer prescribing decisions and places emphasis on careful monitoring when patients are simultaneously exposed to multiple drug classes (de Cuevas et al., 2022). Toxicology thus deals not only with single drugs but also with the nuances of combined drug effects (Figure 12.1). At its core, toxicology unites scientific investigation and clinical application to meet the challenge of drug overdose. The scientific inquiry techniques used by the disciplines allow for the determination of toxic levels and the creation of antidotes, finally revolutionizing treatment protocols for overdose. For instance, the transition from a three-bag to a two-bag regimen of acetylcysteine in paracetamol poisoning is illustrative of how toxicological science maximizes therapeutic intervention through the minimization of unwanted effects and preservation of efficacy (Nakatsu et al., 2025). In addition, toxicology influences risk assessment and policymaking for the minimization of incidence of overdoses by teaching and regulating. Such interdisciplinary practice ensures that efforts in public health response and clinical guidelines continue to improve. By merging molecular understanding with patient-centered care, toxicology remains pivotal in addressing the ongoing global burden of drug overdose and poisoning.

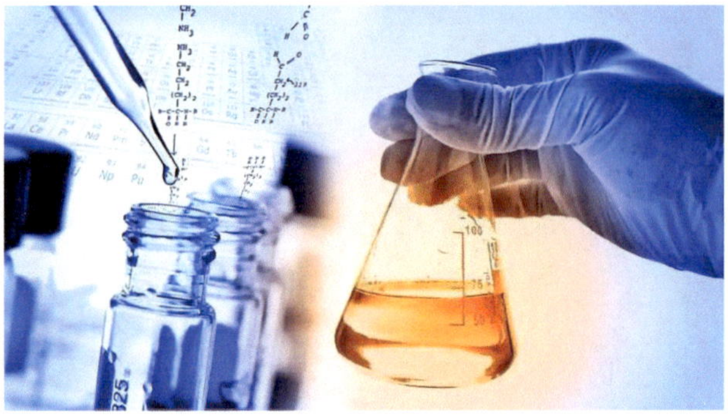

Figure 12.1. Toxicology.

Source: **Lansdowne, L. E.** (2017). *4 Toxicology Approaches in Drug Discovery*. Technology Networks. https://assets.technologynetworks.com/production/dynamic/images/content/294488/4-toxicology-approaches-in-drug-discovery-294488-960x540.jpg?cb=9565137.

Definition of Toxicology

Chemical agents acting upon living things span numerous fields, with toxicology becoming a paramount discipline focused on elucidating the effects. Toxicology investigates how chemicals, ranging from medicines to environmental contaminants, engage biological systems to produce deleterious effects. Toxicology involves the systematic study of dose-response relations, mechanisms of toxic action, and factors that determine an organism's susceptibility. The importance of this field has become stronger in the wake of growing cases of drug overdoses, when the clarification of the toxic character of many substances is necessary to create successful therapies. Through determining the mechanisms by which toxins inflict their harm, toxicologists provide support for both prevention and therapy, thus playing a key role in public health and clinical care. In medical settings, toxicology is the basis for diagnosing and treating poisonings, especially drug overdoses that often baffle healthcare practitioners. The scientific field is not only concerned with identifying the toxic substances but also entails thorough investigations into their physiological disruption and evolution of toxicity. For example, in drug poisonings that are severe, e.g., those caused by nephrotoxic substances, timely intervention by extracorporeal detoxification methods can significantly enhance patient chances of survival (Natalia et al., 2024a). This shows how toxicology integrates empirical evidence and clinical methods, providing a systematic approach toward preventing drug-induced injury. Toxicology, therefore, goes beyond theoretical expertise, becoming absolutely crucial in acute medical scenarios where rapid, accurate responses dictate patient success or failure. In addition, the field of toxicology covers not only the immediate physiological responses but also the long-term effects of toxic exposure, particularly on the brain and nervous system. Overdose of drugs may result in chronic neurological disorders, such as apallic syndrome, which is defined by extended coma and long-lasting vegetative states due to extensive toxic injury (Kurdil et al., 2024b). In-depth neuropathological examinations uncover particular brain areas—like the basal ganglia and cortical gray matter—are susceptible to such toxic insults, reflecting the sophistication of toxic effects at molecular and cellular levels. As a result, toxicology not only educates acute care but also prognostic assessment and rehabilitation of patients who have experienced a severe overdose. This dual emphasis on acute and chronic effects makes toxicology a critical field for fully grasping and addressing the multidimensional burdens of drug overdoses.

Importance of Toxicology in Public Health

Its inclusion in public health practice is critical for the identification and prevention of the harmful consequences of chemical exposure on populations (Figure 12.2). Its application is more than knowing individual poisonings, but it includes the evaluation of environmental poisons, prescribed drugs, and illicit drugs that cause collective health threats. Toxicological testing supplies fundamental information to establish regulatory policy toward the prevention of overdoses and drug safety management, which leads to fewer cases of morbidity and mortality. In addition, toxicology educates the clinical management of victims of drug overdose through an explanation of mechanisms of toxicity and antidote administration, ultimately saving lives. Such a dynamic science relies on multidisciplinary cooperation, including epidemiological monitoring and molecular toxicology to predict emerging threats and tailor interventions. The significance of toxicological know-how comes strongly into view in dealing with multifaceted drug interactions and vulnerabilities across heterogeneous populations, underscoring its absolute value addition to public health practices (Zeppenfeld et al., 2022). Knowledge of biochemical and molecular pathways underlying drug toxicity allows public health practitioners to implement focused prevention and intervention strategies. For example, the development in understanding mutant enzymes and their effect on drug metabolism exemplifies how genetic aspects determine susceptibility to toxicity in individuals. Treatment advances like azacitidine and ivosidenib combined for the treatment of certain cancers exemplify the importance of toxicological analysis to guarantee therapeutic outcomes and reduce unwanted effects. The vigilant tracking of adverse effects, such as severe occurrences like electrocardiogram QT prolongation and differentiation syndrome, is an example of how toxicology supports the safe drug development and clinical use. Such knowledge is important in supporting risk assessment procedures and guides policy that safeguards patients with maximum therapeutic gain. Therefore, toxicology not only assists in the treatment of drug overdoses but also promotes safer pharmaceutical usage that benefits public health in general (Courtney et al., 2020). Outside of regulatory and clinical realms, toxicology serves a preventive purpose by guiding public information and awareness strategies on drug abuse and overdose. By explaining the toxic effects of substances, toxicologists offer evidence that informs educational content advocating for safer behavior and knowledgeable use of medication. In addition, toxicological monitoring is able to identify trends in drug use and novel toxins in a population to allow for timely public health responses that can reduce harm. The discipline also supports forensic analysis, allowing for the identification of substances in overdose fatalities that can inform policy changes and resource allocation for treatment programs for addiction. With these diverse activities, toxicology functions as a linchpin for the construction of robust public health systems equipped to address the complexity of issues inherent in drug overdose epidemics, highlighting its increased societal significance (Courtney et al., 2020; Zeppenfeld et al., 2022).

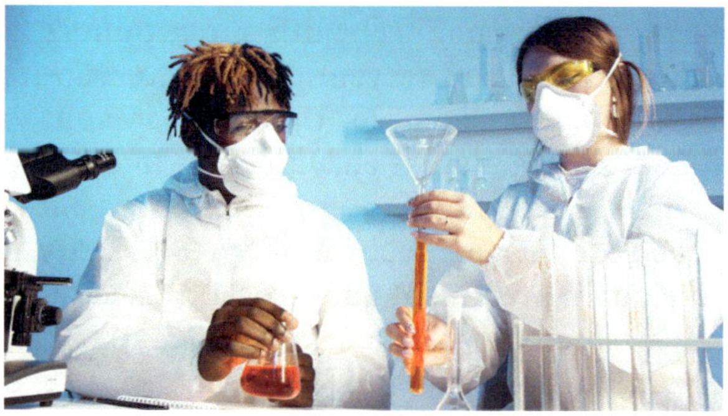

Figure 12.2. Toxicology in public health.

Source: Witness Experts. (n.d.). *14 Fascinating Facts About Toxicologist*. https://witness-experts.com/hubfs/14-fascinating-facts-about-toxicologist-1695747877-1.jpg.

Overview of Drug Overdose as a Toxicological Issue

The pharmacology of drug overdose is more than a set of individual case studies to illustrate larger toxicological issues that overlap with problems in public health. Toxicology as a field examines how chemicals interact with biological systems, and drug overdoses are acute presentations of poisoning both at the molecular and systemic level. For such overdoses, varied pharmaceutical substances, such as opioids, stimulants, and sedatives, interfere with normal physiological processes, usually resulting in multi-organ failure or death. These results highlight the need to appreciate dose-response mechanisms and metabolic pathways that determine toxicity. Also, drug intoxication often involves polydrug administration, which makes toxicological examinations and treatment more challenging. This complexity demands multidisciplinary solutions involving clinical toxicology, pharmacology, and epidemiology for successful management of overdose risks and body toxic insults (Zeppenfeld et al., 2022). Knowledge of these mechanisms is vital to design preventive strategies and specific therapeutic interventions. The drug overdose epidemiology demonstrates changing patterns that emphasize the toxicological load on society and health infrastructures. Longitudinal data over almost four decades document an unsettling rise in unintentional drug overdose deaths, fueled by changing trends in drug use and synthetic opioid proliferation. Most notably, the rise is not one of a monolithic wave but rather the effect of several sub epidemics of various substances, with prescription opioids, heroin, and more potent synthetic analogues leading the way. Geographic and demographic differences also contribute to the toxicology profile, where regional "hotspots" bear a disproportionate burden of overdose fatalities and are typically associated with socioeconomic and healthcare inequities (Jalal et al., 2018). These trends highlight not only the chemical toxicity of drugs but also the complex dynamic interactions between toxicological variables and social determinants of health. Recognition of these multifaceted aspects is necessary for developing effective public health interventions. From a clinical perspective, drug overdose as a toxicological emergency requires swift identification and intervention to avoid morbidity and mortality. The toxic action of most drugs is reflected in depression of respiration, cardiovascular collapse, or impairment of the nervous system, with specific antidotes or supportive therapy. Naloxone therapy for opioid overdose is a paradigm of specific toxicological treatment in reversal of receptor-mediated toxicity. Difficulty still arises in the diagnosis of overdoses from less common or new psychoactive substances (NPSs) because limited toxicological testing capabilities are available. In addition, long-term polydrug exposure can camouflage or potentiate acute presentations, requiring extensive toxicological knowledge and diagnostic skill (Zeppenfeld et al., 2022). Successful overdose care blends toxicological principles, clinical experience, and pharmacodynamics knowledge to inform treatment strategies that reduce systemic toxicity and enhance patient outcomes.

12.1. Types of Drugs Involved in Overdoses

Learning Outcome

1. Prescription Medications
2. Over-the-Counter Drugs
3. Illicit Substances

The nature of drug overdose events is highlighted by the range of drugs that lead to such deadly events (Figure 12.3). Among the most common are opioids, including synthetic opioids like fentanyl, which have become much more prevalent in terms of their presence because of their potency and widespread illicit market availability. Opioids bind with the nervous system to cause pain alleviation but can readily suppress respiratory function, resulting in death. Aside from opioids, other substances frequently involved in cases of overdose include benzodiazepines, which are frequently prescribed for conditions such as anxiety and insomnia. Benzodiazepines, when taken with other central nervous system (CNS) depressants, pose a greater risk of overdose since the drug combination enhances their depressive effects. Current statistics point to the changing patterns of drug use, necessitating ongoing observation and specific intervention to meet the changing drugs involved in overdoses (Spencer et al., 2022). Aside from opioids and benzos, drugs with stimulating effects on the CNS like cocaine and methamphetamine are major contributors to overdose fatalities. The stimulating effects of these substances on the CNS increase heart rate and blood pressure, which can induce cardiovascular collapse among susceptible individuals. Stimulants generally present distinctive toxicological challenges due to the fact that their overdoses can appear differently than those of depressants and call for different therapeutic management. Polysubstance use, wherein a combination of drugs is consumed together, further obscures clinical presentation and treatment approach. Such practice is increasingly widespread and forms a key aspect of the overdose crisis that should not be ignored during toxicological workup and public health interventions. Overall awareness of all drugs involved is paramount for successful overdose prevention and response activities (Spencer et al., 2022). Overdose case diversity involving various drugs is additionally compounded by involvement of NPSs and non-opioid and non-stimulant prescription drugs. Synthetic cannabinoids and other new drugs typically fall outside standard toxicology assays, rendering detection and analysis infeasible using traditional methods by forensic and clinical toxicologists. Additionally, drugs like antidepressants and antipsychotics, although less frequently implicated in lethal overdoses, can also significantly contribute to toxicological findings, particularly in the context of deliberate self-poisoning or accidental overdose. Expert opinions from toxicologists worldwide, such as Vedran Velagic and Sami Viskin, highlight the need for changing toxicological methods to match the dynamic drug scenario and enhance the detection and management of overdoses. This changing aspect of drug activity requires constant research and adaptive measures in the field of toxicology.

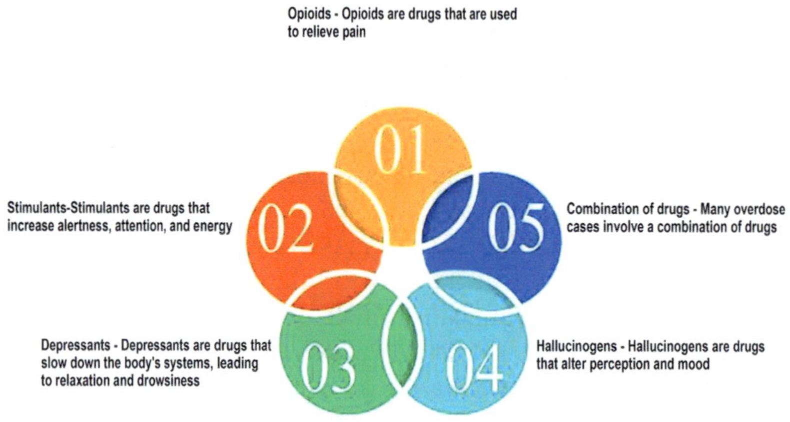

Figure 12.3. Types of drugs involved in overdoses.

Source: **Verywell Health.** (n.d.). *Types of Drugs Involved in Overdoses. https*://encrypted-tbn0.gstatic.com/images?q=tbn:ANd9GcSIyuYjF4zLXHd65LqMHQpbeulbo0MiHxhmcw&s.

12.1.1. Prescription Medications

With the rise in usage of prescription drugs, particularly opioids, in treatment has come with a proportionate rise in drug toxicity and overdose challenges. Despite the imperative role of these drugs in pain management and other medical disorders, their potential for abuse and drug interaction remains a top toxicological concern. For example, buprenorphine, one drug commonly used for treating opioid use disorder because of its safety profile, has been detected in a small but significant proportion of drug-related fatalities. Even though it is effective, cases where buprenorphine is used in combination with other drugs like benzodiazepines, methamphetamine, or fentanyl greatly increase the risk of life-threatening overdose. These mixtures make clinical management more difficult and underscore the subtle role of prescription drugs in overdose situations (Dai et al., 2022). This subtlety requires cautious prescription habits and surveillance to reduce unwanted toxic effects. Demographic considerations also cross over with prescription drug use and risk of overdose in ways that go beyond typical cases of poisoning. Studies investigating opioid positivity in suicide victims find that high percentages of them tested positive for opioids even though their deaths were the result of non-poisoning. This result puts into perspective the larger context of prescription drugs in mental illness and substance abuse, as it demonstrates how opioid positivity relates to physical and mental health issues like depression and substance use disorder. Furthermore, the demographic patterns indicate that widowed, older individuals, especially of white race, are more likely to be opioid-positive, implying that prescription drug management among vulnerable populations demands increased concern and intervention mechanisms (Mason et al., 2020). This information allows us to have a deeper insight into how prescription drugs affect patterns of mortality beyond the direct incidences of overdoses. The contribution of prescription drugs to drug overdose is compounded by comorbidities and polydrug consumption that enhance toxicological hazards. Research shows that most overdose fatalities with prescription drugs take place in persons with predisposing cardiovascular or pulmonary conditions, enhancing the physiological effects of the substances. Furthermore, polydrug use, specifically the use of five or more agents in overdose situations with drugs such as buprenorphine, illustrates the way in which simultaneous substance use enhances overdose risk. These observations serve to emphasize the need for thorough patient evaluation prior to prescribing drugs, combining medical history and possible drug interactions in order to reduce risks of overdose effectively. Such an approach is paramount in clinical toxicology to avoid fatal consequences through guaranteeing the safe use of prescription drugs in the realm of the patient's overall health conditions (Dai et al., 2022).

12.1.2. Over-the-Counter Drugs

One frequently underappreciated variable in the field of toxicology is the ready availability and utilization of over-the-counter (OTC) medications, which can initiate accidental toxic exposure and overdose (Figure 12.4). These drugs, available without prescription, comprise many agents such as antihistamines, decongestants, and analgesics. Their pharmacodynamics and pharmacokinetics are multifaceted, making them a challenge to toxicological analysis. Especially in children, OTC medications employed for the management of common conditions such as cough and cold symptoms have inherent risks because of their multiple formulations and the fragile physiology of children. The fact that these combined products contain more than one active ingredient enhances the risk of adverse effects and accidental overdose, making it imperative to have a complete understanding of their toxicity profiles. Clinical toxicology acts as a fundamental resource in determining and counteracting such risks, highlighting the acute need for constant research and strict public health policy to ensure the safety of susceptible populations (Diantini et al., 2024). Misuse and unintentional overdose related to OTC antihistamines present a pertinent concern in toxicological research. Of these, first-generation H1 antihistamines like diphenhydramine are especially significant because of their anticholinergic activity, including significant sedation. Sedative potential can be synergistically enhanced to a harmful extent when used with other CNS depressants, including opioids. Evidence has shown that diphenhydramine is occasionally utilized as a diluent in illicit drug preparations, inflicting further hazards by imparting modifications to the pharmacological profiles of such compounds. In addition, surveillance data indicate that overdose deaths involving antihistamines are not rare, presenting a pivotal juncture at which access to OTC medication meets public health hazard. The pharmacological interplay of effect and risk for intentional or accidental overdose serves as a compelling reason to incorporate toxicological understanding into clinical and policy structures that work toward prevention of overdose (Amanda et al., 2022). Toxicological risk assessment of OTC medications extends from drug toxicity in an individual to public health and clinical practice implications. Case studies reveal serious consequences, including death, due to accidental overdose and abuse of OTC medications, especially among children where dosing mistakes and ingredient redundancy can quickly increase the level of toxicity. The pharmacokinetic attributes of absorption, distribution, metabolism, and excretion (ADME) differ by age and among individuals, making it difficult to manage overdoses. In addition, OTC medications' multi-component nature maximizes the probability of drug-drug interactions (DDIs) and cumulative toxicities, particularly upon concomitant administration or at supratherapeutic doses. These complexities call for an interdisciplinary effort from clinicians, toxicologists, and policymakers to facilitate safer utilization through education, regulation, and informed clinical decision-making. Finally, its progression in knowledge of OTC drug toxicology is crucial in curbing overdose rates and protecting public health (Amanda et al., 2022; Diantini et al., 2024).

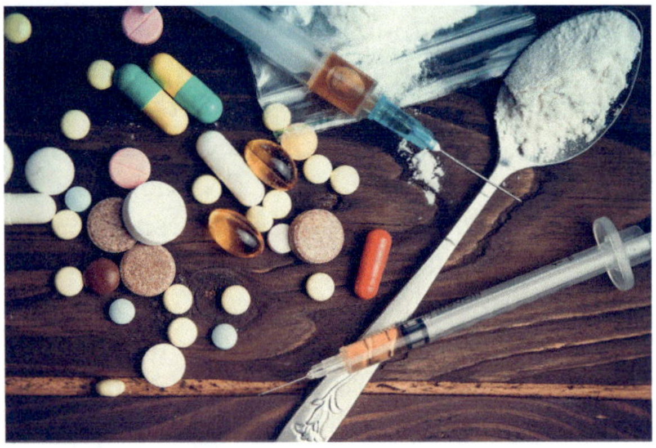

Figure 12.4. Over-the-counter drugs.

Source: Encyclopedia Britannica. (n.d.). *Drug Concept: Drug Abuse, Addiction, Heroin Injection, Doping, Opium Epidemic.* https://cdn.britannica.com/05/213705-050-4331A79A/drug-concept-drug-abuse-addition-heroin-injection-doping-opium-epidemic.jpg.

12.1.3. Illicit Substances

The issues of illegal drugs also reach beyond pharmacology to involve the detection and monitoring issues of clinical toxicology. Development of better analytical methods has played a critical role in helping to deal with these challenges, especially during the investigation of drug overdoses. More recent advances utilizing advanced mass spectrometry methods, including quadrupole orbitrap analyzers paired with paper spray cartridges that incorporate solid phase extraction, have greatly enhanced the selectivity and sensitivity of drug detection in biological samples. These advances allow for screening of a wide range of both classic and emerging illicit drugs, including many fentanyl derivatives and synthetic cannabinoids, commonly involved in overdose deaths. The capacity to screen for drugs at sub nanogram concentrations in plasma is a crucial advancement for emergency rooms where precise and timely detection guides treatment choices and public health responses. It plays a crucial role in elucidating overdose causality and trends, particularly since the ongoing creation of NPSs in the illicit market poses a challenge (Zimmerman-Federle et al., 2024). Illicit drugs commonly include sympathomimetic agents, a chemically heterogeneous group whose actions are mediated predominantly by stimulation of the sympathetic nervous system.

The drugs, either naturally occurring or synthetic, produce significant physiological effects on cardiovascular and CNS function that can enhance toxicological crises in the event of abuse. The general category comprises classical drugs such as cocaine and ephedrine, in addition to more recent synthetic derivatives that mimic or enhance endogenous catecholamine effects. An understanding of the pharmacodynamics of these drugs is crucial, especially the function of trace amine-associated receptors (TAARs), which control sympathomimetic activity and contribute to toxicity profiles. Natural sympathomimetic agents' misconception as safe highlights the need to identify their potential for dangerous side effects, especially when abused or taken with other psychoactive drugs, complicating overdose treatment even further (Costa et al., 2022). Treatment of the dangers of illegal drugs requires a multiple-component solution that combines toxicological detection, pharmacological insight, and clinical management principles. Since synthetic drug analogs are constantly changing, their uncharacterized potency and interaction patterns increase the risk of lethal overdose, necessitating ongoing modification of analytical methods and treatment programs.

The detection of new fentanyl analogs and designer benzodiazepines in overdose samples is a prime example of the changing nature of illicit drug use and its impact on public health surveillance. In addition, the crossover between illicit sympathomimetics and prescription medications requires caution to prevent misdiagnosis and maximize patient outcomes.

Continued research on the mechanisms of toxicology and the enhancement of detection capacity continue to be vital to the prevention of morbidity and mortality due to overdose from illicit substances in various healthcare facilities (Costa et al., 2022; Zimmerman-Federle et al., 2024).

Test Your Knowledge

1. What is a prescription medication?
2. Can prescription drugs become OTC medications?

12.2. Mechanisms of Drug Action

Learning Outcome

1. Pharmacokinetics and Pharmacodynamics
2. Interaction with Biological Systems
3. Factors Influencing Drug Toxicity

The complex interaction between drugs and biological systems is the basis of their therapeutic activity and also their toxic potential. Drugs act at the molecular level by interacting with specific targets, including enzymes, ion channels, or receptors, to modulate cellular function. These mechanisms can either activate or suppress physiological functions depending on the type of drug and desired effect. For example, agonists stimulate receptors to simulate endogenous compounds, while antagonists inhibit receptor activity. Knowledge of these interactions is important, especially in the case of toxicology and overdose, where overstimulation or inhibition can upset homeostasis, resulting in harmful consequences. In addition, the drug's affinity and effectiveness at its receptor impact the extent of the response, and the subtle interplay between therapeutic effect and toxickop—the balance that has to be well regulated in the clinical setting (Zeppenfeld et al., 2022). Pharmacokinetic properties significantly impact drug action and toxicity by the mechanisms of ADME. Changes in any one of these can result in higher plasma levels, thus enhancing a drug's pharmacological or toxic effects. For instance, route of administration influences onset and potency; intranasal administration has been a potential route, particularly for CNS drugs, because of its quick absorption and delivery advantages. Yet, although this pathway has benefits like non-invasiveness and targeted delivery, it also brings with it distinct toxicological considerations like local tissue irritation and formulation-related toxicity. These highlight the need to appreciate both systemic and localized drug behaviors, particularly in overdose situations where drug accumulation can lead to profound toxicity (Keller et al., 2021). On the cellular level, drug toxicity mechanisms typically disrupt normal signaling, oxidative stress, or interference with mitochondrial function. For example, certain toxic drugs can uncouple oxidative phosphorylation, causing energy loss and cell death. Some others cause excessive calcium influx, which causes apoptosis or necrosis. These pathways need to be identified so that antidotes can be formulated and overdose cases can be treated effectively. In addition, genetic differences among people can influence drug metabolism pathways in a way that leads to varying susceptibility to toxicities. Therefore, understanding the mechanisms of drug action not only aids in designing safer drugs but also informs clinical interventions to counteract toxicity in overdose situations, underscoring its pivotal position in the practice of toxicology (Zeppenfeld et al., 2022).

12.2.1. Pharmacokinetics and Pharmacodynamics

Appreciation of how drugs interact in the body is key to explaining the processes of toxicity and overdose. Pharmacokinetics (PK) includes the ADME of drugs, which governs the levels reaching target tissues with time. This dynamic process governs the onset, peak, and duration of action of a drug, which is pivotal to forecasting therapeutic as well as toxic effects. Differences in PK profiles due to genetic variability or organ dysfunction can result in unforeseen accumulation and toxicity. As an example, *in vitro* PK/PD models evaluation of voriconazoles activity on *Candida albicans* showed how drug exposure's dose-dependent nature influences the inhibition of fungal growth directly and how accurate drug concentrations become critical in controlling toxic outcomes (Abdalwahd et al., 2024). Such facts highlight the importance of comprehensive PK evaluations in toxicology to control overdose hazards. Pharmacodynamics (PD) is a complement to pharmacokinetics and indicates how drugs affect the body's biochemical and physiological processes, including drug concentration versus effect (Figure 12.5).

It describes how drugs bind to receptors, enzymes, or cellular pathways to cause therapeutic or toxic effects. This interaction establishes the dose-response relationship, which is an important factor in assessing overdose toxicity. Narrow therapeutic index compounds could cause significant toxic effects even at minimal rises in plasma levels due to sharp dose-response curves. The toxicological investigation of substances such as phenibut and kratom demonstrates this phenomenon, where their pharmacodynamic pattern shows opioid-like and CNS activity, magnifying the toxicity potential upon overdose situations (Samantha et al., 2023). Thus, the combination of PK with PD information yields a more holistic description of drug behavior essential for toxicity evaluation. The balance between pharmacokinetics and pharmacodynamics provides the basis for the prediction and control of drug toxicity and overdose. Reliable PK/PD modeling allows clinicians and toxicologists to model drug behavior under different dosing regimens, maximizing therapeutic effects while minimizing side effects.

\The *in vitro* PK/PD model utilized to investigate voriconazoles activity against resistant and sensitive *Candida* isolates illustrates how such models can inform dosing regimens through the demonstration of dose-dependent efficacy for inhibition (Abdalwahd et al., 2024). Further, knowledge of the PK/PD profiles of drugs with abuse liability like mitragynine from kratom serves to predict drug interaction and overdose effects (Samantha et al., 2023). Together, these strategies lead to more secure clinical practice and evidence that shapes policy addressing increasing complexities of drug-related toxicology and overdose management.

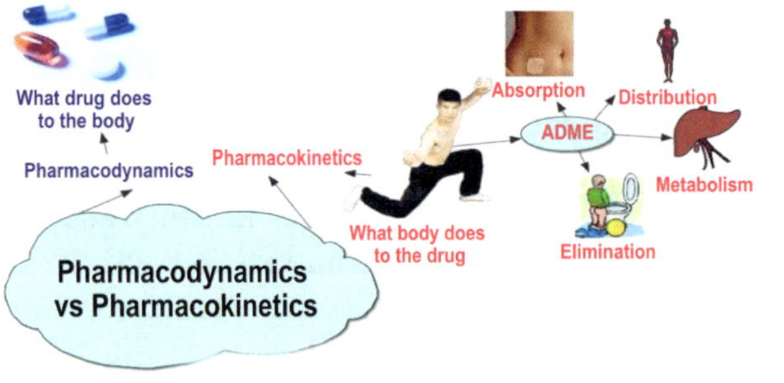

Figure 12.5. Pharmacokinetics and pharmacodynamics.

Source: **The Med Note.** (n.d.). *Pharmacodynamics vs. Pharmacokinetics.* https://www.themednote.com/wp-content/gallery/basic-science/pharmacoloy/pharm-basic/pharmacodynamics-vs-phar.jpg.

12.2.2. Interaction with Biological Systems

Knowledge of the intricate interactions between drugs and biological processes is crucial in understanding the mechanisms of toxicology and drug overdoses (Figure 12.6). As a drug is administered, its passage through the body includes ADME, each process affecting its final biological action. The route of administration has a profound influence on these interactions, as intranasal delivery provides a non-invasive route that provides quick systemic and CNS access with avoidance of first-pass metabolism and possible diminution of systemic toxicity. Nevertheless, this route also comes with unique toxicological challenges involving local tissue irritation and formulation stability. Assessment of these factors is essential to maximize drug effectiveness and reduce side effects, particularly in overdose situations where modified pharmacokinetics can increase toxicity (Keller et al., 2021). Thus, the subtleties of drug interaction with biological systems need to be thoroughly examined in therapeutic as well as toxicological contexts. Biological systems react to drugs not only by specific therapeutic action, but also by unwanted toxic effects, which are produced by the interaction of active constituents with different physiological processes. Natural compounds, like *Salvia officinalis*, display a variety of pharmacological activities such as anti-inflammatory and antioxidant activity, yet the same complicated bioactivities may affect biological systems in an unpredictable manner. These chemical constituents are responsible for their effects, which act on cellular receptors, enzymes, and genetic material and bring about beneficial therapeutic responses or toxic effects depending on dosage and individual susceptibility. Thus, knowledge of pharmacodynamics of such substances is necessary in the context of toxicology to forecast and monitor anticipated overdose hazards and adverse drug reactions (ADRs) (Ghorbani et al., 2017). This equilibrium of therapeutic effect and toxicity underscores the essential requirement of detailed assessment of drug interactions within biological systems. Additionally, toxicological profiles of drugs and compounds are influenced by the dynamic relationship between their chemical properties and physiological surroundings. Metabolic processes, especially those related to hepatic enzymes, exercise a determining influence in regulating drug toxicity by converting substances into more or less toxic entities. When overloaded, in cases of overdose, these systems may be unable to neutralize the toxins properly, and thus, build up and cause extensive biological harm. Further, the distinctive features of the route of delivery, like the intranasal route, can affect the disposition and toxicity profile of the drugs by modifying absorption kinetics and tissue local exposure (Keller et al., 2021). Therefore, identification of these interactions at a molecular and body system level is essential for progressing the field of toxicology, enhancing treatments for overdose, and designing safer pharmaceuticals.

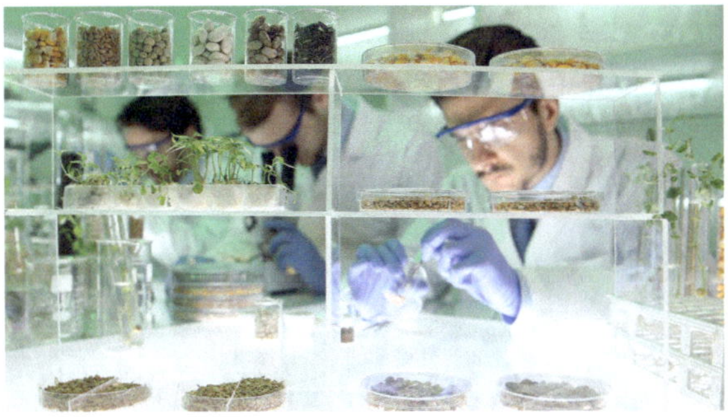

Figure 12.6. Interaction with biological systems.

Source: Biology Online (2020). *Regulation of Biological Systems.* https://www.biologyonline.com/wp-content/uploads/2020/02/Regulation-of-Biological-Systems.jpg.

12.2.3. Factors Influencing Drug Toxicity

The multifactorial complexity of drug toxicity is determined by a myriad of factors that become intertwined to determine the severity and outcome of poisoning events. Patient factors like age, genetic profile, and presence of existing illnesses determine the metabolism and elimination of a drug from the body. An example is the hepatic function, which becomes important because most drugs are biotransformed in the liver. A compromised liver reduces the body's capacity to detoxify toxic metabolites, thus enhancing the risk of toxicity. Furthermore, polypharmacy, or the simultaneous use of several drugs, may result in adverse drug interactions, either amplifying toxic effects or hindering clearance. These variables highlight the need for individualized evaluation in management of overdose, typically comprising difficulties in diagnosis and treatment because of different patient responses and unpredictable clinical behavior (Aki et al., 2018). Pharmacokinetics and the biochemical mechanisms by which drugs are metabolized significantly influence toxicity profiles. Paracetamol is an example of such drugs, which are safe within therapeutic doses but lethal on excessive consumption. Paracetamol is usually metabolized in the liver, where the toxic intermediates are quenched through conjugation with glutathione; in the case of overdose, however, glutathione stores are exhausted, causing hepatotoxic metabolites to accumulate. This causes extensive liver injury, which is fatal if not immediately treated with antidotes that replenish glutathione stores. These mechanisms serve to emphasize the fine line between therapeutic effect and toxic risk, supporting the requirement for pharmacologic expertise and education of the patient to reduce risk from overdose (Forte et al., 2002). Environmental and behavioral considerations also have a major contribution to risk and severity of drug toxicity. Voluntary or accidental abuse, involving errors in dose and abuse of substances, reflects the human factor involved in causing poisoning episodes. Socioeconomic determinants and access to health care also influence outcomes in overdose cases by impacting timely intervention and support. In addition, formulation and route of administration impact absorption and bioavailability of drugs, potentially exacerbating or lessening toxic effects. It is critical for clinicians to understand these variables to create effective prevention strategies, rapid identification, and treatment of toxic exposures. Therefore, toxicology is an essential field in emergency medicine, with the aim of combining patient history, physical examination, and familiarity with frequent toxic agents to minimize morbidity and mortality (Aki et al., 2018).

Test Your Knowledge

1. How does age affect drug toxicity?
2. What role do enzymes play in drug interactions?

12.3. Signs and Symptoms of Drug Overdose

Learning Outcome

1. Physical Symptoms
2. Psychological Symptoms
3. Variability Based on Substance Type

Clinical presentations of drug overdose are varied, depending upon the pharmacological properties of the drugs involved (Figure 12.7). Patients typically arrive with altered mental status, which varies from agitation or aggressive behavior to deep coma. Agitation and hallucinations are significantly found with the stimulant-type drugs like cocaine, cathinones, and amphetamines, which may require sedation to control these extreme behavioral disturbances. On the contrary, opioids and sedative drugs like benzodiazepines are responsible for respiratory depression and loss of consciousness, often necessitating advanced airway management or reversal agent administration like Naloxone and Flumazenil. This heterogeneity highlights the difficulty of determining intoxication on clinical grounds alone, since more than one drug can be present, each producing unique signs and symptoms, with opioids still the leading causes of morbidity and mortality in overdose (Zellner et al., 2024). The difficulty of diagnosing drug overdose is further exacerbated by the common underreporting or incomplete histories given by patients. Analytical toxicology shows that patients tend to consume more than one substance, significantly more than they admit to, which makes it difficult to clinically assess and emphasizes the need for detailed toxicological investigation. For instance, the use of Pregabalin and THC is regularly underreported but prominently identified in laboratory tests, indicating the trends towards polysubstance misuse. Such mismatches between history and toxicology results require a high level of suspicion on the part of clinicians and highlight toxicological testing as a crucial tool for directing effective intervention and guiding prognosis in overdose situations (Zellner et al., 2024). Advances in forensic toxicology make important contributions to the identification of new and potent drugs involved in overdoses, which in turn affect symptom recognition and management strategies. The introduction of synthetic opioids, such as nitazene analogues isotonitazene and metonitazene, has been increasingly identified by more sensitive monitoring methods since 2021. These compounds have strong opioid activity, sometimes associated with lethal overdose presentation with respiratory arrest. Preliminary detection by advanced ion monitoring systems, while not definitive, allows for the anticipation of clinical presentation and guide emergent management. This interdisciplinary interface of forensic chemistry and toxicology units is essential in appreciating emerging drug trends and their related clinical manifestations, hence enhancing treatment outcomes and patient recovery in cases of overdose.

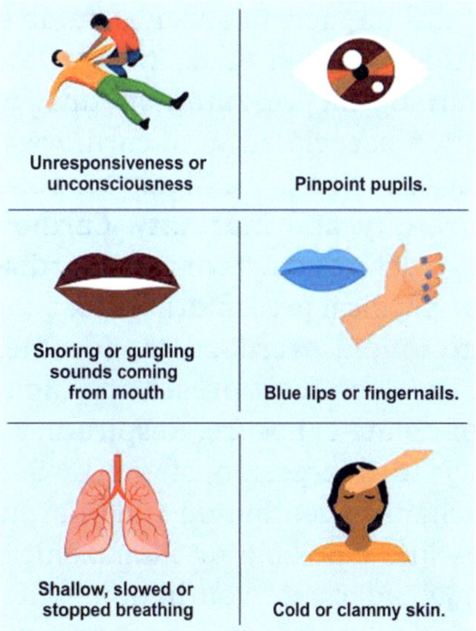

Figure 12.7. Signs and symptoms of drug overdose.

Source: Cleveland Clinic. (n.d.). *Opioid Overdose.* https://my.clevelandclinic.org/-/scassets/images/org/health/articles/24583-opioid-overdose.

12.3.1. Physical Symptoms

Clinical presentation in patients who are suffering from drug overdose includes a broad range of physical findings that frequently confound initial diagnosis and management (Figure 12.8). Most of the patients have nonspecific presentations such as altered mental status, varying from agitation to coma, necessitating immediate clinical assessment to identify the offending toxic agents. Symptoms such as agitation, anxiety, hallucinations, and psychosis are most commonly associated with stimulants like cocaine and amphetamines, usually requiring sedation to treat these acute neuropsychiatric presentations efficiently. In contrast, depressant drugs like opiates and benzodiazepines most frequently cause respiratory depression and coma and raise the risk of hypoxia and requiring high-level airway support. These divergent patterns of symptoms highlight the sophistication of the challenges for healthcare workers in emergency presentations, where it is essential to recognize promptly distinctive toxicological impacts in order to guide effective interventions (Zellner et al., 2024). Outside the acute neurological presentations, drug overdose is also often associated with cardiorespiratory complications, which are highly responsible for both morbidity and mortality. Cardiovascular instability, such as arrhythmia and cardiac arrest, is a major physical presentation most commonly related to opioid overdose, as documented by cases of cardiac arrest presenting alone in the setting of opiate exposure. Respiratory distress secondary to depression of the CNS can also need mechanical ventilation and pharmacologic antidotes like naloxone or flumazenil to effect a return to adequate ventilation. These signs and symptoms, in addition to representing the pharmacodynamic properties of the drugs in question, demonstrate the value of prompt toxicological screening to direct targeted therapy. Furthermore, polysubstance use common in the overdose patient confounds symptomology, with concurrent ingestion of substances such as pregabalin contributing to CNS depression and adverse outcome risk (Zellner et al., 2024). The more general social and occupational determinants of drug overdose death also have an impact on the physical symptom burden seen in clinical practice. Variations in drug overdose deaths by industry have been demonstrated in recent research, with service sectors being more vulnerable during pandemic lockdowns. Such demographic and occupational changes influence the profile of physical symptoms seen, as some populations will present more commonly with complications of certain drugs or combinations of drugs. For instance, heightened stress and limited access to healthcare facilities during emergencies can worsen the severity of overdose, with increased physical signs like longer-lasting hypoxia or multi-organ failure. It is important to understand these trends in epidemiology in order to make public health interventions and clinical action more suited to counteracting the catastrophic physical effects of drug overdose among different populations.

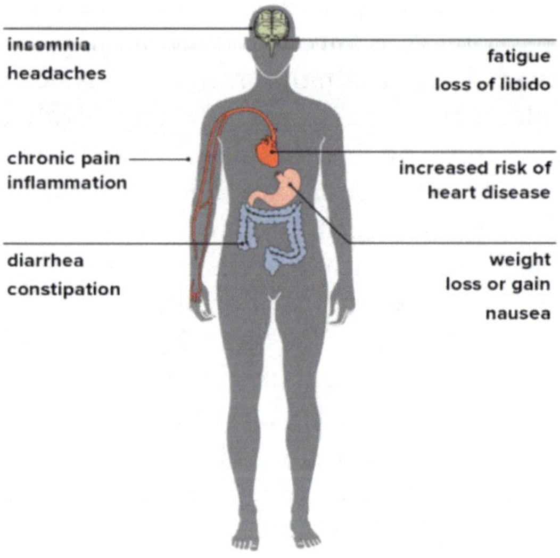

Figure 12.8. Physical symptoms.

Source: Medical News Today. (2021). *Depression Physical Symptoms. https*://i0.wp.com/post.medicalnewstoday.com/wp-content/uploads/sites/3/2021/07/1100823-Depression-physical-symptoms-1296x1296-body-1024x969.jpg?w=1155&h=2576.

12.3.2. Psychological Symptoms

The expression of psychological manifestations during drug overdose commonly makes assessment and management at the clinical level challenging (Figure 12.9). Acute recreational drug toxicity is commonly presented by patients who are agitated, anxious, hallucinated, and psychotic and can be explained by the drug's pharmacological actions, including cocaine, cathinones, and amphetamines. Such symptoms not only limit communication but also contribute to aggressive tendencies, and therefore sedation and observation are required. Such psychological disturbances are an indication of the complex effect of toxicants on the CNS and underscore the relevance of extensive clinical assessment over patient self-reporting. According to research, patient histories also underreport some drug classes, especially benzodiazepines and newer psychoactive drugs, and hence toxicological screening is critical to make an accurate diagnosis and develop appropriate treatment plans in such complex presentations (Zellner et al., 2024). In prison environments, the psychiatric symptoms of drug overdose are complicated in a deep way by underlying mental health vulnerabilities. Prison populations have notoriously high rates of psychiatric conditions, and events of acute intoxication during prison riots heighten them.

The disorganized environment and attendant psychological distress occurring during the event can lead to a range of pathological reactions including extreme anxiety, psychosis, and suicidal thoughts. Toxicological analysis in these acute environments usually shows poly-substance misuse, with drugs such as methadone, benzodiazepines, and antidepressants playing a role in the psychological and behavioral distress seen. The concurrence of toxicological effect and mental illness disorders presents difficulties in forensic and clinical assessment, particularly in differentiating accidental overdose, deliberate self-injury, or compulsive use under psychosis or extreme stress (Tomassini et al., 2024). Psychological symptomatology of drug overdose is also a key indicator of trends in drug abuse, mirroring drug availability and legislative effects. For instance, the decrease of new psychoactive drugs like cathinones and synthetic cannabinoids parallels decreases in their prevalence of use as well as incidence of related psychological disturbances. On the other hand, increased drug abuse of drugs such as Pregabalin heralds new challenges manifesting in sedation, confusion, and depression that complicate acute presentations, particularly when used with opioids or benzodiazepines. Awareness of the subtleties of psychological impact benefits not only acute management of overdose but also public health strategies to prevent substance abuse and its psychiatric ramifications. These findings highlight the critical role of toxicological information in the recognition and response to changing drug-induced psychological damage trends (Zellner et al., 2024).

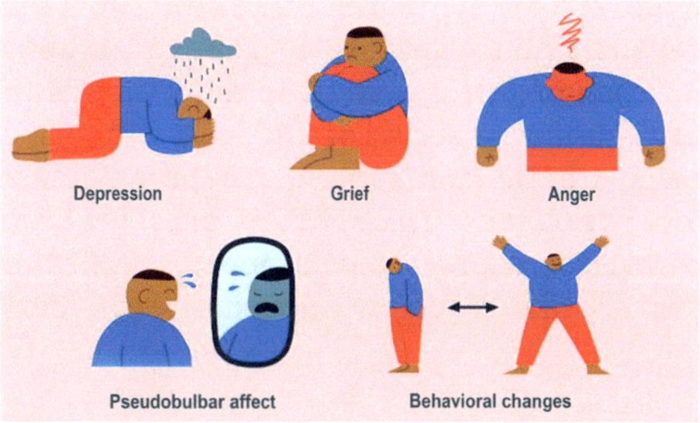

Figure 12.9. Psychological symptoms.

Source: Verywell Health. (n.d.). *Emotional Symptoms in Multiple Sclerosis.* https://www.verywellhealth.com/thmb/WK3gv8db2cdLHP642Vs7GOH0iKU=/1500x0/filters:no_upscale():max_bytes(150000):strip_icc()/emotional-symptoms-in-multiple-sclerosis-4588077_v2-012-c40c2f3b4adc478e85f08d4d2a418323.png.

12.3.3. Variability Based on Substance Type

The clinical presentation and toxicological effects of drug overdoses are highly variable based on the substance, reflecting the challenge of precise diagnosis and successful treatment in toxicology. Patient histories tend to underestimate the number and variety of substances consumed, making clinical evaluation difficult. Analytical screening demonstrates that polysubstance use is prevalent, with a median of three classes of substances identified, versus the median of one in patient histories. Particular drugs like opiates/opioids, benzodiazepines, and pregabalin have leading roles in morbidity and mortality. For instance, opiate exposure is often associated with coma and cardiac arrest, requiring urgent measures such as naloxone administration. Stimulants like cocaine and amphetamines, on the other hand, cause agitation, hallucinations, and psychosis, which may need sedation. This diversity emphasizes the necessity of thorough toxicological examination beyond patient history to inform proper clinical management (Zellner et al., 2024). Temporal trends in substance prevalence also disclose legislative influence and changing drug trends. Initially, within the period under observation, NPS like cathinones and synthetic cannabinoid receptor agonists were prevalent in overdose presentations; however, their prevalence dropped significantly after specific regulatory actions. At the same time, drugs like pregabalin have shown rising rates of abuse and detection, which reflects changing patterns of substance use. These trends immediately affect toxicological priority screening and healthcare resource management, as shifts in availability and popularity of substances can create changes in clinical presentations and necessary interventions. Awareness of such temporal variation is essential to modify overdose prevention strategies and accommodate patient care in accordance with the prevailing drug climate (Zellner et al., 2024). Demographic analyses of overdose fatalities also demonstrate how substance type dictates toxicological outcome and opportunity for interventions. Substance use behaviors and risks of overdose among older adults differ by social connectedness, health status, and healthcare access. For instance, patients involved in pain management treatment regimens are more accessible via healthcare settings, while socially isolated individuals may avoid conventional medical treatment. Substance-related fatalities also occur heterogeneously in terms of alcohol consumption and co-morbid conditions, corresponding to differential toxicological harms and differing opportunities for prevention according to exposure to substances and environmental circumstances. An appreciation of these complexed profiles enables specific harm reduction interventions and highlights the relevance of the combination of toxicological information and patient characteristics toward maximizing interventions for overdose.

Test Your Knowledge

1. What physical symptom is associated with stimulant overdoses?
2. What physical sign indicates a potential drug overdose?

12.4. Risk Factors for Drug Overdose

Learning Outcome

1. Demographic Factors (Age, Gender, etc.)
2. Pre-Existing Health Conditions
3. Patterns of Drug Use

The susceptibility of subjects to drug overdose can be multifariously intertwined with the drug use environments in which it is practiced, more so in a hospital context (Figure 12.10). Patients hospitalized on medical or psychiatric grounds for abusing opioids illicitly are at elevated risk of overdoses, with increased risk of overdoses following and during hospitalization. Variables such as zero-tolerance will force patients into hiding drug practice, most frequently in unsafe environments such as sealed bathrooms for their consumption. Also, the patients might self-treat with illegal opioids or bring their own medication because of fears of undertreated withdrawal or pain management. Discharge to unstable environments like short-term hostels or homelessness further adds to this risk. The multifaceted nature of these factors emphasizes the importance of having hospital policies that are cognizant of the substance use reality, integrating harm reduction strategies and promoting continuity of care to counteract post-discharge overdose death (Lewer et al., 2023). Poly-sedative use significantly aggravates the risk of drug overdose death in opioid users, especially in cases of acute illness or mental health emergencies. Concurrent use of sedatives like benzodiazepines with opioids enhances respiratory depression, a major contributor to overdose death. Hospitalization usually involves patients escalating their sedative intake to alleviate acute symptoms, while changes in physiology during treatment, such as loss of opioid tolerance, render individuals more vulnerable to overdose when they return to typical drug doses. Further, multiple CNS depressants' interaction makes clinical handling and risk assessment problematic. This trend of risky drug combinations underscores the urgent need for increased monitoring and specific interventions against poly-substance use, both in clinical settings and after patient discharge (Lewer et al., 2023). Outside the clinical setting, demographic and psychosocial determinants also play an important role in overdose risk. Forensic toxicology evidence indicates specific patterns in drug use and suicide mechanisms with implications for identifying overdose vulnerability. Males, more commonly engaged in drugs of abuse such as opioids and stimulants, exhibit a greater prevalence of overdose attributed to intentional and accidental situations. On the other hand, females typically use prescription medications, for example, benzodiazepines and antidepressants, associated with self-injury and suicide attempts. Alcohol is found to be a frequent co-factor, mixed with other drugs, thus enhancing overdose potential through dynamic pharmacological interactions. These gendered trends and concurrent toxics highlight the necessity of extensive toxicological testing and focused prevention efforts accounting for sociodemographic factors in preventing drug overdose.

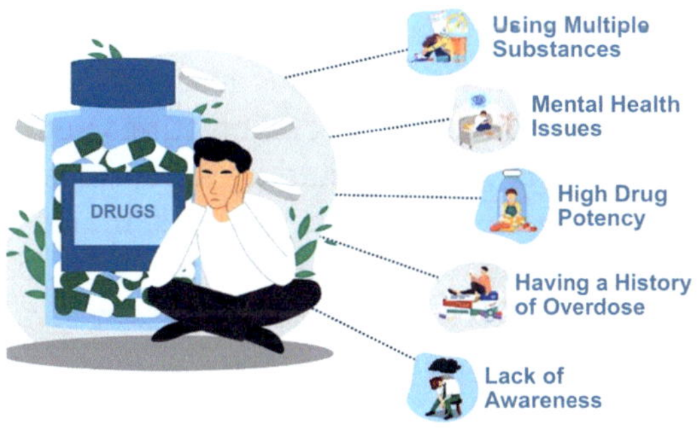

Figure 12.10. Risk factors for drug overdose.

Source: ChoicePoint Health. (2024). *BP-222-Optimized. https*://www.choicepointhealth.com/wp-content/uploads/2024/01/BP-222-optimized.jpg.

12.4.1. Demographic Factors (Age, Gender, etc.)

Grasping the heterogeneity of drug toxicity and metabolism requires an investigation of demographic effects, Shift more specifically the age factor and gender. The pharmacodynamics and pharmacokinetics of most drugs are influenced by these factors, which can have marked effects on toxicity risk and therapeutic efficacy (Figure 12.11). For example, research into phenytoin, a prevalent antiepileptic, has found that blood concentration levels differ significantly among various ethnic groups. Women have higher levels of serum phenytoin than men, which suggests a possible added risk of toxicity if dosing is not well controlled. Additionally, older patients have changed ability to process drugs as a result of the physiological changes of aging. These differences highlight the need for personal treatment monitoring in order to avoid the accumulation of drugs to toxic levels and overdose, particularly in patients with other risk factors including intensive care unit admission or comorbid chronic disease, whose pharmacological effects can be further confounded (Uskur et al., 2025). Gender differences in toxicology are more than just differences in drug metabolism rates, affecting susceptibility to overdoses of some drugs and response to treatment. Evidence from epidemiology shows that males are more likely to have poor outcomes for severe infections needing intensive drug therapy, including tuberculosis. In cases of drug-resistant tuberculosis, males not only have higher susceptibility to multidrug-resistant and extensively drug-resistant strains but also usually present with resistance at the median age of about 40 years. This population trend mirrors underlying biological, behavioral, and potentially socioeconomic determinants predisposing to worse disease courses and complicating pharmacological treatment, thus leading to increased risks of toxicity from complex regimens. This interaction between demographic factors and drug resistance emphasizes the importance of taking gender into account in the evaluation and treatment of drug toxicity and overdose situations (Tariq et al., 2024). Age remains a critical determinant in the landscape of toxicology and overdose risk, influencing both the pharmacological profile of substances and the vulnerability of individuals to adverse effects.

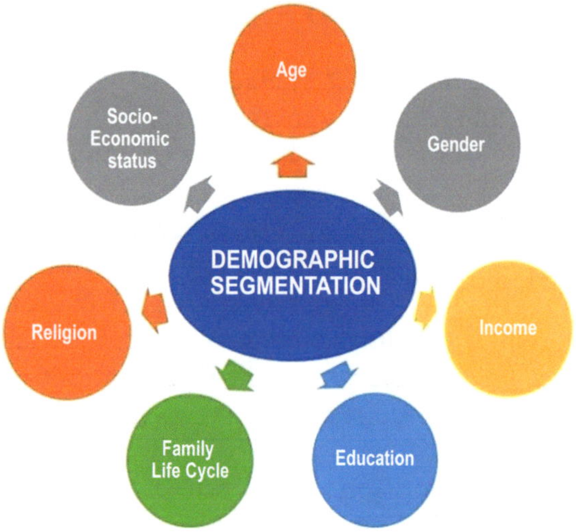

Figure 12.11. Demographic factors.

Source: Cleveland Clinic. (n.d.). Opioid Overdose. https://media.licdn.com/dms/image/v2/D5612AQGNZfTx6xFkRQ/article-cover_image-shrink_720_1280/article-cover_image-shrink_720_1280/0/1687906208798?e=2147483647&v=beta&t=14Ha8uhgUy17ovBxZgK4YAA0YcXJt8WQNhauKw-z8pM.

Younger patients may metabolize drugs more efficiently, albeit with different sensitivities to toxicity, while older adults face increased risks due to diminished organ function and polypharmacy, which raises the propensity for drug interactions and toxic accumulation. As seen in phenytoin treatment, even though age had no statistically significant direct relationship with blood drug concentrations in one investigation, the clinical relevance of changes due to age cannot be dismissed, particularly when combined with gender and comorbidities. Comprehensive toxicological evaluations must thus incorporate demographic factors to ensure that drug dosing and monitoring guidelines are adjusted to minimize overdose rates and enhance therapeutic efficacy in various patient populations (Uskur et al., 2025).

12.4.2. Pre-Existing Health Conditions

The complexity of drug overdose cases is usually compounded by the existence of pre-existing health conditions, which can greatly modify the pharmacokinetics and pharmacodynamics of toxic substances (Figure 12.12). Such underlying conditions, including chronic liver or kidney disease, can compromise the body's capacity to metabolize and eliminate drugs, resulting in increased toxicity or extended drug action. For instance, impaired liver function can decrease the biotransformation of drugs that undergo hepatic metabolism, leading to an increase in plasma drug levels and the risk of toxicity. Pre-existing heart or lung disease can, in a similar manner, potentiate the cardiotoxic or respiratory depressant action of some drugs or toxic substances. This interaction highlights the importance of proper clinical evaluation and personalized treatment plans in the management of overdoses in patients with underlying medical illnesses (Zeppenfeld et al., 2022). Patient history is, therefore, key to maximizing therapeutic intervention and outcomes in toxicological emergencies. Apart from organ pathology, systemic illnesses like immunodeficiency and metabolic syndromes can also affect the severity and outcome of drug overdoses. These health problems commonly weaken the body's ability to recover homeostasis following toxic insult. Oxidative stress is a central factor in this weakness, causing damage to cellular constituents and promoting tissue damage. In this context, the importance of compounds such as N-acetylcysteine (NAC) comes into play, as they inhibit oxidative damage through the replenishment of intracellular glutathione stores, an essential antioxidant. NAC's multi-pronged activities, such as its application in acetaminophen overdose, underscore the ways in which underlying biochemical imbalances influence drug toxicity and overdose treatment (Raghu et al., 2020). Thus, therapeutic drugs acting on oxidative stress pathways are potential adjuncts in the treatment of overdoses with underlying illnesses. The challenge posed by underlying diseases in toxicology goes beyond physiological changes, extending to clinical decision-making and prediction. Chronic neuropathic pain, psychiatric illness, and addictions are conditions that pose both pharmacological and behavioral challenges. Comorbid patients tend to have drug metabolism altered, risk of polypharmacy, and possible drug interactions that heighten the risk of overdose. Chronic illnesses also mask or mimic overdose symptoms, making early diagnosis and intervention difficult. Appreciation of these subtleties necessitates thorough evaluation of the patient and an interdisciplinary approach, including toxicologists, psychiatrists, and other experts to provide optimum care. As explained in new clinical evidence, individualized interventions based on the patients overall health condition improve survival rates and diminish long-term morbidity in overdose situations (Raghu et al., 2020; Zeppenfeld et al., 2022).

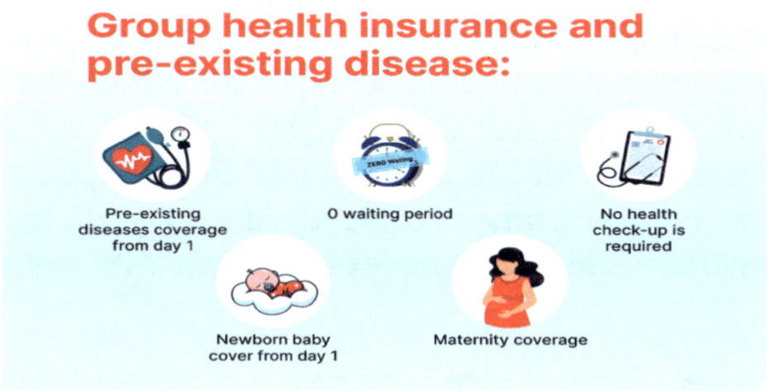

Figure 12.12. Pre-existing health conditions.

Source: https://cdn.prod.website-files.com/6145f7156a1337613524d548/62419fd8c16fe585927601d0_Pre-existing_Infographic02-01.jpg.

12.4.3. Patterns of Drug Use

The knowledge of patterns of drug consumption is of significance in toxicology and managing cases of drug overdose. Trends of substance use identify opioids as the most significant cause of overdose deaths, reflecting prevailing prescription rates and availability of illicit drugs. Such drugs high potential for lethality is compounded by their pharmacologic characteristics such as rapid onset and extreme potential for respiratory depression. This incidence highlights the critical necessity of evidence-based, targeted interventions that acknowledge demographic risk, including unique age cohorts and gender-specific risks, to maximize prevention efforts. In-depth examination of these trends educates clinicians and policymakers regarding evolving drug scenes and the onset of polysubstance use, which makes clinical toxicology and management of overdose challenging. A detailed understanding of usage patterns allows for more effective resource allocation for treatment and harm reduction activities, which can help reduce these increasing public health issues. Knowledge of these changing trends is the foundation for all initiatives to stem the devastating effects of drug overdose in society (Zeppenfeld et al., 2022). No less important is an understanding of the subtlety of interaction between drug and usage context, particularly in high-risk groups such as children. Research indicates that fatal poisonings in children frequently involve opioids, often linked to household exposure rather than direct use. This scenario highlights a pattern where prescription drugs meant for adult therapeutic use inadvertently become deadly in pediatric environments. The complexity deepens with cases involving benzodiazepines, amphetamines, and antidepressants, which contribute significantly to poisoning incidents through either accidental ingestion or intentional misuse. In addition, the analysis highlights that these deaths sometimes entail homicide-suicide dynamics, representing the intense psychosocial correlates of drug use patterns. These findings call for a comprehensive response integrating toxicological surveillance with education at the community level on safe storage of medication, highlighting prevention of accidental exposure in children and acknowledging the wider societal implications of these patterns (Amy et al., 2021). Drug use patterns also mirror more general socio-environmental determinants, including socioeconomic status, availability, and cultural perceptions of drugs. These determinants influence the manner and reasons why specific groups use particular drugs, affecting rates of overdose and toxicological findings. For instance, the transition from solitary prescription abuse to polysubstance abuse patterns demonstrates shifting user patterns based on availability and tolerance. As drug combinations rise, so does the complexity in diagnosing and managing overdoses, calling for robust toxicological models that can cope with multi-agent exposure. The uniform reduction in risk of fatal poisoning with the increment in age of the children also further illustrates the way exposure and use are entangled with phases of growth and family life. A complete understanding of these complex patterns, including intended and unintended administration settings, plays a key role in the development of successful public health policies and creating drug-free environments to lower drug-related morbidity and mortality (Amy et al., 2021).

Test Your Knowledge

1. What is a pre-existing health condition?
2. What is a significant risk factor for drug overdose?

12.5. Diagnosis of Drug Overdose

Learning Outcome

1. Clinical Assessment Techniques
2. Laboratory Tests and Toxicology Screens
3. Differential Diagnosis

The patient's clinical presentation when drug overdose is suspected usually prompts the diagnostic process, necessitating extensive evaluation of history and symptoms (Figure 12.13). Because signs may be uncharacteristic and widely diverse depending on the offending substance, clinicians have to utilize a methodical approach to discern toxic versus non-toxic cause. Initial evaluation typically comprises assessment of vital signs, mental status, and physical examination that aid in the identification of life-threatening conditions and prioritization of treatment interventions. History, if available, gives important information on the type, amount, and time of drug intake but is usually confounded by patient unconsciousness or unreliability. Laboratory tests, such as blood chemistry, arterial blood gas, and levels of certain drugs, add to the clinical scenario by establishing exposure and detecting complications like metabolic acidosis or renal failure. This multi-modal approach reflects the intricacies involved in the diagnosis of drug overdose and the need for combining clinical observations with ancillary investigations to make an accurate judgment (Zeppenfeld et al., 2022). Toxicological screening is an integral part of drug overdose diagnosis but is subject to practical and technical limitations. Immunoassays, which are a common tool for use in emergency situations, provide quick preliminary results to identify drug classes like opioids, benzodiazepines, or amphetamines. The screens, however, can yield false positives or miss identification of some substances, and additional confirmatory testing by more advanced techniques like gas chromatography-mass spectrometry (GC-MS) is required. Proper identification of the causative compound helps guide directed therapy and predict possible complications. In spite of the progress made, the toxicology tests may not indicate the clinical severity or yield quantifiable information adequate for predicting the prognosis. Therefore, it is essential to interpret them cautiously by correlating with clinical presentation as well as other diagnostic results, proving that laboratory investigation compliments but not supersedes thorough clinical assessment in the context of overdose (Zeppenfeld et al., 2022).

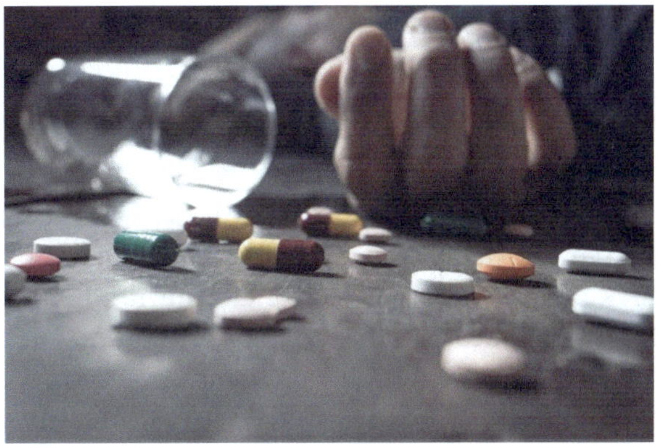

Figure 12.13. Diagnosis of drug overdose.

Source: White River Manor. (n.d.). *Medical complications of drug use disorder*. https://external-content.duckduckgo.com/iu/?u=https%3A%2F%2Fwww.whiterivermanor.com%2Fwp-content%2Fuploads%2FMedical-complications-of-drug-use-disorder-1200x800.jpeg&f=1&nofb=1&ipt=d4648f95083da71c7b28e81c6109e43ed49e76e32677058d017f656a67d92fba.

The need for the multidisciplinary management is witnessed in the overdose diagnosis and management, where toxicology overlaps with other specialties of medicine in managing related complications like musculoskeletal pain due to protracted immobilization or rhabdomyolysis. Musculoskeletal conditions are not the central concern in the event of overdose, yet their assessment is important, especially in altered consciousness or prolonged immobilization patients, possibly adding to morbidity. Early identification of these secondary conditions through physical examination and laboratory indicators advances overall patient care. Furthermore, interaction with toxicologists, pharmacists, and critical care professionals maximizes the diagnostic and therapeutic specificity needed. Therefore, drug overdose diagnosis transcends mere detection of toxins, including thorough clinical and supportive care evaluations that advance outcomes and minimize long-term sequelae.

12.5.1. Clinical Assessment Techniques

In emergency situations, the initial response in treating suspected drug overdose cases is a quick but thorough clinical examination (Figure 12.14) to determine the toxic substance and the physiological status of the patient. One of the common challenges faced by clinicians is the incomplete or unreliable patient history since patients can be unconscious, confused, or resistant to revealing substance use. Hence, clinical evaluation methods must blend observational data, vital signs, and physical examination results with lab analyses to create a cohesive evaluation model. High-throughput mass spectrometry offers improved toxicologic assays that enable rapid and accurate detection of multiple substances, enabling clinicians to distinguish among many ingested agents even if histories are suspect. Such diagnostic improvements have been pivotal in tailoring patient management strategies to individual toxic profiles, particularly as poisoning presentations become increasingly complex due to poly-drug use and NPSs (Siddiqui, 2025; Zellner et al., 2024). Beyond initial identification, clinical assessment encompasses continuous monitoring of neurological and cardiovascular parameters, which are critical in determining the severity of intoxication and guiding therapeutic interventions. For instance, agitation and psychosis are frequently associated with stimulant overdoses such as cocaine and amphetamines, for which sedation is required, while opioid and benzodiazepine poisoning can manifest as respiratory depression with a need for immediate antidote and advanced airway management. The use of scoring systems and clinical decision aids facilitates the stratification of the severity and prognosis of overdose to provide patients with corresponding levels of care ranging from general monitoring to intensive care. Such techniques highlight the necessity of systematic clinical evaluation not merely for the diagnosis of drug overdose but also to predict complications and optimize resource distribution in acute environments (Zellner et al., 2024).

Latest developments in the application of clinical evaluation methods have involved precision medicine and artificial intelligence to improve predictive accuracy and therapy customization of overdoses. Through the incorporation of patients' genetic profiles and metabolic markers with clinical information, patient outcomes can be enhanced and side effects minimized with personalized detoxification regimens. Machine learning patterns are increasingly applied to interpret massive toxicology datasets, enabling forecasts of patient courses and optimising antidote dosing regimens. Telemedicine platforms also bring distant access to toxicology knowledge, especially useful in regions that do not possess specialised facilities, thus greatly enhancing expert clinical evaluation reach. These advances constitute a paradigm change in toxicology from the reactive symptom handling towards proactive individualized intervention, which emphasizes the changing role of clinical evaluation as both diagnostic and prognostic pillar of care in overdoses (Siddiqui, 2025).

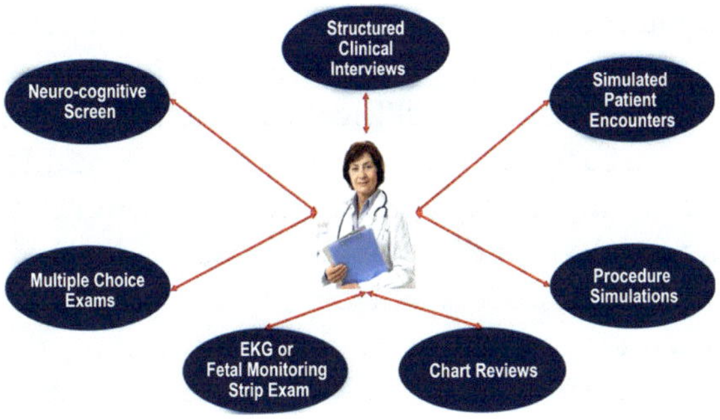

Figure 12.14. Clinical assessment techniques.

Source: Center for Personalized Education for Physicians (CPEP). (n.d.). Revised assessment flowchart. https://www.cpepdoc.org/wp-content/uploads/2018/05/Revised-Assessment-Flowchart-1-1030x541.png.

12.5.2. Laboratory Tests and Toxicology Screens

Differential diagnosis of toxin exposures is essential for efficient patient management in the emergency environment. Laboratory analysis and toxicology screens offer invaluable tools to identify and measure substances in body fluids and tissue samples and hence influence clinical decisions. Such tests, usually conducted on blood, urine, or other body fluids, assist in distinguishing the presence of both ordinary drugs and novel psychoactive substances. In older trauma patients, for instance, identification of polypharmacy by urine toxicology screens within 24 hours of admission has clarified associations between drug use and poor outcomes like hospital stays longer than expected and unplanned intubations. Laboratory confirmation of drug exposure thus not only allows for directed intervention but also increases knowledge about the effects of polypharmacy on prognosis in trauma (Alser et al., 2024). This diagnostic clarity is vital given the nuanced presentation of intoxication symptoms, which can often overlap with other medical conditions. The increasing prevalence of NPS further complicates the toxicological landscape, challenging traditional laboratory screening methods. Standard drug tests frequently fail to detect NPS, which often remain unclassified and are chemically modified to evade regulatory controls. Systematic toxicological examinations using sophisticated analytical methods, such as mass spectrometry and chromatography, are thus needed to determine these substances precisely (Figure 12.15). Initiatives such as Sweden's STRIDA project demonstrate the efficiency of coordinated, systematic toxicology screening combined with clinical data monitoring in responding to and controlling NPS-related intoxications successfully.

By analyzing a broad range of drugs, both traditional illicit drugs and recently produced analogs, such programs reflect the fluidity of drug abuse patterns and emphasize laboratories' need to change constantly in order to offer timely, useful diagnostic information (Helander et al., 2020). When it comes to toxicology and the management of drug overdose, laboratory analyses also have an important role to play in guiding pharmacological and behavioral interventions. Early identification of poly-substance use by sensitive toxicology screens in hospitalized patients enables healthcare providers to predict complications such as respiratory depression or the need for prolonged mechanical ventilation. This is particularly important in at-risk populations such as elderly trauma patients, where co-ingestion of benzodiazepines and opioids has been associated with poor outcomes such as higher rates of unplanned intubation. By combining toxicological information with clinical findings, healthcare teams can individualize treatment regimens to reduce risks and maximize recovery pathways. Furthermore, the continuous improvement of testing protocols in response to new drug trends enhances ongoing public health initiatives to treat substance use disorders more effectively (Alser et al., 2024; Helander et al., 2020).

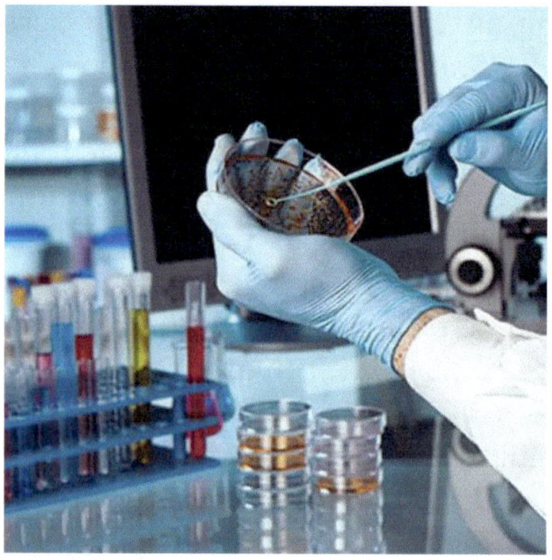

Figure 12.15. Laboratory tests and toxicology screens.

Source: Ganesh Diagnostic and Imaging Centre. (2022). *Toxicology Screen Body Test. https*://www.ganeshdiagnostic.com/admin/public/assets/images/product/1665659450-Toxicology%20Screen%20Body%20Test.webp.

12.5.3. Differential Diagnosis

Correct diagnosis in instances of suspected drug overdose and toxicology calls on clinicians to pay close attention in distinguishing among an array of medical conditions with simulating symptoms of intoxication. Altered mental status, respiratory depression, or cardiovascular instability may be caused by various etiologies such as metabolic abnormalities, infection, neurological conditions, and drug abuse. Separating overdose from other life-threatening illnesses requires a detailed patient history, where available, physical exam, and appropriate laboratory testing. This is compounded by the differences in pharmacodynamics of drugs involved and their effects on comorbid conditions. For instance, individuals with serious substance abuse backgrounds frequently have superimposed psychiatric and medical complications, further clouding the clinical picture. Decisions about treatment, for example, whether to start opioid substitution therapy with methadone or buprenorphine, are dependent on proper diagnosis and knowledge of patient factors underpinning retention and relapse outcomes in clinical experience (Holland et al., 2010). Postmortem toxicology adds a further layer of complexity in differential diagnosis when diagnosing cause of death due to drug overdose. Analysis of drug levels after death must consider variables including drug redistribution, tolerance, and the individual's pathological findings, which can make it difficult to identify the association between substances detected and death. Traditionally, depending on static reference tables in the absence of broad contextual understanding has resulted in diagnostic ambiguity. Recent developments using probabilistic models, such as Bayesian networks, provide a more sophisticated method by combining drug concentration information and pathological condition to quantitatively predict the probability of overdose as a cause of death. Such methods work to enhance the precision of forensic diagnostic estimates, ultimately improving mortality rates and informing public health responses to toxicological emergencies (Bolton et al., 2015). Clinically, differential diagnosis in toxicology highlights the need for the combination of subjective patient reports and objective data with expert systems. Determining the exact substance in an overdose is critical for directing antidotal treatment and estimating patient outcomes. Overlapping presentations and polypharmacy, though, usually render direct diagnosis problematic. The addition of knowledge about the differing drug potencies, half-lives, and susceptibility to dependence makes targeted interventions possible. Further, not excluding alternative diagnoses like acute metabolic or infectious causes prevents misattribution of symptoms to toxic substances alone. In combining clinical acumen, laboratory results, and new analytical techniques, health practitioners can improve the accuracy of diagnosis, enhance the effectiveness of treatment, and limit morbidity and mortality for drug overdose situations (Bolton et al., 2015; Holland et al., 2010).

Test Your Knowledge

1. What is a toxicology screen?
2. Which of clinical assessment techniques?

12.6. Treatment and Management of Overdose

Learning Outcome

1. Immediate Medical Interventions
2. Use of Antidotes
3. Long-Term Rehabilitation Strategies

Successful management and treatment of drug overdose necessitate a clear understanding of the drugs involved as well as their clinical presentations (Figure 12.16). Patients usually present with multifaceted toxicological profiles that baffle traditional diagnostic approaches. Of particular interest, dependence on patient history is not always reliable due to the tendency of patients to underreport the quantity and quality of drugs taken. Analytical urine testing identified a greater median number of classes of substances being used than patient reports, suggesting polysubstance use that complicates treatment. Healthcare providers need to be aware of symptoms like agitation, aggression, hallucinations, and coma that are associated with certain drug detections such as cocaine, opioids, and benzodiazepines. Treatment usually requires immediate sedation, intubation, and administration of antagonists such as Naloxone and Flumazenil to counteract opioid and benzodiazepine toxicity. These interventions are essential in the prevention of morbidity and mortality, especially among patients with multi-drug ingestion patterns and changing substance use patterns (Zellner et al., 2024). New challenges in managing cases of overdose also arise from new substances that are increasingly found in the drug supply. For example, xylazine, a veterinary tranquilizer, has been identified in unregulated opioid supplies, making diagnosis and treatment more difficult. Clinical presentations with xylazine may involve unusual psychoactive symptoms and characteristic cutaneous injury at the sites of injection, which indicate a new pattern of harm. Treatment for xylazine-associated toxicity is not yet well defined, and thus the need for multidisciplinary care including wound care, dermatology, infectious disease, and addiction medicine is a priority. Optimizing medication-assisted treatment of opioid use disorder is a key harm reduction approach that decreases exposure frequency to drug-contaminated xylazine.

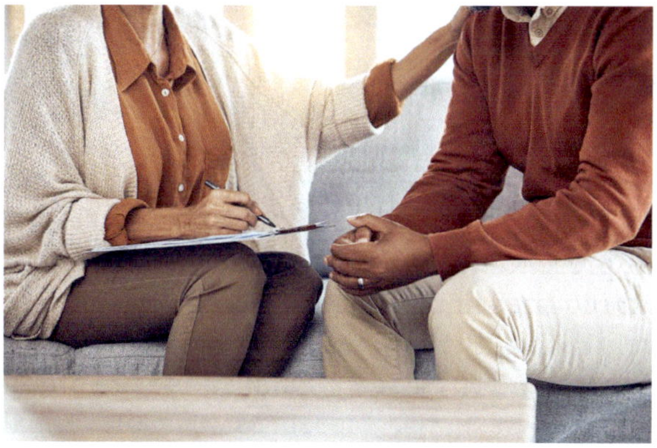

Figure 12.16. Treatment and management of overdose.

Source: San Antonio Recovery Center. (2020). *Stages of Substance Abuse Treatment.* https://www.sanantoniorecoverycenter.com/wp-content/uploads/2020/01/Stages-of-Substance-Abuse-Treatment-.jpg.

This all-encompassing management strategy manages both the acute toxic consequences and the overall setting of substance use disorder to enhance patient outcomes (Dowton et al., 2023). The shifting legislative environment directed at NPSs also affects clinical treatment policies. Decreases in cathinone and synthetic cannabinoid overdoses after legislation suggest the dynamic nature of drug exposure, necessitating ongoing adaptation in clinical practice.

In parallel, the increasing incidence of such substances as Pregabalin in cases of overdose requires increased vigilance and individualized management strategies. Practitioners need to combine toxicological screening with prompt intervention and supportive management, taking into consideration the multifarious pharmacodynamics of novel drugs. Furthermore, the tendency for polysubstance abuse requires multidisciplinary engagement, including psychiatric referral and harm reduction counseling. Optimal overdose care thus depends on reliable toxicological evaluation, timely and targeted medical intervention, and long-term measures to prevent recurrence and enhance survival rates (Zellner et al., 2024).

12.6.1. Immediate Medical Interventions

The presentation of a drug overdose can be abrupt and requires immediate medical intervention to avoid mortality. Airway management, respiratory support, and circulatory stabilization are among the rapid response measures to avoid anoxic brain injury and organ failure. Just as important is the provision of specific antidotes if the toxic substance is known, as it can be used to reverse life-threatening effects. For opioid overdoses, early administration of naloxone has been linked to dramatic decreases in fatality rates. The COVID-19 pandemic emphasized the urgency of instant intervention; emergency medical services and harm reduction measures such as naloxone delivery increased, which was a testament to their role in slowing the surge of overdose fatalities amid times of healthcare disruption and social isolation (Dickson-Gomez et al., 2024). Prompt treatment not only enhances individual survival but also reduces the overall public health burden by limiting the occurrence of severe complications and subsequent healthcare costs. Pharmacologic measures to reverse pathophysiologic processes caused by toxic agents are key to urgent medical management. In overdose with agents causing coagulopathy or hyperfibrinolysis, rapid reversal of bleeding complications is crucial. Conventional antifibrinolytic medications like tranexamic acid (TXA) have been used to stabilize clot development and avert hemorrhage but are being overtaken by newer agents with more favorable potency and safety profiles. BT-114143, an emerging small-molecule plasminogen inhibitor, for example, has demonstrated significantly better affinity and efficacy compared to animal models, holding great promise for larger clinical use in emergency situations presenting with excessive bleeding (Tang et al., 2023).

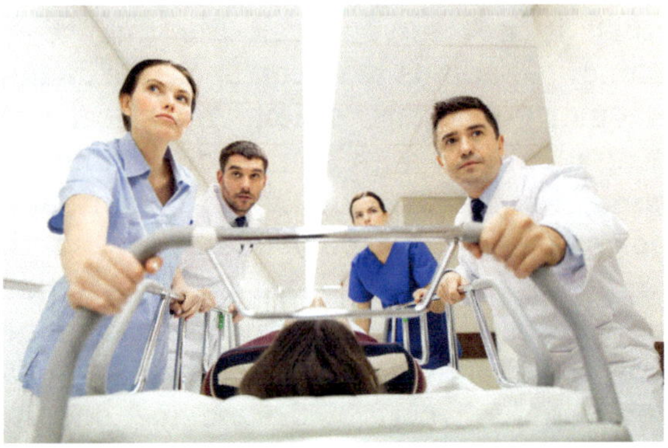

Figure 12.17. Immediate medical interventions.

Source: Hope ER. (2018). *Emergency Medical Care Services in Lufkin.* https://hopeer911.com/wp-content/uploads/2018/01/Emergency-Medical-Care-Services-Lufkin--1024x682.jpg.

Development of such agents highlights the need for pharmacologic advancements to aid in timely care for multifactorial overdose situations with toxic effects. Beyond therapy, timely medical interventions include coordinated system responses that maximize results for victims of overdose. Declines in traditional addiction treatment services during the initial pandemic phase emphasized service availability vulnerabilities, worsening overdose threat. Yet, rising emergency transport requests and Naloxone distribution activities illustrate adaptive measures ensuring a continuum of care through disruptions in healthcare (Dickson-Gomez et al., 2024). Such evidence emphasizes the need for coordinated, elastic emergency response systems that can quickly mobilize resources, provide timely antidote delivery, and continue making addiction treatment accessible. Early intervention, in this context, is a multi-faceted strategy involving clinical expertise, access to specialized drugs, and strong public health infrastructure to minimize mortality and morbidity resulting from toxic exposures and drug overdoses (Figure 12.17).

12.6.2. Use of Antidotes

The antidote's crucial function in treating toxicology cases and drug overdoses cannot be overemphasized. Antidotes are specific agents that reverse the toxic effects of certain poisons, usually by neutralizing the toxins or reversing their physiological effects. The quick administration of such substances can be life-saving, especially in the case of overdoses with opioids or acetaminophen. For instance, treatment of opioid overdose is greatly dependent on using antagonists that act at opioid receptors to effectively reverse normal respiration. The choice of an antidote is based on the type of toxin involved, how it causes toxicity, and clinical presentation, and therefore, their application is a staple in emergency and critical care environments. Their role in toxicologic emergencies is truly invaluable as timely identification and treatment with an antidote tend to decrease morbidity and mortality. The best-known antidotes for opioids include naloxone, which has been the workhorse of opioid reversal for over four decades. Nalmefene, introduced as a strong competitor to naloxone in recent times, has greater receptor affinity and action duration than the latter. Nevertheless, despite the pharmacologic benefit of nalmefene, its application continues to be disputed by virtue of its ability to precipitate prolonged and severe withdrawal syndromes as well as limited clinical evidence confirming its effectiveness within existing synthetic opioid environments. Toxicology professionals suggest that naloxone be continued as a standard opioid antidote until comparative trials confirm the safety and effectiveness of nalmefene. This conservative stance illustrates the delicate deliberations involved when adopting new antidotes in clinical practice to guarantee patient safety always comes first (Stolbach et al., 2023). Another landmark antidote in toxicology is N-acetylcysteine (NAC), mostly utilized to prevent acetaminophen overdose, which is among the most frequent drug toxicities globally. NAC acts by replenishing liver stores of glutathione to detoxify the toxic metabolites generated in the metabolism of acetaminophen. In addition to its antidotal function, NAC's antioxidant activities allow it to shield cells against oxidative stress-mediated damage, further expanding its therapeutic use to respiratory and neurological diseases. The versatile mechanisms of NAC highlight the changing scene in antidotal therapy, where antidotes not only counteract toxicity but also assist in cellular repair and recovery. This clinical extension underlines the necessity for continued research aimed at taking maximum advantage of current antidotes across a variety of toxicological settings (Raghu et al., 2020).

12.6.3. Long-Term Rehabilitation Strategies

Successful recovery from drug overdose goes far beyond emergency medical treatment and requires integrated long-term rehabilitation programs addressing the physical as well as psychological aspects. Survivors of toxicological emergencies frequently struggle with residual complications like chronic pain, neurological deficits, or organ dysfunction, which need cautious handling to avoid relapse or secondary illness. The integration of multi-disciplinary strategies that incorporate pharmacological treatment, physical therapy, and psychological counseling has the potential to regain functional capacity and improve quality of life. The use of multimodal analgesia and interventional therapies can specifically enhance chronic musculoskeletal pain management, frequent overdose sequelae, thereby enabling their return to normal activities and minimizing dependence on potentially dangerous medications (Salah et al., 2021). This integrated strategy recognizes that long-term rehabilitation is not a one-time process but a dynamic and adaptive process demanding individualized and dynamic interventions. The integration of emerging technology is central to maximizing long-term rehabilitation protocols for drug overdose recovery. Wearable electrochemical biosensors, developed for real-time and noninvasive drug monitoring, are a hallmark of personalized medicine by allowing minute-by-minute evaluation of drug levels and metabolic responses. They enable accurate dose control, eliminating side effects and overdose recurrence through faithful adherence to prescribed regimens of therapy (Teymourian et al., 2020). All such advancements allow for dynamic personalization of treatment by clinicians according to real-time pharmacokinetic information, enhancing efficacy of treatment and patient safety. In addition, incorporating these wearable sensors into rehabilitation treatment is in support of autonomous closed-loop systems able to adapt medication administration in reaction to physiological alterations, forecasting a future where long-term rehabilitation grows more data-driven and attuned to unique patient requirements. Successful long-term rehabilitation results must be maintained by a complex balance of continuous medical management and psychosocial support to treat multifactorial difficulties in overdose survivors. Chronic pain management, mental health treatment, and lifestyle change are essential elements that require long-term focus to avoid relapse and encourage functional recovery. The balance between physical recovery and psychological strength is essential; unaddressed chronic pain or outstanding mental health issues can weaken rehabilitation efforts and enhance potential future toxic exposures (Salah et al., 2021). Furthermore, the incorporation of technological innovations like wearable drug monitoring can facilitate continuous monitoring, allowing clinicians to identify early warning signs of nonadherence or withdrawal symptoms (Teymourian et al., 2020). Finally, long-term rehabilitation approaches need to be adaptive, integrating evidence-based clinical interventions with novel technologies and psychosocial interventions to maximize recovery pathways in toxicology settings.

Test Your Knowledge

1. Why is immediate medical intervention critical in cases of drug overdose?
2. What are common conditions requiring long-term rehabilitation?

SUMMARY

The complexity of drug overdose and toxicology necessitates a multi-faceted management and prevention strategy. The diversity of drug interactions, metabolic processes, and patient factors underscores the need for individualized medical interventions and thorough clinical evaluations. Resolution of the causes of overdose, accidental or intentional, necessitates cooperation among healthcare providers, toxicologists, and public health officials. Furthermore, approaches that include education, early intervention, and support systems enhance patient outcomes dramatically. While new therapeutic modalities and drug delivery mechanisms continue to emerge, it is critical that toxicological issues be kept at the front of both research and clinical practice to provide patient safety and effective treatment. The integration of emerging drug delivery systems, including intranasal delivery, displays the directions in the future for overdose management and pain treatment modalities. This approach holds great promise with decreased systemic side effects and the ability to produce a quick therapeutic effect, essential in acute overdose situations. Nonetheless, these new technologies introduce novel toxicological issues that need to be thoroughly assessed to avoid undesirable outcomes. The synergy between innovation and safety highlights the value of aggressive toxicological screening and evidence-guided guidelines, with the goal of ensuring that both pharmacologic innovation and patient-oriented care come together for best recovery and reduced harm in the case of overdoses (Keller et al., 2021). Lastly, the role of multidisciplinary strategies in treating toxicological emergencies, particularly drug overdoses, cannot be emphasized enough. Multimodal analgesia and interventional treatments are the quintessential holistic approaches to managing chronic pain and its risks, such as overdose potential (Salah et al., 2021). Preventative measures in combination with individualized interventions improve recovery and quality of life while mitigating societal burdens. Ultimately, ongoing research, public health action, and clinical surveillance are necessary to counter the catastrophic effect of drug overdose, underpinned by a sophisticated appreciation of toxicological concepts and a dedication to patient-focused care.

Summary of Key Points

Appreciation of the complexity of drug overdose death involves the recognition of wide differences in outcomes based on geographic and demographic variables. Current analysis identifies significant disparities in pregnancy-related deaths between states, where homicide, suicide, and drug overdose as causes vary in contributing to mortality. The influence of firearms adds to violent death among pregnant and postpartum women, highlighting the complexity of variables involved in maternal safety. These results highlight the need for site-specific policy intervention specific to filling in the separate epidemiological landscapes of each state. Developing responses that are evidence-based on statewide trends can provide better outcomes with respect to more effective public health efforts to slow down deaths from overdose and other external causes of death, toward safer environments among at-risk individuals (Maeve et al., 2025). The difficulties in properly identifying and reporting overdose deaths further complicate the efforts to comprehend and fight the opioid crisis. Differences in death investigation practices and resource availability between states lead to substantial underreporting of opioid-related deaths, which in turn impacts the allocation of prevention and treatment funds. A case study of Indiana's legislative changes provides evidence of better surveillance in toxicology and fatal overdose classification, showing the positive effect of organized improvements in coroners' offices. Differences remain, though, due to decentralized systems and limited budgets, suggesting ongoing investment in standardizing death investigations in order to have reliable data collection and policies based on strong data (Meredith et al., 2025). In bringing these findings together, it is clear that responding to drug overdose death requires a multifaceted strategy combining valid surveillance, context-dependent interventions, and ongoing resource investments. Policy informed by data that addresses regional inequities and attacks the root social determinants of overdose, such as violence and mental health, holds the best chance of decreasing fatalities. In addition, enhancing forensic toxicology infrastructure allows for more accurate identification of overdose cases, which subsequently informs public health responses and funding. This integration of epidemiological trends, reporting, and policy implications provides the basis for moving forward with toxicology and overdose prevention initiatives, emphasizing the important convergence of clinical, legal, and social spaces in preventing this chronic public health crisis (Maeve et al., 2025; Meredith et al., 2025).

KEY TERMS FROM THIS CHAPTER

- Polypharmacy
- Toxicology
- Central nervous system (CNS)
- Over-the-counter (OTC)
- Biological Systems
- Dynamic relationship
- Drug Toxicity
- Clinical presentation
- Pharmacodynamics
- Physiological
- Toxicological Issue
- Prescription Medications
- Pharmacokinetics and Pharmacodynamics
- Mechanisms
- New psychoactive substances (NPSs)
- Physical Symptoms
- Blood chemistry
- Drug Overdose

CRITICAL THINKING QUESTIONS

1. **Which of the following is the most commonly used antidote for acetaminophen (paracetamol) overdose?**
   a. Atropine
   b. Naloxone
   c. N-acetylcysteine (NAC)
   d. Flumazenil
2. **What is the mechanism of action of naloxone in opioid overdose?**
   a. Enhances opioid metabolism
   b. Inhibits GABA receptors
   c. Opioid receptor agonist
   d. Opioid receptor antagonist
3. **Which of the following symptoms is characteristic of anticholinergic toxicity?**
   a. Bradycardia
   b. Miosis
   c. Diaphoresis
   d. Dry skin and hallucinations
4. **A patient presents with salicylate (aspirin) overdose. What is the primary acid-base disturbance likely to be seen?**
   a. Respiratory acidosis
   b. Metabolic acidosis
   c. Respiratory alkalosis followed by metabolic acidosis
   d. Metabolic alkalosis
5. **Which drug is used to treat benzodiazepine overdose?**
   a. N-acetylcysteine
   b. Naloxone
   c. Flumazenil
   d. Activated charcoal

Short Answer Questions

1. Differentiate between the toxicological of Types of Drugs Involved in Overdoses?
2. Explain about the Mechanisms of Drug Action?
3. Which of Signs and Symptoms of Drug Overdose?
4. How does a history of mental health disorders increase the risk of intentional and unintentional drug overdose?
5. What Diagnosis of Drug Overdose?
6. What do you understand Treatment and Management of Overdose?

Answers to Multiple choice Questions

1. (c) 2 (d) 3. (d) 4. (c) 5. (c)

REFERENCES

1. Abdalwahd, N., Al-Humadi, H. W., & Al-Saigh, R. J. (2024). Using an *in vitro* pharmacokinetics/pharmacodynamics model to simulate and assess the pharmacodynamic characteristics of voriconazole against some *Candida albicans* isolates in humans. *Review of Clinical Pharmacology and Pharmacokinetics–International Edition.* https://www.semanticscholar.org/paper/444e303533a65e7088f31a6e42e51f4315a9eb35 (accessed on 9 May 2025).
2. Aki, E., Said, E., Alessai, J., Salem, J., & Awad, W. (2018). *Toxicology in Emergency Medicine.* https://core.ac.uk/download/322437837.pdf (accessed on 9 May 2025).
3. Alser, O., Gallastegi, A. D., El Moheb, M., Raybould, T., DePesa, C., Gervasini, A., Flaherty, M., et al. (2024). Outcomes of combined opioids and benzodiazepines consumption in elderly trauma: A retrospective cohort study. *The American Surgeon.* https://www.semanticscholar.org/paper/cbbbe5732ed7776729d81d78e151c14228ad6dbc (accessed on 9 May 2025).
4. Bolton, J., Carlin, M., Langford, A., & Palmer, et al. (2015). *Post-Mortem Toxicology: A Pilot Study to Evaluate the Use of a Bayesian Network to Assess the Likelihood of Fatality.* https://core.ac.uk/download/41072180.pdf.
5. Bunn, T., Costich, J., Mirzaian, M., Daniels, L., Wang, D., & Quesinberry, D. (2023). Interrupted time series analysis of drug overdose fatalities in service-related industries versus non-service-related industries during the COVID-19 pandemic, 2018–2021. *Injury Prevention, 29,* 511–518. https://www.semanticscholar.org/paper/810e089530978a0e6231ab471f80e76ad2b2c291 (accessed on 9 May 2025).
6. Canada, M. L., Farnworth, M. D., Keyes, K. A., Cunningham, R., Ray, B., & Buchanich, J. M. (2025). Unspecified drug overdose deaths and state policy changes: A case study of local coroners. *Journal of Forensic Science and Medicine.* https://www.semanticscholar.org/paper/95775dceb979211a0fae662c5f4176dee9d60182 (accessed on 9 May 2025).
7. Collados-Ros, A., Magarinos Torres, C., Pérez-Cárceles, M. D., Luna Maldonado, A., & Legáz, I. (2022). Suicidal behavior and its relationship with postmortem forensic toxicological findings. *Toxics, 10,* 319. https://doi.org/10.3390/toxics10060319.
8. Costa, V. M., Grando, L. G. R., Milandri, E., Nardi, J., Teixeira, P., Mladěnka, P., Remião, F., et al. (2022). Natural sympathomimetic drugs: From pharmacology to toxicology. *Biomolecules, 12.* https://www.semanticscholar.org/paper/4eb77f95a85553c9cbfd32f38fc255a2db12fec1 (accessed on 9 May 2025).
9. Dai, Z., Limen, G. N., Abate, M., Kraner, J., Mock, A. R., & Smith, G. S. (2022). Characterization of unintentional deaths among buprenorphine users. *Journal of Studies on Alcohol and Drugs, 84*(1), 171–179. https://www.semanticscholar.org/paper/0bf2d1db1f6f3bcb9349b397ab109a800c4fc448 (accessed on 9 May 2025).
10. de Las Cuevas, C., Sanz, E., & de Leon, J. (2022). Respiratory aspiration during treatment with benzodiazepines, antiepileptic and antidepressant drugs in the pharmacovigilance database from VigiBase. *Expert Opinion on Drug Metabolism & Toxicology, 18,* 541–553. https://www.semanticscholar.org/paper/51fc5b47787c5165a17f2b8e325eafae50ceb735 (accessed on 9 May 2025).
11. Diantini, A., Alfaqeeh, M., Permatasari, L. I., Nurfitriani, M., Durotulailah, L., Wulandari, W., Sitorus, T. D., et al. (2024). Clinical toxicology of OTC cough and cold pediatric medications:

A narrative review. *Pediatric Health Medicine and Therapeutics, 15*, 243–255. https://doi.org/10.2147/phmt.s468314.

12. Dickson-Gomez, J., Moran, L., Henriques, S., Brown, C. H., Johnson, K. A., Hills, H. A., Vermeer, W., et al. (2024). Overdose deaths before and during the COVID-19 pandemic in a US county. *Frontiers in Public Health, 12*. https://www.semanticscholar.org/paper/6dc3f1bf95a4dab057d2d1f04e0df4db974d4aa8 (accessed on 9 May 2025).
13. DiNardo, C. D., Stein, A. S., Stein, E. M., Fathi, A. T., Frankfurt, O., Schuh, A. C., Döhner, H., et al. (2020). Mutant isocitrate dehydrogenase 1 inhibitor ivosidenib in combination with azacitidine for newly diagnosed acute myeloid leukemia. *Journal of Clinical Oncology, 39*, 57–65. https://doi.org/10.1200/jco.20.01632.
14. Dinwiddie, A. T., Tanz, L. J., & Bitting, J. (2022). Notes from the field: Antihistamine positivity and involvement in drug overdose deaths—44 jurisdictions, United States, 2019–2020. *MMWR Morbidity and Mortality Weekly Report, 71*, 1308–1310. https://doi.org/10.15585/mmwr.mm7141a4.
15. Dowton, A., Doernberg, M., Heiman, E., Barelli, P. J., Golden, M., Wang, H., Leventhal, J., et al. (2023). Recognition and treatment of wounds in persons using xylazine: A case report from New Haven, Connecticut. *Journal of Addiction Medicine.* https://www.semanticscholar.org/paper/62abba8e2bdfd95ba74163598bbe137eb5f0a80b (accessed on 9 May 2025).
16. El-Tallawy, S. N., Nalamasu, R., Salem, G. I., LeQuang, J. A., Pergolizzi, J. V., & Christo, P. J. (2021). Management of musculoskeletal pain: An update with emphasis on chronic musculoskeletal pain. *Pain and Therapy, 10*, 181–209. https://doi.org/10.1007/s40122-021-00235-2.
17. Forte, S., & John, J. (2002). *Paracetamol: Safety Versus Toxicity.* https://core.ac.uk/download/83019627.pdf (accessed on 9 May 2025).
18. Ghorbani, A., & Esmaeilizadeh, M. (2017). Pharmacological properties of *Salvia officinalis* and its components. *Journal of Traditional and Complementary Medicine, 7*, 433–440. https://doi.org/10.1016/j.jtcme.2016.12.014.
19. Gray, A., Douglas, S., Tiller, M., & Bleakley, M. (2024). Using forensic intelligence as a model for determining future toxicology methods: TBI forensic toxicology and forensic drug chemistry nitazene identification. *Journal of Analytical Toxicology.* https://www.semanticscholar.org/paper/6ae6830a968811c0ff8682116767f6fb8efa8bb5 (accessed on 9 May 2025).
20. Helander, A., Bäckberg, M., & Beck, O. (2020). Drug trends and harm related to new psychoactive substances (NPS) in Sweden from 2010 to 2016: Experiences from the STRIDA project. *PLoS ONE, 15.* https://www.semanticscholar.org/paper/1390facd2399bde9585b429b4b91146a1d1acdae (accessed on 9 May 2025).
21. Holland, R., Maskrey, V., Pinto, H., Rumball, L., et al. (2010). The SUMMIT trial: A field comparison of buprenorphine versus methadone maintenance treatment. https://core.ac.uk/download/2774301.pdf (accessed on 9 May 2025).
22. Hunter, A. A., Schwab-Reese, L. M., DiVietro, S., & McCollum, S. (2021). An examination of fatal child poisonings in the United States using the National Violent Death Reporting System (NVDRS), 2012–2017. *Clinical Toxicology, 60*, 342–347. https://doi.org/10.1080/15563650.2021.1955913.
23. Jalal, H., Buchanich, J. M., Roberts, M. S., Balmert, L. C., Zhang, K., & Burke, D. S. (2018). Changing dynamics of the drug overdose epidemic in the United States from 1979 through 2016. *Science, 361*. https://doi.org/10.1126/science.aau1184.

24. Keller, L. A., Merkel, O. M., & Popp, A. (2021). Intranasal drug delivery: Opportunities and toxicologic challenges during drug development. *Drug Delivery and Translational Research, 12*, 735–757. https://doi.org/10.1007/s13346-020-00891-5.
25. Klein, S. S., Bloom, J., Gnirke, M., & Howland, M. (2023). Comment on: Are antimuscarinic effects common in hydroxyzine overdose? A cohort analysis of antimuscarinic effects in hydroxyzine and diphenhydramine poisoned patients. *Clinical Toxicology, 61*, 562–563. https://www.semanticscholar.org/paper/24251edcde3c6b79a75818f34aed4c9e0715d3a3 (accessed on 9 May 2025).
26. Kurdil, N. V., Andriushchenko, V. V., Ivashchenko, O. V., Volosovets, A., Sheyman, B. S., Bobkovych, K. O., & Palamar, B. (2024a). The modern view of the use of extracorporeal detoxification in the treatment of drug poisoning (overdose). *Polski Merkuriusz Lekarski, 52*(5), 522–528. https://www.semanticscholar.org/paper/2fd78112ff0d218422dc4f693b8a614e25125286 (accessed on 9 May 2025).
27. Kurdil, N., Volosovets, A., Ivashchenko, O. V., Lisovska, V., Balan, H. M., Rozhkova, O. M., & Andriushchenko, V. (2024b). Apallic syndrome of toxic origin: The diagnostic criteria. *Emergency Medicine*. https://www.semanticscholar.org/paper/30d97deb93656107ba810a6eddff0cd1b19aa9b1 (accessed on 9 May 2025).
28. Lewer, D., Brothers, T. D., Harris, M., Rock, K. L., & Copeland, C. S. (2023). Opioid-related deaths during hospital admissions or shortly after discharge in the United Kingdom: A thematic framework analysis of coroner reports. *PLoS ONE, 18*, e0283549. https://doi.org/10.1371/journal.pone.0283549.
29. Mason, M., Mclone, S., Bartell, T. R., Welch, S. B., Sheehan, K., & Post, L. (2020). A cross-sectional study of opioid involvement in non-poisoning suicide–Risks and prevention opportunities. *BMC Public Health, 21*. https://www.semanticscholar.org/paper/ed8a883e5d268ad3f9a1c036eae6b69e8766676b (accessed on 9 May 2025).
30. Mason, M., Pandya, K., & Lundberg, A. L. (2024). Older adult drug overdose: An application of latent class analysis to identify prevention opportunities. *Harm Reduction Journal, 21*. https://www.semanticscholar.org/paper/1188c8eaf9163a518878ac05ac0ef903cde4e3b4 (accessed on 9 May 2025).
31. Nakatsu, L., Lopez, J. R., Garcia, C. M., Cherian, M., Nash, J., Tofighi, D., Seifert, S. A., et al. (2025). Comparison of two-bag and three-bag acetylcysteine regimens in the treatment of paracetamol poisoning: A systematic review and meta-analysis. *Clinical Toxicology*. https://www.semanticscholar.org/paper/9a0d105f1c704c6134af1260110275c930bf7743 (accessed on 9 May 2025).
32. Raghu, G., Berk, M., Campochiaro, P. A., Jaeschke, H., Marenzi, G., Richeldi, L., Wen, F., et al. (2020). The multifaceted therapeutic role of N-acetylcysteine (NAC) in disorders characterized by oxidative stress. *Current Neuropharmacology, 19*, 1202–1224. https://doi.org/10.2174/1570159x19666201230144109.
33. Siddiqui, N. (2025). Advances in medical toxicology: Innovative approaches for poisoning and overdose management. *Asian Journal of Pharmaceutics*. https://www.semanticscholar.org/paper/b550f36549aea70ea4285fbad4d821f31452d4b3 (accessed on 9 May 2025).
34. Spencer, M., Miniño, A. M., & Warner, M. (2022). Drug overdose deaths in the United States, 2001–2021. https://doi.org/10.15620/cdc:122556.

35. Stolbach, A., Mazer-Amirshahi, M., Nelson, L. S., & Cole, J. B. (2023). American College of Medical Toxicology and the American Academy of Clinical Toxicology position statement: Nalmefene should not replace naloxone as the primary opioid antidote at this time. *Clinical Toxicology, 61*, 952–955. https://doi.org/10.1080/15563650.2023.2283391.

36. Tang, J., Ji, S., Hu, X., Wang, Y., Qi, J., Wang, X., Wang, H., et al. (2023). Discovery of BT-114143, a novel and potent small-molecule plasminogen inhibitor for hyperfibrinolysis. *Blood*. https://www.semanticscholar.org/paper/2f015771ee068b09bb95ed1e07b0a435226fb2dc (accessed on 9 May 2025).

37. Tariq, A., & Fazal, S. (2024). Exploring genomic patterns to identify drug-resistant TB: A comprehensive study of age, gender, lineage, and outcome. *Advancements in Life Sciences*. https://www.semanticscholar.org/paper/447ef737e79f67e073c6fe0e638fce302f16063b (accessed on 9 May 2025).

38. Teymourian, H., Parrilla, M., Sempionatto, J. R., Montiel, N. F., Barfidokht, A., Van Echelpoel, R., De Wael, K., et al. (2020). Wearable electrochemical sensors for the monitoring and screening of drugs. *ACS Sensors, 5*, 2679–2700. https://doi.org/10.1021/acssensors.0c01318.

39. Tomassini, L., Giuli, G., Bottoni, E., David, M. C., & Scendoni, R. (2024). Drug overdose deaths during prison riots and mental states of prisoners: A case study. *Frontiers in Psychiatry, 15*. https://www.semanticscholar.org/paper/541d2b9e657bca97acfe68067bc3138c22f120b6 (accessed on 9 May 2025).

40. Uskur, T., Guven, O., Kartal, Y., Tat, M., & Onal, B. (2025). Phenytoin blood levels and their relationship with physiological and demographic factors: A retrospective analysis of gender, age, and drug interactions. *Medicine Science | International Medical Journal*. https://www.semanticscholar.org/paper/8bd8275a90906bf079372d73b6cf70c567c22d48 (accessed on 9 May 2025).

41. Wallace, M. E., & Jahn, J. L. (2025). Pregnancy-associated mortality due to homicide, suicide, and drug overdose. *JAMA Network Open, 8*. https://www.semanticscholar.org/paper/c199d46333cb870b421538014d898e4756b906d4 (accessed on 9 May 2025).

42. Zellner, T., Eyer, F., Rabe, C., Geith, S., Haberl, B., & Schmoll, S. (2024). Recreational drug overdose—Clinical value of toxicological analysis. *Toxics, 12*. https://www.semanticscholar.org/paper/e702cea3ab910fae858a570f90754b57a0152e62 (accessed on 9 May 2025).

43. Zeppenfeld, K., Tfelt-Hansen, J., Riva, M., Winkel, B. G., Behr, E. R., Blom, N. A., Charron, P., et al. (2022). 2022 ESC Guidelines for the management of patients with ventricular arrhythmias and the prevention of sudden cardiac death. *European Heart Journal, 43*, 3997–4126. https://doi.org/10.1093/eurheartj/ehac262.

44. Zimmerman-Federle, H., Ren, G., Dowling, S., Warren, C., Rusyniak, D., Avera, R., & Manicke, N. E. (2024). Plasma drug screening using paper spray mass spectrometry with integrated solid phase extraction. *Drug Testing and Analysis, 17*, 138–151. https://www.semanticscholar.org/paper/1dca8a0c052c37cb2dec68bf6fef49961c4349ff (accessed on 9 May 2025).

PHARMACOGENOMICS

13

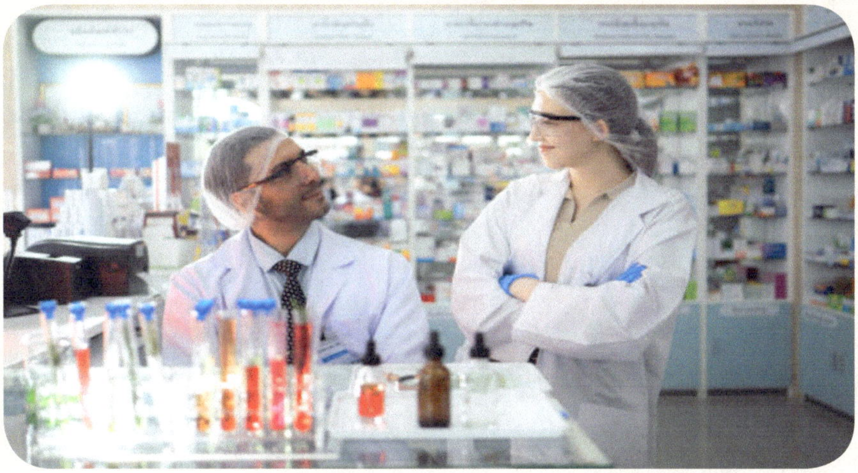

Introduction

The rapid progress of genomic technologies has fueled a paradigm change in biomedical research and medicine, allowing an in-depth analysis of the genetic basis of disease and responsiveness to treatment. Of these developments, next-generation sequencing (NGS) is noteworthy for the fast and inexpensive generation of huge amounts of genetic information, thus speeding up discoveries in genetic diversity and its clinical correlates. This technological shift lends the basis on which the science of pharmacogenomics has developed—a new field that attempts to personalize drug treatment with respect to each person's genetic makeup. By way of in-depth genomic investigations, scientists are able to determine genes that affect drug metabolism, drug action, and drug toxicity, with a final aim to maximize therapeutic outcomes and reduce side effects. The scientific advancements provided by high-throughput sequencing platforms and the related bioinformatics challenges highlight the challenge but promise of mainstreaming genomics in daily clinical practice (Abdi et al., 2024). Complex diseases

LEARNING OBJECTIVES

After studying this chapter, you will be able to:

1. Explain historical background
2. Identify the mechanisms of pharmacogenomics
3. Discuss applications in medicine
4. Define challenges and limitations
5. Describe future directions
6. List of case studies

like diabetes mellitus show the importance of precision in the medical treatment paradigm, showing the shortcomings of traditional "one-size-fits-all" models. Genetic variation between individuals frequently governs variable drug response, making some drugs ineffective or even toxic to specific patient groups. Personalized medicine, especially pharmacogenomics (Figure 13.1), presents a powerful vehicle to contend with such variability through correlating genetic data with personalized drug therapy choices. This not only enhances efficacy but also minimizes the potential for adverse drug reactions (ADRs)—a significant issue in diabetes management of multifactorial diseases.

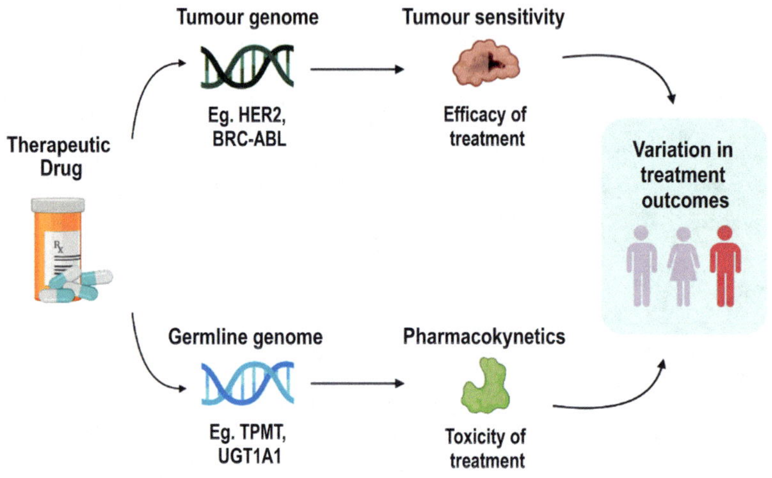

Figure 13.1. Pharmacogenomics of genomic.

Source: Jeyang259. (2020). *Cancer Pharmacogenomics.* Wikimedia Commons.https://upload.wikimedia.org/wikipedia/commons/1/1c/Cancer_pharmacogenomics.png.

The integration of genetic screening and pharmacogenomic testing makes patient-specific risk factors and drug metabolism profiles identifiable, allowing clinicians to develop targeted treatment strategies. Combined with lifestyle change and behavioral interventions, individualized medication regimens can dramatically improve patient outcomes and quality of life across a wide range of disease conditions (Sugandh et al., 2023). Pharmacogenomics is a convergence of genomics, pharmacology, and clinical medicine and uses genetic information to drive the choice, dosage, and combination of medications for specific patients. Its development has been driven by high-density genomic mapping technologies and the increasing availability of large datasets explaining genotype-phenotype associations. Through the explanation of the molecular basis of variable drug response, pharmacogenomics is poised to revolutionize therapeutic practice from reactive to anticipatory and preventive. The assimilation of this information into clinical practice must consider ethical issues, patient privacy, and testing and implementation logistics. In spite of these obstacles, the continued cross-disciplinary collaboration between researchers, clinicians, and bioinformaticians continues to drive the advancement of pharmacogenomic knowledge into everyday healthcare. This overlap has the promise not only to enhance the efficacy of treatment but also to initiate a new generation of precision medicine based on the genomic individuality of every patient (Abdi et al., 2024; Sugandh et al., 2023).

Definition of Pharmacogenomics

The comprehension of how genetic variation impacts personal responses to drugs has emerged as an essential priority in contemporary biomedical research. Pharmacogenomics is a multidisciplinary endeavor that examines how an individual's genetic composition impacts their response to medicines, both in terms of therapeutic effects and side effects. Through the examination of genetic profiles, pharmacogenomics seeks to maximize drug choice and dosing, ultimately improving drug safety and efficacy. This strategy diverges from the one-size-fits-all approach and instead opens up the door for individualized medicine. The use of genomics information to inform clinical choices hinges on sophisticated computational technology, which enables the gathering, storing, and analysis of large-scale biological data. The cross-disciplinary interplay between genetics and pharmacology requires a collaborative effort from different scientific disciplines, underscoring pharmacogenomics place in the larger umbrella of bioinformatics and molecular medicine (Mahanayak, 2024). The introduction of NSG technologies has greatly increased the breadth and depth of pharmacogenomic research. NSG technologies enable the creation of large genomic datasets that reflect variation responsible for varying drug response at unprecedented scales of detail. Accumulation of such data calls for high-value bioinformatics tools to properly process, analyze, and interpret intricate genomic data. Pharmacogenomics uses these resources to detect genetic markers associated with drug metabolism, effectiveness, and toxicity, thereby informing treatment choices. Notwithstanding its potential, the discipline is challenged by integrating data, interpreting them, and communicating results in medical practice. Overcoming these traps involves implementing standardized procedures in data handling and multidisciplinary cooperation between computational biologists and physicians to provide scientific worth and clinical utility (Barrot et al., 2019). Pharmacogenomics can thus be envisioned as a precision technology to individualize pharmacotherapy according to the genetic makeup of a patient. It integrates genomics, molecular biology, and drug development to forecast drug response heterogeneity, reducing ADRs and enhancing therapeutic efficacy. Pharmacogenomics informs mechanistic approaches to personalized therapy by determining the genetic polymorphisms that govern pharmacokinetics and pharmacodynamics. The discipline also interlinks with structural bioinformatics, which helps explain molecular interactions between drugs and their targets at an atomic level, further addressing drug design and optimization (Mahanayak, 2024). With the ongoing development of pharmacogenomics, the discipline has the capability to transform medicine by changing therapeutic decision-making from generalized protocols to individualized regimens based on genetic information.

Importance in Personalized Medicine

The changing landscape of contemporary medicine increasingly places importance on the use of individualized care to maximize therapeutic responses. Pharmacogenomics, through the study of genetic variation among human beings, enables customization of medication types and dosages according to an individual's personalized genetic profile. The approach reduces ADR risks and increases efficacy by going beyond the conventional one-size-fits-all model. For example, applying genomic information into clinical practice supports accurate drug metabolism and response prediction, eventually making patient care more secure and efficient at a healthcare cost perspective. The efficacy of this practice does rely to some extent, nonetheless, on both the existence of complete genetic databases and the community's contribution in biobanking, promoting collecting varied genetic sources needed for viable research and development (Al-Delaimy et al., 2019). Thus, the convergence of pharmacogenomics and personalized medicine is a revolutionary step towards safer and more effective medicines that meet individual requirements. Traditional therapeutics have long been bogged down by challenges arising out of drug response variability across populations, which pharmacogenomics aims to resolve with population-specific information. Particularly in the context of genetic diversity, knowledge about allele frequencies and how these affect drug metabolism can assist clinicians in prescribing the right drugs. Yet, variations in access to resources and genomic knowledge restrict the utilization of pharmacogenomics globally. Programs like the Pharmacogenetics for Every Nation Initiative (PGENI) attempt to offset such variations by aggregating pharmacogenomic marker profiles and developing country-specific guidelines that enable the incorporation of genetic information into clinical practice. This international strategy identifies the role of pharmacogenomics in personalized care by facilitating balanced and well-informed drug therapy choices, thus ensuring that the patient receives medicines that account for their individualized genetic profile (Borg et al., 2012).

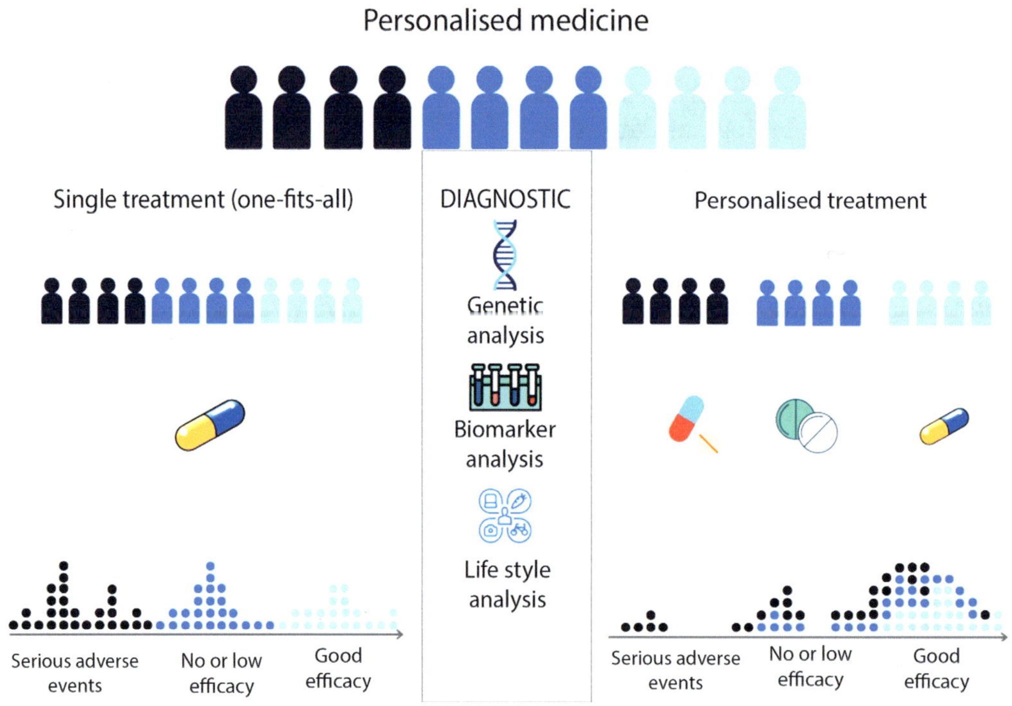

Figure 13.2. Personalized medicine.

Source: Genosalut. (2022). *Genosalut Personalized Medicine.* https://www.genosalut.com/wp-content/uploads/2022/05/Genosalut_Personalised_medicine-1024x683.png.

Increasing awareness between healthcare providers and patients is also key to optimizing the potential offered by precision medicine. In addition to clinical efficacy, pharmacogenomics-based personalized medicine also emphasizes ethical and social factors, important in the maintenance of public trust and engagement (Figure 13.2). Volunteer participation in donating biological samples to biobanks is essential for the advancement of pharmacogenomic research, but this is affected by the diverse sociocultural beliefs of individuals such as age, educational level, and religious factors. Privacy protection, confidentiality, and protecting participant autonomy are indispensable in responding to fears that could discourage participation. Positive public sentiment offers a platform upon which ethical biobanking practices can thrive, thus enabling continued advancement in personalized medicine (Al-Delaimy et al., 2019). Ultimately, awareness and integration of these social forces promote the Responsible use of pharmacogenomics, creating a climate that promotes innovation while maintaining ethical requirements for long-term achievement in personalized healthcare.

13.1. Historical Background

Learning Outcome

1. Early Discoveries in Genetics
2. Development of Pharmacogenomics as a Field
3. Key Milestones in Pharmacogenomic Research

This path to deciphering the genetic mechanisms of drug response started well before the development of contemporary molecular biology, with roots in early observations of widely varying reactions to drugs between individuals. Early intuitions arose from recognition of the role of inherited characteristics in determining susceptibility to certain diseases and to toxicities of drugs. Advances in genetic technology progressively enabled scientists to extend beyond phenotypic observation to the molecular definition of genes involved in drug metabolism. A milestone in this evolution was the development of a holistic strategy that would be able to combine individual genomic information to forecast therapeutic responses. This futuristic concept—encompassing the sequencing and analysis of complete genomes—predicted a future where personalized medical treatment could become commonplace, as suggested by the idea of newborns having a genomic map to guide clinical choices (Felice et al., 2002). Such vision highlighted the revolutionary role of pharmacogenomics in individualized medicine. Developments in the late 20th and early 21st centuries were a defining period for pharmacogenomics, propelled by technological advances in genotyping and DNA sequencing. The breakthroughs facilitated the detection of polymorphisms in drug-metabolizing enzymes, like those in the cytochrome P450 family, which are of paramount importance in pharmacokinetics. A striking example is that of CYP2B6 enzyme, whose genetic forms have been associated with various metabolic phenotypes in diverse populations. Studies of CYP2B6 polymorphisms among African populations identified unique haplotype patterns together with convergent metabolic abilities, reporting strong interaction between genes and drug metabolism (Dongho et al., 2018).

Not only did this create more focus on population genetics during pharmacogenomic studies, but it also reaffirmed the need for ethnic diversity to be taken into consideration while formulating precision medicine treatment schedules. The historical basis of pharmacogenomics is also complemented by its global health implications. Inter-individual variation in drug response has been vital to solve diseases with high morbidity and mortality around the world, such as malaria and HIV. Research carried out in Botswana has been a case in point regarding how knowledge about genetic variation within drug-metabolizing enzymes may explain variable treatment outcomes in disease-burdened areas (Dongho et al., 2018). This geographically and culturally situated strategy constitutes a break with one-size-fits-all medicine, promoting genetic profile-guided individualized treatment strategies. By historical standards, the incorporation of pharmacogenomics into clinical medicine is a turning point from experience-based treatment toward evidence-based precision medicine, supported by decades of clinical and genetic research that develops further today.

13.1.1. Early Discoveries in Genetics

The roots of contemporary pharmacogenomics have their origins in groundbreaking observations on heredity predating the era of molecular biology. Early experiments, including Gregor Mendels experiments with pea plants, provided the basis for the idea of inheritable characteristics directed by distinct units of inheritance, today referred to as genes (Figure 13.3). They led the way to insights into the ways genetic variation affects individuals response to biology. Later, scientists came to realize that genetic differences could account for differences in drug metabolism and response among patients, and that was a milestone. The determination of chromosomal theory and the development of cytogenetics further explained how genes are structured and passed on and gave needed outlines for relating genetics to phenotypic characteristics. Breakthroughs in the characterization of phenotypes—subsequently formalized by the development of tools like the Human Phenotype Ontology—provided foundation for genotype-phenotype correlation, a relationship central to pharmacogenomics discovery (Sebastian et al., 2020). This marriage of genetics to the clinical information created early paradigms that continue to influence personalized medicine.

The breakthrough in early genetic studies came with the discovery of hereditary patterns in complex diseases, which unveiled the multifactorial nature of gene-environment relationships. Studies of neurodevelopmental disorders, including attention deficit hyperactivity disorder (ADHD), emphasized the large heritability factor, approximated at 74%, based on family and twin studies. They confirmed that genetic effects extend beyond Mendelian patterns of inheritance, with polygenic and rare variant contributions. Genome-wide association scans (GWAS) and copy number variant analyses revealed the subtle but additive impact of many genetic sites on disease risk, substantiating the complex interplay of genes in human health. These findings highlighted the need to analyze whole genomic patterns instead of individual genes, an approach that spurred pharmacogenomic strategies to forecast varying responses to drugs attributed to genetic variation (Stephen et al., 2018).

It has been critical to understand such sophisticated genetic foundations to be able to personalize treatment approaches to an individual's specific genetic profile. Systematic enumeration of phenotypicucky" abnormalities and their genetic basis has played a key role in driving the science of pharmacogenomics. With such tools as the Human Phenotype Ontology, accurate, computationally tractable descriptions of clinical characteristics have been made possible to enable cross-species phenotype comparisons and improve the discernment of gene-phenotype associations. This methodical strategy allows researchers and clinicians to associate genetic variants with particular clinical outcomes more precisely, enhancing diagnostic yield and therapeutic choices (Sebastian et al., 2020). With early genetic findings shedding light on the mechanisms of inheritance and gene expression variation, incorporation of precise phenotypic information was essential for translating genomic data into the clinic. In turn, these developments have influenced contemporary pharmacogenomic designs by facilitating more accurate genotype-phenotype correlations that direct individually tailored medication choice and dosing to optimize efficacy and limit side effects.

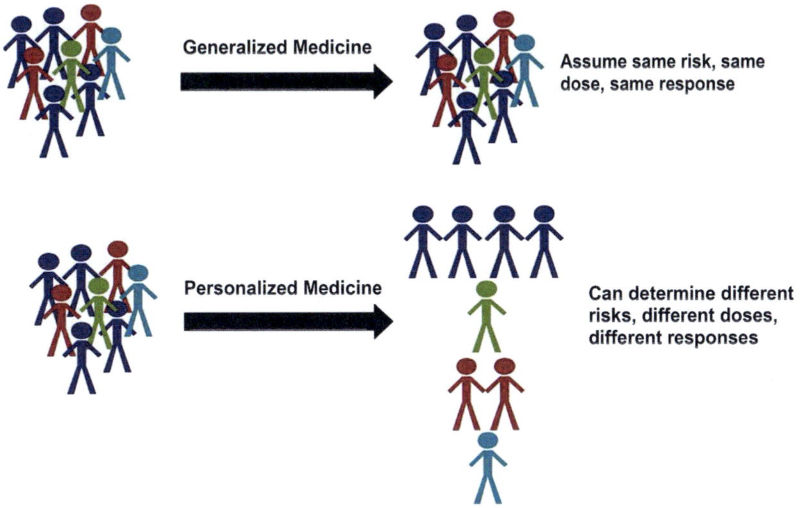

Figure 13.3. Early discoveries in genetics.

Source: https://1.bp.blogspot.com/-20COc2fk96w/UXsbsegtqbI/AAAAAAAAA-g/9BO8Y3WO6yk/s1600/Personalized+medicine.jpg.

13.1.2. Development of Pharmacogenomics as a Field

The evolution of medicine from a one-size-fits-all to more tailored treatments represents a big step forward in medicine, closely linked to the emergence of pharmacogenomics. The science developed as researchers aimed to figure out how variations in genes affected response to medications and tried to reduce unwanted side effects while maximizing therapeutic effect (Figure 13.4). The Human Genome Project's completion formed the building block, cracking the intricate blueprint of human genetics and allowing researchers to discover certain genetic variants of drug metabolism and action. It created precision medicine, which extends beyond historical evidence-based care by stratifying patients into biologically defined groups for precise treatments. Pharmacogenomics, as a cornerstone of this movement, focuses on tailoring medication regimens based on individual genetic profiles, advancing the goal of more effective and safer healthcare interventions (Wang et al., 2023). Technological advancements have been instrumental in accelerating the development of pharmacogenomics. The introduction of NGS revolutionized genomic analysis by allowing rapid, large-scale, and cost-effective sequencing of DNA and RNA. This technology opened up unparalleled access to rich genetic data, revealing variations that affect drug response at a much more nuanced resolution. NGS has broadened pharmacogenomic studies from single-gene studies to whole-genome and transcriptome analysis that allows overall identification of genetic markers indicative of drug efficacy and toxicity. Accordingly, the incorporation of high-throughput sequencing has allowed for the discovery of novel therapeutic targets, design of new drug development protocols, and more tailored treatment strategies based on molecular understanding (Satam et al., 2023). In spite of these developments, the evolution of pharmacogenomics as a discipline still encounters challenges that define its path. To reach its full potential, it needs to overcome technical and analytical challenges, including enhancing the sensitivity and accuracy of genomic information and designing stable algorithms to decipher intricate interactions among genes. In addition, the effective clinical application of pharmacogenomic information is contingent on defining standard protocols for genetic testing and incorporating the information into standard healthcare systems. As the discipline evolves, interdisciplinary coordination among clinicians, researchers, and policymakers becomes essential to improve disease subtype classification and extend targeted therapies, realizing the two major goals of precision medicine. Pharmacogenomics is therefore set to revolutionize clinical practice by providing tailored treatments that mirror individual genetic variability (Satam et al., 2023; Wang et al., 2023).

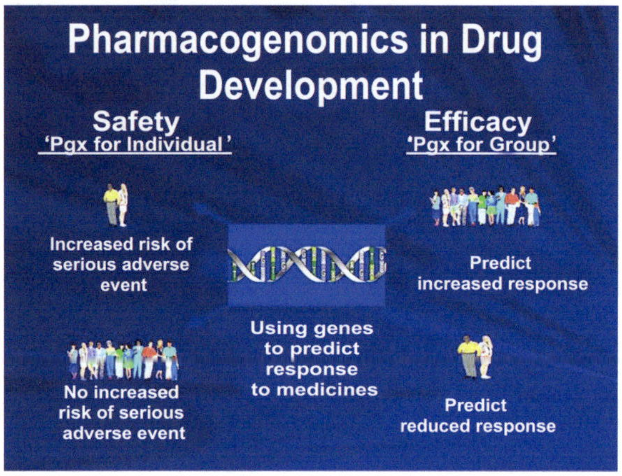

Figure 13.4. Development of pharmacogenomics as a field.

Source: Walker, M. G. (n.d.). *Pharmacogenomics in Drug Development.* https://slideplayer.com/slide/9404695/28/images/3/Pharmacogenomics+in+Drug+Development.jpg.

13.1.3. Key Milestones in Pharmacogenomic Research

The path to discovery of how genetic variation affects drug response has been characterized by a series of landmark advances that set the stage for contemporary pharmacogenomics. Early advances in the middle of the 20th century, including the detection of genetic polymorphisms in drug-metabolizing enzymes such as cytochrome P450, highlighted the biological origin of variability in drug efficacy and toxicity between individuals. As molecular techniques advanced, researchers began to characterize the genetic variants responsible for altered drug metabolism, enabling the prediction of ADRs and individual drug responses. This shift from empirical treatment to a more personalized approach catalyzed the evolution of pharmacogenomics from a theoretical concept into a clinical science. The coming together of large-scale genomic data sets and bioinformatics has since speeded up clinically applicable gene-drug interactions, ultimately resulting in better therapeutic outcomes and decreased costs of healthcare. These achievements are a landmark change in the comprehension of human genetics within pharmacotherapy. Building on the initial biochemical and molecular findings, contemporary pharmacogenomic studies have explored population-based genetic variations, a field with far-reaching implications for global health equity. The appreciation of genetic diversity among populations has led to large-scale genomic studies, especially among underrepresented populations, to ensure that pharmacogenomic interventions are maximally effective and inclusive globally. Indeed, translational research and applications in genomics in Africa have accentuated the continent's unique genetic landscape and how it contributes to variability in drug response. These efforts encourage interdisciplinary work among geneticists, clinicians, and bioethicists to direct scientific findings in accordance with regional health needs, tackling infectious and non-communicable diseases that are common in these areas. These achievements highlight the importance of integrating varied genetic profiles in pharmacogenomics studies as a central move toward just healthcare and better patient outcomes worldwide (David et al., 2024). The process of translation of research results to clinical and commercial use is another noteworthy achievement in pharmacogenomic research. The application of laboratory breakthroughs into useful diagnostic tools and therapeutics is an example of how university innovation can have a direct impact on clinical practice. Technology transfer case studies highlight the challenges and successes of doing this process, particularly in life sciences where there are regulatory, technical, and market obstacles. For example, the creation and validation of targeted pharmacogenomic prototypes illustrate how scientific understanding of gene-drug interactions can be converted into marketable products that enable personalized medicine. These developments not only confirm the technical viability of pharmacogenomic tools but also illustrate their potential for enhancing laboratory medicine practice on a large scale. These gains underscore the significant role played by translational science in bringing pharmacogenomics to bedside from the bench, delivering improved patient outcomes through precision treatment and diagnostics (Cariati et al., 2020).

Test Your Knowledge

1. What early genetic discoveries laid the foundation for pharmacogenomics?
2. What is the future direction of pharmacogenomics research?

13.2. Mechanisms of Pharmacogenomics

Learning Outcome

1. Role of Genetic Variations in Drug Metabolism
2. Influence of Single Nucleotide Polymorphisms (SNPs)
3. Impact of Gene Expression on Drug Response

Progresses in molecular genetics have dramatically transformed our ability to explain individual differences in drug response, largely via the analysis of pharmacogenomics. Fundamentally, pharmacogenomics investigates how genetic variation affects the metabolism, effectiveness, and toxicity of drugs. Key mechanisms include genetic variation in genes coding for drug-metabolizing enzymes, transporters, and receptors, which together define a patient's pharmacokinetic and pharmacodynamic profiles (Figure 13.5). For instance, polymorphisms within cytochrome P450 enzymes have the potential to cause variations in drug metabolism, hence influencing drug concentrations and therapeutic outcomes. The application of NGS methods has greatly improved the capacity to investigate these variants quickly and more accurately, facilitating extensive genetic characterization. But even with growing sequencing capability, problems persist in deciphering the complex genetic information and placing it in clinical decision-making processes owing to problems with quality, ethics, and a lack of standardized procedure for implementation (Paepe et al., 2013). Realizing how complex genetic factors affect drug response underscores the need for personalized medicine, especially in the management of complex diseases such as hypertension. The traditional one-size-fits-all strategy frequently does not take into account the heterogeneity of patients' genetic background and disease manifestation. Mechanistically, pharmacogenomic differences may influence both the pharmacokinetics of drugs—how drugs are absorbed, distributed, metabolized, and excreted by the body—and pharmacodynamics—how drugs interact with biological targets. These differences are responsible for variable therapeutic effects and ADRs, making it difficult for clinicians to provide optimal dosing. Through the integration of genetic risk factors, phenotype characterization, and molecular profiles, pharmacogenomics facilitates personalized therapies that improve drug efficacy with less toxicity. This is a paradigm shift from empirical treatments to precision medicine, which is particularly important for diseases with variable etiologies such as hypertension (Borghi et al., 2017). The use of pharmacogenomics in clinical practice depends predominantly on identifying the particular molecular pathways disrupted by genetic variants. Mechanisms including modified enzyme activity, binding affinity at receptors, and drug transporter function directly impact the pharmacological response.

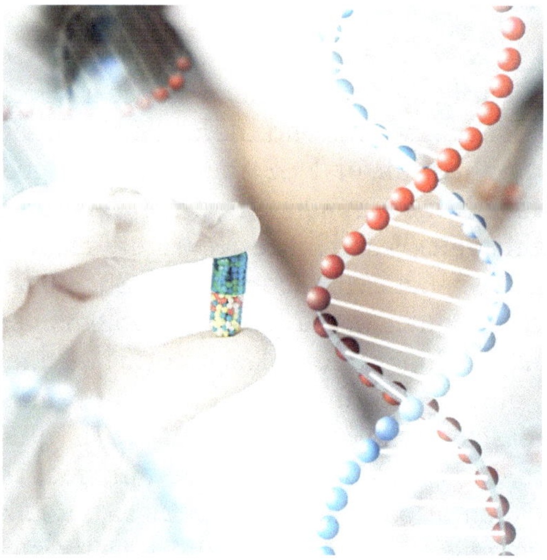

Figure 13.5. Mechanisms of pharmacogenomics.

Source: Scion Lab Services. (n.d.). *What is Pharmacogenomics?* https://scionlabservices.com/assets/images/what-is-pharmacogenomics-square.jpg.

For example, loss-of-function mutations in metabolic enzymes lead to drug accumulation and elevate the risk of toxicity, while gain-of-function variants promote accelerated clearance, lowering therapeutic effectiveness. Transporter proteins influenced by genetic polymorphisms can alter drug absorption and distribution, further making response variability more complex. In spite of the potential of NGS technologies to facilitate quick and extensive genotyping, bridging these mechanistic findings into routine clinical practices is a hurdle because of heterogeneity in the reproducibility of genetic correlations and the ethical implications of genomic screening. Consensus-based recommendations and further studies are needed to overcome these limitations and realize the full potential of pharmacogenomic mechanisms for tailored therapy (Paepe et al., 2013).

13.2.1. Role of Genetic Variations in Drug Metabolism

This interindividual variability in drug response has been a conundrum for clinicians for many years, leading investigators to seek explanations in underlying biological, as opposed to environmental, factors. Of these factors, genetic differences play a central role in determining drug metabolism, and consequently the therapeutic effect, as well as the risk of adverse drug reactions. Drug metabolism is largely regulated by enzymes that are coded by genes having polymorphic variants, resulting in variations in enzymatic activity between individuals. Such genetic polymorphisms have the potential to influence rates of drug biotransformation, affecting active drug levels and, therefore, clinical response. Variations in cytochrome P450 enzymes, for instance, have been demonstrated to heavily influence drug clearance. Knowledge of such genetic variation is important in optimizing drug dosing and enhancing patient safety, setting the stage for pharmacogenomics-directed personalized medicine (Barrese et al., 2014). Further explaining the role of genetic variations, studies on β-blockers in the treatment of heart failure illustrate how pharmacogenomics can guide individualized therapy. The adrenergic receptor system, which mediates the pharmacodynamics of β-blockers, has polymorphisms that affect variability in patients' drug response. Research on adrenergic receptor genes and proteins shows that some polymorphisms can increase or decrease β-blocker efficacy, indicating the requirement for genotype-directed dosing regimens. Additionally, genetic differences influencing the metabolism of β-blockers per se play a pivotal role in deciding the drug's bioavailability and therapeutic effect. Incorporation of such genetic data in clinical practice is likely to aid in maximizing treatment regimens based on individual genetic backgrounds, thus enhancing prognosis in heart failure therapy (Barrese et al., 2014). As pharmacogenetics matures from initial observational studies to a strong scientific field, the clinical uses of genotyping technologies have grown enormously. The discovery of several gene polymorphisms that affect both pharmacokinetics and pharmacodynamics forms the basis of the development of pharmacogenetic tests that can predict drug response. Such tests allow clinicians to predict therapeutic efficacy and adverse effects, thereby enabling more accurate drug selection and dosing. This patient-specific strategy minimizes trial-and-error prescribing and maximizes the benefit-risk ratio in drug treatment. The growing accessibility and cost-effectiveness of genetic screening are propelling pharmacogenomics to the center of personalized medicine, ushering in an era of therapies tailored to unique genetic compositions (Fenech et al., 2014).

13.2.2. Influence of Single Nucleotide Polymorphisms (SNPs)

Genomic technology advances have dramatically influenced our comprehension of how personal genetic variation impinges on drug response. Single nucleotide polymorphisms (SNPs), the most prevalent type of genetic variation, are important in affecting pharmacological treatment efficacy and toxicity. Single-base variations can modify drug metabolism, transport, and receptor binding, thereby affecting therapy (Figure 13.6). For example, enzyme gene variants controlling drug biotransformation may accelerate or inhibit metabolism, requiring dosage adaptation to maximize efficacy and reduce toxicities. As pharmacogenomics guides more clinical decisions, SNP profiling has the potential for tailored medicine by predicting patients most responsive to a given treatment or in danger of adverse side effects. Such accuracy in drug treatment would improve rates of treatment success, particularly in conditions such as hepatitis C, where response to treatment is affected by SNPs in important host genes (Caputo et al., 2017). Implementation of SNP analysis in clinical practice depends not only on identifying pertinent variants but also on correctly interpreting their clinical implications. Technologies of high-throughput genotyping are now available that can simultaneously screen thousands of SNPs and thereby present an exhaustive genetic picture to guide therapy. With this advance in the capacity for genetic testing, challenges also arise in data interpretation: finding a variant is not always an inevitable precursor to clinical phenotype, and high-quality genotype-phenotype correlation studies are required. In addition, economic and logistical imperatives inherent to the introduction of extensive SNP testing into clinical labs need to be weighed against cost-effectiveness and the potential for enhanced patient care. The complex recognition of the way SNPs affect drug response heightens the need for multidisciplinary collaboration in the translation of genetic discoveries into useful clinical guidelines (Schrijver et al., 2011). Aside from their implications on the management of individual patient care, SNPs carry important consequences for public health policies, especially in populations with dissimilar genetic backgrounds. Allele frequency differences among ethnic groups influence drug response profiles, emphasizing the need for population-specific pharmacogenomic studies. For instance, American populations with Native American backgrounds exhibit dissimilar SNP profiles related to drug metabolism, requiring customized treatment regimens to ensure maximum therapeutic gain and reduced side effects. This population-centered approach is crucial in resource-limited settings where universal access to new therapeutics is constrained. Assessing SNP markers could offer a cost-effective method for prioritizing treatment and managing healthcare resources more efficiently. Thus, pharmacogenomics, through SNP analysis, offers a pathway to equitable, individualized treatment paradigms that consider both genetic diversity and socioeconomic realities (Caputo et al., 2017).

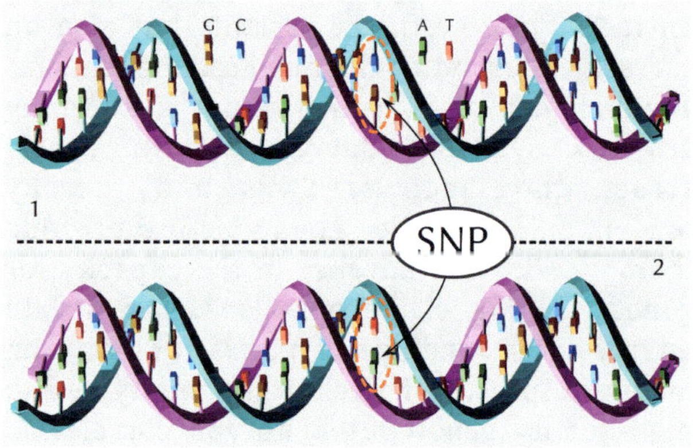

Figure 13.6. Influence of single nucleotide polymorphisms (SNPs).

Source: Wikipedia contributors. (n.d.). *DNA Single Nucleotide Polymorphism (SNP)*. Wikimedia Commons. https://upload.wikimedia.org/wikipedia/commons/thumb/2/2e/Dna-SNP.svg/1200px-Dna-SNP.svg.png.

13.2.3. Impact of Gene Expression on Drug Response

The heterogeneity of patient responses to drugs is a key problem in clinical pharmacology, which is usually due to the differential expression of genes that are responsible for drug metabolism, transport, and targets. Gene expression affects the concentration and activity of enzymes that are responsible for drug biotransformation, thus modifying the pharmacokinetics and pharmacodynamics of drugs. This dynamic pattern can result in tremendous variability in drug efficacy and toxicity profiles between individuals, making standardized dosing regimens challenging. By comprehending these molecular differences, one can better predict drug response, thus enabling personalized treatment. Pharmacogenomics as a field merges patterns of gene expression with clinical pharmacology to enhance therapeutic action. Multidisciplinary educational platforms and research meetings like the Golden Helix Pharmacogenomics Days have helped distribute knowledge in these areas with a focus on the importance of gene expression in maximizing drug response and promoting personalized medicine (Borg et al., 2012). Immunosuppressive therapy in organ transplantation best illustrates the importance of gene expression on drug response as a result of narrow therapeutic index and intricate pharmacokinetics. Genetic variations in the expression of genes for drug-metabolizing enzymes, transport proteins, and immune-related targets underlie marked interpatient variability in immunosuppressant blood concentrations and clinical response. Thus, deficient gene expression can lead to patients becoming at risk for transplant rejection or for toxicities like nephrotoxicity or enhanced susceptibility to infections. Though therapeutic drug monitoring (TDM) continues to be the cornerstone of personalized care, it never fully addresses the pharmacodynamic complexity influenced by gene expression patterns. The combination of pharmacogenetic information with biomarker-guided strategies holds the promise of optimizing dosing regimens and risk stratification, thereby revolutionizing immunosuppressive regimens and enhancing graft survival rates (Abboudi et al., 2012). Advances in high-throughput technologies have made precise characterization of gene expression patterns possible, creating essential information on how these molecular signatures shape drug responses in heterogeneous populations. This knowledge holds practical utility in optimizing drug development and clinical decision-making for targeted therapies according to genetic and transcriptomic profiles. In addition, differential expression of drug targets and transporter proteins directly influences treatment efficacy and resistance mechanisms, uncovering new therapeutic targets. Pharmacogenomics harmonizes these intricate biological variables to develop better and safer drug regimens, minimizing ADRs and enhancing patient compliance. As continuing research identifies further gene expression biomarkers, the discipline is set to provide more accurate and mechanistically guided pharmacotherapy, underpinning the shift towards the genuine personalized medicine paradigm (Abboudi et al., 2012; Borg et al., 2012).

Test Your Knowledge

1. What is a Single Nucleotide Polymorphism (SNP)?
2. How do genetic variations influence drug metabolism and response?

13.3. Applications in Medicine

Learning Outcome

1. Tailoring Drug Therapies for Individual Patients
2. Case Studies of Successful Pharmacogenomic Interventions
3. Integration into Clinical Practice

Development in molecular diagnostics and genomic technologies has driven a revolutionary change in clinical practice, facilitating more precise and personalized methods of healthcare. This revolution makes it possible for doctors to customize treatments according to a patient's individual genetic makeup, making therapeutic interventions both more effective and safer. Pharmacogenomics is one of the key drivers of this personalized medicine approach by determining genetic variations that impact drug metabolism, response, and toxicity (Figure 13.7). For example, patients with certain genetic markers may be treated with drugs that optimize therapeutic benefit and reduce side effects, thus enhancing clinical outcomes. This type of precision therapy not only improves chronic disease management but also guides preventive interventions that address individual risk profiles. This ability to tailor medical treatment to the genetic complexities of a given patient illustrates the increased potential and use of pharmacogenomics in current medicine (Borro et al., 2017). Financial implications are an intrinsic part of the wider introduction of pharmacogenomic testing to health systems. New cost-effectiveness analyses demonstrate that pharmacogenomic screening usually means a sound financial investment compared to standard treatment strategies. Numerous reviews of studies illustrate that the application of these genetic tests can save healthcare dollars by lowering ADRs, preventing wasteful treatment, and maximizing drug choice at initiation. Nevertheless, the heterogeneity of testing charges and the inconsistency of reporting on the internal value of pharmacogenomic tests pose challenges in evaluating their economic effect comprehensively. In spite of these constraints, most existing assessments concur with the cost-saving potential of pharmacogenomics, highlighting the necessity for strong clinical evidence and well-designed economic models for future healthcare policy and reimbursement decisions (Annemans et al., 2016). Introducing pharmacogenomics into healthcare practice is not without issue, specifically in terms of standardization and validation of genetic tests used to inform therapeutic choices. Ensuring the clinical utility of pharmacogenomic information requires strict validation of test accuracy and the development of clear guidelines for the interpretation of genetic information in the context of treatment choice.

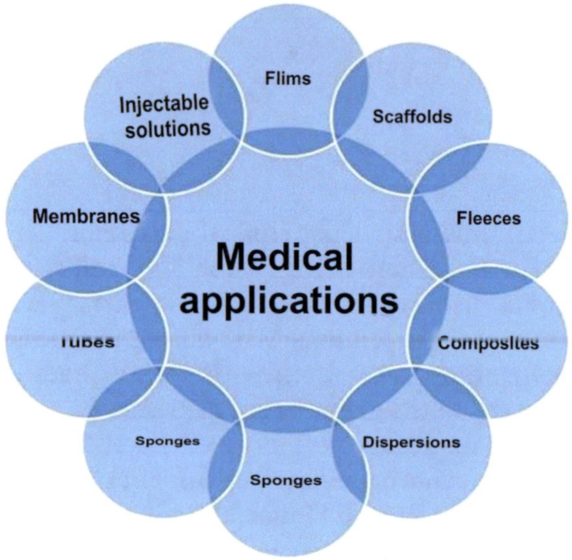

Figure 13.7. Applications in medicine.

Source: Kulkarni, P., & Maniyar, M. G. (2020). *Medical Applications of Collagen* [Figure 3]. In *Utilization of Fish Collagen in Pharmaceutical and Biomedical Industries: Waste to Wealth Creation*. Research Journal of Life Sciences, Bioinformatics, Pharmaceutical and Chemical Sciences, 6(3), 1–10.

In addition, the complexity of gene-drug interactions necessitates continued research to increase the scope of actionable markers and to define how multiple genetic factors together affect drug response. The success of these challenges will depend on interdisciplinary teamwork between clinicians, geneticists, and health economists to maximize implementation plans. As pharmacogenomics keeps developing, its use holds a future where therapy is not just more efficient but also economically viable and accessible to everyone, finally improving personalized patient care (Annemans et al., 2016; Borro et al., 2017).

13.3.1. Tailoring Drug Therapies for Individual Patients

The progress of personalized medicine has revolutionized the field of therapeutic interventions significantly, promoting innovations that emphasize the individual variability in drug response. At the center of this transition is the integration of pharmacogenomics, which explains how genetic variation affects drug metabolism, efficacy, and toxicity. Through polymorphism analysis in drug-metabolizing enzymes, transporters, and receptor targets, clinicians can better anticipate patient-specific responses, reducing side effects and enhancing therapeutic success. This genomic understanding, coupled with advancements in other "omics" sciences like proteomics and metabolomics, allows for a multi-faceted appreciation of patient biology. These integrated biomarker panels provide a nuanced method for customizing therapies beyond genetic code to include environmental and personal elements for maximizing patient care. Even with the promise, issues such as ethnic heterogeneity and healthcare biases remain, emphasizing the necessity of continued research and validation to facilitate fair application in heterogeneous populations (Sad Wée et al., 2023). Recent advances in diagnostic tools simultaneously improve the accuracy of customized treatments (Figure 13.8). Implementation of next-generation sequencing (NSG) and high-end proteomic and metabolomic assays enables a detailed investigation of cellular and subcellular functions in patients. These instruments allow the discovery of specific molecular signatures for disease states and thus direct the choice and dosage of drugs with greater specificity. The increasing application of assays combining genomic information with clinical parameters is an example of the advance toward actionable, individualized therapeutic strategies. Additionally, advances in software and analytical platforms make it possible to interpret sophisticated datasets, ushering in a new era of artificial intelligence-directed clinical decision-making. Effective cooperation between disciplines and international industries is needed to move these developments into everyday clinical use, because they have the promise of improving outcome by delivering treatment to the genetic and molecular nature of each patient's illness (Samuel et al., 2020). The day-to-day implementation of pharmacogenomics in the clinical environment illustrates the shift away from a one-size-fits-all approach towards a more tailored, patient-oriented practice. Molecularly targeted therapies, especially in cancer, illustrate the advantages of this paradigm, in which drugs are chosen according to the genetic profile of tumors and not merely by histological type. This specificity diminishes trial-and-error prescribing, lowers exposure to ineffective medication, and shortens response times. But the application of extensive genomic information to prescribed drug regimens demands strong clinical guidelines, regulatory systems, and economic factors. The embedding of multifactorial panels of biomarkers with environmental and lifestyle information illustrates the intricacy of personalized medication management. As these factors come together, clinicians can more accurately predict adverse reactions and drug resistance, thus personalizing interventions responding to individuality at various biological levels (Sad Wée et al., 2023).

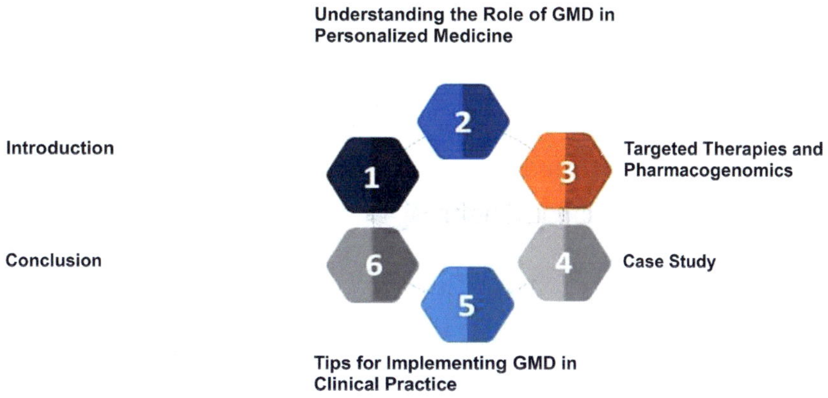

Figure 13.8. Tailoring drug therapies for individual patients.

Source: FasterCapital. (n.d.). *Tailoring Treatments to Individual Needs.* https://fastercapital.com/topics/tailoring-treatments-to-individual-needs.html.

13.3.2. Case Studies of Successful Pharmacogenomic Interventions

The implementation of pharmacogenomics in the clinical setting has been characterized by a number of well-known case studies illustrating its ability to maximize therapeutic benefit. A prime example has been the application of genetic screening to inform warfarin dosing, a commonly used anticoagulant with a narrow therapeutic margin. By examining gene variation in the CYP2C9 and VKORC1 genes, physicians can individualize doses of warfarin to each patient, decreasing the risk of adverse bleeding complications and enhancing efficacy. Individualized dosing not only maximizes patient safety but also eliminates the trial-and-error phase inherent in conventional dosing regimens. Other analogous interventions in oncology have applied genetic profiling to choose targeted therapies, illustrating how pharmacogenomic information is converted into treatment regimens that enhance response rates substantially and reduce toxicity, reflecting a hopeful turn towards personalized medicine. Additionally, the successful use of pharmacogenomics can be seen in the therapy of psychiatric illness, where genetic variants guide patients' response to antidepressants and antipsychotics. For example, patient stratification by CYP450 enzyme polymorphisms enables psychiatrists to forecast metabolic rates and drug clearance and accordingly modify dosages and medication. Such decisions minimize ADRs and maximize treatment compliance and outcomes. Research following such interventions has documented enhanced symptom control and decreased hospitalization rates among patients on genotype-guided therapies. These case studies indicate the significant position of pharmacogenomics in narrowing the gap between genetic data and clinical action, pointing to its applicability in sophisticated disease care involving sensitive medication regimens. In addition, success with implementation in pharmacogenomics is also affected by system-based aspects like healthcare infrastructure and practitioner training, as exemplified in multidisciplinary collaborative frameworks. Application of pharmacogenomic testing in the clinical environment is frequently dependent on technological infrastructure and experts to respond to genetic information. Programs prioritizing ongoing professional education and organizational support have reflected significant improvements in the adoption of pharmacogenomic guidelines. Integrative models, which couple genetic knowledge with patient reflective practice and personalized education, have been associated with improved clinical outcomes and an open culture to personalized medicine (Naz et al., 2024; Ruşen, 2024). These holistic case studies set a roadmap for expanding pharmacogenomic interventions, pointing to the interplay between scientific innovation and pragmatic healthcare delivery.

13.3.3. Integration into Clinical Practice

The introduction of whole genome sequencing (WGS) has opened unprecedented avenues for transforming clinical practice in many areas of medicine. WGS provides a full genome analysis of the human genome, generating massive quantities of genetic information that can be used to support individualized treatment regimens. Interpreting such abundance, though, requires advanced computational algorithms, incorporating machine learning software and large-scale genotype–phenotype databases to provide clinically useful information (Figure 13.9). This incorporation of genomics into regular healthcare allows the subdiscipline of pharmacogenomics, whereby patient individual genetic profiles direct medication selection and dosage. With the use of this strategy, physicians can predict drug response variability and reduce ADRs, which are still considerable issues in standard prescribing strategies. Therefore, incorporating WGS-driven pharmacogenomics into clinical routines is an essential step toward achieving genuinely individualized medicine, increasing therapeutic efficacy, and optimizing patient outcomes (Brlek et al., 2024). The move from bench to bedside for pharmacogenomics is especially important in areas like anesthesia, where accurate dosing and medication selection can literally make or break patient safety and recovery. Precision medicine approaches utilize genetic data to personalize anesthetic treatment, minimizing the risk of perioperative complication due to variable drug metabolism or adverse reactions. For example, patients possessing certain genetic variants might need different dosages of anesthetics or associated drugs to obtain the intended therapeutic effect without toxicity. Pharmacogenomics implementation in surgical protocols requires the creation of strong genetic databases and clinical decision support systems so that anesthesiologists can obtain genomic-related information in an efficient manner. Ethical issues and cost-benefit assessments also have implications for successful implementation. However, with advancing technology and mounting evidence, the application of pharmacogenomics in anesthesia is an exciting horizon to improve individualized patient management as well as healthcare quality (Malviya et al., 2024). Although it has great potential, the large-scale clinical implementation of pharmacogenomics faces several hurdles in the form of requisite standardized guidelines, education of providers, and infrastructure to facilitate genomic information interpretation. The integration of genetic testing into standard clinical practice involves not just technological commitment but agreement regarding when and how to use pharmacogenomic information in medication prescription. It will take coordination among geneticists, pharmacologists, and clinicians at the point of care to convert genomic findings into useful tools that enhance drug safety and effectiveness. In addition, the ethical concerns of handling genetic data, patient consent, and data privacy should be addressed cautiously to enhance trust and acceptance. With increasing numbers of multi-omics data integrated and reducing costs of sequencing, implementation barriers are slowly decreasing, making pharmacogenomics an integral part of individualized healthcare and clinical decision-making (Brlek et al., 2024; Malviya et al., 2024).

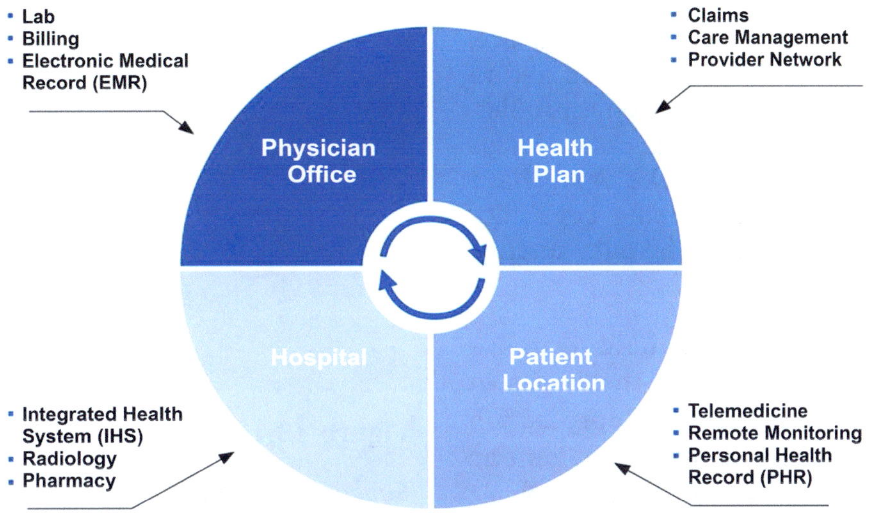

Figure 13.9. Integration into clinical practice.

Source: Impetus Digital. (2019). *Integration into Clinical Practice.* https://www.impetusdigital.com/wp-content/uploads/2019/01/Screen-Shot-2019-01-21-at-12.28.59-PM.png.

Test Your Knowledge

1. What is the primary goal of tailoring drug therapies to individual patients?
2. What is Whole Genome Sequencing (WGS)?

13.4. Challenges and Limitations

Learning Outcome

1. Ethical Considerations in Genetic Testing
2. Variability in Patient Responses
3. Regulatory and Accessibility Issues

Even with the potential of pharmacogenomics in tailoring medicine, its integration into regular clinical practice is still limited. A major hindrance is the inconsistent and at times contradictory results with specific genetic variants, which makes it difficult to develop concrete treatment guidelines. In the absence of standardized procedures, clinicians are left uncertain in the interpretation of pharmacogenomic results, thus reluctant to implement widespread use. In addition, the comparatively sluggish nature in acquiring in-depth pharmacogenomic profiles, particularly in emergency clinical cases, delays decision-making. Advances like NSG have nonetheless increased sequencing capability but with still-existing issues of data quality, interpretation, and ethics.

These new technologies hold promise but, at the same time, present challenges in guaranteeing effective utilization, protection of privacy, and ethical handling of genetic information in medical settings (Paepe et al., 2013). Aside from technical and interpretive challenges, ethical and social factors pose considerable hurdles in the realization of pharmacogenomics (Figure 13.10). The storage, handling, and use of genetic information pose privacy and confidentiality issues among patients, affecting their participation in genetic testing or biobanking programs. Confidence in healthcare institutions and the protection of sensitive genomic information are topmost in fostering acceptance. Sociodemographic considerations also shape public opinion about involvement in pharmacogenomic studies, including age, education, and religious or cultural beliefs. Resolution of these issues entails open communication and culturally appropriate policies that respect participant rights while creating an enabling environment for genomic research (Al-Delaimy et al., 2019). In addition, the intricacies of pharmacogenomics also involve scalability and cost-effectiveness of incorporating genomic information into healthcare systems.

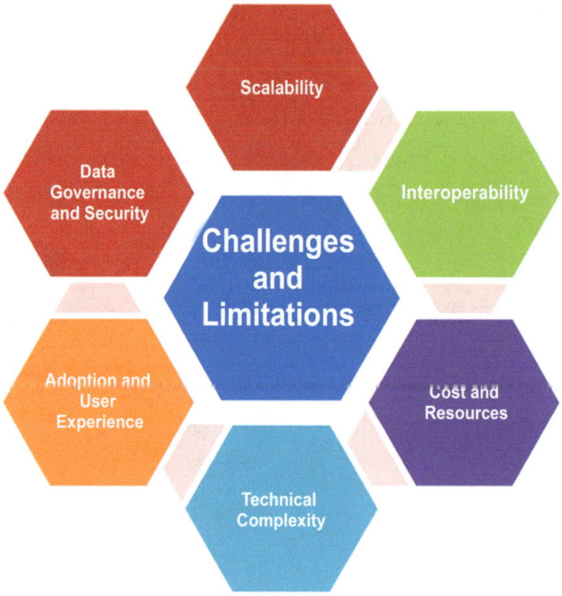

Figure 13.10. Challenges and limitations.

Source: Alsamarai, B., & Morato, J. (2023). *Navigating Challenges and Limitations in Educational Blockchain Integration: Scalability, Integration, and Data Privacy*. In *The Use of Blockchain Technology in the Educational Field in Bahrain.*

Most healthcare professionals are not well trained to interpret and use pharmacogenomic information in a meaningful way, and there are gaps in clinical implementation. Furthermore, the cost of comprehensive genotyping and the resultant individualized therapies could pose a barrier to access, particularly in resource-limited environments. Regulatory and reimbursement concerns also must be addressed by laboratories and clinics, further hindering routine use. Until such economic, educational, and policy constraints are resolved, the complete clinical potential of pharmacogenomics will continue to be limited, hampering its translation from investigation to common practice (Paepe et al., 2013).

13.4.1. Ethical Considerations in Genetic Testing

The speedy evolution of gene-testing technologies, led mainly by NGS, has uncovered new horizons of targeted medicine and pharmacogenomics. While these technologies hold out the hope of more effective and targeted treatment, they also introduce multifaceted ethical concerns that need to be resolved in order to protect individual rights. The ability to screen large amounts of genetic data on NGS platforms raises the likelihood of revealing incidental findings outside the scope of the initial diagnostic purpose, creating issues regarding disclosure, patient consent, and psychological burden. Additionally, handling such sensitive information requires strict privacy measures and security controls to avoid unauthorized use or exposure, which are paramount in sustaining patient trust.

These issues underpin the need to incorporate ethical frameworks (Figure 13.11) in the use of pharmacogenomic testing to maintain that increased therapeutic effectiveness does not require a compromise in either patient autonomy or confidentiality (Bature et al., 2024). In the application of pharmacogenomic testing to clinical practice, informed consent becomes a key ethical issue. In view of the inherent complexity of genetic information and its potential implications, patients should be provided with clear, detailed information regarding the scope, the limits, and the potential consequences of testing. Such a process should enable individuals to make informed choices about having genetic analysis, such as the right to refuse or opt out from ascertaining certain genetic risks. Clinicians are also confronted with ethical obligations to reduce disparities in access to these new diagnostic technologies, since unequal availability threatens to widen healthcare disparities. Such challenges need to be addressed through organized guidelines and policies that encourage fair access, transparency, and patient education. Through the integration of these ethical principles, pharmacogenomic testing can develop in a way that honors patient rights and promotes fair improvement in medication safety and efficacy (Abdi et al., 2024).

A second vital ethical concern crosses over with potential for genetic discrimination based on pharmacogenomic information. Employers, insurers, and other third parties would attempt to use the results of genetic tests to inform employment or coverage decisions, which could result in stigmatization or denial of opportunity. Legislative safeguards such as the Genetic Information Nondiscrimination Act (GINA) in the United States provide some protection; however, there are issues regarding enforcement and the scope of such protection, particularly as genetic testing becomes more prevalent and a part of standard healthcare. In addition, application of pharmacogenomics in ethnically diverse populations requires attention to cultural values and possible mistrust based on past abuses. Ethical application in pharmacogenomics thus has to incorporate constant monitoring, regulation, and culturally appropriate counseling to avoid discrimination and ensure social justice for genomic medicine (Abdi et al., 2024; Bature et al., 2024).

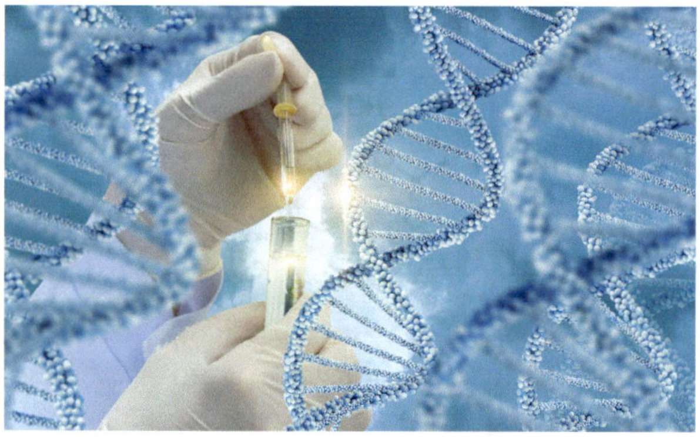

Figure 13.11. Ethical considerations in genetic testing.

Source: Shutterstock. (2021). *Ethical Considerations in Genetic Testing*. https://d1dbgh6ga9ets8.cloudfront.net/wp-content/uploads/2021/07/shutterstock_656140189.jpg.

13.4.2. Variability in Patient Responses

The drug response is determined by the complexity of multiple factors that go beyond the obvious clinical variables. Among them, genetic heterogeneity plays a role that is increasingly well understood in determining why individuals respond differently to the same drug. This heterogeneity can be explained by genetic differences inherited through their effects on drug-metabolizing enzymes, transporters, and drug targets, which in turn affect drug pharmacokinetics and pharmacodynamics. Especially in children, the intersection of developmental change and genetic constitution, including age-related gene expression, also makes dosing accuracy even more challenging. This ontogeny-pharmacogenomics interaction clearly points to the need for individually designed therapies because genetic considerations alone cannot always accurately predict drug action without integrating developmental physiology (Hoshitsuki et al., 2021). These observations highlight the way personalized therapy requires combining genetic information with individual patient data to achieve optimal efficacy and reduce harm. Aside from developmental parameters, a major role in differential drug reactions among populations is played by ancestral genetic heterogeneity. Drug metabolic genes that harbor variants have frequencies differing among ancestral groups, and some polymorphisms are found to be specific to a population. Pharmacogenomic studies historically have disproportionately studied individuals of European and East Asian descent, creating a knowledge gap regarding genetic variants most common in other groups, such as minority groups within the United States. This gap emphasizes health disparities by restricting the predictive value and clinical utility of pharmacogenomic testing to diverse populations. Consequently, there is increasingly the awareness of the necessity of incorporating different ancestries in research to reveal population-specific genetic determinants of drug response and to produce fair precision medicine strategies (De et al., 2018).

Closing this gap is necessary to guarantee that pharmacogenomics is accessible to all patients regardless of their genetic makeup. The heterogeneity of patient responses is further confounded by the multi-factorial aspect of drug reaction, with genomics intersecting with environmental, physiological, and developmental factors. Whereas genetic attributes inherited through a fixed blueprint serve as a reference point, extrinsic variables like diet, co-morbid conditions, intercurrent medications, and organ function continuously alter drug impact. Particularly in susceptible populations such as children, the interaction of changes due to maturation and genetic polymorphisms requires sophisticated dosing algorithms that also consider genetic and age-related variables. Even with progress, complete data across the wide range of life stages are lacking, and longitudinal pharmacogenomic studies following patient responses over time are needed. By integrating this whole-person approach, pharmacogenomics can move toward more accurate, personalized therapy, minimizing ADRs and improving therapeutic outcomes across patient groups (Hoshitsuki et al., 2021).

13.4.3. Regulatory and Accessibility Issues

Pharmacogenomic advances hold the potential to transform individualized medicine by adapting drug treatments to a person's unique genetic makeup. Yet this breakthrough is faced with serious regulatory challenges that complicate its integration in the clinical setting. Regulatory bodies have to create systems that reconcile strict standards of safety and efficacy with nimble approval mechanisms needed by fast-changing genomic technologies. The difficulty of interpreting genomic information and obtaining proper, replicable results complicates things further for regulatory agencies, which must devise good guidelines for testing validation, quality control, and reporting. Inconsistent country-to-country regulatory policy also hinders the international rollout of pharmacogenomic tests. All these regulatory issues come on top of ethical issues of data privacy and informed consent, which require good governance frameworks to safeguard patient information while promoting innovation. Successful regulation, then, demands subtle policies that balance technological advance with measures not stifling accessibility or clinical use (Kraus et al., 2020). Apart from regulatory guidelines, accessibility presents another deep challenge within pharmacogenomics. Genomic testing is prohibitively expensive and not covered by insurance, which limits patient access, especially among vulnerable populations, and deepens already existing healthcare inequalities. Geographic inequities also hinder fair delivery of healthcare, including rural and poor communities often not having the facilities and expert staff to adopt pharmacogenomic services. In addition, obstacles like narrow health literacy and suspicion of genetic technologies limit patient uptake and acceptability. These problems need to be tackled through interlinked interventions of policy changes, educational programs, and investment in healthcare facilities. Absent such interventions, pharmacogenomics threatens to be an elite weapon, accessed solely by a privileged minority of patients instead of being a generative force for widespread population health gains (Kraus et al., 2020). Where data science and pharmacogenomics intersect, regulatory and access landscapes are further complicated. Although machine learning and artificial intelligence may improve the prognostic capabilities of pharmacogenomic models, their implementation is hindered by challenges in the interpretation of advanced algorithmic outputs and proving clinical value through intense trials. The regulatory bodies must struggle with how to assess these dynamic, data-driven devices for accuracy and patient safety without curtailing innovation. At the same time, the incorporation of large-scale genomic information poses deep privacy and ethical concerns, necessitating high levels of data protection that inadvertently limit sharing of data critical to scientific advances. Accessibility on a larger scale therefore requires not only affordable testing and informed regulation but also technological literacy and building confidence between clinicians and patients. Resolution of these complex issues is essential to the realization of the full potential of pharmacogenomics in precision medicine.

Test Your Knowledge

1. What is Ethical considerations in genetic testing?
2. What is the impact of drug interactions on patient response?

13.5. Future Directions

Learning Outcome

1. Ethical Considerations in Genetic Testing
2. Variability in Patient Responses
3. Regulatory and Accessibility Issues

Pharmacogenomics breakthroughs promise to transform personalized medicine through the ability to conduct large-scale, high-throughput genetic testing. With increasing need for rapid and extensive genetic information, clinical labs are employing new molecular technologies that can screen thousands of genetic variants in an economical manner. These advancements will make it possible for healthcare professionals to customize drug regimens to unique genetic profiles precisely, maximizing therapeutic efficiency while reducing side effects. Yet, the increasing ability to identify genetic variants also raises substantial interpretative hurdles, since clinical relevance for most identified mutations is still unclear. Closing this knowledge gap will take a collaborative effort to bring genetic information together with clinical outcomes so that pharmacogenomic testing yields useful information. Future studies will need to center on the validation of new biomarkers and optimization of testing strategies, developing strong frameworks for integrating genomic data into treatment decisions (Schrijver et al., 2011).

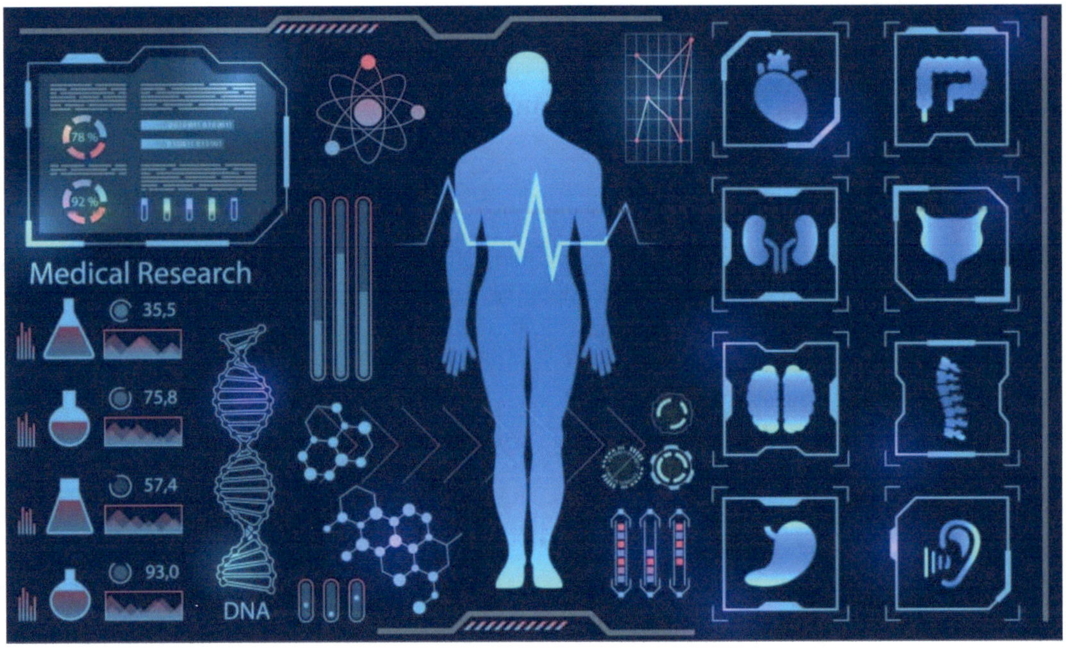

Figure 13.12. Future directions.

Source: **Shutterstock.** (n.d.). *Doctor and Patient Discussing Medical Information. https*://getreferralmd.com/wp-content/uploads/2018/05/shutterstock_783381802-1024x614.jpg.

The development of targeted therapies is a classic example of the exciting future applications of pharmacogenomics, most notably in the field of oncology. The creation of antibody-drug conjugates, including trastuzumab emtansine (T-DM1), is an example of how pharmacogenomic findings inform the design of therapies with specificity coupled with cytotoxicity. This precision strategy not only improves treatment outcomes with HER2-positive breast cancer but also has lower toxicity than traditional chemotherapy regimens. However, mechanisms of resistance to targeted drugs are still a significant challenge, calling for further research that brings together pharmacogenomic understanding with tumor biology. Research on these pathways of resistance will guide second-generation treatments as well as combination regimens and how they can overcome treatment failure and enhance patient outcomes. In addition, the extension of the use of such targeted therapies to other cancers promises wider clinical benefit (Hurvitz et al., 2014). In the future, the integration of pharmacogenomics into standard clinical practice will be contingent upon the surmounting of economic, infrastructural, and educational obstacles. Healthcare systems will need to invest in scalable technologies and bioinformatics tools facilitating the interpretation of complex genetic information. Aside from this, standardized guidelines must be adopted to harmonize testing protocols and provide equal access to pharmacogenomic services. Clinicians will need special training to evaluate genomic reports and advise patients properly, paving the way for interdisciplinarity. Issues of genetic privacy and data security will become paramount as testing becomes more prevalent. As these issues are resolved, the futures of pharmacogenomics will include the widening of individualized therapeutic opportunities, enhancing healthcare results, and promoting a more accurate, patient-focused method of medicine (Figure 13.12) (Schrijver et al., 2011).

13.5.1. Advances in Genomic Technologies

Advances in sequencing technologies over recent times have transformed the capacity for the examination of genetic variations and have provided unprecedented information about drug response variability, the underlying complexity. Population-scale NSG initiatives have identified millions of variants in pharmacogenes, including single-nucleotide variants, indels, and structural changes. These informative datasets, compiled in repositories such as the Genome Aggregation Database, provide a basis for the elucidation of the genetic determinants of pharmacokinetics and pharmacodynamics (Figure 13.13). Nonetheless, traditional short-read sequencing methods have limitations in mapping complicated pharmacogenetic loci owing to segmental duplications and homologous pseudogenes, hindering detailed variant detection. The emergence of long-read sequencing technologies with the ability to generate continuous reads across whole gene regions holds the key to overcoming these limitations by allowing for accurate haplotype resolution of genes like CYP2D6 and HLA. This technical advancement is central to the forward movement of pharmacogenomics and individualized drug therapy based on genetic profiles. Understanding the functional implications of the enormous number of rare pharmacogenetic variants found is still a major challenge. Conventional epidemiological research and *in vitro* experiments have low throughput, and it is not practical to systematically functionally annotate large numbers of variants. Computational prediction models, using attributes like sequence conservation, protein structure, and physicochemical properties, provide scalable options but typically have reduced accuracy for pharmacogenes, which evolve under low selective pressure and often harbor common functionally significant polymorphisms incorrectly classified as benign. To improve predictive ability, new algorithms tailored to pharmacogenetic variant effect prediction are arising, incorporating experimental information from multiplexed high-throughput functional assays. These assays, such as deep mutational scanning and massively parallel reporter assays, enable the assessment of variant impact on protein activity or level simultaneously, thus creating rich datasets to improve computational models. This synergistic application of experimental and computational approaches represents a critical milestone in closing the gap between variant discovery and clinical usefulness (Sad Wée et al., 2023). Artificial intelligence and machine learning technologies further expand the reach of genomic advances by allowing advanced analysis of complex pharmacogenomic data. These techniques allow for pattern detection in large, multidimensional data sets, enabling both supervised learning with labeled phenotype data and unsupervised methods that uncover new variant-phenotype associations. Through the use of training sets based on deep mutational scanning and large biobank data, machine learning algorithms can optimize variant effect predictions to enhance individualized treatment decisions. AI also facilitates the integration of heterogeneous data types—genomic, environmental, and clinical—to create multicomponent biomarker panels that account for drug response's multifactorial nature. While there are still challenges in applying these findings to standard clinical practice, the intersection of NSG, high-throughput functional assays, and AI-powered analytics augurs well for a new era of pharmacogenomics to enhance therapeutic efficacy and reduce ADRs (Sad Wée et al., 2023).

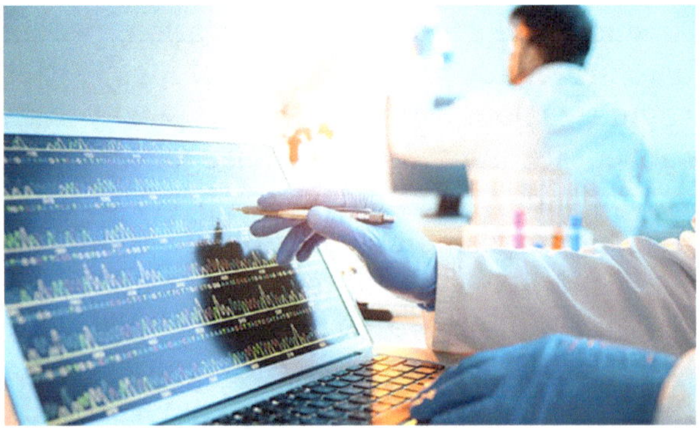

Figure 13.13. Advances in genomic technologies.

Source: SingHealth (2023). *Advances in Genomic Technologies.*

13.5.2. Potential for New Drug Development

Dramatic improvements in genomic technologies and data integration have opened unprecedented doors to drug discovery and development (Figure 13.14). The marriage of pharmacogenomics with large databases has greatly widened the scope of discovering new drug targets customized to genetic profiles. Tools such as DrugBank have been upgraded to contain enormous surges in data on investigational drugs, drug interactions, and SNP-related drug effects, which are key indicators of individual response to therapeutics. This abundance of molecular and clinical data allows researchers to make more precise predictions of drug efficacy and side effects, thereby streamlining the pipeline from target discovery to clinical trial design. Furthermore, the incorporation of pharmacometabolomic, pharmacotranscriptomic, and pharmacoproteomic data increases the comprehension of drug action at various biological levels, enabling precision in drug development approaches and increasing the probability of successful, personalized treatments (David et al., 2017). The advent of large health data has also revolutionized drug development to an even greater extent by facilitating a more comprehensive appreciation of disease mechanisms and patient heterogeneity. Massive genomic sequencing accompanied by long-term electronic health records makes possible real-time assessment of drug targets and therapeutic responses across heterogeneous populations. These integrated datasets are useful for the identification of new biomarkers and sub-phenotypes that can guide the development of drugs, which diminishes the trial-and-error nature of pharmacotherapy. Further, the infusion of pharmacogenomic data into hospital systems facilitates pre-emptive pharmacogenomics to enable clinicians to choose or avoid drugs according to genetic risk before adverse reactions can occur. These innovations mark a paradigm shift where drug development is supplemented by ongoing feedback loops from population-level data to generate more efficient and effective therapeutics (Hemingway et al., 2017). Notwithstanding such encouraging developments, challenges persist to unlock the entire potential of pharmacogenomics to facilitate new drug development. Matters like data quality, standardization, ethical aspects, and compatibility across varied health databases require concerted efforts to make research infrastructures optimal. Overcoming these obstacles will allow for improved aggregation and interpretation of multi-dimensional data that are essential for improving drug target validation. The potential of big data pharmacogenomics is that it has the ability to uncover new disease pathways and mechanisms of action for drugs, thereby allowing the development of new therapeutic agents with enhanced safety and individualized efficacy. With ongoing technological advancement and interdisciplinarity, the drug discovery process can further use genetic understanding to develop revolutionary medical treatments (Hemingway et al., 2017).

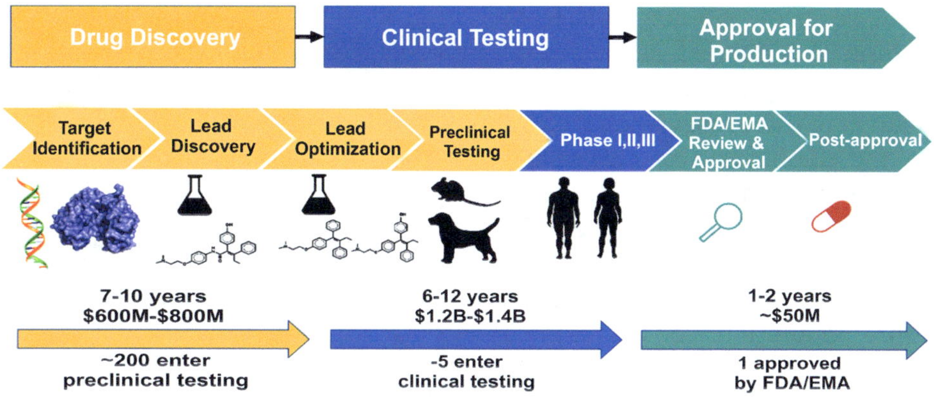

Figure 13.14. Potential for new drug development.

Source: **Zhang, Y et al.** (2022). *Figure 1. The Process of Drug Research and Development.* In *Application of Computational Biology and Artificial Intelligence In Drug Design. International Journal of Molecular Sciences, 23*(21), 13568.

13.5.3. Expanding the Role of Pharmacogenomics in Healthcare

Genetic breakthroughs have made it possible for revolutionary shifts in personalized medicine, and specifically by incorporating pharmacogenomics in healthcare. This novel field examines the individual genetic profile to forecast how one will react to drugs in an effort to maximize therapeutic effects with reduced side effects. Pharmacogenomics' extension is important in the prescription of medications, particularly in difficult diseases such as cancer, cardiovascular disease, and psychiatric illness where genetic differences have a tremendous bearing on the success of treatment. Technology is costly, and challenges are present, but the hope of enhanced patient care and resource efficiency drives research and clinical implementation forward. In addition, the integration of pharmacogenomic information into electronic health records may enable real-time clinician decision-making through the use of genetic information to inform viable treatment plans (Figure 13.15). Breaking down barriers of limited clinician knowledge and data interpretation guidelines continues to be necessary for pharmacogenomic methods to be incorporated into standard healthcare practice (Bartlett et al., 2012). Healthcare systems need to adapt to the increasing importance of pharmacogenomics through policies that promote regular genetic testing and data sharing. The growth entails not just technological infrastructure but also ethical and educational systems addressing patient privacy, informed consent, and fair access. As the applications of pharmacogenomics increase, multidisciplinary collaboration between geneticists, pharmacists, clinicians, and bioinformaticians becomes critical to providing complete care. Secondly, reimbursement systems have to be remodeled to facilitate pharmacogenomic services, avoiding cost from limiting integration. The changes also need to account for future challenges laid out by earlier projections regarding laboratory medicines evolution, with the implication of embracing versatile and future-oriented strategies towards evolving technologies (Fortina et al., 2015). This is done with the purpose of democratizing pharmacogenomics in order to open up its utilization to more populations for customized treatment while driving healthcare systems to innovate. Lastly, broadening pharmacogenomics holds the promise of transforming drug development pipelines by allowing more accurate selection of drug targets and patient subgroups that will be most likely to benefit from certain treatments. The strategy can mitigate the excessive attrition rates frequently encountered in clinical trials by stratifying volunteers on the basis of genetic markers, thereby making new drugs more cost-effective and efficient to bring to market. In addition, real-time pharmacogenomic information can contribute to post-market monitoring of medicines, enabling earlier detection of ADRs and the adaptation of dosage recommendations in a wide variety of populations. Through the incorporation of pharmacogenomic concepts throughout all aspects of clinical practice and pharmaceutical development, healthcare can be transformed into a predictive and preventive model, thus enhancing patient outcomes as a whole and maximizing public health investments (Bartlett et al., 2012; Fortina et al., 2015).

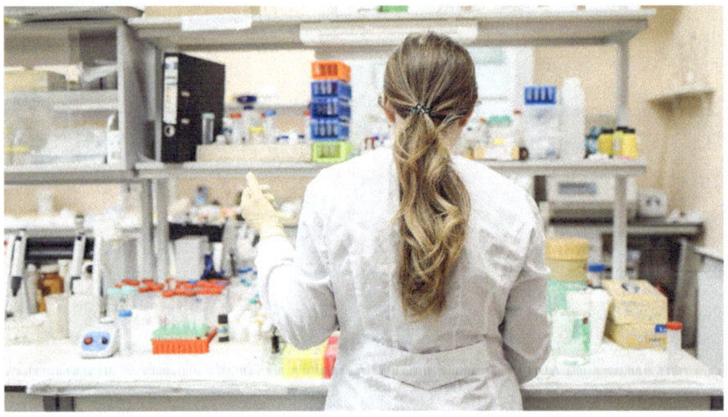

Figure 13.15. Expanding the role of pharmacogenomics in healthcare.

Source: The Daily Dispatches (2023). *Expanding the Role of Pharmacogenomics in Healthcare.* *https*://www.thedailydispatches.com/wp-content/uploads/2023/05/Pharmacogenomics.jpg.

Test Your Knowledge

1. What is Advances in Genomic Technologies?
2. How do organ-on-chip technologies contribute to drug development?

13.6. Case Studies

Learning Outcome

1. Pharmacogenomics in Oncology
2. Pharmacogenomic Testing in Psychiatry
3. Cardiovascular Drug Response and Genetics

Clinical use of pharmacogenomics has been made progressively more advanced through rigorous case studies that illustrate the importance of genetic heterogeneity in drug response. A high-profile case is the study of carbamazepine-induced cutaneous adverse drug reactions in the Han Chinese population. Case-control studies pooled in a meta-analysis showed compelling associations between individual human leukocyte antigen (HLA) alleles and severe adverse drug reactions, including Stevens-Johnson syndrome and toxic epidermal necrolysis. The designation of HLA-B*15:02 as a risk factor for these reactions highlights the potential for genetic screening to avoid life-threatening consequences through influencing prescription choices. Furthermore, specific alleles such as HLA-A*31:01 and HLA-B*38:02 were associated with other carbamazepine-associated eruptions, highlighting the heterogeneity of drug hypersensitivity in genetic subpopulations. Such outcomes of intensive case studies highlight the promise of pharmacogenomics to customize medication decisions according to specific genetic profiles and enhance therapeutic safety (Meng et al., 2023). Case studies also offer valuable information regarding unusual genetic variants influencing drug metabolism and disease susceptibility, thus extending pharmacogenomics clinical application. As an illustration, the identification of a new frameshift mutation in the OFD1 gene by whole-exome sequencing in a subject with primary ciliary dyskinesia (PCD) shows how genetic diagnosis can shed light on underlying conditions with implications in pharmacology. While OFD1 mutations are generally expected to be coupled with syndromic dysmorphias, this presentation showed one with the phenotype largely characterized by PCD symptomatology, without related renal or morphological findings. By analyzing the functional impact of this mutation on ciliary function using high-speed video microscopy and electron microscopy, the case study indicates how genetic variation affects disease processes and responses to treatment. These close clinical-genetic correlations form the basis in the development of pharmacogenomics from frequent polymorphisms into precision medicine for multifactorial disorders (Yang et al., 2022). Case studies are a vital part of the incorporation of pharmacogenomics in research for translation of genomic data into practical therapeutic approaches. These studies not only confirm genetic markers linked with ADRs or disease phenotypes but also offer an avenue for adopting preemptive genetic testing into clinical practice. By systematic case examination, clinicians could create guidelines for genotype-based prescribing, decreasing trial-and-error prescriptions and improving patient safety. In addition, case studies tend to unveil population-specific genetic variants, highlighting the importance of representing diverse populations in pharmacogenomic studies. In general, the comprehensive examination of instances where drugs are affected by genetics or become toxic is a foundation for customized medicine, so pharmacogenomics is an essential component of healthcare models to come. Such inclusion promotes better, safer treatment tailored to the individual patient's genetic blueprint (Meng et al., 2023; Yang et al., 2022).

13.6.1. Pharmacogenomics in Oncology

Advances in precision medicine have revolutionized the cancer therapy paradigm by individualizing drugs according to the genetic constitution of patients. In cancer medicine, the use of pharmacogenomics (PGx) allows clinicians to anticipate the response of patients to specific anticancer therapies based on inherited genomic difference (Figure 13.16). This reduces toxicities while maximizing therapeutic benefits, leading to better clinical outcomes. Yet, translation of PGx to standard oncology practice has been patchy. Numerous PGx findings have long concentrated on individuals of European descent, and as a result, there has been a gap in knowledge that has the potential to worsen racial and ethnic minorities' health disparities. Identifying this bias is important in the quest for providing fair access to individualized cancer therapy and the prevention of mislabeling of genetic influences on drug response. To solve these challenges, there is a need for inclusive PGx research and incorporation of germline variant testing that captures the diversity of patient populations (Sharon et al., 2024). Clinical trials have more and more integrated pharmacogenetic and pharmacogenomic data to improve the assessment of the safety and efficacy of oncological treatments. The increased incidence of PGx in clinical research, especially in oncology, highlights its significant role in driving personalized treatment approaches. Genes like CYP2D6 and CYP2C9, often characterized in these trials, have an effect on the metabolism of a number of chemotherapeutic drugs and supportive medications that influences drug dosing and toxicity profiles. In spite of this expansion, there is still a lag in clinician training and interpreting data, which can discourage the maximum use of PGx knowledge in clinical decision-making. Improving education for healthcare professionals in PGx will lead to better-informed prescribing, ultimately better patient outcomes and facilitating the wider adoption of personalized oncology care (Nogueiras, 2023). In spite of the potential of pharmacogenomics for better cancer treatment, its integration into routine clinical practices remains challenging. As somatic genetic testing has become standard practice for the majority of solid tumors, germline PGx testing has not yet seen comparable clinical uptake. Barriers are restricted provider awareness, inadequate access to integrated genetic testing, and the difficulty of interpreting PGx information across heterogeneous populations. To overcome these issues, changes are needed at the systemic level, such as extending the representativeness of genomic databases, revising drug labeling to incorporate PGx results, and creating guidelines that encourage fair testing. Ensuring that PGx applications are available and applicable to all patients irrespective of ancestry will be the key to fully achieving the advantages of personalized oncology care and enhancing safety and survival (Sharon et al., 2024).

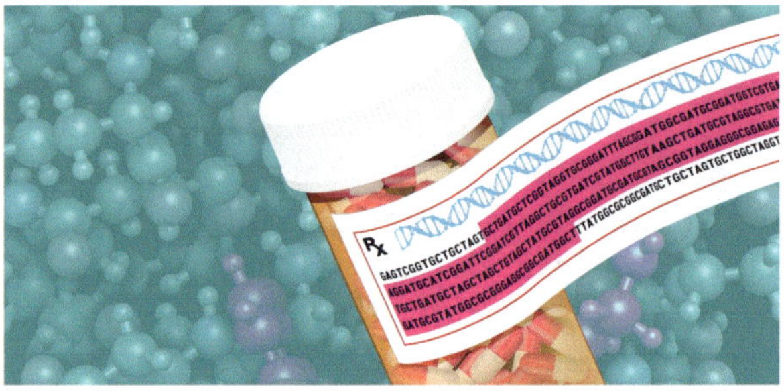

Figure 13.16. Pharmacogenomics in oncology.

Source: DrOmics Labs. (2024, May). *Genetic Testing Infographic. https://*external-content.duckduckgo.com/iu/?u=https%3A%2F%2 Fdromicslabs.com%2Fwp-content%2Fuploads%2 F2024%2F05%2F3_20240502_174056_0001.jpg&f=1&nofb=1&ipt=fb08d1217bb6703d7190d79a992d74b853d92e50db466b57d3cd55893a2facae.

13.6.2. Pharmacogenomic Testing in Psychiatry

Personalized medicine advances have transformed many medical disciplines, especially psychiatry, whose conventional treatment methods usually suffer from overriding challenges owing to the heterogeneity of the response of patients. Psychiatric illnesses like major depressive disorder often defy initial medication treatments, leading to long durations of symptom chronicity and drug trial-and-error practice. Pharmacogenomic screening becomes a central solution to these challenges by pointing to genetic differences that affect an individual's metabolism of drugs and response to treatment. Through matching medication with an individual's genetic makeup, clinicians can better focus effective treatments, minimize side effects, and shorten the course to remission. Studies have shown that pharmacogenomic-guided therapy significantly enhances response and mood improvement in treatment-resistant depression, underscoring the pragmatic utility of this method in the field of psychiatry (Velazquez et al., 2021). The inclusion of this presents a significant step towards precision psychiatry, with more educated and patient-specific practice. The application of pharmacogenomic testing by nursing is becoming widely acknowledged as a key component of successful clinical practice. Nurses who have knowledge in pharmacogenomics can advance the therapeutic process by doing genetic tests, interpreting results, and teaching patients about how genetic influences affect drug response. This empowered nurse role promotes safer dispensing of medicines, careful monitoring of adverse reactions, and effective patient-centered advocacy for pharmacotherapy. Additionally, the integration of pharmacogenomic literacy in nursing practice enables further comprehensive conceptuality of individualized care, complementing nursing theories that focus on knowledge translation and patient advocacy. Such integration not only contributes to minimizing adverse effects but also ensures enhanced compliance and overall patient well-being (Nguyen et al., 2021). Nursing experts, therefore, significantly advance the optimization and convergence of pharmacogenomic testing in psychiatric treatment protocols. Although it holds promise, the application of pharmacogenomic testing in psychiatry on a large scale is hindered by low provider familiarity and a requirement for ongoing education, as well as economic and systemic barriers. The motivation of healthcare providers to adopt this technology is critical in that it entails changing clinical workflows and deciphering complex genetic information. Educational interventions have been shown to be effective in raising provider confidence and intention to implement pharmacogenomics in everyday care, ultimately enhancing patient outcomes in treatment-resistant disorders. The evidence base for better depressive symptom outcomes after pharmacogenomic-guided therapy highlights the return on investment in provider training and infrastructure building (Velazquez et al., 2021). Multidisciplinary cooperation, continuous research, and institutional support are crucial to achieve the full potential of pharmacogenomic testing in psychiatry. These interacting factors altogether might culminate in a holistic, evidence-based care model based on genomic accuracy and personalized treatment plans.

13.6.3. Cardiovascular Drug Response and Genetics

Progress in genetic studies has profoundly changed the field's comprehension of how people react to cardiovascular drugs (Figure 13.17). Genetic variations involved in drug transport and metabolism may cause significant differences in treatment responses among patients. For example, polymorphisms in SLCO1B1 gene affect the pharmacokinetics of statins rosuvastatin and atorvastatin, affecting efficacy and risk of side effects such as myopathy. Furthermore, cytochrome P450 enzymes, particularly CYP2C19 and CYP2D6, regulate antiplatelet drug activation and clearance of beta-blockers, influencing cardiovascular drug response. The awareness of these genetic effects allows clinicians to personalize treatment modalities more accurately, maximizing efficacy while reducing toxic side effects. This incorporation of genetic information into prescribing is a hallmark of the potential of pharmacogenomics in cardiovascular disease therapy (Andhi et al., 2024). The therapeutic implications of pharmacogenomics go beyond enhanced efficacy, with the promise of safer profiles via customized therapeutic approaches. Genetic variations in VKORC1 and CYP2C9, the primary enzymes for the metabolism of anticoagulants warfarin and acenocoumarol, illustrate how genetic testing can predict dosing needs and bleeding hazards. Such accuracy minimizes trial-and-error therapy and the occurrence of ADRs, a key issue in the treatment of chronic cardiovascular diseases. Further, the pharmacogenomic information can assist in the identification of patients who would respond poorly to conventional treatments, suggesting an alternative drug or dose. As this personalized medicine continues to mature, it has the potential to improve patient compliance and maximize long-term cardiovascular outcomes by matching treatment protocols to an individual's genetic blueprint (Andhi et al., 2024). Although cardiovascular pharmacogenomics has made great progress, genetic information must continue to be combined with clinical and environmental variables in order to achieve optimal treatment. Lifestyle, comorbidities, and concomitant drugs, in addition to genetic analysis, can further optimize therapeutic choice. This integrated paradigm is parallel to advances in other areas of medicine, including psychiatry, where personalized therapy plans that combine pharmacogenomics and drug monitoring are being used to maximize efficacy and tolerability. The future of cardiovascular therapy therefore hinges on ongoing research into gene-environment interactions and the creation of cost-efficient, accessible genetic testing. Eventually, these pursuits will render personalized cardiovascular pharmacotherapy an integral component of clinical practice, enhancing patient outcomes across a wider scope.

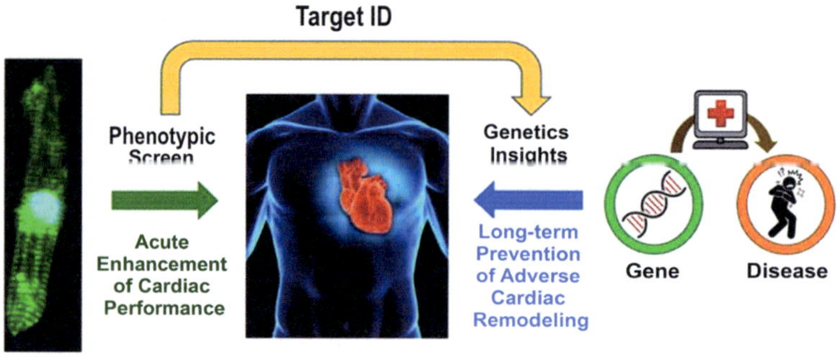

Figure 13.17. Cardiovascular drug response and genetics.

Source: Frontiers. (n.d.). *Cardiovascular Drug Response and Genetics* [Image]. *Frontiers in Drug Delivery.* https://www.frontiersin.org/files/Articles/1027401/fddsv-02-1027401-HTML/image_m/fddsv-02-1027401-g002.jpg.

Test Your Knowledge

1. How do genetic variations impact cardiovascular drug metabolism?
2. What is pharmacogenomic testing in psychiatry?

CONCLUSION

The application of pharmacogenomics to contemporary medical practice represents a major milestone in the customization of medicine. It is part of a wider movement toward tailoring treatment to individual genetic characteristics, thus maximizing therapeutic effectiveness and reducing side effects. Ongoing expansion of biobanks and genomic databases is crucial to this effort, as they supply the essential materials required to decipher genetic diversity between populations. Public attitudes and trust significantly influence the success of these initiatives, with demographic factors such as age, education, and cultural beliefs playing pivotal roles in shaping participation in biobanking activities. These considerations underscore the necessity of ethical frameworks and transparent communication strategies to foster public engagement and safeguard patient confidentiality, ensuring that pharmacogenomic research progresses responsibly and inclusively (Al-Delaimy et al., 2019). In addition, the interdisciplinary character of pharmacogenomics demands concerted actions among clinical, bioinformatics, and research communities. Scientific conferences and knowledge-sharing forums are critical areas for sharing novel ideas and pushing the frontier of the fields. Conferences such as the Golden Helix Pharmacogenomics Days are examples of how global collaboration fosters enhanced comprehension of genetic determinants of drug response, while promoting synergism between novel bioinformatic tools and clinical decision-making. This international discourse not only speeds up research but also assists in harmonizing standards and methodologies, ensuring consistency in the use of personalized medicine across the globe. As a result, these collaborative efforts lead to the mitigation of healthcare disparities and enhanced patient outcomes through precision therapies based on genetic profiles (Borg et al., 2012). In summary, pharmacogenomics has revolutionary potential for transforming therapeutic strategies, but its complete fulfillment relies on multi-dimensional contributions across ethical, social, and scientific spheres. Positive public sentiments for biobanking combined with clear and accountable governance, in turn, building upon sensitivity for the contexts in culture provides grounds for progress going forward. Second, cultivating cross-global scientific interactions as well as ongoing training on focused forums remains instrumental for applying pharmacogenomic findings effectively in practice. As research goes on, an equilibrium between innovation and societal values will be a key to realising personalized medicine's potential for improving healthcare quality and equity within diverse populations (Al-Delaimy et al., 2019; Borg et al., 2012).

Summary of Key Points

Pharmacogenomics advancements have emphasized the vital contribution of genetic variation in drug response, transforming personalized medicine strategies. Incorporating genomic information enables more accurate predictions of drug efficacy and toxicity, reducing unwanted effects and maximizing therapeutic benefit. Significantly, platforms like GSCA have improved our capability to analyze intricate genomic and pharmacogenomic information across different types of cancer, unveiling important correlations among gene set alterations and clinical outcomes that single-gene research might fail to identify (Liu et al., 2022). These observations demonstrate the promise of gene set analysis in optimizing drug targeting approaches, highlighting the significance of integrating multi-dimensional genomic data in pharmacogenomic investigations. Therefore, pharmacogenomics ushers in an era of customized treatment strategies based on thorough molecular profiles instead of universalized therapeutic protocols. In addition, drug repositioning has become a major strategy under pharmacogenomics, using already approved drugs to discover new therapeutic uses. Not only does this maximize drug development timelines but also offset the tremendous cost charges conventionally attributed to de novo drug discovery (Tamer et al., 2020). The rapid emergence of large-scale biological and clinical data, along with high-level computational methodologies, has enabled the prediction of novel alternative drug indications with greater precision. Computational drug repositioning is a prime example of how pharmacogenomics and bioinformatics converge to promote therapeutic discovery. By methodically venturing into drug–gene interactions and disease-associated genetic landscapes, this approach demonstrates a realistic utilization of pharmacogenomic information toward a more effective translation from genomic knowledge to the clinic. Overall, the most essential points in pharmacogenomics highlight how genomic analysis and computer technologies align to propel individualized medicine. Methods that facilitate large-scale gene set analysis unveil patterns and associations relevant for comprehending drug reaction at a molecular level, enhancing the precision of treatment (Liu et al., 2022). Concurrently, the process of computational drug repositioning illustrates attempts to leverage in-place pharmaceutical assets using pharmacogenomic knowledge, lowering barrier development and increasing therapeutic horizons (Tamer et al., 2020). Combined, these advances identify pharmacogenomics as a revolutionary area that converges genetics, computer science, and clinical investigation to maximize drug therapy based on an individualized genetic portrait in order to enhance patient care outcomes on a macro scale.

KEY TERMS FROM THIS CHAPTER

- Medical treatment
- Pharmacogenomics
- Personalized Medicine
- Polymorphisms
- Genetic polymorphisms
- Drug Metabolism
- Genomic technologies
- Whole genome sequencing (WGS)
- Genetic Testing
- Adverse drug reactions (ADRs)
- Molecular medicine
- Genetic mechanisms
- Healthcare
- Mechanisms of Pharmacogenomics
- Single Nucleotide Polymorphisms (SNPs)
- Personalized medicine
- Emergency clinical
- Pharmacogenomics in Healthcare

CRITICAL THINKING QUESTIONS

1. **Which of the following best defines pharmacogenomics?**
   a. The study of how drugs affect the genome
   b. The study of the interaction between diet and genes
   c. The study of how genetic differences influence drug response
   d. The study of drug interactions and side effects
2. **CYP2D6 is involved in the metabolism of all the following drugs EXCEPT?**
   a. Codeine
   b. Tamoxifen
   c. Metoprolol
   d. Warfarin
3. **Poor metabolizers of CYP2C19 are at increased risk of therapeutic failure with?**
   a. Simvastatin
   b.. Clopidogrel
   c. Warfarin
   d. Acetaminophen
4. **A patient with HLA-B*57:01 allele is at high risk of a hypersensitivity reaction to which drug?**
   a. Efavirenz
   b. Abacavir
   c. Zidovudine
   d. Tenofovir
5. **Which gene is most commonly associated with increased warfarin sensitivity?**
   a. CYP3A5
   b. CYP2D6
   c. VKORC1
   d. ABCB1

Short Answer Questions

1. Describe the historical Background development of pharmacogenomics?
2. Explain the mechanisms by which genetic variations can influence drug pharmacokinetics and pharmacodynamics?
3. Discuss the clinical applications of pharmacogenomics in modern medicine?
4. What are some major challenges and Limitations in implementing pharmacogenomics in clinical practice?
5. What is future directions of pharmacogenomics in clinical medicine?

Answer to Critical Thinking Questions

1. (c) 2 (d) 3. (b) 4. (b) 5. (c)

REFERENCES

1. Abboudi, H., & Macphee, I. A. (2012). Individualized immunosuppression in transplant patients: Potential role of pharmacogenetics. https://core.ac.uk/download/17297975.pdf (accessed on 9 May 2025).
2. Abdi, G., Abbasi Tarighat, M., Jain, M., Tendulkar, R., Tendulkar, M., & Barwant, M. M. (2024). Revolutionizing genomics: Exploring the potential of next-generation sequencing. *Advances in Bioinformatics*. https://doi.org/10.1007/978-981-99-8401-5_1.
3. Al-Delaimy, W., Alrabadi, N., Alzoubi, K. H., Khabour, A., et al. (2019). Population's perspectives toward biobanks in scientific research: A study from Jordan. https://core.ac.uk/download/323064955.pdf.
4. Andhi, N., & Darawadi, B. (2024). The genetic blueprint of cardiovascular therapy: Pharmacogenomics for improved efficacy and safety. *Journal of Indian College of Cardiology*. https://www.semanticscholar.org/paper/0f78a65f9bfc3b498c20c24a2f7e4e1d40fe579a (accessed on 9 May 2025).
5. Annemans, L., Berm, E. J. J., Boersma, C., de Looff, A., et al. (2016). Economic evaluations of pharmacogenetic and pharmacogenomic screening tests: A systematic review: Second update of the literature. https://core.ac.uk/download/55807615.pdf (accessed on 9 May 2025).
6. Barrese, V., Femminella, G. D., Ferrara, N., Rengo, C., et al. (2014). Tailoring therapy for heart failure: The pharmacogenomics of adrenergic receptor signaling. https://core.ac.uk/download/29469447.pdf (accessed on 9 May 2025).
7. Barrot, C., Woillard, J., & Picard, N. (2019). Big data in pharmacogenomics: Current applications, perspectives, and pitfalls. *Pharmacogenomics*, *20*(8), 609–620. https://www.semanticscholar.org/paper/57836162cf8990d0ed773361e67decf2c55fe529 (accessed on 9 May 2025).
8. Bartlett, G., Hızel, C., Kahveci, R., Manamperi, et al. (2012). Pharmacogenomics in primary care: A crucial entry point for global personalized medicine? https://core.ac.uk/download/643450591.pdf (accessed on 9 May 2025).
9. Bature, J. T., Eruaga, M. A., & Itua, E. O. (2024). Integrating pharmacogenomic testing into personalized medicine practices in the USA: Implications for medication quality control and therapeutic efficacy. *GSC Biological and Pharmaceutical Sciences*, *26*(3), 019–026. https://doi.org/10.30574/gscbps.2024.26.3.0081.
10. Borg, J. J., Fenech, A. G., Grech, G., Mitropoulos, et al. (2012). Relevance of pharmacogenomics for developing countries in Europe: Implementation in the Maltese population. https://core.ac.uk/download/46602333.pdf (accessed on 9 May 2025).
11. Borg, J. J., Fenech, A. G., Grech, G., Patrinos, et al. (2012). Conference scene: Golden Helix Pharmacogenomics Days: Educational activities on pharmacogenomics and personalized medicine. https://core.ac.uk/download/46603880.pdf.
12. Borghi, C., Grassi, G., Rosei, E. A., Savoia, et al. (2017). Personalized medicine—a modern approach for the diagnosis and management of hypertension. https://core.ac.uk/download/96884785.pdf (accessed on 9 May 2025).
13. Borro, M., Di Sanzo, M., Fineschi, V., Frati, et al. (2017). Clinical applications of personalized medicine: A new paradigm and challenge. https://core.ac.uk/download/80315182.pdf (accessed on 9 May 2025).

14. Brlek, P., Bulić, L., Bračić, M., Projić, P., Škaro, V., Shah, N., Shah, P., et al. (2024). Implementing whole genome sequencing (WGS) in clinical practice: Advantages, challenges, and future perspectives. *Cells, 13*(4). https://www.semanticscholar.org/paper/d9628377273a4ff74a798fc50fd0f8cfa7bc741f (accessed on 9 May 2025).

15. Caputo, M., Corach, D., Flichman, D. M., Hulaniuk, et al. (2017). Hepatitis C virus pharmacogenomics in Latin American populations: Implications in the era of direct-acting antivirals. https://core.ac.uk/download/159296291.pdf (accessed on 9 May 2025).

16. Cariati, F., D'Argenio, V., Izquierdo, R., Tomaiuolo, et al. (2020). From laboratory bench to benchmark: Technology transfer in laboratory medicine. https://core.ac.uk/download/pdf/323187997.pdf (accessed on 9 May 2025).

17. David, B., Mwakilili, A. D., & Mwakilili, A. D. (2024). Harnessing genomics and translational research to improve health in Africa: A report of the 13th African Society of Human Genetics meeting in Dar es Salaam, Tanzania. https://core.ac.uk/download/636759348.pdf (accessed on 9 May 2025).

18. De Paepe, A., & Vanakker, O. (2013). Pharmacogenomics in children: Advantages and challenges of next-generation sequencing applications. https://core.ac.uk/download/55848729.pdf (accessed on 9 May 2025).

19. De, T., Park, C. S., & Perera, M. A. (2018). Cardiovascular pharmacogenomics: Does it matter if you're Black or White? *Annual Review of Pharmacology and Toxicology, 59*, 577–603. https://doi.org/10.1146/annurev-pharmtox-010818-021154.

20. Dongho, G., Djeunang, B. D., Martinelli, A., Motshoge, T., Muthoga, et al. (2018). Human cytochrome P450 2B6 genetic variability in Botswana: A case of haplotype diversity and convergent phenotypes. *Core*. https://core.ac.uk/download/154947683.pdf (accessed on 9 May 2025).

21. Faraone, S. V., & Larsson, H. (2018). Genetics of attention deficit hyperactivity disorder. *Molecular Psychiatry, 24*(4), 562–575. https://doi.org/10.1038/s41380-018-0070-0.

22. Felice, A. (2002). Molecular biology at the bedside: The impact of genomics on the practice of medicine. *Core*. https://core.ac.uk/download/46601830.pdf.

23. Fenech, A. G., & Grech, G. (2014). Pharmacogenetics: The science of predictive clinical pharmacology. *Core*. https://core.ac.uk/download/46602555.pdf (accessed on 9 May 2025).

24. Fortina, P., Kricka, L. J., Park, J. Y., & Polsky, T. G. (2015). The future of laboratory medicine–A 2014 perspective. *Core*. https://core.ac.uk/download/54509579.pdf (accessed on 9 May 2025).

25. Fröhlich, H., Balling, R., Beerenwinkel, N., Kohlbacher, O., Kumar, S., Lengauer, T., Maathuis, M. H., et al. (2018). From hype to reality: Data science enabling personalized medicine. *BMC Medicine, 16*, 122. https://doi.org/10.1186/s12916-018-1122-7.

26. Hemingway, H., Asselbergs, F. W., Danesh, J., Dobson, R., Maniadakis, N., Maggioni, A. P., van Thiel, G. J. M. W., et al. (2017). Big data from electronic health records for early and late translational cardiovascular research: Challenges and potential. *European Heart Journal, 39*(12), 1481–1495. https://doi.org/10.1093/eurheartj/ehx487.

27. Hoshitsuki, K., Fernandez, C. A., & Yang, J. J. (2021). Pharmacogenomics for drug dosing in children: Current use, knowledge, and gaps. *The Journal of Clinical Pharmacology, 61*, 250–258. https://doi.org/10.1002/jcph.1891.

28. Hurvitz, S. A., Olevsky, O., & Sadeghi, S. (2014). Profiling and targeting HER2-positive breast cancer using trastuzumab emtansine. *Core*. https://core.ac.uk/download/323079599.pdf.

29. Jarada, T. N., Rokne, J., & Alhajj, R. (2020). A review of computational drug repositioning: Strategies, approaches, opportunities, challenges, and directions. *Journal of Cheminformatics, 12*, Article 46. https://doi.org/10.1186/s13321-020-00450-7.

30. Köhler, S., Gargano, M., Matentzoglu, N., Carmody, L., Lewis-Smith, D., Vasilevsky, N., Daniš, D., et al. (2020). The Human Phenotype Ontology in 2021. *Nucleic Acids Research, 49*(D1), D1207–D1217. https://doi.org/10.1093/nar/gkaa1043.

31. Kraus, S., Schiavone, F., Pluzhnikova, A., & Invernizzi, A. C. (2020). Digital transformation in healthcare: Analyzing the current state-of-research. *Journal of Business Research, 123*, 557–567. https://doi.org/10.1016/j.jbusres.2020.10.030.

32. Liu, C., Hu, F., Xie, G. Y., Miao, Y. R., Li, X., Zeng, Y., & Guo, A. Y. (2022). GSCA: An integrated platform for gene set cancer analysis at genomic, pharmacogenomic, and immunogenomic levels. *Briefings in Bioinformatics, 24*. https://doi.org/10.1093/bib/bbac558.

33. Mahanayak, B. (2024). Meaning, concept and application of bioinformatics. *International Journal of Scientific Research in Engineering and Management*. https://www.semanticscholar.org/paper/94962088a8e62635fb6efbd4569daf4f63cfc804 (accessed on 9 May 2025).

34. Malviya, A. K., & Khanna, P. (2024). Precision medicine in anesthesia: Pharmacogenomics and personalized care. *National Board of Examinations Journal of Medical Sciences*. https://www.semanticscholar.org/paper/c23339ffda6b32e49ff331b27f7fa9cebe434e60 (accessed on 9 May 2025).

35. Meng, Q., Gu, H., Zhang, Q., Yi, Z., & Jiang, D. (2023). Carbamazepine cutaneous adverse reactions and HLA gene variation in the Chinese population: A systematic review and meta-analysis. *Pharmacogenomics*. https://www.semanticscholar.org/paper/4b1dba7090a3dbdca24ad8dd5c7de9a74c7effd6 (accessed on 9 May 2025).

36. Meylani, R. (2024). An in-depth literature review of remote, online, and hybrid learning with case studies of successful and failed attempts. *International Journal of Studies in Education and Science*. https://www.semanticscholar.org/paper/4cc6aa2aef831f625bf91fb5aa713577b99ded51 (accessed on 9 May 2025).

37. Nassar, S. F., Raddassi, K., Ubhi, B. K., Doktorski, J., & Abulaban, A. (2020). Precision medicine: Steps along the road to combat human cancer. *Cells, 9*(9), 2056. https://doi.org/10.3390/cells9092056.

38. Naz, B., Aftab, M. J., & Sarfraz, A. H. (2024). Impact of reflective practice on the successful implementation of teacher education programs: A case study of Punjab Province. *Global Educational Studies Review*. https://www.semanticscholar.org/paper/0e0b808c3e4bf29fbb221153cd75ce54653e6c12 (accessed on 9 May 2025).

39. Nogueiras-Álvarez, R. (2023). Pharmacogenomics in clinical trials: An overview. *Frontiers in Pharmacology, 14*, 1247088. https://doi.org/10.3389/fphar.2023.1247088.

40. Sadée, W., Wang, D., Hartmann, K. E., & Toland, A. E. (2023). Pharmacogenomics: Driving personalized medicine. *Pharmacological Reviews, 75*(4), 789–814. https://doi.org/10.1124/pharmrev.122.000810.

41. Salatin, S., Shafiee-Kandjani, A., Hamidi, S., Amirfiroozi, A., & Kalejahi, P. (2024). Individualized psychiatric care: Integration of therapeutic drug monitoring, pharmacogenomics, and biomarkers. *Personalized Medicine*. https://www.semanticscholar.org/paper/d75960c852a88ac355231ad59ec68eed23cf7712 (accessed on 9 May 2025).

42. Satam, H., Joshi, K., Mangrolia, U., Waghoo, S., Zaidi, G., Rawool, S., Thakare, R. P., et al. (2023). Next-generation sequencing technology: Current trends and advancements. *Biology, 12*(7), 997. https://doi.org/10.3390/biology12070997.

43. Schrijver, I., & Wiita, A. P. (2011). Clinical application of high throughput molecular screening techniques for pharmacogenomics. *CORE*. https://core.ac.uk/download/323063319.pdf.

44. Shriver, S. P., Adams, D. V., McKelvey, B. A., McCune, J. S., Miles, D., Pratt, V. M., Ashcraft, K., et al. (2024). Overcoming barriers to discovery and implementation of equitable pharmacogenomic testing in oncology. *Journal of Clinical Oncology, 42*(10), 1181–1192. https://doi.org/10.1200/jco.23.01748.

45. Sugandh, F., Chandio, M., Raveena, F. N., Kumar, L., Karishma, F. N., Khuwaja, S., Memon, U. A., et al. (2023). Advances in the management of diabetes mellitus: A focus on personalized medicine. *Cureus, 10*(7), 43697. https://doi.org/10.7759/cureus.43697.

46. Thanh, N. T. D. (2021). Pharmacogenomics in nursing. *Core*. https://core.ac.uk/download/646123841.pdf (accessed on 9 May 2025).

47. Velazquez, I. M. (2021). A quality improvement project to assess the value of pharmacogenomic testing in adults diagnosed with major depression. *Core*. https://core.ac.uk/download/489832313.pdf (accessed on 9 May 2025).

48. Wang, R., & Wang, Z. (2023). Precision medicine: Disease subtyping and tailored treatment. *Cancers, 15*(15), 3837. https://doi.org/10.3390/cancers15153837.

49. Wishart, D. S., Djoumbou-Feunang, Y., Guo, A. C., Lo, E., Marcu, A., Grant, J. R., Sajed, T., et al. (2017). DrugBank 5.0: A major update to the DrugBank database for 2018. *Nucleic Acids Research, 46*, D1074–D1082. https://doi.org/10.1093/nar/gkx1037.

50. Yang, B., Lei, C., Yang, D., Lu, C., Xu, Y., Wang, L., Guo, T., et al. (2022). Identification of a novcl OFD1 variant in a patient with primary ciliary dyskinesia. *Pharmacogenomics and Personalized Medicine, 15*, 697–704. https://www.semanticscholar.org/paper/df5a83529b3fdf76d44d10e98e121211a574505b (accessed on 9 May 2025).

51. Zhou, Y., Tremmel, R., Schaeffeler, E., Schwab, M., & Lauschke, V. M. (2022). Challenges and opportunities associated with rare-variant pharmacogenomics. *Trends in Pharmacological Sciences, 43*(10), 852–865. https://doi.org/10.1016/j.tips.2022.07.002.

DRUG DEVELOPMENT AND CLINICAL TRIALS

14

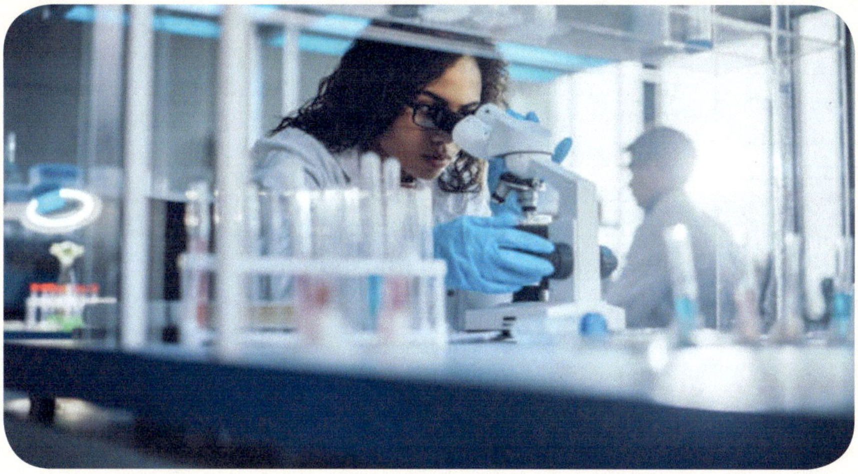

LEARNING OBJECTIVES

After studying this chapter, you will be able to:

1. Explain the drug development process
2. List the types of clinical trials
3. Explain about ethical considerations in clinical trials
4. Define challenges in drug development
5. Explain the role of technology in drug development
6. Discuss post-marketing surveillance

Introduction

The journey from the laboratory to the patient of new therapeutic agents is a multi-faceted and complex process that involves scientific innovation along with diligent regulatory control. New biotechnology has resulted in biological therapeutic agents, which are pharmaceutical products obtained from living organisms with the help of recombinant methods. Such biologics reflect a major break from conventional small-molecule therapeutics, which have opened the door to unprecedented opportunities for addressing a variety of chronic and acute diseases. Innovation in such treatment has required compromises in drug discovery and regulatory pathways to guarantee efficacy, safety, and maximum utilization in the clinical setting. To appreciate how these novel treatments become available to patients under strict scientific and ethical guidelines, it is important to understand the basics of drug development and clinical trials (Fenech et al., 2009) (Figure 14.1). In addition to innovation in therapeutics, the environment of drug development is also more and more shaped by global economic and technological trends, especially with the emergence of biosimilars. As patents on most biologic drugs are running out, a new biosimilar market is opening up with lower-cost versions of proprietary biologics. This has helped to bring about a more competitive marketplace, and this has allowed drug companies in developing nations, particularly India and China, to compete with the traditional players by making biosimilars at lower prices. This transformation has serious repercussions for medication access worldwide, which may reduce the costs of healthcare and increase treatment access in low-resource environments. The shifting market conditions require serious consideration of biosimilar development, regulatory acceptance, and clinical trial designs to uphold therapeutic quality (Huzair et al., 2011). At the core of drug development is the process of conducting clinical trials, which is the most important bridge between research conducted in the lab and general clinical use. Clinical trials are planned systematically to test the safety, dosage, and effectiveness of new medicines or biologics in human patients through phased clinical trials, beginning from small numbers of healthy individuals to large populations suffering from the disease in question. Such a thorough test guarantees that only treatments with proven benefits and acceptable risks go on to be used extensively. The clinical trial process comes under close observation of regulatory agencies, which develop guidelines to protect participants' rights and welfare as well as provide trustworthy scientific evidence. Understanding the clinical trial structure is imperative to value the obstacles and milestones encountered to introduce new therapeutics to the market and finally enhance patient care outcomes.

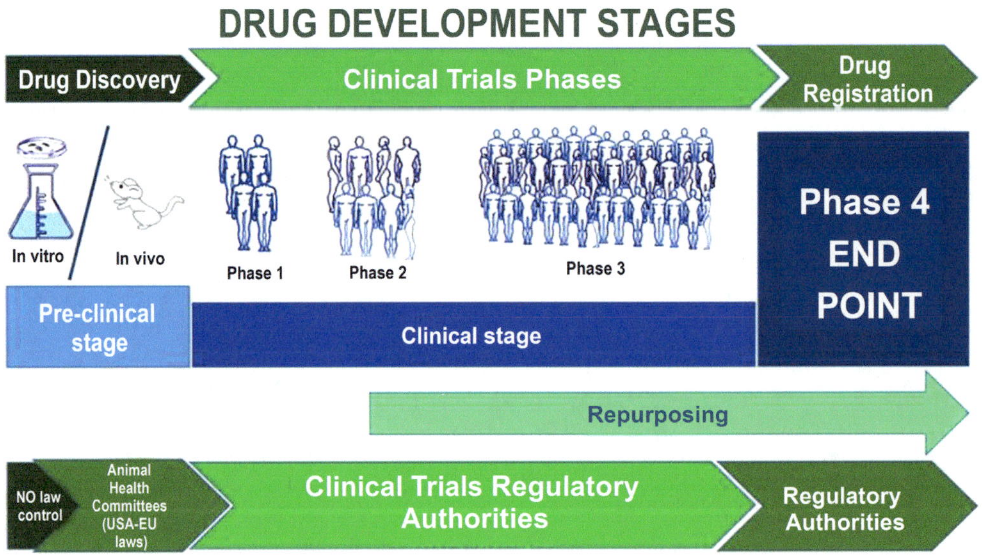

Figure 14.1. Drug development and clinical trials.

Source: Meringolo, M., et al. (2023). *Figure 1. Drug Development and Clinical Trial Stages*. In *Leaflet: Operative Steps for Interventional Studies*. ResearchGate.

Definition of Drug Development

The creation of a new pharmaceutical product from concept to product is a multi-faceted process of preclinical and exploratory and clinical research. A first phase of intense laboratory study and preclinical investigation establishes the biological mechanisms and promises of potential candidate substances and lays the foundation for the studies to come. Drug development entails not only the identification and optimization of pharmacologically active compounds but also cautious evaluation of safety and efficacy through an incremental series of clinical trials. The trials are set up to respond to key questions about dosage, side effects, and therapeutic value, factors fundamental to regulatory acceptance and clinical use. Interestingly, drug discovery is not merely the detection of the biological activity of a compound but also comprises extensive assessments that predict the chances of success in the major clinical trials, thereby allowing making appropriate decisions during drug development (Gasparini et al., 2018). The core of drug development lies in the measurement of efficacy and safety, which involves combining diverse endpoints to assess the aggregate benefit-risk profile of a treatment. Clinical trials utilize several metrics such as mortality rate, hospitalization rate, and patient-reported outcomes (PROs) to gain a holistic overview of the impact of a drug on worsening of disease and quality of life of the patients. Such a multi-faceted evaluation becomes crucial in conditions such as heart failure, in which traditional endpoints such as mortality must be weighed with improvement in functional status and symptom relief in order to derive clinical meaningfulness. As such, the drug development process necessarily entails creating trials involving these diverse endpoints since the definition of what constitutes therapeutic success continues to change (Bozkurt et al., 2022). Drug development is also characterized by iterative decision-making that hugely relies on statistical and quantitative techniques to forecast trial results and maximize development strategies. The composite predictive model of success enables stakeholders to compare potential directions before the start of large-scale pivotal trials. This methodological strategy enhances drug development productivity by reconciling existing evidence with hypotheses of future trial results, ultimately enabling data-based go/no-go decisions. Hence, drug development is a pragmatic, science-driven process which aims to find a balance between scientific excellence and practical concerns where only the best profiles qualify candidates to go further toward approval for use in patients and clinical use (Gasparini et al., 2018).

Importance of Clinical Trials in the Drug Approval Process

The journey from lab discovery to licensed drug is intricate, with numerous critical steps collectively that ensure the efficacy and safety of new drugs. Preclinical studies are conducted rigorously prior to human trials, and these serve as the first sieve to identify potentially useful drug candidates and rule out those that are unacceptably toxic or ineffective. But only through formal execution of clinical trials do researchers obtain ultimate evidence of the therapeutic value and risk profile of a drug in people (Figure 14.2). The trials formally evaluate the drug's pharmacodynamics, pharmacokinetics, and safety across dosing regimens, which will guide opinions regarding its potential clinical use. This stage takes a large amount of time and investment of resources, much like the imperative to safeguard public health and navigate the intricate interstices of human biology and disease variation (Kohli et al., 2018). Disciplined stages like these are the only way drugs would receive the stringent testing necessary to justify widespread use, undermining trust in medicine and regulatory mechanisms. Perhaps the most important aspect of clinical trials is to determine the optimal dosage regimen—a task pivotal to striking a balance between safety and efficacy. The quandary of how to select the appropriate dose is realized when one realizes that excessive doses can lead to serious adverse effects, while subtherapeutic doses are not sufficient to provide sufficient benefit, thus compromising the entire drug approval process. Statistical design breakthroughs, including optimal and efficient dose-finding designs, have been defined to address this problem through efficient estimation of the minimum effective dose. Adaptive techniques and predictive modeling are included in such designs to cope with uncertainties in dose-response curves for enhancing the accuracy and reliability of clinical trial findings. Through focus on dose optimization, clinical trials not only promote patient safety but also minimize regulatory approval pathways, allowing effective therapies to reach the market in an efficient and ethical manner (Bretz and Dette, 2025). This delicate element of dosage acknowledges the important role clinical trials play in advancing experimental agents into successful therapies. Other than dosing and safety, clinical trials are the ultimate testing ground for establishing a drug's true benefits in actual practice, rendering regulatory considerations based on empirical realities rather than theoretical hypothesis. Regulatory bodies rely heavily on the evidence generated during these trials to establish risk-benefit profiles, often requiring multidimensional evidence from diverse populations of patients and clinical environments. The methodical stages of clinical trials—ranging from initial human safety research to large-scale confirmatory studies—progressively seek to build evidence about a drug's effect on disease outcomes, including efficacy, tolerability, and long-term outcomes. Clinical trials in this regard also serve scientific progress by integrating emerging methods and filling methodologic gaps between translational science and the clinic. In addition, the process enables continuous improvement with post-marketing surveillance to guarantee continuous drug quality and patient safety. Finally, clinical trials are required as a public guardian, embodying the stringent scientific assessment required to promote public health and stimulate therapeutic advancement (Kohli et al., 2018).

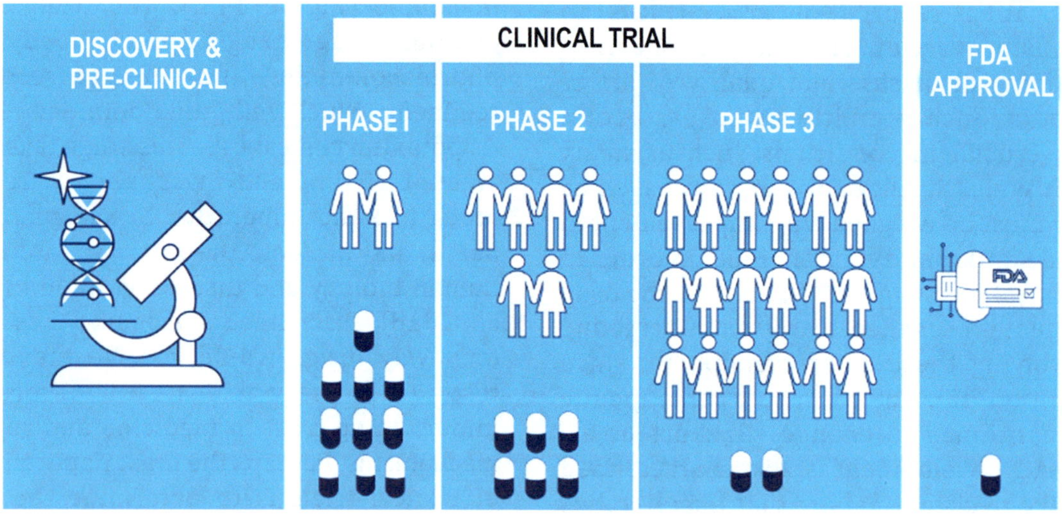

Figure 14.2. Clinical trials in the drug approval process.

Source: SevenPonds (2019). *Clinical Trials Process.* https://blog.sevenponds.com/wp-content/uploads/2019/08/clinical_trials_process.png.

14.1. The Drug Development Process

Learning Outcome

1. Stages of Drug Development
2. Role of Preclinical Research
3. Regulatory Requirements Before Clinical Trials

Before a drug reaches clinical trials, it must undergo rigorous preclinical testing to evaluate its pharmacokinetic properties, including absorption, distribution, metabolism, and excretion (ADME). One critical element during this phase is determining drug absorption, which significantly influences whether a candidate progresses to human testing. Current advances employ molecular dynamics simulations to examine water molecule interaction with the drug compound and allow scientists to estimate permeability metrics independent of parameter tuning. The computational method is highly correlated with traditional assays such as the human colon adenocarcinoma (Caco-2) cell line test, accelerating early-stage assessment and minimizing late-stage failures. Such integration of new modeling approaches optimizes candidate selection in such a way that only compounds with better absorption profiles progress, therefore enhancing the efficiency of the drug discovery pipeline (Milanetti et al., 2015). Having identified a lead drug candidate, clinical trials then become the cornerstone for determining its safety and efficacy in human subjects. Yet, the phase of clinical trials is highly challenging, with high rates of failure commonly caused by poor clinical model building and inefficient trial protocol design (Figure 14.3). Overcoming this requires multi-faceted approaches that improve the simulation models and minimize trial parameters to accurately forecast outcomes. New technologies, including quantum computing, have been suggested to transform this phase by streamlining clinical trial simulation, site selection, and patient cohort identification. These innovations hold the potential to maximize trial design, minimize costs, and expedite timelines. The integration of these new computational tools is vital to overcoming the current limitations and ultimately delivering value to stakeholders throughout the pharmaceutical development pipeline (Andress et al., 2024).

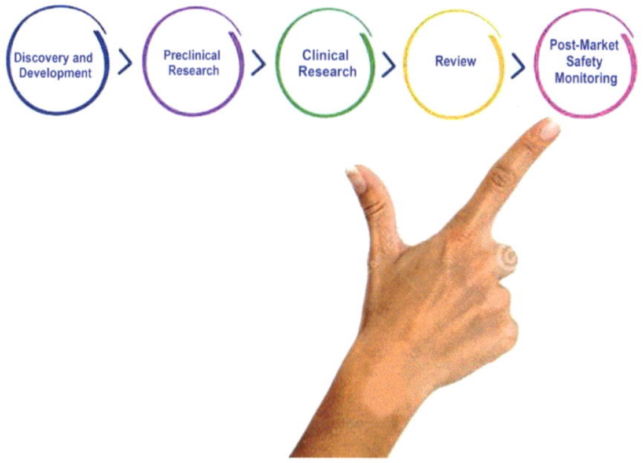

Figure 14.3. Drug development process.

Source: Vaeenma. (2017). *Diagram of Drug Development Process.* Dreamstime. https://thumbs.dreamstime.com/z/drug-development-process-diagram-94366765.jpg.

The drug development process is interdisciplinary by design, requiring coordination between chemists, biologists, data scientists, and clinicians to convert laboratory findings into an effective therapeutic candidate. Computational advances in the prediction of drug behavior and the design of clinical trial architecture have emerged as central to this multi-faceted effort. Predictive techniques of molecular permeability drive early candidate screening, whereas quantum-aided algorithms are able to simulate trial environments dynamically and inform decisions on patient recruitment and site selection. Collectively, these advancements represent a more data-driven and accurate drug development process, remedying past inefficiencies and ethical issues in patient exposure during trials. As therapeutic targets become increasingly complex, incorporating such novel methodologies will be instrumental in progressing the pharmaceutical industry and bringing safe, effective treatments to market.

14.1.1. Stages of Drug Development

The path from a lead compound to an approved drug consists of a series of carefully crafted steps, each necessary for the validation of the final therapeutic product's safety and efficacy (Figure 14.4). First, drug discovery aims at finding and validating molecular targets of a disease, which requires extensive biological investigation and advanced screening methods. After target validation, lead compounds need to be chosen and optimized for their intended biological activity. This step is specifically resource-hungry and involves optimization of the chemical properties in order to enhance efficacy and diminish probable toxicity. The process of drug development combines a blend of experimental information and computational models with the intention of cutting down on the lengthy time and money spent on drug discovery. Maximizing this initial phase is key to simplifying downstream development phases and prevents wasting funds on compounds with little chance of advancement (Gabbert et al., 2008).

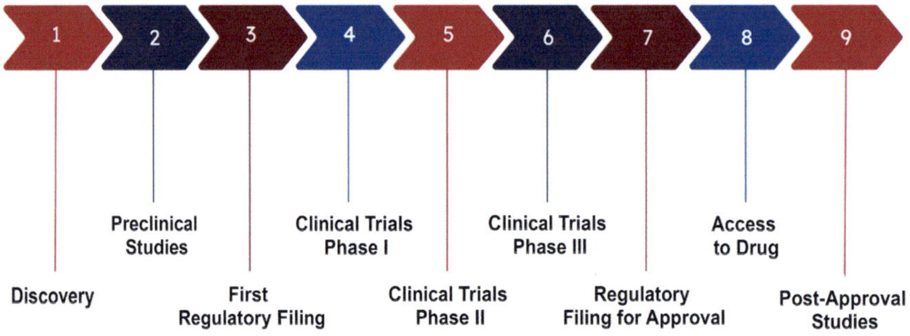

Figure 14.4. Stages of drug development.

Source: Friedreich's Ataxia Research Alliance. (2024). *Stages of Drug Development. https*://www.curefa.org/wp-content/uploads/2024/03/STAGES-OF-DRUG-DEVELOPMENT_block1.png.

Once a lead compound shows significant biological activity, nonclinical evaluation and early clinical studies take over, aimed at determining safety, dosing, and pharmacokinetics. Preclinical tests employ *in vitro* assays and animal models to extrapolate human responses, but such models do not replicate human physiology at all. New technologies such as *ex vivo* metrics hold new promise through the utilization of ethically donated human organs to model drug effects with enhanced biological relevance and bridge the translational gap to facilitate improved assessment of efficacy and toxicity in a closer-to-human setting. This advancement facilitates better decision-making regarding which drug candidates to send into clinical trials, thereby minimizing late-stage failure and optimizing overall drug productivity (Gabbert et al., 2008). The clinical trial stage is further divided into several stages—Phases I, II, and III—each of which is aimed at increasing knowledge on the safety profile of the drug, best dosing, therapeutic effectiveness, and possible adverse effects in human subjects. Phase I trials are mainly concerned with the determination of safety and tolerability within a small number of volunteers, whereas Phase II tests therapeutic effectiveness as well as additional safety in a larger population. Phase III trials consist of large-scale, randomized controlled trials across heterogeneous populations to establish clinical benefit as well as track adverse effects over longer periods. Success within these phases leads to regulatory filing and marketing authorization. The whole drug development process needs not only strict scientific research but also compliance with ethical principles and regulatory guidelines to protect patients and confer therapeutic benefit (Marashi et al., 2005).

14.1.2. Role of Preclinical Research

Before human testing, a rigorous preclinical research period is required to establish the safety, efficacy, and mechanism of action of a prospective drug (Figure 14.5). Preclinical investigations consist of *in vitro* experiments and animal models that mimic conditions of human disease to predict therapeutic effects and identify possible adverse effects. Preclinical screening is important in the reduction of risks such that only lead drugs make it to clinical trials.

For example, the identification of therapeutics modulating viral entry and replication pathways capitalizes on extensive amounts of laboratory data that enable the identification of molecular mechanisms such as TMPRSS2 participation in viral infections to have a reason to target some proteins in an attempt to maximize treatment (Jonathan et al., 2020). In the absence of upstream anchoring studies, unforeseen toxicities or inefficacies may result in costly clinical trial failure. Thus, preclinical studies are the gateway that determines clinical protocols, dosage regimens, and safety parameters, ultimately deciding the direction of drug development and clinical evaluation. Besides establishing initial efficacy and safety, preclinical studies are important in exploring pharmacodynamic and pharmacokinetic properties of drug candidates. It allows scientists to establish how a drug is absorbed, distributed, metabolized, and excreted, which guides dosage and administration strategies. The results thus achieved can inform if modifications should be made to enhance bioavailability or reduce toxicity. Further, preclinical studies stand first in addressing comorbidities and patient vulnerabilities. For instance, patients with compromised lung function or conditions that predispose them to substance abuse disorders may be under greater risk when infected with certain viruses, further justifying the use of patient-specific treatments based on preclinical data (Nora, 2020). By mimicking different physiological conditions, these investigations make it possible to determine patient-specific responses and potential drug interactions, thereby making personalized medicine programs feasible even before clinical trials. Besides mechanistic and safety assessments, preclinical investigation presents a valuable platform for drug repurposing and combination therapy strategies, especially in emerging health crises. Because long timescales are typically required for the creation of new medicines, established drugs have a safety profile and can be tested in preclinical models for efficacy against novel pathogens or diseases. TMPRSS2 inhibitors and antiviral drugs, for example, were preclinically evaluated to determine whether they could block viral entry and replication, with the aim of developing useful cocktails as therapies (Jonathan et al., 2020). These studies also help to define potential synergistic or adverse interactions, which are vital to be considered prior to clinical trial planning. While accelerated clinical assessment may be necessary for some critical situations, comprehensive preclinical data remain at the center of ensuring that drug development is proceeding on a sound scientific basis, with the greatest chance of clinical success and benefit to patients.

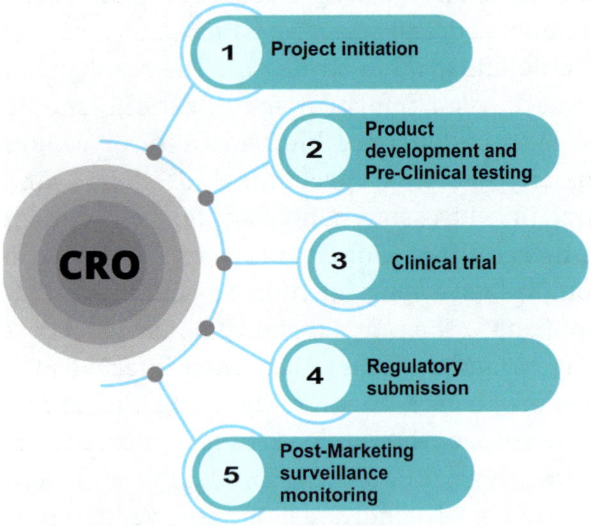

Figure 14.5. Role of preclinical research.

Source: **LIDE Biotech.** (2023). *Preclinical and Clinical Research Pipeline. https*://www.lidebiotech.com/sites/default/files/2023-08/preclinical_clinical_research.png.

14.1.3. Regulatory Requirements Before Clinical Trials

Before proceeding to clinical trials, a drug undergoes a rigorous regulatory examination to ensure safety and efficacy standards are adequately met (Figure 14.6). The first step involves extensive preclinical investigations, including *in vitro* and *in vivo* experiments, which provide key information on pharmacodynamics, pharmacokinetics, and toxicological profiles. Regulatory bodies insist on thorough documentation demonstrating that a drug candidate has been rigorously tested for toxic effects and metabolic fate. Such findings establish that the drug being tested is tolerably safe for initial human exposure. Meeting such conditions is of utmost significance because it provides the basis upon which clinical trial designs are laid out. Without this critical regulatory clearance, one cannot obtain clearance to start human trials, and this clearly shows high priority for safety considerations for drug candidates in the early phases of drug development (Deore et al., 2019). Besides preclinical data, regulatory requirements demand the submission of an Investigational New Drug (IND) application or comparable dossier, depending on geographical region. It should comprehensively summarize the drug's chemical and production information, descriptions of preclinical results in detail, protocols for studies, and qualifications of investigators. Oversight agencies review justifications for human experimentation and clinical trial design that is intended in order to protect against ethical impropriety and trial integrity. The strict scrutiny process aims for minimizing risk in favor of optimal therapeutic benefit and thereby safeguarding participants and verifying the scientific legitimacy of the trial. These processes highlight the intricate regulatory process that governs drug development, emphasizing that advancement to clinical trials needs an objective and open assessment process with set standards (Deore et al., 2019). Innovative therapeutic approaches, such as phage therapy, emphasize evolving regulatory barriers that must be surmounted before commencing clinical trials. As demand for novel therapies to combat antimicrobial resistance (AMR) grows, regulators are adapting standards to incorporate novel modalities while maintaining robust safety and efficacy expectations. In recent years, these advancements include clinical trials in compliance with Good Manufacturing Practice (GMP) and good medical practice standards, which reflect heightened scrutiny when introducing new biologics to human patients. The changing regulatory environment is constantly adding new scientific information, such as immunomodulatory effect of experimental therapies, thereby expanding traditional paradigms. This innovation ensures that all investigational medicines, representing either established medicines or innovative biologics, comply with regulatory standards aimed at protecting patients as well as ensuring successful clinical development.

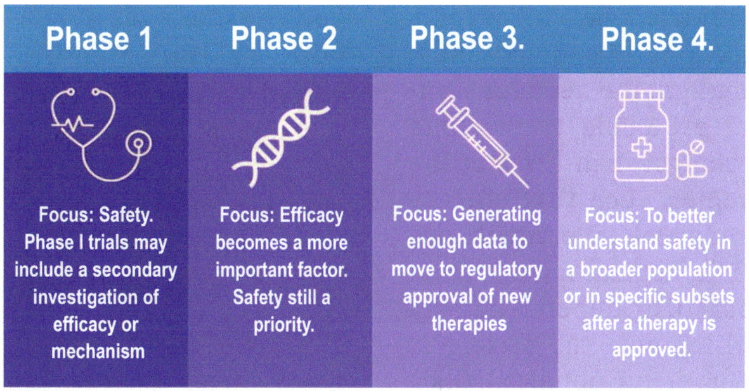

Figure 14.6. Regulatory requirements before clinical trials.

Source: Lustgarten Foundation (2022). *Infographic Clinical Trials.* https://lustgarten.org/wp-content/uploads/2022/05/infographic-clinical-trials-1-1024x683.png.

Test Your Knowledge

1. What follows after discovery in the drug development process?
2. What is the purpose of regulatory requirements before clinical trials?

14.2. Types of Clinical Trials

Learning Outcome

1. Phase I Trials: Safety and Dosage
2. Phase II Trials:, Efficacy and Side Effects
3. Phase III Trials: Comparison with Standard Treatments

The development from discoveries made in the laboratory to successful medical therapy requires strict testing by clinical trials that vary in design based on their goals and stages (Figure 14.7). Phase I, among early-phase trials, is basically designed to test the safety, dosing, and pharmacokinetics of experimental drugs in a limited number of healthy volunteers or patients. These trials offer benchmark data important for deciding if a drug is allowed to proceed to subsequent testing phases. Phase II trials increase the number of participants to test the drug's effectiveness and ideal dosing while maintaining safety evaluations. Both phases focus on controlled settings to track precise biological responses, something especially important for emerging therapeutic modalities such as microRNA-based therapies that are known for their complicated cellular interactions and risk of off-target effects (Diener et al., 2022). Such a phased, structured process guarantees thorough vetting of each candidate therapy prior to exposure in larger populations. Later clinical trials, Phase III studies, involve more extensive and varied patient populations to establish efficacy, track side effects, and test the new therapy against standards or placebos. These randomized controlled trials (RCTs) are regarded as the gold standard to determine clinical benefit and risk profiles. Their methodical design consists of random allocation to treatment or control groups and frequently employs blinding to reduce bias. In chronic and complicated conditions like hemophilia, changing guidelines highlight the need for well-designed clinical trial protocols to evaluate new therapies like prolonged half-life clotting factors and gene therapies, such that efficacy is balanced with safety as well as practical use (Srivastava et al., 2020). Regulatory approval and subsequent clinical use depend heavily on Phase III trials, which give the strongest evidence for a drugs therapeutic potential. Once regulatory approval is given, Phase IV or post-marketing trials still test the performance of the drug in actual conditions. These trials track long-term safety, efficacy, and possible rare side effects not seen during previous phases. They can also investigate other indications, varying populations, or combination therapy.

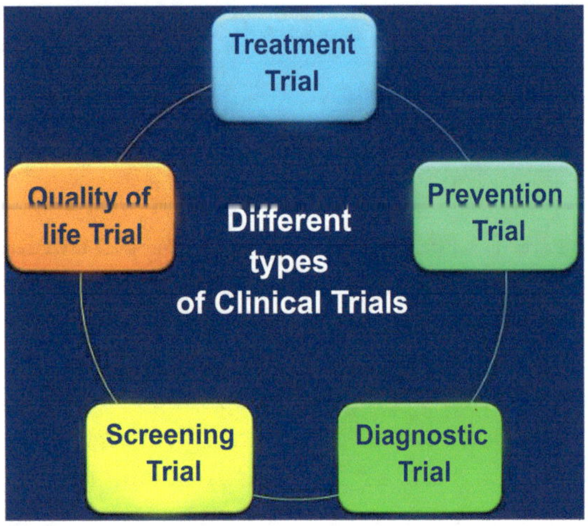

Figure 14.7. Types of clinical trials.

Source: https://3.bp.blogspot.com/-EWsv0Yp3nh8/VmJCTY8EgyI/AAAAAAAAAsw/_TqCi8GJq8Y/s1600/Clinical%2Btrial.jpg.

For example, the use of novel therapies calls for continued monitoring to identify unexpected immune reactions or delayed complications, a requirement that is underscored in chronic conditions that need to be treated lifelong (Srivastava et al., 2020). Adaptive trial designs and pragmatic trials are also gaining stature as powerful methods to speed up drug development with safety maintained. Together, these varied categories of clinical trials constitute a complementary and sequential system that supports evidence-based drug development and guides clinical practice.

14.2.1. Phase I Trials: Safety and Dosage

Early drug development requires careful attention to patient safety and reliable dosing strategies to provide a basis for subsequent clinical investigation. Phase I trials fulfill this important function by recruiting a small number of healthy volunteers or patients to assess how a drug is broken down, its pharmacokinetics, and possible side effects. Instead of progressing treatment effectiveness, these studies focus on determining the maximum tolerated dose alongside watching for toxicity levels to guarantee patient safety. This process of determining the optimal dose is instrumental in developing a therapeutic window that strikes an efficacy-risk balance. Regulatory policies also highlight that clinical judgment and compliance with predetermined safety procedures are essential during such trials since each subject's response is quite variable (Visseren et al., 2021). These precautions not only safeguard individual subjects but also prevent expensive failures in subsequent trial stages. Phase I trials' determination of the correct dosage is a gradual increase in drug levels under controlled conditions, allowing researchers to monitor dose-dependent effects and side effects in real-time. This stepwise design enables scientists to determine not only the maximum tolerated dose but also to set pharmacodynamic markers that indicate therapeutic potential. Since the human response is complex, particularly in treatments that address new pathogens or mechanisms, Phase I studies usually include biochemical and immunological assays to determine safety in depth. For example, knowledge about immune system interactions, as presented in viral pathophysiology and immune dysfunction studies, guides decisions on dosage and risk reduction in initial trials (Tay et al., 2020). Through the incorporation of such mechanistic understanding, Phase I trials facilitate the optimization of dosing regimens to minimize toxicity while opening the door for efficacy testing in later phases. Safety monitoring throughout Phase I trials is ongoing and multidimensional, including both clinical observation and laboratory analysis to identify any indication of acute or cumulative toxicity.

Adverse event reporting schemes have to be strict, as early detection of harmful impacts can lead to prompt dose corrections or even trial termination to safeguard participants. The multidisciplinary aspect of these analyses frequently calls for coordination among clinical pharmacologists, toxicologists, and regulatory specialists in the interpretation of data in the overall context of patient well-being and regulatory law. Notably, even when Phase I trials have been completed, medical professionals still have the duty to use trial results responsibly, considering changing regulatory requirements and patient-specific factors in developing therapeutic plans (Visseren et al., 2021). Such constant watchfulness identifies the critical role of Phase I trials in providing assurance that drug development continues with maximized safety and scientifically appropriate dosing principles.

14.2.2. Phase II Trials:, Efficacy and Side Effects

Development of a drug candidate from first safety assessments through evaluation of therapeutic benefit requires Phase II clinical trials of high intensity, in which efficacy and side effect profiles are carefully scrutinized. Such trials typically include a larger group of patients with the targeted disease to enable more reliable estimation of drug effectiveness and continued assessment of side effects. Phase II trials represent a critical transition phase; they not only validate dose ranges but also provide insight into identifying biomarkers of response or resistance. This phase is able to elucidate intricate interactions between drug and biology, at times uncovering unexpected off-target effects, especially with drugs that target mechanisms that are broad regulatory in nature like microRNAs. The complex function of microRNAs in modulating multiple genes makes widespread side effects a cause for concern, a fact that has come to fore in the earliest miRNA-targeted therapeutics where dose control and delivery remain paramount in harmonizing therapeutic response with toxicity (Diener et al., 2022).

Successful outcomes from Phase II trials are seen with advancements in targeted immunomodulatory pharmaceuticals, while outcomes in different disease contexts and drug specificity may yield mixed results. In inflammatory disorders such as Crohn's disease, Janus kinase inhibitor trials showed divergent results: tofacitinib failed to achieve primary efficacy measures in Phase II CD trials, but its selectivity and systemic effects were reportedly responsible for variable responses and side effect profiles. In contrast, more stringent JAK1 inhibitors and newer drugs with better intestinal targeting showed encouraging outcomes, validating the importance of patient stratification and drug design in maximizing efficacy and reducing side effects. This heterogeneity highlights the need for thorough Phase II studies to identify the subtleties of drug activity beyond initial safety confirmation, directing additional clinical development choices (Rogler, 2019). Phase II trial side effects frequently appear as a double-edged sword, unmasking potential toxicities but allowing mitigation measures prior to initiating larger Phase III studies. As an example, miRNA therapies like MRX34, a miR-34a mimic for cancer therapy, exhibited strong antitumor activity but caused serious immune-related adverse effects, prompting the termination of trials early. This parallels the intrinsic challenges in modulating intricate regulatory RNAs, such that pleiotropic effects elicit unwanted disturbances in immune and organ function, highlighting the necessity of delivery technology, dosing regimens, and molecular targeting accuracy, requiring Phase II trials to carefully enumerate not only benefit but also mechanism-based toxicities. Finally, this step offers a necessary risk-benefit assessment, informing the direction of drug candidates throughout the pipeline of clinical development (Diener et al., 2022).

14.2.3. Phase III Trials: Comparison with Standard Treatments

As a novel therapeutic agent progresses towards regulatory sanctioning, movement out of early-stage phases and into Phase III trials represents a point of great distinction marked by exhaustive comparison against comparative therapies. These studies enroll large numbers of participants and are intended not simply to prove safety and efficacy, but to determine comparative effectiveness compared to established treatments in use. The comparative framework is necessary for placing the new intervention's value in the context of established practice and informing decision-making at the bedside.

By comparing with established therapeutic standards, investigators can identify incremental advantage or disadvantage, thus informing clinicians and policymakers. This stage also considers more general patient populations and a range of clinical settings to maximize findings' generalizability. The rich data accumulated in Phase III trials therefore become the evidentiary foundation for later regulatory assessment, health technology appraisals, and clinical guideline development to ensure that any new treatment at least matches or surpasses the current standard of care. Phase III trial design usually involves randomization, blinding, and multi-center involvement to reduce bias and provide strong comparisons with control therapies. Parallel-group and active-control trial designs are used most frequently to compare differences in efficacy, safety profiles, and PROs directly. Trials that test treatments for prevalent and life-affecting conditions like cardiovascular diseases (CVDs) commonly use these standards for accurate assessment, as evidenced by influential bodies promoting evidence-based guidelines (Williams et al., 2018). The strategic choice of comparators is critical; a recognized effective treatment instead of placebo is usually used as the control to ethically balance patient interest with scientific integrity. In addition, trials often evaluate long-term effects and side effects, variables essential for establishing the clinical usefulness of the test product. This integrated scheme guarantees that outcomes from Phase III can have an impact on therapeutic protocols and coverage determinations and thus speed up the incorporation of better interventions into standard practice. Even with methodological strength, Phase III comparisons against control treatments are not without some challenges, such as heterogeneity in patient populations, variability in treatment compliance, and changing clinical practice.

The fluid nature of medical knowledge, as illustrated by quickly arising conditions like the recent global COVID-19 pandemic, highlights the necessity for responsive trial designs that can accommodate changing standards (Hu et al., 2020). Additionally, making inferences from comparative efficacy requires subtle statistical methods to control for confounding and bias in large studies. Ethical concerns are also important, especially when available treatments provide considerable benefit, limiting equipoise. However, the careful exercise of benchmarking new agents against standard therapies in Phase III trials continues to be invaluable; not only does it ensure that incremental innovation is beneficial to patient care, but also it promotes the equitable distribution of healthcare resources. In the end, such comparisons underlie evidence-based medicine, guaranteeing that new drugs enhance or supplement current treatment paradigms.

Test Your Knowledge

1. What is the primary objective of Phase I clinical trials?
2. How do Phase III trials contribute to regulatory approval?

14.3. Ethical Considerations in Clinical Trials

Learning Outcome

1. Informed Consent and Patient Rights
2. Institutional Review Boards (IRBs)
3. Ethical Dilemmas in Trial Design

The incorporation of new technologies within clinical trials has greatly improved the effectiveness and accuracy of drug discovery processes. Yet, these new technologies raise serious ethical issues that should be properly managed to safeguard the rights of participants and ensure scientific integrity (Figure 14.8). Ensuring informed consent, particularly with the influence of artificial intelligence systems on patient selection and data interpretation, is a high-priority issue. Volunteers need to have a complete comprehension of the impact of AI-based approaches on their participation, such as risks and benefits. In addition, transparency in trial design and analysis algorithms is crucial to prevent bias and unfair treatment outcomes. Failure to have proper controls can undermine fairness through automated decision-making, eroding public trust in clinical studies. The delicate balance between availing the progress of technology and ensuring ethical compliance requires stringent regulatory mechanisms and close monitoring (Roy et al., 2022; Singh et al., 2023). Data privacy and security are yet another critical ethical consideration in contemporary clinical trials, especially as they become more reliant on large amounts of biomedical data and machine learning algorithms. The sensitive nature of participant data calls for strong controls against unauthorized disclosure or misuse. Even though AI can hasten research and tailor treatments, mismanagement of data can result in confidentiality breaches and worsening healthcare access inequities. In addition, the issue of algorithmic bias must be addressed because biased data sets can lead to discriminatory practices that can influence trial results and subsequent drug approvals unfairly among different groups of people. Ethical stewardship of data needs transparency, accountability, and the use of explainable AI to enable auditing by researchers and participants (Roy et al., 2022; Singh et al., 2023). The intervention of human oversight continues to be necessary in the ethical operation of clinical trials despite increasing use of machine learning and AI resources. Although technology provides new capacity to handle intricate data sets and forecast therapeutic effectiveness, human discernment is critical in interpreting results and ensuring participant well-being. Ethical frameworks need to place paramount importance on the participants safety, respect, and agency throughout the trial life cycle. Moreover, interdisciplinary synergy between scientists, ethicists, regulators, and patient advocates is necessary to cope with ethical challenges from technological adoption. Such collaboration has the potential to develop holistic guidelines that balance innovation with ethical responsibility, in the end strengthening the credibility and social legitimacy of drug development efforts (Roy et al., 2022; Singh et al., 2023).

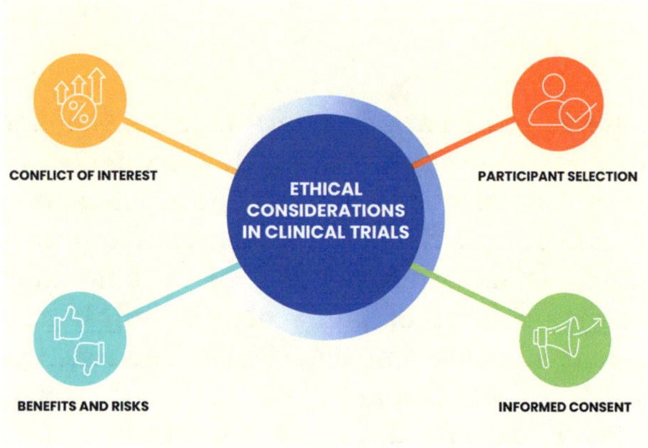

Figure 14.8. Ethical considerations in clinical trials.

Source: **ZoomRx.** (2023). *Ethical Considerations in Clinical Trials. https*://blog.zoomrx.com/content/images/2023/05/Ethical-Considerations-in-clinical-trials.png.

14.3.1. Informed Consent and Patient Rights

The sophistication of contemporary drug development and clinical trials has amplified the moral obligations researchers have to their subjects. Central to this endeavor is ensuring the informed consent, which is a keystone that protects patient autonomy and rights (Figure 14.9). Patients need to be given adequate, understandable information about the nature of the trial, risks, benefits, and other treatment alternatives prior to consent. This openness is essential to building trust and encouraging ethical integrity, especially when trials investigate new treatments whose outcomes are unknown. Recent trials of potentially groundbreaking immunotherapy combinations, for example, like atezolizumab and bevacizumab in hepatocellular carcinoma (Richard et al., 2020), require straightforward explanation so participants understand the experimental nature and possibility of unknowns that lie within these new treatments. Informed consent also has an important function in ensuring that patient safety and scientific progress are balanced during clinical trials. Patients are not objects for research but participants who have rights that need to be preserved in the interest of medical advances. This ethical principle has become increasingly important in multi-phase clinical trials in which survival advantages and safety endpoints are repeatedly assessed, e.g., trials of nivolumab and ipilimumab in stage III/IV melanoma (Jedd et al., 2017). In these cases, the shifting evidence regarding efficacy and safety profiles necessitates that consent forms be fluid, presenting changing information to participants. This constant discussion guarantees respect for the patient's right to make fully informed choices as new evidence accumulates and reaffirms the value of their voluntary involvement throughout the trial period. Additionally, protection of patient rights goes beyond first consent to post-trial access and confidentiality concerns. Personal health information protection must be strictly upheld to avert exploitation and discrimination, especially with the increased data generation in precision medicine and immunotherapy trials. Participants need to be made aware of their rights to withdraw at any point without penalty, which is a key aspect that ensures autonomy is retained even during advanced trial conditions. By integrating these principles into the entire drug development life cycle, investigators pay homage to ethical responsibilities while enabling trust-based relationships necessary for scientific advancement. Accordingly, full informed consent and abiding respect for patient rights are not only ethical requirements but cornerstones to successful and ethically conducted clinical research (Jedd et al., 2017; Richard et al., 2020).

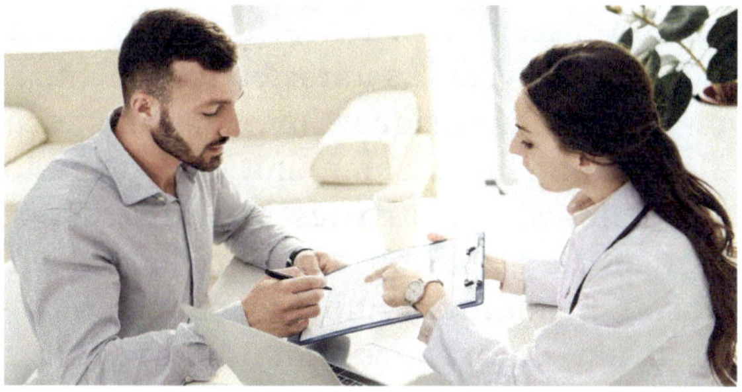

Figure 14.9. Informed consent and patient rights.

Source: Healthline (2019). *Patient Doctor Signing. https*://post.healthline.com/wp-content/uploads/2019/10/Patient_Doctor_Signing_1200x628-facebook.jpg.

14.3.2. Institutional Review Boards (IRBs)

Ethical monitoring of clinical trials plays a pivotal role in protecting participant well-being while maintaining scientific integrity. Institutional Review Boards (IRBs) play this protective role by meticulously examining study protocols to evaluate risk, benefit, and informed consent procedures (Figure 14.10). Their function becomes increasingly important with the changing trial methods, including decentralized and virtual trials fueled by recent global pandemics. The COVID-19 pandemic, for instance, catalyzed rapid adaptations in trial conduct, prompting IRBs to navigate unprecedented challenges related to remote monitoring, telemedicine, and patient data confidentiality. Such shifts require IRBs to balance innovation with compliance, ensuring that expedited trial processes do not compromise participant safety or data validity. The need for streamlined but intensive IRB reviews is a prime example of the changing regulatory climate around drug development, where ethics review has to keep pace with innovation in clinical research methodologies (Sessa et al., 2021). The embedding of digital technologies in clinical trials highlights the increased role of IRBs today. Mobile health devices, wearable sensors, and artificial intelligence drive digital clinical trials, improving recruitment, data collection, and patient participation, potentially beyond the conventional clinic. This new direction calls for IRBs to review not just the science but also the technology aspects of data protection, privacy, and distant consent processes. Ensuring confidentiality for sensitive health data in digital media calls for IRBs to be familiar with evolving cybersecurity standards and regulations. Also, more use of algorithms and machine learning in data analysis leads IRBs to assess potential biases and confirm the validity of digital endpoints. Therefore, IRBs act as important intermediaries, ensuring innovative methodologies meet ethical standards and regulatory guidelines while supporting the future-proofing of clinical trials (Omer et al., 2020). Effective IRB and other trial stakeholder collaboration is crucial to maximize the balance between research progress and participant protection. The pandemic underscored the potential for expedited protocol review and accelerated regulatory approval without sacrificing ethical principles. Harmonized IRB processes, possibly via centralized or single IRB models, can streamline administrative tasks and accelerate trial initiation, particularly for multi-site and global studies. These changes can facilitate the use of patient-focused trial designs that minimize participant burden through telemedicine assessments and decentralized processes. Challenges like varying regional needs and data privacy regulations, though, require sophisticated IRB oversight. Promoting stakeholder involvement—such as sponsors, investigators, regulators, and patients—with IRBs can enable a collaborative environment that maintains ethical integrity while facilitating nimbleness in drug development and clinical trials (Sessa et al., 2021).

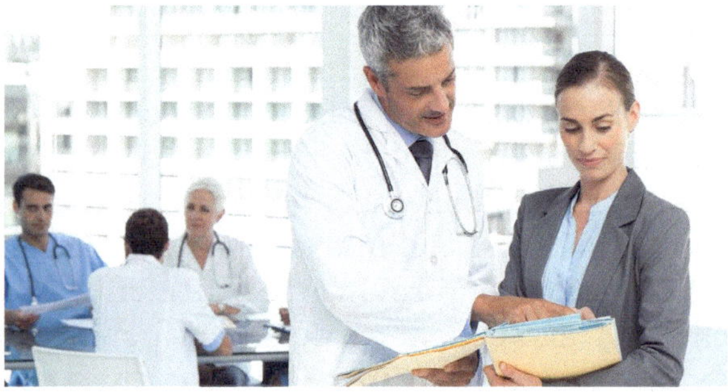

Figure 14.10. Institutional review boards (IRBs).

Source: **Versiti Clinical Trials.** (n.d.). *Salus IRB Review Services.* https://media.versiticlinicaltrials.org/versiti/clinicaltrials/media/page/services/ct-services-card-salus-review-1200x630.jpg.

14.3.3. Ethical Dilemmas in Trial Design

The need to create effective treatments amid large-scale health emergencies frequently compels researchers to face deep ethical challenges in clinical trial design (Figure 14.11). When new diseases spread quickly, as with COVID-19 and Ebola outbreaks, the need to identify therapies that can save lives clashes with the need for strict scientific testing. Rapid trial protocols and compassionate use of unregistered interventions bring in challenges in striking a balance between patient safety and the requirement for generating quick data. Under such circumstances, standard randomized controlled trials might not always prove feasible or ethical, particularly when withholding potentially life-saving interventions from control groups could lead to deaths that could have otherwise been avoided. This tension calls on investigators and regulatory agencies to develop novel trial designs that maintain the scientific integrity of evidence while being sensitive to patient autonomy and well-being, without compromising ethical principles at the cost of needlessly postponing access to interventions (Krech et al., 2014; Tomasz et al., 2020). Complicating these are issues of informed consent and disclosure, especially among populations beset by health crises. Clear communication of benefits and risks becomes absolutely essential when evidence for safety and efficacy is weak, as untested treatments are given under compassionate use. The conundrum is also extended to community participation, where cultural sensitivities and mistrust can influence participation and compliance with protocols. In addition, vulnerable populations—most often disproportionately impacted by outbreaks—need special protections to avoid exploitation or coercion. Confirming that patients or their representatives are able to make authentically informed choices requires sensitivity to ethical considerations like respect for persons and justice.

These issues require trial designs that blend ethical structures with community outreach strategies in order to establish trust and openness (Krech et al., 2014). An added level of complexity comes in the requirement to gather and provide data produced under emergency interventions, even beyond conventional trial environments. Although having a strong set of safety and efficacy data is important for ascertaining treatment effect, there may be pressure to put patient care needs ahead of systematic data collection in the short term. The ethical conflict in this scenario is managing the need to deliver care quickly with the obligation to advance generalizable knowledge that can inform future treatment. Open reporting and data sharing are important to maximize overall benefit and avoid duplication of effort, but practical and regulatory barriers can slow these processes. Therefore, trial designs need to have mechanisms that ensure all the information generated during crisis responses are ethically handled and released, sustaining the integrity of the drug development process (Krech et al., 2014).

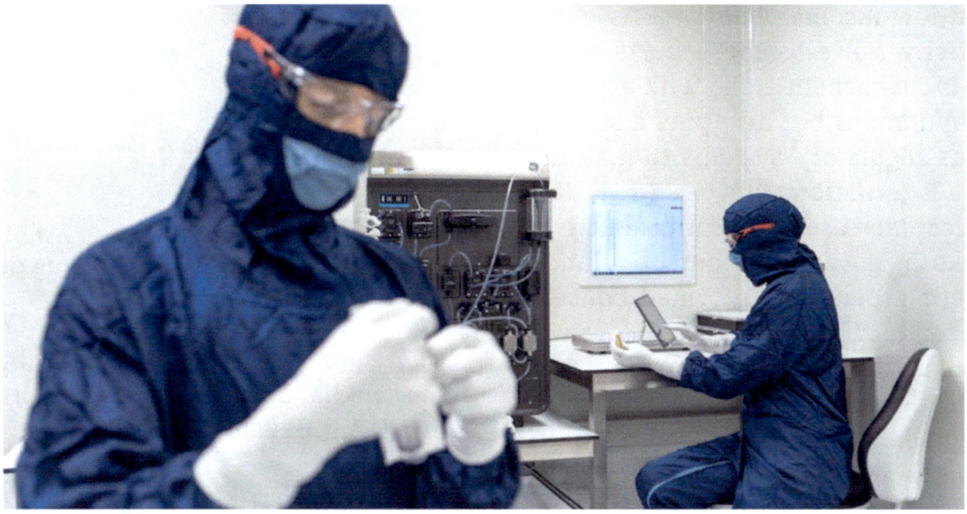

Figure 14.11. Ethical dilemmas in trial design.

Source: Bit2Geek. (2023). *The Ethical Dilemmas of Human Clinical Trials*. https://www.bit2geek.com/wp-content/uploads/2023/09/the-ethical-dilemmas-of-human-clinical-trials.jpg.

Test Your Knowledge

1. What is ethical considerations in clinical trials?
2. What is the primary purpose of an Institutional Review Board (IRB)?

14.4. Challenges in Drug Development

Learning Outcome

1. High Costs and Funding Issues
2. Time Constraints and Regulatory Hurdles
3. Patient Recruitment and Retention Difficulties

One of the major challenges in drug development is the timely recruitment and maintenance of trial participants. Success with these trials not only requires enrolling enough numbers in a timely fashion but also meeting a representative and satisfactory sample. When recruitment is slow, drug development timelines are extended, costs rise proportionally, and therapeutic benefits for patients are delayed. In addition, under-enrollment or biased sampling can undermine trial validity and generalizability, and may conceal the actual efficacy or safety profile of the investigational drug. This is a particularly serious challenge in diseases as complex as Alzheimer's, in which patient entry criteria are rigorous and recruitment bases are narrow. Meeting these challenges necessitates strategic trial design and patient participation strategies to achieve speed and accuracy in balance, thus maximizing the quality and relevance of trial outcomes (Grill et al., 2010). In addition to recruitment, globalisation in drug development presents special regulatory and ethical challenges when clinical trials are performed in low-income countries. As global research activity flows to these parts of the world, there is cost benefit along with exposure to diverse populations but also puts a squeeze on indigenous regulatory systems to maintain standards at international levels. In nations such as Mexico, increased clinical trial activity reveals cracks in governance and regulation, putting patient protection, informed consent, and ethical conduct into question. Moreover, technological and infrastructural limitations may result in uneven data quality, making it difficult for global acceptance of trial results. Such challenges highlight the balancing act between taking advantage of global assets and upholding demanding ethical and scientific standards throughout drug development (Santiago-Rodriguez, 2025.).

In addition, the complex nature of contemporary drug development includes overcoming complex scientific, logistical, and cost impediments. Drug candidates are often confronted by high rates of attrition resulting from unanticipated safety problems or lack of sufficient therapeutic impact, which creates cycles of testing and discovery repeatedly utilizing enormous resources. The diseases that have multifactorial causes are highly demanding of advanced biomarkers and endpoints that are inadequately present or underdevelopment. Regulatory paths of approval also continue to grow stronger, mandating heavy documentation and validation. Collectively, these drivers are responsible for delayed timelines and increasing expense, deterring innovation and restricting the velocity at which therapies arrive in the patient population. While bringing these challenges to heel requires constant interaction between researchers, regulators, and industry stakeholders, streamlining development while maintaining patient safety and efficacy is necessary (Figure 14.12).

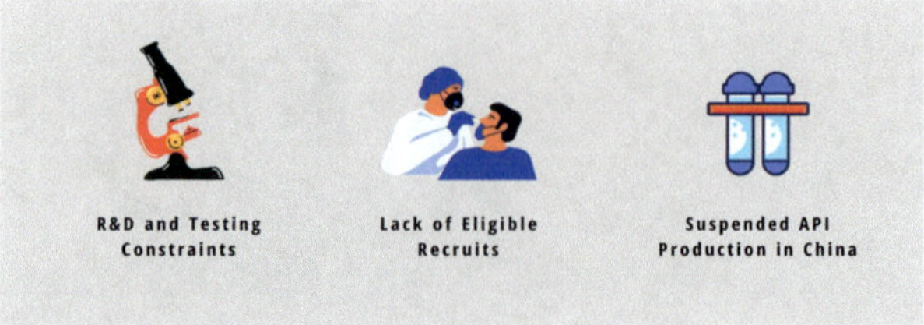

Figure 14.12. Challenges in drug development.

Source: Business Wire (2020). *Challenges in Drug Development.* https://mms.businesswire.com/media/20200904005279/en/818573/5/New_Drug_Development_PR.jpg.

14.4.1. High Costs and Funding Issues

The process of drug discovery to market authorization is usually beset by economic barriers that heavily influence the speed and extent of pharmaceutical innovation. Large amounts of money are needed at the different stages of drug development, such as preclinical research and large-scale clinical trials, to establish safety and efficacy. These stages are not only time-consuming but also expensive due to the necessity of specialized staff, sophisticated equipment, and regulatory requirements.

The cost is also increased by the high attrition rates, with numerous compounds failing during clinical trials, incurring sunk costs without marketable returns. As a result, the rising costs have rendered the drug development process only accessible to large pharmaceutical firms with strong funding, potentially excluding smaller organizations or academic institutions from playing a role in bringing novel therapies. This gatekeeping by finance highlights systemic impediments to innovation that cause delays and limit the diversity of research projects in therapeutics (Matthew et al., 2021). The problem of investment in drug development is further exacerbated by overdependence on complicated and uncertain sources of financial investment, such as venture capital, government funding, and private investment. While public funding is intended to encourage research in underdeveloped or high-risk fields, it frequently fails to cover the entire costs, particularly as trials move into later and more costly stages. Private investors, however, are inclined to focus on projects with well-defined commercial prospects, which can result in underfunding for the treatment of rare diseases or diseases that strike low-income groups. Additionally, the greater regulatory demands on clinical trials add further financial pressure, with greater protocols and data monitoring driving up operating costs. All of these combined create a funding climate both short in resources and mismatched to public health requirements, thus shaping the kinds of drugs that are given priority for development (Cara et al., 2019). Initiatives to meet the exorbitant expense and funding issue in drug development have involved innovative financing structures and policy changes with the aim of improving efficiency and minimizing financial risk. Adaptive trial designs and the utilization of biomarkers have been encouraged to facilitate streamlined clinical trials, which may reduce timelines and lower costs. Collaborative efforts by industry, government, and academia aim to consolidate resources and exchange information to reduce duplication and capitalize on pooled expertise. Furthermore, policy interventions like tax breaks, patent term extensions, and public-private partnerships are increasingly being used to promote investment and finance innovation. In spite of these measures, the underlying challenge of balancing financial sustainability with equitable access to new therapies is not resolved. Treating high expenditures and funding challenges involves ongoing conversation and planning in order to make drug development work in the interests of broad society without sacrificing scientific standards or patient safety (Cara Mack et al., 2019; Matthew et al., 2021).

14.4.2. Time Constraints and Regulatory Hurdles

The drug development process to market approval is notoriously long, taking more than a decade on many occasions owing to rigorous regulatory procedures and thorough clinical testing. Time pressures within drug development are compounded by ensuring thorough evaluation of safety and efficacy, which cannot be hurried without jeopardizing patient well-being (Figure 14.13). Regulatory bodies require several stages of clinical trials, sequentially larger and more complicated, involving extensive data gathering and analysis. The complexity is such that the trials must adhere to strict criteria to pick up adverse effects and establish therapeutic gains over available drugs. The net effect is a long production cycle that can result in a time lag before potentially life-saving medicines become accessible, highlighting a conflict between urgency and careful examination. Technologies like organ-on-a-chip platforms have the potential to simplify initial testing stages, potentially decreasing dependency on slower, less predictive animal models, and speeding up early-stage drug assessment (Donald, 2022). Overcoming regulatory challenges is a complex problem that significantly affects drug development timelines. Regulatory agencies require meticulous specifications for only safe and effective drugs to reach the marketplace, but processes tend to require intricate documentation, multiple submissions, and lengthy reviews that prolong project timelines. In addition, pending issues like antimicrobial resistance and the necessity of new antimicrobials necessitate the demand for new therapy, but regulatory routes for such essential drugs continue to be convoluted. The multidisciplinary character of antibiotic development, which incorporates synthetic biology and genomic research, places additional layers of regulatory oversight, frequently requiring subsequent cycles of validation to achieve standards changing over time (Uddin et al., 2021). Developers are therefore required to weigh innovation against compliance, a tension that regularly extends clinical pipeline development and adds substantial financial and temporal costs. Apart from the procedural strictness, regulatory challenges also affect the translation of laboratory results to clinical use. Promising preclinical models, including technological advances like human organ chips, meet regulatory skepticism as agencies demand substantial validation to embrace these novel methodologies as credible substitutes for conventional animal testing (Donald, 2022). This conservative stance, while imperative for patient safety, hinders the accelerated deployment of technologies that might shorten development times and lower costs. The increasing complexity of infectious diseases and AMR also forces drug developers to seek novel approaches under strict regulatory regimes intended to avoid unintended risks. Consequently, time pressures are added on top of the mechanics of phases of trial plus the need to harmonize new scientific discoveries with established standards, highlighting a perpetual conflict between regulatory caution and the need for faster therapeutic progress (Uddin et al., 2021).

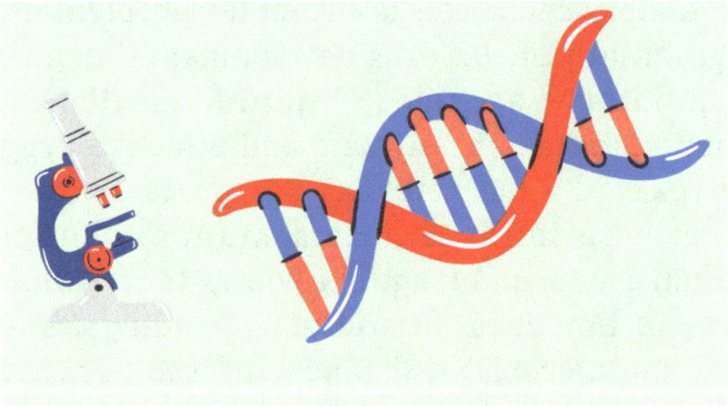

Figure 14.13. Regulatory hurdles.

Source: https://media.licdn.com/dms/image/v2/D4E12AQGiRdixDkQ_pg/article-cover_image-shrink_720_1280/article-cover_image-shrink_720_1280/0/1684492255234?e=2147483647&v=beta&t=0-PCOY4IAYBHdDreHV7jVwt4yfQ9eJG-c94tGXPQ7RY.

14.4.3. Patient Recruitment and Retention Difficulties

Successful conduct of clinical trials is crucial to effective drug development, and patient recruitment is a key element (Figure 14.14). Even with improvements in trial design and technology, enrolling an adequate and representative patient population is still a daunting challenge. This is due to several reasons, such as strict eligibility criteria, patient distrust, and practical issues like travel distance and time required. Ineffective recruitment delays trial times, increases expense, and potentially weakens the study's statistical power. Further, the variability of diseases, particularly in chronic illness such as inflammatory bowel disease, makes it challenging to identify and recruit appropriate candidates. New technologies, especially artificial intelligence, hold great promise to improve patient recruitment by processing complex data and identifying trial eligibility more precisely; however, these technologies need to overcome data integration and privacy issues to achieve maximum potential (Sedano et al., 2025). It is therefore necessary to address recruitment challenges to streamline drug development and provide equitable access to new therapies. Retention of study participants in clinical trials is another equally important, but commonly underestimated, hurdle to effective drug development. Patient dropout rates may be affected by side effects, lack of perceived benefit, or inconvenient trial protocols that interfere with daily life. Retention problems not only diminish sample size but also introduce bias, compromising the validity and generalizability of results. Clear communication and long-term engagement strategies are crucial to ensure participant motivation and retention. Clinical trial management experiences from healthcare facilities highlight the significance of stakeholder collaboration, patient-centric methodologies, and clear communications to battle retention challenges (Sappor et al., 2025). Retention is also closely linked to recruitment since early clarity regarding trial requirements might avoid premature withdrawal. In order to maximize retention, trials have to strike a balance between scientific intensity and patient ease, using digital means and customized interaction to build engagement over the course of the study. The dual challenges of recruitment and retention highlight the need for broad, flexible strategies suiting the varied needs of trial populations. The use of sophisticated predictive analytics can make it easier to identify promising participants most likely to sign up and stay through the trial, maximizing trial efficiency. Yet, these technological innovations need to be paired with ethical guidelines and inclusive trial designs to respond to imbalances in participant representation and trust. Organizational changes in healthcare environments, such as improved communication and collaborative participation among staff, patients, and regulators, are essential to surmount regulatory and operational challenges that hinder patient engagement (Sappor et al., 2025). Finally, the optimization of recruitment and retention procedures not only shortens the timelines of drug development but also leads to stronger, more stable clinical results that capture true real-world patient experiences, thus enhancing the overall effectiveness of new treatments (Sedano et al., 2025).

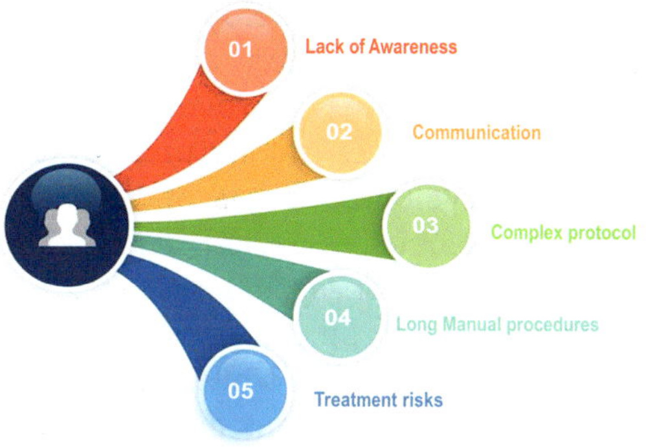

Figure 14.14. Patient recruitment and retention difficulties.

Source: https://www.cloudbyz.com/resources/wp-content/uploads/2018/11/Screenshot-2019-07-03-at-5.12.17-PM.png.

Test Your Knowledge

1. What role does regulatory approval play in drug development challenges?
2. Which of Patient Recruitment and Retention Difficulties

14.5. The Role of Technology in Drug Development

Learning Outcome

1. High Costs and Funding Issues
2. Time Constraints and Regulatory Hurdles
3. Patient Recruitment and Retention Difficulties

Technology advances have profoundly impacted the drug development landscape, especially by enabling more targeted and advanced therapeutic strategies. Generally, and as illustrated by historical orphan drug development in the realm of rare lysosomal storage diseases, individual technological platforms, like enzyme replacement therapies and substrate reduction methodologies, have transformed therapeutic opportunities for intricate multisystemic diseases. These advances not only enhance the drug's biological effectiveness but also overcome issues that come with orphan diseases, where the smaller populations and strict clinical endpoints make it difficult to conduct trials. The potential to personalize treatment by molecular and genetic characteristics highlights the critical role technology can play in facilitating regulatory approval and clinical success, particularly when combined with design of biomarkers and endpoints strategic to the distinct nature of the disease (Hoffmann et al., 2015). This technological convergence drives precision and achievability of clinical development programs, critical to the conversion of rare disease drug candidates into approved drugs. The infrastructure that underpins drug discovery and clinical development has also developed through the efforts of varied organizational models, such as the conventional pharmaceutical corporations and smaller, more nimble biotechnology companies. While the established pharmaceutical corporations have the size and resources to pursue high-risk, complicated clinical projects, the newer biotechnology companies make valuable contributions at the discovery phase, investigating new compounds with novel mechanisms of action. This complementary dynamic is made possible by technological innovations in molecular screening, data analytics, and collaborative research platforms, which improve productivity and minimize early-stage attrition. Furthermore, technology allows these entities to change their development strategies, with big firms retaining dominance in clinical trial execution because of their better capabilities and resource mobilization, whereas small firms excel in exploratory research through concentrated innovation (Arora et al., 2025). This synergy underscores the manner in which technology and institutional functions together further improve the efficiency and scale of drug development pipelines. Additionally, disease prevalence and regulatory precedence crucially affect the use and success of particular technological platforms in drug development. Technologies with the ability to use quantifiable biological markers or somatic endpoints, including enzyme replacement, can often offer smaller clinical trials with better-defined outcomes, therefore enhancing approval prospects. Conversely, neurological disorders, which frequently do not have quantifiable clinical endpoints, have experienced slower technological advancements and lesser treatment approvals. This contrast highlights the relationship between technological viability and trial design, illustrating that even innovative solutions have to deal with regulatory and methodological paradigms in order to become clinically relevant (Hoffmann et al., 2015). Eventually, the function of technology in drug development is not just invention but has a close relationship with disease nature, regulatory climate, and trial practices and hence goes on to determine the fate and success of novel therapeutic agents (Figure 14.15).

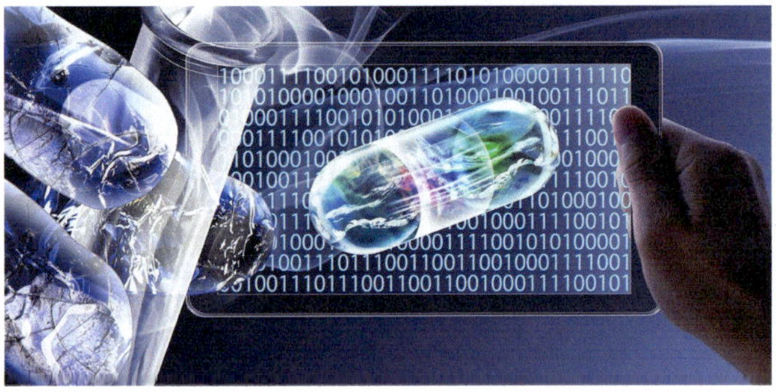

Figure 14.15. The role of technology in drug development.

Source: Lab Manager (2022). *Research Boosts 'Game-Changing' Technology to Strengthen Drug Development.* https://cdn.labmanager.com/assets/articleNo/28140/aImg/50919/research-boosts-game-changing-technology-to-strengthen-drug-development-l.jpg.

14.5.1. Advances in Biotechnology

Over the last several years, unprecedented speed has been accelerated in the incorporation of biotechnology into drug development pipelines, redefining conventional paradigms in therapeutic progress. Newer molecular technologies, including monoclonal antibody technology, have presented novel windows to address drug-resistant infections, which are an increasing worldwide health issue. Their use not only offers increased target specificity but also promises options for individualized treatment approaches that traditional small molecules cannot fulfill. Yet, even with encouraging laboratory and initial clinical trial data, challenges related to large-scale manufacturing, cost-effectiveness, and regulatory approval continue to hinder their broadened clinical use. The growing prominence of multidrug-resistant bacterial strains during the COVID-19 pandemic has amplified the need to discover new antibacterial agents, emphasizing the need for sustained biotechnological advances in drug development (Chen et al., 2024). Such developments are a turning point in transitioning conventional treatments to address current medical needs. Concurrent with advancements in antibacterial agents, RNA-based therapeutic agents have cropped up as a sophisticated class of drugs, especially in the treatment of cancer. The function of microRNAs (miRNAs) in gene regulation and disease pathogenesis has driven research into their therapeutic applications, particularly following recent successes with mRNA vaccines for infectious disease. These advances have renewed enthusiasm for RNA-based immunotherapies, with the use of advanced delivery and chemical modification approaches to improve efficacy and minimize toxicity. In spite of all these technological advancements, miRNA-based therapeutics are still essentially experimental, and repeated failures during clinical trials continue to highlight the necessity for precision targeting, optimum dosing, and immunogenicity control. Additionally, the lack of mature mechanistic understanding of miRNA action makes them difficult to translate into effective therapeutics. Yet, the redundancy and versatility embodied in RNA therapy hold the key to an increased role in drugs of the future, subject to overcoming existing constraints (Attila, 2024). Along with molecular innovation, refinements in biotechnological tools have optimized clinical trial approaches, thus facilitating the bench-to-bedside transition at a faster pace. Combining high-throughput screening with bioinformatics and artificial intelligence facilitates faster identification of candidate drugs and accurate stratification of patients. Integration here minimizes timelines and cost barriers conventionally linked with clinical trials, promoting regulatory involvement through enhanced robustness and reproducibility of data. In addition, biotechnological advancements enable the creation of new biomarkers for tracking treatment response and side effects in real time, improving trial designs and individualized therapies. Together, these advances highlight the synergistic partnership between biotechnology and clinical research, enabling a more responsive and adaptive drug development environment to address unmet medical needs with greater accuracy and effectiveness.

14.5.2. Use of Artificial Intelligence in Drug Discovery

In the last ten years, the growing cost and complexity of oncology drug development have highlighted the critical necessity for innovative approaches. Classical paradigms, weighed down by inefficiencies and constrained target populations because of personalized medicine, have increasingly become unsustainable on a worldwide level. This is where artificial intelligence has come in as a revolutionary instrument that will solve such challenges by optimizing the accuracy and speed of drug discovery processes. With the use of sophisticated machine learning methods, AI enables more efficient data organization in drug repurposing and target identification, allowing researchers to better cope with large and intricate biological data (Figure 14.16). Such integration not only streamlines the initial phases of drug development but also has the potential to enhance clinical trial designs, thus potentially overcoming time and cost hurdles in oncology therapeutics. The application of artificial intelligence in drug discovery is not limited to oncology, with impacts across various areas of pharmaceutical research. The major challenges including data heterogeneity, resource management, and necessary expertise have long affected AIs full potential in drug development. However, recent surveys show increased faith in the deployment of AI, with almost 60% of the respondents expecting enhanced staffing to complement these technologies. AI's capability to model complex biological systems and predict compound efficacy accelerates the identification of viable drug candidates, enhancing productivity and minimizing human error. Importantly, AI fosters interdisciplinary collaboration by bridging the gap between medicinal chemistry and computational sciences, streamlining the pathway from theoretical design to laboratory validation (Keerthana et al., 2022).

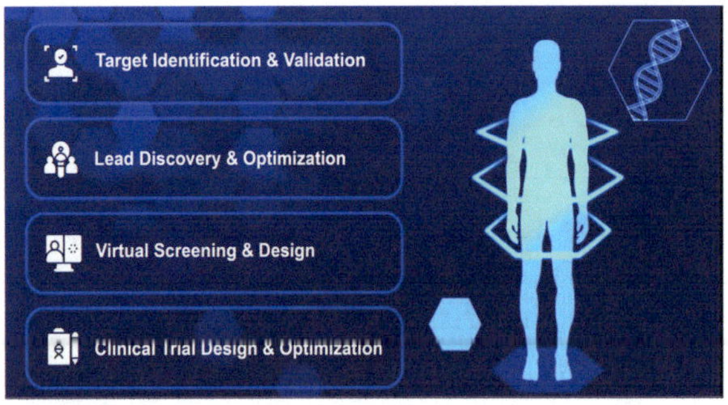

Figure 14.16. Use of artificial intelligence in drug discovery.

Source: Bacancy Technology. (2024). *Role of Artificial Intelligence in Drug Discovery. https://* assets.bacancytechnology.com/blog/wp-content/uploads/2024/05/01083614/Role-of-Artificial-Intelligence-in-Drug-Discovery.webp.

In spite of the promise, uptake of AI within drug discovery also continues to suffer from data quality, interpretability, and integratability in current workflows. Well-organized and well-curate datasets of high scope still underlie the predictive precision and reliability of AI. Further, as AI-informed approaches penetrate deeper into phases of clinical trials, algorithmic decision-making with regard to patients and ethics has become a subject of rising salience. Overcoming these challenges will need to be an integrated effort aimed at improving AI models and confirming transparency and trustworthiness all along the drug development process. As such, the strategic use of AI not only speeds up drug discovery but also is a part of the development of a more sustainable and patient-centric model in pharmaceutical innovation.

14.5.3. Impact of Data Analytics on Clinical Trials

Computational advances have transformed many areas in drug development, and clinical trials are no exception. Of these advances, data analytics stands out as a revolutionary technology that maximizes the capacity to handle and analyze large volumes of clinical data. Such an ability not only expedites the recruitment of patients by locating the correct subjects more quickly but also facilitates real-time tracking of trial performance. Therefore, data analytics have helped shorten timelines and costs related to clinical trials. Additionally, the use of predictive modeling helps in predicting patient responses and side effects, thus enabling more adaptive and personalized trial designs. These innovations overcome some of the traditional hurdles of clinical trial operations, ultimately leading to quicker, safer, and more tailored drug development pathways that harmonize well with changing regulatory expectations (Matthew et al., 2021). The application of advanced analytics also enhances the reliability and transparency of clinical trial results, which are essential for regulatory approval and clinical uptake. By using strict statistical techniques and machine learning models, scientists can reveal patterns and associations that may otherwise be hidden in intricate data sets. This level of analysis aids in more precise efficacy estimates and risk assessments, strengthening the scientific foundation for evidence-based decision-making. Data visualization tools also assist in communicating the results to stakeholders, enabling easier interpretation and cultivating confidence among healthcare providers, regulators, and patients. Such methodological strength guarantees adherence to increasingly sophisticated guidelines for systematic reviews and meta-analyses, essential for the reproducibility and generalizability of clinical trial outcomes (Matthew et al., 2021). Data analytics, in turn, bolster the underpinning for evidence-based clinical and therapeutic planning in drug development. With these advantages notwithstanding, application of data analytics in clinical trials has to be met with professional and ethical balance to guarantee patient safety and data integrity. Healthcare professionals and scientists are reminded by authoritative guidelines to use their clinical judgment in interpreting the outputs of analysis since analytical models cannot substitute for personalized decision-making. Additionally, compliance with regulatory guidelines regulating the use of data, privacy, and reporting standards is still of utmost importance to maintain validity and acceptability of trial results. The continuous interaction of statisticians, clinicians, and regulators is crucial to streamline analytical techniques, mitigate potential biases, and ensure conformance to local and global regulations. This sensitive alignment of data analysis with the proven clinical framework ensures that innovation supports but does not undermine the ethical and scientific foundations of drug development.

Test Your Knowledge

1. How does AI accelerate drug development?
2. How does data analytics enhance patient recruitment in clinical trials?

14.6. Post-Marketing Surveillance

Learning Outcome

1. Importance of Phase IV Trials
2. Monitoring Long-Term Effects and Safety
3. Reporting Adverse Events and Drug Recalls

Aside from the finalization of clinical trials, ongoing assessment of a drug's safety and efficacy is still very important to public health. Post-marketing surveillance (PMS) performs this important function by detecting adverse events and unintended effects that might not have yet appeared within controlled clinical environments. This stage usually identifies complex and unusual adverse events related to actual practice, including a wide variety of patient populations and co-morbidities. For instance, the launch of sodium-glucose co-transporter-2 (SGLT2) inhibitors in the treatment of diabetes brought to the forefront the role of PMS when new side effects like ketoacidosis and dehydration were seen after launch. The aggregation of such information prompted the establishment of specialized committees and revised clinical guidelines to ensure safer use, highlighting PMS's dynamic role in responding to regulatory guidelines based on new evidence. This phase thus transitions clinical trial end points with the long-term concern for patient safety in routine clinical practice. Elaborate adverse event tracking and analysis in PMS demand exacting methodologies often combining both *in silico* prediction tools and clinical observations. Molecular docking, a structure-based computational method, has matured beyond its early function in early drug discovery to play a role in predicting possible adverse effects and off-target interactions following a drug's market launch. Through the simulation of drug candidate interactions with various biological targets, molecular docking can detect unexpected binding affinities that are associated with unwanted side effects. This growing use enhances the ability of post-marketing surveillance systems to actively signal risks before they become prevalent clinical issues, adding to conventional pharmacovigilance. The merging of *in silico* predictions with clinical safety information is a new promising area for optimizing risk evaluation and therapeutic outcomes (Pinzi et al., 2019). As such, the integration of empirical and in silico methodology reinforces the overall strength of the post-marketing phase. Additionally, post-marketing surveillance entails active cooperation between regulatory agencies, pharmaceutical industries, healthcare professionals, and patients. Open data collection and prompt release of results facilitate informed risk management options, including dose modification or contraindication in certain groups. SGLT2 inhibitors are a prime example, wherein PMS data guided dose reduction recommendations when used with insulin secretagogues and warnings for older adults or comorbid patients. Such monitoring also raised the alarm among clinicians to dangers such as severe skin reactions and urinary tract infections, which induced revised patient education and monitoring practices. These practices illustrate how ongoing monitoring manifests into tangible clinical recommendations that ensure patient safety long after a drug has been approved. Finally, PMS is an integral part of drug development, ensuring therapeutic benefits remain greater than risks over the life span of a drug.

14.6.1. Importance of Phase IV Trials

Post-marketing surveillance is a critical augmentation of the clinical trial process to ensure ongoing monitoring of a drug's safety and efficacy post-regulatory approval. Early trials, such as Phases I to III, largely determine a drug's safety profile, optimal dosage, and initial efficacy in highly controlled settings. Such studies typically entail small population sizes and short study periods and might not be able to capture infrequent or delayed adverse effects. Phase IV trials overcome this drawback by tracking the drugs performance under real-world conditions in various patient populations. Longer observation is necessary to identify unusual electrolyte derangements or other side effects that were overlooked initially, as evidenced by findings demonstrating the prognostic role of severe electrolyte disturbances in clinical trial enrollees (Ameratunga et al., 2018). As a result, Phase IV trials are critical to further defining our knowledge of drug safety and patient welfare. Clinical assessment techniques can significantly influence the apparent efficacy of treatments in post-marketing investigations. In contrast to previous trial phases, which tend to employ structured and controlled evaluation protocols, Phase IV trials can employ more flexible or creative techniques to measure real-world therapeutic effects. For example, more recent studies into facial erythema treatments illustrated how the addition of baseline comparison via standardized images increased the accuracy of efficacy determination, minimizing distortions like hyperbole in the placebo effect (Alvandi et al., 2019). Such a methodological step-up in Phase IV trials corroborates not just the results from previous phases but also enhances data reliability, which allows clinicians and regulators to base informed decisions about the continued prescription of a drug. This critical assessment guarantees that therapies are effective outside the controlled environment and conform to the realities of routine clinical practice. Other than safety and efficacy, Phase IV trials further contribute significantly to the fine-tuning of therapeutic practice by way of long-term follow-up and subgroup comparisons. Data generated under this phase can identify differences in drug response due to patient demographics, comorbidities, or concomitant medications, which were underrepresented or excluded from the pre-approval studies. Further, continuous monitoring identifies delayed adverse reactions or interactions that only become evident with prolonged usage. Such information informs clinicians in the customization of treatments to a patient's individual needs, finally improving clinical outcomes. Furthermore, Phase IV information can result in revised prescribing details, dosage, or even drug withdrawal if critical risks are realized. Therefore, Phase IV trials are absolutely crucial to the ongoing development of drug therapy, creating an active feedback cycle among research, regulators, and clinical practice.

14.6.2. Monitoring Long-Term Effects and Safety

The drug development process goes well beyond early efficacy trials, as the long-term consequences and safety profiles of new drugs must be continually and critically assessed (Figure 14.17). Monitoring is important because early clinical trials are typically short in duration and involve controlled populations that do not necessarily represent diversity in the general population. Post-marketing surveillance is then a critical mechanism to identify adverse events once a drug has been approved that could only be seen after long-term exposure or among subpopulations that have comorbidities. All of these long-term data are collected through registries, observational studies, and pharmacovigilance systems, which collectively give a complete picture of safety. Patient safety over the long term is especially crucial in chronic diseases, where prolonged therapy is typical and unplanned toxicities have a substantial effect on patient quality of life and public health outcomes as a whole (Mary et al., 2023). Moreover, managing long-term effects includes not just the physical safety but also the wider effects such as efficacy durability and unintended interactions. In multicomponent diseases such as advanced breast cancer, in which treatment regimens are changing and usually consist of combinations of treatments, the interplay between efficacy and cumulative toxicity requires careful longitudinal studies. Such studies need to include endpoints other than survival, like quality of life and control of treatment-related side effects, in order to obtain a comprehensive impression of drug action over time. The adaptive clinical trial design and integration of real-world evidence can facilitate the identification of late-emerging safety signals and improvement in treatment approaches accordingly.

The inclusion of PROs enhances the interpretation of long-term safety further, highlighting the significance of patient-centric therapy in drug development (Fátima et al., 2018). Regulatory bodies across the globe also require stringent post-approval safety assessments for the ongoing safeguarding of public health. These assessments demand cooperation between stakeholders, such as clinicians, researchers, pharmaceutical industries, and patients, to report and examine adverse effects in a systematic manner. Technological advances, like electronic health records and big data analytics, are being used more and more to improve monitoring capacity, enabling quicker identification of potential risks. Nevertheless, there are challenges, such as underreporting, heterogeneity of data quality, and difficulty in attributing causality to the drug vs. confounding variables. Therefore, strong regulatory frameworks and open lines of communication are essential to providing valid and actionable risk-benefit evaluations on an ongoing basis. Extended safety monitoring eventually leads to confidence in therapeutic innovations and aids informed clinical decision-making (Fátima et al., 2018; Mary et al., 2023).

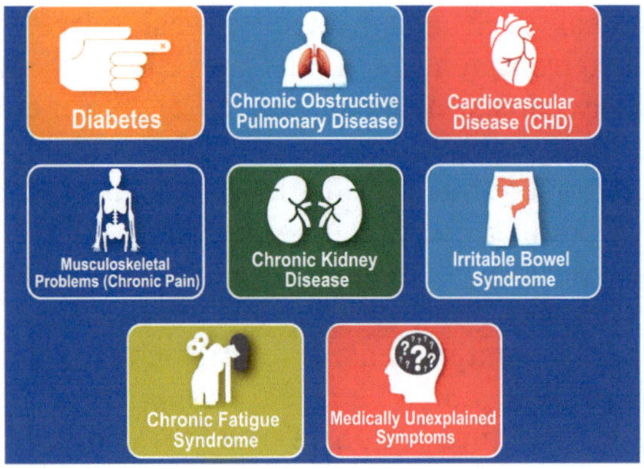

Figure 14.17. Monitoring long-term effects and safety.

Source: https://livingwellconsortium.com/wp-content/uploads/2019/12/lt-info2.png.

14.6.3. Reporting Adverse Events and Drug Recalls

The sophistication of drug development requires a continued commitment to safety monitoring far beyond the early clinical trials. Post-marketing surveillance is important in detecting adverse events that were not otherwise fully apparent in pre-approval periods because of small sample sizes or trial lengths. All stakeholders including healthcare providers, manufacturers, and regulatory agencies need to have in place strong mechanisms for timely reporting and data sharing on any adverse reactions. Transparent reporting systems promote the prompt identification of safety signals so that timely interventions like drug recalls or labeling changes can reduce patient risk. Systematic documentation and reporting of such events promote trust and maintain ethical standards in pharmaceutical science, ensuring that medications' benefits continue to exceed their risks in larger patient populations. Successful management of drug recalls relies on the integrity and completeness of adverse event reporting. Well-designed recall programs benefit not only consumers but also public trust in the healthcare system and the pharmaceutical sector. Technologies like electronic databases, such as large-scale drug information repositories, offer significant real-time knowledge about a drug's safety profile by collating molecular data, interaction risks, and trial records. These assets, such as sites listing drug-related facts on molecular processes and trial statuses, are essential building blocks for detecting patterns that need recalls or closer examination. Having access to comprehensive drug information empowers regulatory decision-making and informs ongoing refinements throughout the life cycle of drugs. Toward making adverse event reports more reliable and useful, there must be clear instructions and standardized reporting schemes. The function of systematic frameworks guarantees that information gathered from various sources is able to be synthesized and analyzed in a proper manner to give actionable insights. This process follows the same principles used in systematic reviews in clinical research, whereby clear, full, and accurately reported results are necessary for the production of credible evidence (Matthew et al., 2021). Adopting similar rigor in pharmacovigilance promotes consistency and comparability across reports, facilitating quicker recognition of safety concerns and enhancing patient protection. By integrating evolving drug data repositories with structured reporting protocols, the field of drug development can better anticipate risks and respond with informed, evidence-based recall practices (David et al., 2017).

Test Your Knowledge

1. Why is Post-marketing surveillance (PMS) important for public health?
2. What is an adverse event in the context of drug use?

SUMMARY

The intricacies involved in drug development and clinical trials require new approaches to bypass conventional inefficiencies. New developments, including seamless clinical trial designs and master protocols, have been instrumental in speeding up the assessment of therapeutic agents. By enabling phase transitions without disruption and the exploration of multiple treatments within a single paradigm, these approaches save time and money. Especially in oncology, where progress is hindered by extremely high attrition, such strategies offset regulatory hurdles and allow for earlier access to life-saving therapies by patients. The flexibility of these designs then promotes an even more dynamic drug development landscape that ensures promising compounds can move through the pipeline with enhanced efficiency and diminished redundancy (Baird et al., 2024). This transformation represents a pivotal milestone in meeting the urgent demand for timely innovations in clinical practice. Furthermore, the strategic creation of combination therapies is further evidence of advances in optimizing clinical trial design. With an awareness that most diseases, particularly pediatric malignancies, need to be treated with multi-agent regimens to avoid resistance and increase efficacy, investigators now focus on strict preclinical testing and mechanistically guided combinations. Early-stage trials are more often framed to validate dosing and schedules instead of discovering them from first principles, accelerating the trajectory to approval. Including randomized comparisons between new agents and usual treatments provides greater insight into therapeutic benefits and risks. Stakeholder collaboration across regulators, investigators, and patient advocates is necessary to align expectations and advance drug development outcomes in highly vulnerable populations like children and adolescents (Bird et al., 2023). Such integrated efforts are exemplary examples of how sophisticated trial designs allow for effective translation of scientific knowledge into clinical progress. Finally, the future of drug development is contingent upon unified, adaptable clinical trial frameworks with focus on benefit to the patient and scientific integrity. The confluence of seamless trials, master protocols, and carefully constructed combination studies is a paradigm shift from the conventional, isolated model. This paradigm not only speeds the provision of novel therapies but also maximizes resource utilization and regulatory interaction. Having early and frequent communication with regulatory agencies and enrolling broader populations of patients maximizes the generalizability and utility of trial results. These innovations envision a more responsible and effective process of development in the end to create better therapy options and therapeutic outcomes for the patient in case of different diseases. Adopting these revolutionary steps is still of paramount importance for overcoming the complexities involved in present-day drug development (Baird et al., 2024; Bird et al., 2023).

Summary of Key Points

Within the sophisticated drug development environment, clinical trials are a crucial component for the confirmation of new drug safety and efficacy. Extensive data collection and validation methods ensure the accuracy of data, as illustrated in the reanalysis of the RECORD trial using rigorous event reascertainment and readjudication to respond to concerns raised by regulators. This activity emphasized the value of rigorous follow-up processes and application of both automated and manual approaches for identifying possible adverse events, including cardiovascular endpoints. Such stringent methodologies are essential in retaining scientific integrity and offering regulatory bodies with strong evidence required for sound decision-making, improving the accountability of clinical trials conducted under a variety of worldwide conditions (Bigelow et al., 2013). This paradigm highlights the critical balance between methodological excellence and regulatory compliance in drug development. PROs (PROs) have become an important area in clinical trials, providing richness to the assessment of therapeutic effect from the patient's viewpoint. Regulatory filings to the European Medicines Agency from 2008–2012 demonstrate that laboratory-reported results continue to be the most frequently used endpoints; however, PROs are significantly represented as primary or secondary endpoints in close to half of the products under review. The presence of PROs is particularly evident in nervous system and cancer treatment, mirroring a growing focus on patient experiences and quality of life metrics. Although they are valuable, trends in PROs usage have been surprisingly stable, suggesting increased integration and transparency in the report to better guide stakeholders and facilitate holistic benefit-risk assessments (Bansal et al., 2015). Integrating these findings, then, it is apparent that drug development and clinical trials rely on a multi-dimensional evidence base involving the use of rigorous event verification and heterogeneity in the endpoint evaluation. The use of robust adjudication designs, as evident in milestone trials, enhances credibility of data and reduces biases embedded in open-label studies. In parallel, greater use of PROs augments conventional clinical measurements by offering in-depth information regarding treatment effects under real-world scenarios. Transparent reporting of all outcome types is important for regulatory authorities and industry partners to ensure credibility and ease regulatory approvals. In combination, these components provide the foundation of a successful drug development paradigm that focuses on patient safety, scientific precision, and significant therapeutic progress (Bansal et al., 2015; Bigelow et al., 2013).

KEY TERMS FROM THIS CHAPTER

- Biotechnology
- Drug Development
- Clinical assessment
- Good Manufacturing Practice (GMP)
- Patient safety
- Standard Treatments
- Personal health
- Public health
- Methodologies
- Patient-reported outcomes (PROs)
- Human testing
- Antimicrobial resistance (AMR)
- Safety and Dosage
- Immunomodulatory
- Clinical Trials
- Institutional Review Boards (IRBs)
- Clinical trial
- Artificial Intelligence

CRITICAL THINKING QUESTIONS

1. **What is the primary objective of Phase I clinical trials?**
   a. To test the efficacy of the drug
   b. To identify long-term side effects
   c. To evaluate safety and dosage in healthy volunteers
   d. To compare the new drug with existing treatments
2. **Which regulatory body approves new drugs in the United States?**
   a. WHO
   b. EMA
   c. FDA
   d. CDC
3. **What does "double-blind" mean in clinical trials?**
   a. Neither the researcher nor the participant knows which group they're in
   b. Only the researcher knows the treatment group
   c. Only the participant knows the treatment group
   d. The trial has two treatment groups
4. **What is the purpose of a placebo in a clinical trial?**
   a. To replace the active drug
   b. To improve drug absorption
   c. To serve as a control for comparison
   d. To cause adverse effects
5. **During which phase of clinical trials is the drug tested on a large number of patients (usually 300–3,000)?**
   a. Phase I
   b. Phase II
   c. Phase III
   d. Phase IV

Short Answer Questions

1. What is the difference between preclinical and clinical drug development?
2. What are the main types of clinical trials used in medical research?
3. What is the role of an Institutional Review Board (IRB) or Ethical Considerations in Clinical Trials?
4. What are the major scientific challenges encountered during the early stages of drug Development?
5. What is The Role of Technology in Drug Development?
6. What is post-marketing surveillance, and why is the drug development process?

Answer to Critical Thinking Questions

1. (c) 2 (c) 3. (a) 4. (c) 5. (c)

REFERENCES

1. AI4Cancer Research Group. (2025). *Artificial Intelligence in Oncology Drug Discovery and Development.* https://core.ac.uk/download/362225656.pdf (accessed on 9 May 2025).
2. Alvandi, N., Baldwin, H. E., Del Rosso, J. Q., Eichenfield, L. F., et al. (2019). Use of an alternative method to evaluate erythema severity in a clinical trial: Difference in vehicle response with evaluation of baseline and post dose photographs for effect of oxymetazoline cream 1.0% for persistent erythema of rosacea in a phase IV study. https://core.ac.uk/download/323310735.pdf.
3. Ameratunga, M., Ang, J. E., Banerji, U., Chénard-Poirier, M., et al. (2018). A study of 1088 consecutive cases of electrolyte abnormalities in oncology phase I trials. https://core.ac.uk/download/237406398.pdf.
4. Andress, A., Bettencourt-Silva, J., Blankenberg, D., Bose, R., et al. (2024). Towards quantum computing for clinical trial design and optimization: A perspective on new opportunities and challenges. *Trends in Pharmacological Sciences, 45*, 880–891. https://arxiv.org/abs/2404.13113 (accessed on 9 May 2025).
5. Arora, A., Gambardella, A., Pammolli, F., Riccaboni, M., et al. (2025). The nature and the extent of the market for technology in biopharmaceuticals. https://core.ac.uk/download/pdf/6381764.pdf (accessed on 9 May 2025).
6. Baird, R., Burdon, A., Chen, X., Jaki, T., et al. (2024). Next generation clinical trials: Seamless designs and master protocols. *Preprint.* https://arxiv.org/abs/2405.06353 (accessed on 9 May 2025).
7. Bansal, D., Bhagat, A., Cudala, K., & Schifano, F., et al. (2015). Role of patient-reported outcomes and other efficacy endpoints in the drug approval process in Europe (2008–2012). https://core.ac.uk/download/287582647.pdf (accessed on 9 May 2025).
8. Bigelow, R., Burns, S., Dickerson, S., Hafley, G., et al. (2013). Methodology of a reevaluation of cardiovascular outcomes in the RECORD trial: Study design and conduct. https://core.ac.uk/download/42359786.pdf (accessed on 9 May 2025).
9. Bird, N., Buenger, V., DuBois, S., Glade Bender, J., et al. (2023). Combination early-phase trials of anticancer agents in children and adolescents. https://core.ac.uk/download/581115289.pdf (accessed on 9 May 2025).
10. Bozkurt, B., Hussain, A., & Misra, A. (2022). Endpoints in heart failure drug development. https://core.ac.uk/download/643778626.pdf (accessed on 9 May 2025).
11. Bretz, F., & Dette, H. (2025). Optimal designs for dose finding studies. https://core.ac.uk/download/pdf/6785966.pdf (accessed on 9 May 2025).
12. Cardoso, F., Senkus, E., Costa, A., Papadopoulos, E., Aapro, M., André, F., Harbeck, N., et al. (2018). 4th ESO–ESMO International Consensus Guidelines for Advanced Breast Cancer (ABC 4). *Annals of Oncology, 29*, 1634–1657. https://doi.org/10.1093/annonc/mdy192.
13. Chen, H. C., Pan, Y. L., Chen, Y., Yang, T. H., Hsu, E. T., Huang, Y., & Chiang, M. H. (2024). Monoclonal antibodies as a therapeutic strategy against multidrug-resistant bacterial infections in a post-COVID-19 era. *Life, 14*(2), 246. https://doi.org/10.3390/life14020246.

14. Deore, A. B., Dhumane, J. R., Wagh, R., & Sonawane, R. (2019). The stages of drug discovery and development process. *Asian Journal of Pharmaceutical Research and Development, 7*(6), 62–67. https://doi.org/10.22270/ajprd.v7i6.616.

15. Diener, C., Keller, A., & Meese, E. (2022). Emerging concepts of miRNA therapeutics: From cells to clinic. *Trends in Genetics, 38*(7), 613–626. https://doi.org/10.1016/j.tig.2022.02.006.

16. Fenech, A. G., & Grech, G. (2009). *Biotech Drugs: Biological Therapeutic Agents.* https://core.ac.uk/download/46603869.pdf.

17. Finn, R. S., Qin, S., Ikeda, M., Galle, P. R., Ducreux, M., Kim, T. Y., Kudo, M., et al. (2020). Atezolizumab plus bevacizumab in unresectable hepatocellular carcinoma. *New England Journal of Medicine, 382*(20), 1894–1905. https://doi.org/10.1056/NEJMoa1915745.

18. Gabbert, H., Geddert, H., Haas, R., et al. (2008). *Ex Vivo Metrics™, a Preclinical Tool in New Drug Development.* https://core.ac.uk/download/pdf/7942754.pdf.

19. Gasparini, M., Robert, V., & Saint-Hilary, G. (2018). *Decision-Making in Drug Development Using a Composite Definition of Success.* https://core.ac.uk/download/234923872.pdf (accessed on 9 May 2025).

20. Górski, A., Międzybrodzki, R., Węgrzyn, G., Jończyk-Matysiak, E., Borysowski, J., & Weber-Dąbrowska, B. (2019). Phage therapy: Current status and perspectives. *Medicinal Research Reviews, 40*(1), 459–463. https://doi.org/10.1002/med.21593.

21. Grill, J. D., & Karlawish, J. (2010). *Addressing the Challenges to Successful Recruitment and Retention in Alzheimer's Disease Clinical Trials.* https://core.ac.uk/download/pdf/8521880.pdf.

22. Guzik, T. J., Mohiddin, S., Dimarco, A., Patel, V., Savvatis, K., Marelli-Berg, F. M., Madhur, M. S., et al. (2020). COVID-19 and the cardiovascular system: Implications for risk assessment, diagnosis, and treatment options. *Cardiovascular Research, 116*(10), 1666–1687. https://doi.org/10.1093/cvr/cvaa106.

23. Hoffmann, G. F., Mechler, K., Mountford, W. K., Ries, M., et al. (2015). *Pressure for Drug Development in Lysosomal Storage Disorders–A Quantitative Analysis Thirty Years Beyond the US Orphan Drug Act.* https://core.ac.uk/download/32585968.pdf (accessed on 9 May 2025).

24. Hu, B., Guo, H., Zhou, P., & Shi, Z. L. (2020). Characteristics of SARS-CoV-2 and COVID-19. *Nature Reviews Microbiology, 19*(3), 141–154. https://doi.org/10.1038/s41579-020-00459-7.

25. Huzair, F., & Kale, D. (2011). *Emergence of the Biosimilar Sector and Opportunities of Developing Country Suppliers.* https://core.ac.uk/download/109590.pdf.

26. Inan, O. T., Tenaerts, P., Prindiville, S. A., Reynolds, H. R., Dizon, D. S., Cooper-Arnold, K., Turakhia, M. P., et al. (2020). Digitizing clinical trials. *npj Digital Medicine, 3,* Article 101. https://doi.org/10.1038/s41746-020-0302-y.

27. Ingber, D. E. (2022). Human organs-on-chips for disease modelling, drug development and personalized medicine. *Nature Reviews Genetics, 23,* 467–491. https://doi.org/10.1038/s41576-022-00466-9.

28. Keerthana, V., Kumar, M. S., Mohaideen, S. S., Vigneshwaran, V., et al. (2022). *Role of Artificial Intelligence in Drug Development.* https://core.ac.uk/download/524981029.pdf (accessed on 9 May 2025).

29. Kohli, S. (2018). *Integrated Approach to Nature as Source of New Drug Lead.* https://core.ac.uk/download/322437176.pdf (accessed on 9 May 2025).

30. Krech, R., & Kiény, M. P. (2014). The 2014 Ebola outbreak: Ethical use of unregistered interventions. *Bulletin of the World Health Organization, 92*(9), 622. https://doi.org/10.2471/BLT.14.145789.

31. Mach, F., Baigent, C., Catapano, A. L., Koskinas, K. C., Casula, M., Badimón, L., Chapman, M. J., et al. (2019). 2019 ESC/EAS Guidelines for the management of dyslipidaemias: Lipid modification to reduce cardiovascular risk. *European Heart Journal, 41*, 111–188. https://doi.org/10.1093/eurheartj/ehz455.

32. Mack, C. L., Adams, D. H., Assis, D. N., Kerkar, N., Manns, M. P., Mayo, M. J., Ling, S. C., et al. (2019). Diagnosis and management of autoimmune hepatitis in adults and children: 2019 practice guidance and guidelines from the American Association for the Study of Liver Diseases. *Hepatology, 72*(2), 671–722. https://doi.org/10.1002/hep.31065.

33. Marashi, S. A. (2005). *The Necessity of Extraction of Ligand Binding Data from Literature*. https://core.ac.uk/download/46908448.pdf (accessed on 9 May 2025).

34. Milanetti, E., Raimondo, D., & Tramontano, A. (2015). Prediction of the permeability of neutral drugs inferred from their solvation properties. https://core.ac.uk/download/54529803.pdf (accessed on 9 May 2025).

35. Page, M. J., Moher, D., Bossuyt, P. M., Boutron, I., Hoffmann, T., Mulrow, C. D., Shamseer, L., et al. (2021). PRISMA 2020 explanation and elaboration: Updated guidance and exemplars for reporting systematic reviews. *BMJ, 372*, n160. https://doi.org/10.1136/bmj.n160.

36. Pinzi, L., & Rastelli, G. (2019). Molecular docking: Shifting paradigms in drug discovery. *International Journal of Molecular Sciences, 20*, 4331. https://doi.org/10.3390/ijms20184331.

37. Rinella, M. E., Neuschwander-Tetri, B. A., Siddiqui, M. S., Abdelmalek, M. F., Caldwell, S. H., Barb, D., Kleiner, D. E., et al. (2023). AASLD practice guidance on the clinical assessment and management of nonalcoholic fatty liver disease. *Hepatology, 77*, 1797–1835. https://doi.org/10.1097/hep.0000000000000323.

38. Rogler, G. (2019). Efficacy of JAK inhibitors in Crohn's Disease. *Journal of Crohn's and Colitis, 14*(S1), S746–S754. https://doi.org/10.1093/ecco-jcc/jjz186.

39. Roy, S., Meena, T., & Lim, S. J. (2022). Demystifying supervised learning in healthcare 4.0: A new reality of transforming diagnostic medicine. *Diagnostics, 12*(10), 2549. https://doi.org/10.3390/diagnostics12102549.

40. Santiago-Rodriguez, F. (2025). *Facing the Trial of Internationalizing Clinical Trials to Developing Countries: Some Evidence from Mexico*. https://core.ac.uk/download/pdf/6941422.pdf (accessed on 9 May 2025).

41. Sappor, E. E., & Chakraborty, R. (2025). Exploring staff perceptions of the management of clinical trials and its impact on enhancing health service delivery. *Hospitals*. https://www.semanticscholar.org/paper/ba1b2e4b9c0cac8a740bdae4a7c265d6b92343fa (accessed on 9 May 2025).

42. Sedano, R., Solitano, V., Vuyyuru, S., Yuan, Y., Hanzel, J., Ma, C., Nardone, O., et al. (2025). Artificial intelligence to revolutionize IBD clinical trials: A comprehensive review. *Therapeutic Advances in Gastroenterology, 18*, 175628482412513. https://www.semanticscholar.org/paper/fad70cd30a9614b0de195680cfa8c78b03e65c79 (accessed on 9 May 2025).

43. Sessa, C., Cortés, J., Conté, P., Cardoso, F., Choueiri, T. K., Dummer, R., LoRusso, P., et al. (2021). The impact of COVID-19 on cancer care and oncology clinical research: An experts' perspective. *ESMO Open*, *7*, 100339. https://doi.org/10.1016/j.esmoop.2021.100339.

44. Seyhan, A. A. (2024). Trials and tribulations of microRNA therapeutics. *International Journal of Molecular Sciences*, *25*(3), 1469. https://doi.org/10.3390/ijms25031469.

45. Singh, S., Kumar, R., Payra, S., & Singh, S. K. (2023). Artificial intelligence and machine learning in pharmacological research: Bridging the gap between data and drug discovery. *Cureus, 15*(10), e44359. https://doi.org/10.7759/cureus.44359.

46. Srivastava, A., Santagostino, E., Dougall, A., Kitchen, S., Sutherland, M. L., Pipe, S. W., Carção, M., et al. (2020). *WFH Guidelines for The Management of Hemophilia* (3rd ed., *26*, pp. 1–158). *Haemophilia*. https://doi.org/10.1111/hae.14046.

47. Strope, J. D., Chau, C. H., & Figg, W. D. (2020). TMPRSS2: Potential biomarker for COVID-19 outcomes. *The Journal of Clinical Pharmacology, 60*(6), 801–807. https://doi.org/10.1002/jcph.1641.

48. Tay, M. Z., Poh, C. M., Rénia, L., MacAry, P. A., & Ng, L. F. P. (2020). The trinity of COVID-19: Immunity, inflammation and intervention. *Nature Reviews Immunology, 20*, 363–374. https://doi.org/10.1038/s41577-020-0311-8.

49. The Committee on the Proper Use of SGLT2 Inhibitors. (2019). Recommendations on the proper use of SGLT2 inhibitors. *Journal of Diabetes Investigation, 11*(2), 257–261. https://doi.org/10.1111/jdi.13160.

50. Uddin, T. M., Chakraborty, A., Khusro, A., Zidan, B. M. R. M., Mitra, S., Emran, T. B., Dhama, K., et al. (2021). Antibiotic resistance in microbes: History, mechanisms, therapeutic strategies and future prospects. *Journal of Infection and Public Health, 14*(12), 1750–1766. https://doi.org/10.1016/j.jiph.2021.10.020.

51. Visseren, F. L. J., Mach, F., Smulders, Y. M., Carballo, D., Koskinas, K. C., Bäck, M., Bénétos, A., et al. (2021). 2021 ESC Guidelines on cardiovascular disease prevention in clinical practice. *European Heart Journal, 42*, 3227–3337. https://doi.org/10.1093/eurheartj/ehab484.

52. Volkow, N. D. (2020). Collision of the COVID-19 and addiction epidemics. *Annals of Internal Medicine, 173*(1), 61–62. https://doi.org/10.7326/M20-1212.

53. Williams, B., Mancia, G., Spiering, W., Rosei, E. A., Azizi, M., Burnier, M., Clement, D. L., et al. (2018). 2018 ESC/ESH Guidelines for the management of arterial hypertension. *European Heart Journal*, *39*(33), 3021–3104. https://doi.org/10.1093/eurheartj/ehy339.

54. Wishart, D. S., Djoumbou-Feunang, Y., Guo, A. C., Lo, E., Marcu, A., Grant, J. R., Sajed, T., et al. (2017). DrugBank 5.0: A major update to the DrugBank database for 2018. *Nucleic Acids Research*, *46*(D1), D1074–D1082. https://doi.org/10.1093/nar/gkx1037.

55. Wolchok, J. D., Chiarion-Sileni, V., González, R., Rutkowski, P., Grob, J. J., Cowey, C. L., Lao, C. D., et al. (2017). Overall survival with combined nivolumab and ipilimumab in advanced melanoma. *New England Journal of Medicine, 377*, 1345–1356. https://doi.org/10.1056/nejmoa1709684.

PHARMACOLOGY IN SPECIAL POPULATIONS

15

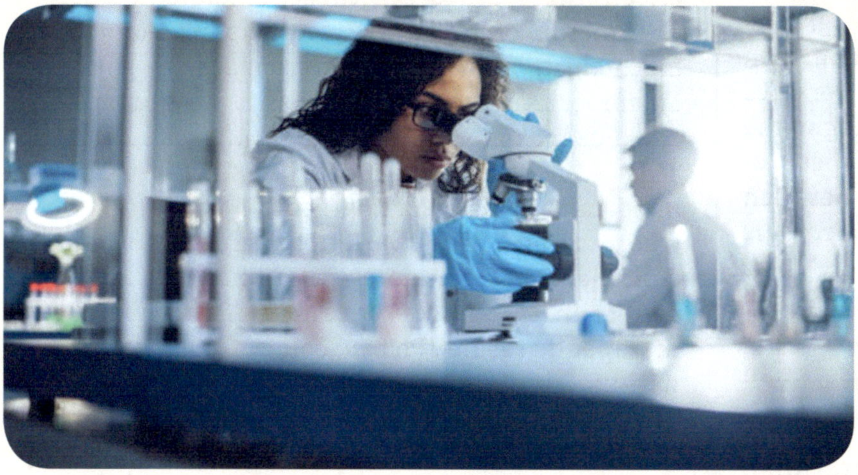

LEARNING OBJECTIVES

After studying this chapter, you will be able to:

1. Understand pediatric pharmacology
2. Define geriatric pharmacology
3. Explain the pharmacology in pregnant women
4. Describe the pharmacology in patients with renal impairment
5. Discuss the pharmacology in patients with hepatic impairment
6. Identify the pharmacogenomics and personalized medicine

Introduction

The sophistication of pharmacology goes beyond routine therapeutic regimens in special populations like pediatrics, geriatrics, and pregnant women. These populations present with resultant individualized physiological and biochemical characteristics that complicate the absorption, distribution, metabolism, and excretion (ADME) of drugs and impact efficacy and safety. With drug development encountering increasing efficiency and cost-effectiveness challenges, incorporating specialized pharmacologic insights within these groups is essential to maximize clinical outcomes. Meeting these complexities needs a multidimensional approach that combines clinical experience with current technological advances in pharmacokinetics and pharmacodynamics. The need is highlighted by the pharmaceutical research crisis, which calls for innovative approaches like modeling and simulation to step up understanding and prediction of drug behaviors across different populations (Hunt et al., 2013). Finally, a specific pharmacological paradigm for special populations is necessary to counteract risk and enhance therapeutic success. Insight into the myriad factors that modulate drug response in special populations is a starting point for designing more effective and tailored medical therapy. Physiological changes like altered enzyme activity, declining organ function, or hormonal alterations can have a significant impact on drug action and tolerability. Such variations require precise dose adjustment and monitoring measures to prevent harmful effects. Additionally, the moral and pragmatic problems embedded in clinical research among vulnerable groups complicate drug data collection even further. Educational curricula, e.g., those of universities such as Wright State University, highlight the significance of these factors, with a focus of awareness on the critical interaction between patient-specific factors and pharmacologic guidelines (Wright State University, 2016). These scholarly frameworks are crucial for equipping future healthcare practitioners to respond to the subtle demands of special populations within clinical environments.

Current progress in computational pharmacology and data science offer bright prospects for the refinement of drug development in special populations. Model and simulation approaches provide powerful tools to anticipate drug performance without the ethical limits of extensive human studies, thereby hastening research with improved safety profiles. These techniques allow for the assembly of biological, chemical, and clinical information into dynamic, changing knowledge bases that can inform decision-making in individualized medicine. Widespread adoption of these technologies will play a key role in reversing the pharmaceutical productivity slump by filling knowledge gaps for characterizing drug interactions in various patient populations (Hunt et al., 2013). Therefore, the synergy between innovative informatics and conventional pharmacological strategies is an important step towards the best therapy for special populations.

Definition of Pharmacology

Grasping the complex mechanisms through which chemicals interact with biological systems is central to the field of pharmacology (Figure 15.1). The scientific field covers the investigation of drug ADME, all of which lead to a drug's final impact on the human organism. Pharmacology is more than learning about the chemical composition of drugs; it examines the therapeutic as well as harmful effects these drugs can cause. Since it lies at the junction of disciplines including physiology, biochemistry, and pathology, pharmacology gives an important understanding into how drugs could be maximized for efficacy as well as safety. This elementary knowledge becomes notably important when handling special populations where physiological variations and comorbid conditions necessitate specific pharmacologic considerations to preempt suboptimal therapeutic results. Pharmacology also includes within its domain the comprehension of variability in drug response between different populations, such as those having their own special physiology or pathology. For example, patients with malabsorption syndromes pose special difficulty for drug therapy, since compromised nutrient absorption frequently accompanies drug bioavailability alteration. Diseases like cystic fibrosis and Crohn's disease demonstrate how gastrointestinal (GI) tract diseases require meticulous pharmacologic adjustment to attain proper therapeutic levels. This emphasizes the need to appreciate malabsorption not only as a nutritional issue but also as a critical determinant of drug distribution and effect. Therefore, understanding pharmacokinetics and pharmacodynamics in these settings assists clinicians in creating effective treatment regimens that take into account these complexities (Lenti et al., 2025). Additionally, pharmacology incorporates the investigation of drug interactions in different cardiovascular conditions, with a focus on individualized strategies for special populations with arrhythmias and other cardiac abnormalities. Pharmacological management of patients with compromised cardiac physiology must involve an in-depth understanding of the involved pathophysiological mechanisms as well as the influence of the pharmacological agents on cardiac rhythm and function. Innovative therapies and diagnostic technology in the treatment of arrhythmias document the evolving role of pharmacology in the treatment of various patient populations, including vulnerable ones like the elderly or pregnant women. This context responsiveness underscores the vital contribution of pharmacology to personalized medicine, in which therapeutic plans are optimized on the basis of patient-specific factors to achieve optimum efficacy and least possible harms (Anmol et al., 2024).

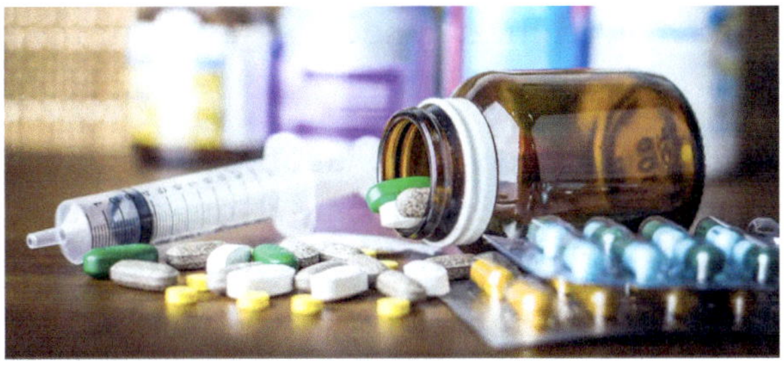

Figure 15.1. Pharmacology.

Source: SGT University. (n.d.). *Pharmacology. https*://sgtuniversity.ac.in/assets/images/faculty/medicine-health-science/programme/pharmacology.webp.

Importance of Studying Special Populations

Patient variability in drug response poses a major challenge in clinical pharmacology, calling for targeted research in special populations. Age, genetics, comorbid conditions, and ethnoracialities may influence pharmacokinetics and pharmacodynamics and hence drug efficacy and safety. For example, elderly patients commonly show changes in the metabolism and excretion of drugs as a result of physiological alterations, which enhance their susceptibility to adverse drug reactions (ADRs). Lacking thorough investigations specific to such populations, common dosing schedules could be suboptimal or even toxic. In addition, the variation of social determinants of health influencing the management of chronic diseases demands patient-specific solutions in pharmacotherapy. Recommendations of teamwork-oriented collaborative care address the requirement by merging evidence from varied populations of patients to maximize therapeutic benefits and prevent harm across differing medical conditions (Salim et al., 2023). The increasing incidence of certain medical conditions in underrepresented ethnoracial groups also highlights the need to examine special populations in pharmacology. Conditions such as Alzheimer's disease (AD) and associated dementias disproportionately impact some ethnic communities, but studies commonly avoid these groups, which restricts the applicability of results. It is essential to realize how genetic heterogeneity and cultural factors affect disease expression and drug response to bring about effective, fair treatments. Absent this attention, health disparities continue, perpetuating systemic inequities in healthcare provision. The international community acknowledges this deficit, motivating a concerted push to incorporate ethnoracial considerations into research models, thus enhancing a more encompassing scientific agenda that responds to the distinct requirements of diverse groups and enhances therapeutic specificity (Ganesh et al., 2018). Special population research is critical not only for the customization of drug treatments but also for the orientation of clinical practice and policy development. Clinical guidelines and regulatory agencies increasingly promote the use of evidence based on heterogeneous groups to assure safety and effectiveness through the lifespan and demographics. For instance, cardiovascular disease (CVD) treatment guidelines currently specifically recognize differences in patient characteristics, facilitating shared decision-making and cost-saving interventions tailored to personal risk profiles (Salim et al., 2023). Such interventions minimize treatment failure and adverse events and maximize patient compliance and quality of life. Therefore, investment in pharmacological research with special populations as a priority promotes a comprehensive understanding of drug action, stimulates innovation in therapeutic approaches, and ultimately encourages health equity by bridging knowledge gaps that traditionally marginalized groups have faced in clinical trials.

15.1. Pediatric Pharmacology

Learning Outcome

1. Developmental Considerations in Drug Metabolism
2. Dosage Adjustments for Children
3. Common Pediatric Medications and Their Uses

The complexities of drug development are further magnified when considering pediatric populations, whose physiological and developmental differences impact pharmacokinetics and pharmacodynamics profoundly. Unlike adults, children possess dynamic organ function and metabolic capacities that evolve with age, making dosing regimens less predictable and necessitating careful adjustment to ensure efficacy and safety. Historically, pediatric patients have been underrepresented in clinical trials, and thus the field has had to rely on extrapolated adult data instead of specific studies. More recent efforts stress the necessity for inclusive clinical trial designs that can handle variability, using quantitative translational sciences like physiologically-based pharmacokinetic (PBPK) modeling to predict drug behavior in children. This transition fits with wider initiatives to adopt diversity in intrinsic characteristics throughout drug development, yielding more relevant and generalizable information to maximize pediatric pharmacotherapy (Figure 15.2) (Venkatakrishnan et al., 2021). Concurrent to the inclusive trial design is the alignment with rapidly developing methodologies that enable targeted therapy in children. Model-based precision medicine platforms leverage sophisticated population pharmacology and disease course models to tailor treatment regimens to pediatric patients based on their individualized developmental stages. These models are essential considering the paucity of evidence base for most children's medications, highlighting the need for adaptive study designs that can effectively investigate dosing in a safe manner across age groups. In addition, real-world evidence and artificial intelligence are increasingly used to enhance insight into drug response in pediatric subpopulations, resulting in stronger clinical guidelines and improved health outcomes.

The technological collaboration underpins the overarching aspiration set out by recent guideline activities, which focuses on evidence-based therapeutic approaches that fit the complex needs of vulnerable populations, such as children (Bhimraj et al., 2020). In spite of progress, there are some issues in pediatric pharmacology, notably related to ethical issues, recruitment difficulties, and extrapolation hazards. There is a call for ongoing collaboration between clinical pharmacologists, regulatory agencies, and industry partners to create designs that reconcile scientific discipline with patient safety. An understanding of pediatric populations as unique populations that need individually adapted pharmacological research allows for a culture of inclusivity that can respond to historical deficits. In addition, methodologies like adaptive safety lead-in studies and exposure-matched dosing regimens are exemplary examples of pragmatic solutions to reduce risks in pediatric trials. Adopting these methods is in line with current appeals to reconsider conventional paradigms in special population drug development, thereby fostering trust and fair access to evidence-based drugs for children globally (Venkatakrishnan et al., 2021).

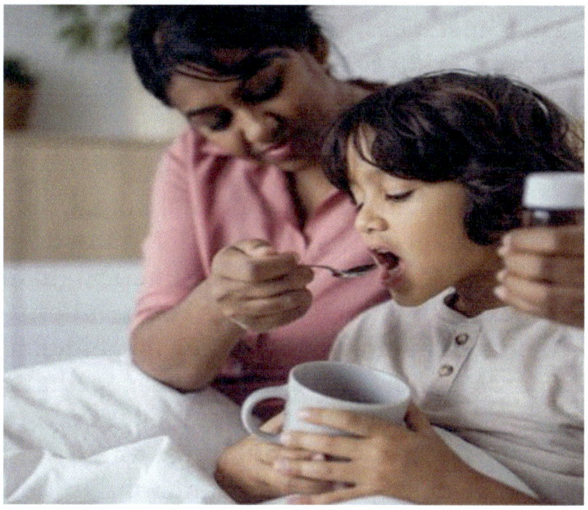

Figure 15.2. Pediatric pharmacology.

Source: Frontiers in Pharmacology. (n.d.). *Pediatric Pharmacology.* https://www.frontiersin.org/files/special%20topics/52621/thumb_400.jpg.

15.1.1. Developmental Considerations in Drug Metabolism

Grasping the intricacies of drug metabolism among children necessitates an understanding of the dynamic physiological developmental changes (Figure 15.3). There are great differences in enzymatic activity in neonates and infants compared to adults, which plays a major role in drug clearance and effectiveness. These developmental changes impact the absorption, distribution, metabolism, and excretion (ADME) processes collectively that determine drug level and response in the body. As a result of these variabilities, administration of dosing regimens derived from adult data is clinically inappropriate and possibly dangerous. The development of population pharmacokinetic analysis makes it now possible for researchers to assess intra- and interindividual variability in neonatal populations more accurately, allowing for personalized therapeutic intervention. Interindividual differences are still significant during early stages of life and result in unanticipatable clinical responses to typical drug dosages. These challenges highlight the need for the integration of developmental pharmacokinetics and pharmacodynamics in pediatric drug development and dosing regimens to maximize efficacy and minimize risks in these susceptible populations (Mutwalli et al., 2022). The complex interaction between growth and development and drug effect is at the heart of developmental pharmacology, which includes both pharmacokinetics and pharmacodynamics throughout the pediatric age range. Maturation not only affects drug metabolism but also the inherent sensitivity of target tissues and organs to therapeutic drugs. Pediatric drug development pipelines increasingly take these into account by utilizing novel, noninvasive sampling methods and sophisticated preclinical models specific to neonatal and pediatric physiology. These allow for invaluable information on drug disposition and metabolite profiling, which identifies novel pharmacokinetic behaviors that are specific to immature organ systems. In addition, developmental pharmacodynamics encourages consideration of the significance of drug response and receptor function variations unique to age and requires specialized instruments of assessment integrated with pediatric pathophysiology. These strategies are supportive of exhaustive knowledge of development physiology coupled with therapeutic approach enhancement, increasing precision in drug therapy in children, as well as reducing risks involving broad assumptions for dosing (Allegaert et al., 2022). Addressing pediatric heterogeneity in drug metabolism also requires a paradigm shift in trial design and regulatory strategies. The traditional sequential age-based subgroup enrollment is increasingly being superseded by more scientifically sensible designs that account for the continuum of maturation and its drug-interactive effect. This change encourages the involvement of pediatric subpopulations with diverse characteristics in early stages of drug development to allow the identification of dosing regimens optimal for developmental stage, not for arbitrary age. Additionally, sustained cooperation between pharmaceutical firms, regulatory authorities, and academic investigators ensures the incorporation of developmental pharmacology knowledge into guidelines and clinical practice. With focused research efforts and expert agreement, more importance is given to the identification of pediatric-specific pharmacodynamic targets and safety profiles so that safer and more effective therapeutic interventions can be made at different developmental stages (Allegaert et al., 2022; Mutwalli et al., 2022).

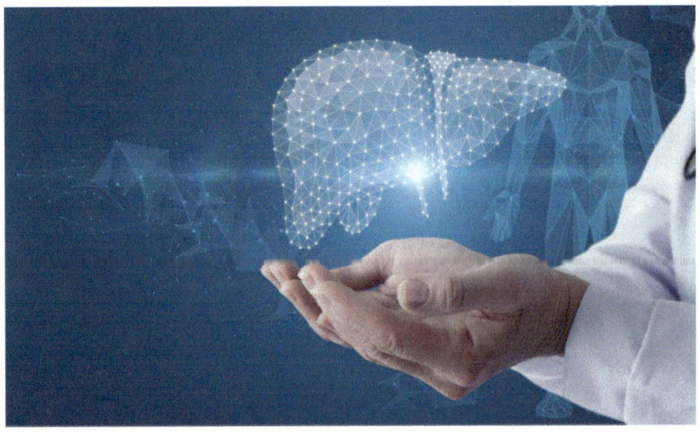

Figure 15.3. Developmental considerations in drug metabolism.

Source: WuXi AppTec. (2023). *Metabolic Stability.* https://labtesting.wuxiapptec.com/wp-content/uploads/2023/10/Metabolic-stability-Feature-ImageLinkedIn.jpg.

15.1.2. Dosage Adjustments for Children

Finding suitable drug dosages in children poses special challenges because of the dynamic body changes that occur during childhood. Unlike adults, children have variability in organ maturation, enzyme activity, and body composition that can greatly affect drug ADME. Successful dosing regimens must limit toxicity and, at the same time, provide therapeutic effect, which frequently requires the extrapolation of adult exposure-response relationships to children when direct efficacy information is unavailable. In such instances, pediatric pharmacokinetic information are the key to determining dosing regimens that provide drug exposures equivalent to those of adults, thus allowing effective and safe therapy. Complications arise mainly in instances where renal impairment crosses with pediatrics, due to the relative lack of strong clinical and pharmacokinetic data for this subgroup. Therefore, clinicians tend to fall back on modified adult renal dosing guidelines or sparse empirical data to inform pediatric prescriptions, highlighting the necessity for more specific research to address these voids (Khurana, 2021). A consideration of body size and composition is most important when dosages are being adjusted in children but one that demands more sophisticated methods than mere weight-based calculations. While drug clearance and volume of distribution are often normalized for body weight, such an approach ignores the complexity of the effects of size, as well as age, gender, and developmental stage, on body composition. More inclusive measures using variables such as height and age yield better normalization for pharmacokinetic parameters. The traditional standard of the "70-kg man" illustrates the shortcomings of established reference values that do not capture the variability of body sizes in clinical practice, particularly in pediatric populations where growth patterns vary widely. As such, dosing regimens need to address these individualized traits, highlighting the pharmacological tenet that dosing in kids cannot be extrapolated from adult norms directly but must be supported by a working knowledge of physiological maturation and heterogeneity (David, 2013). Additionally, the specific pathophysiologic states experienced by children are not the same as those for adults, making it even more challenging to adjust dosages. Considerations like renal function, which can be acutely or chronically impaired by conditions specific or more common in childhood, significantly influence drug clearance and risk of toxicity. For example, whereas adults with renal impairment typically have well-established guidelines for dose adjustment, similar evidence in pediatric patients is limited. Renal impairment is defined differently, and the interaction between developing kidney function and disease makes pharmacokinetic predictions even more difficult. In addition, since most drugs are eliminated through the kidneys, the failure to factor in the altered clearance in pediatric patients with renal impairment can result in inadequate dosing recommendations. This scenario underscores the urgent necessity both for accurate biomarkers of renal function in children and for the establishment of evidence-based recommendations that incorporate pharmacokinetic and pharmacodynamic information to maximize drug dosing in children (Khurana, 2021).

15.1.3. Common Pediatric Medications and Their Uses

The management of pediatric patients is in itself challenged uniquely by the respective physiological and developing features of the child (Figure 15.4). Adult patients, compared to their counterparts in pediatric stages, display uniformly different absorption, metabolism, distribution, and elimination rates for drugs, calling for accurate dose manipulations to obviate the risk of either toxicity or insufficiency. Standard pediatric medications, including acetaminophen and ibuprofen, are often utilized to alleviate pain and fever; yet their administration schedules need to be accurately gauged by age and weight. Besides analgesics, antibiotics such as amoxicillin are used extensively to combat infection, yet the danger of resistance and ill effects exists, so stressing careful prescription is essential. Sedative drugs also demand close scrutiny in the pediatric environment, where the procedural demands have to be weighed against the risks of sedation, again underlining the role of medical control and safe usage guidance as established by professional organizations (Charles et al., 2019). In pediatric pharmacodynamics, there has to be an appreciation of nuance when dealing with medication given for chronic disorders, such as asthma or attention-deficit hyperactivity disorder (ADHD), where maintenance therapy is not unusual. Bronchodilators and corticosteroids are cornerstones in treating childhood asthma, enhancing respiratory function while reducing exacerbations. Likewise, medication for ADHD stimulants require careful monitoring to maximize therapeutic benefit and avoid cardiovascular or neuropsychiatric adverse effects. Off-label prescription, commonly found in the pharmacotherapy of children because of limited clinical trials, likewise adds to the challenges in making treatment decisions and the need for clinical judgment and available data to avoid dangers. The intricacy of pediatric dosing is further compounded in special populations with developmental delays or comorbidities, where individual response can range widely, and requires continuous reassessment and titration in medication regimens. The use of sedative and anxiolytic medications in children for medical procedures illustrates the fine balance in pediatric pharmacology. Safety is ensured through systematic pre-sedation assessment to detect underlying conditions that may pose risk, age-based dosing according to pharmacokinetic and pharmacodynamic principles, and the preparedness to address airway complications or adverse reactions (Charles et al., 2019). Outside of the acute care environments, the case for pediatric drug use continues on to holistic management plans for endocrine diseases like polycystic ovary syndrome (PCOS), wherein new evidence-based practice guidelines reinforce individualized, multidisciplinary management strategies involving drug use as well as lifestyle change. In short, generic pediatric drugs have a wide range of therapeutic uses, requiring careful attention to developmental needs, close observation, and strict adherence to evidence-based guidelines in order to maximize efficacy and safety in this susceptible population.

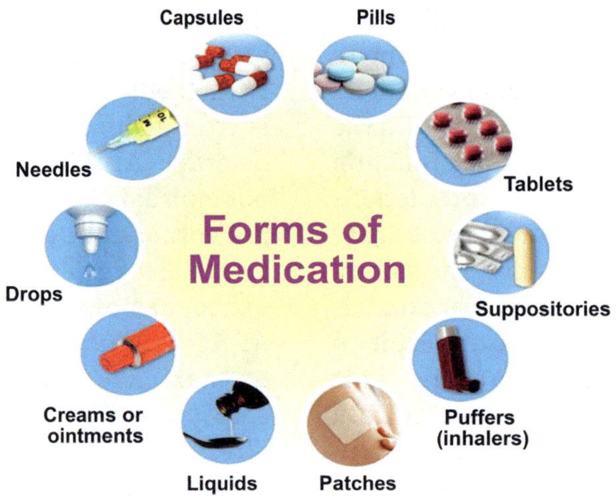

Figure 15.4. Common pediatric medications and their uses.

Source: Canadian Virtual Hospice. (n.d.). *Medications Image*. MyGrief.ca. https://www.mygrief.ca/pluginfile.php/2868/mod_lesson/page_contents/2647/M5%20-%20medications%20image.jpg.

Test Your Knowledge

1. Define pediatric pharmacology?
2. Why are Dosage Adjustments for Children?

15.2. Geriatric Pharmacology

Learning Outcome

1. Age-Related Physiological Changes Affecting Drug Action
2. Polypharmacy and Its Implications
3. Strategies for Safe Medication Management in Older Adults

The complexities of prescribing medications in the older adult involve more than considerations of age, covering a range of physiological and pathological changes affecting the efficacy and safety of drugs. Age-related pharmacokinetic alterations, such as decreased renal elimination and hepatic metabolism, challenge conventional dosing regimens with the need for individualized treatment strategies. Further, multimorbidity and polypharmacy that characterize the population of the aged also make the situation difficult by enhancing the likelihood of ADRs and drug interactions (Figure 15.5). Identification of these factors necessitates a paradigm shift in drug development and assessment, incorporating frailty assessments with traditional criteria.

Baseline and during-treatment measurement of frailty provides a more complete picture of patient vulnerability, improving translational relevance from preclinical models to the clinic. Sophisticated methods, such as physiologically based pharmacokinetic-pharmacodynamic modeling and artificial intelligence, are potential tools for personalizing therapies that take into consideration the intricate biology of aging and ultimately enhance therapeutic outcomes and quality of life in older patients (Sarah et al., 2024). Proper management of pharmacotherapy in geriatric patients also requires attention to disease-specific factors and procedural hazards, especially in diseases common among this population. For instance, urolithiasis in older patients poses distinct diagnostic and treatment challenges, frequently marked by greater stone burden, increased symptom severity, and higher perioperative risk. Conservative pharmacologic therapy, such as analgesia, can be complicated by associated comorbidities, highlighting the need for individualized interventions. Interestingly, surgical interventions like ureteroscopy exhibit similar safety and efficacy in older adults compared to younger populations, allaying clinicians' concerns regarding their applicability. In addition, new pharmacological agents like sodium-dependent glucose co-transporter 2 inhibitors provide new preventive promise, reflecting the dynamic nature of targeted therapies in geriatric pharmacology. These developments highlight the importance of incorporating age-related clinical knowledge into the therapeutic decision-making process for older patients (Tarek et al., 2024). In addition to drug-by-drug considerations, geriatric pharmacology supports an interprofessional approach with patients, caregivers, and healthcare professionals aimed at maximizing medication management in older adults. Engagement of the patient enables adherence and enables a sophisticated understanding of treatment objectives in harmony with patient values and expectations regarding quality of life. Multidisciplinary coordination ensures thorough assessment of polypharmacy risk and facilitates deprescription when indicated. In addition, the inclusion of frailty assessment improves risk stratification and guides dosage adjustment, notably in clinical trials for this population, and thus boosts external validity. Redressing disparities in aging populations' participation in clinical research in low- and middle-income countries remains key to international health equity. Finally, the convergence of innovative technologies, patient-centered care systems, and contextually appropriate clinical guidelines is a path forward to developing pharmacology that addresses the heterogeneous needs of the elderly (Sarah et al., 2024).

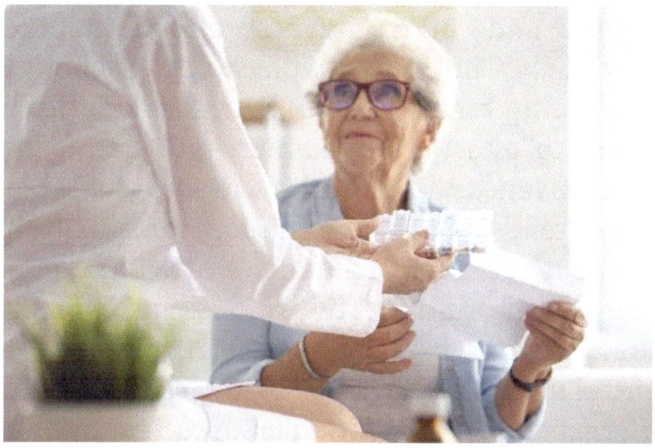

Figure 15.5. Geriatric pharmacology.

Source: https://d2jx2rerrg6sh3.cloudfront.net/image-handler/ts/20240129043345/ri/950/src/images/Article_Images/ImageForArticle_24525_17065208242137026.jpg.

15.2.1. Age-Related Physiological Changes Affecting Drug Action

As patients get older, the body's metabolism of drugs experiences profound changes that complicate traditional pharmacotherapy (Figure 15.6). The changes arise from gradual reduction in the function of organs, such as hepatic and renal systems, with key roles in drug metabolism and excretion. Hepatic metabolic function declines as a result of decreased liver mass and declining activity of cytochrome P450 enzymes, resulting in increased drug half-lives and elevated plasma concentrations. Likewise, renal clearance is also impaired as glomerular filtration rate falls, compromising the removal of renally excreted drugs and increasing the risk of toxicity. Additionally, changes in body composition with age—such as rising fat and falling lean body mass and total body water—impact drug distribution. Lipophilic drugs can be stored in adipose tissue, extending their effects, whereas hydrophilic drugs distribute in a reduced volume, leading to increased plasma concentrations. These physiological changes require meticulous dose individualization to maximize therapeutic benefits and reduce adverse effects in older individuals. The effects of physiological changes with ageing reach beyond pharmacokinetics to extend to pharmacodynamics, modulating the responsiveness of the body to drugs. Ageing tissues tend to have altered receptor sensitivity and post-receptor signaling, which influences drug efficacy and safety profiles. For example, older persons can become more sensitive to central nervous system (CNS) depressants, such as benzodiazepines, with increased sedative and risk of falling. On the other hand, diminished beta-adrenergic receptor responsivity can make beta-blockers less effective, making cardiovascular control more difficult. Furthermore, homeostatic controls like baroreceptor reflexes can be dampened, and hypotensive events will be more likely with antihypertensive medications. The complexity of these pharmacodynamic changes enhances the need for clinicians to be more sophisticated, blending the changed drug activity with individual patient factors and also bringing into account genetic variations that may influence the response to drugs, an increasingly stressed factor in precision medicine practices (Mueller, 2010a). Insights emerging about genetic polymorphisms in association with physiological changes at all stages of life emphasize the complexity of drug therapy in elderly patients. Multifactorial genetic factors regulate drug-metabolizing enzymes, transporters, and receptors and contribute to extensive interindividual differences in drug action. This genotypic variability converges with the aging process, making it difficult to predict drug efficacy and toxicity in the elderly. Systems biology developments indicate that detailed profiling of genetic vulnerabilities in combination with dynamic physiological alterations may enhance customized pharmacotherapy. Novel therapeutic approaches, including protein modification and targeted delivery systems, offer the potential for the circumvention of age-related pharmacokinetic barriers and improvement in drug bioavailability. Such methods may facilitate more accurate and effective treatments suited to the elderly, reducing the risks of polypharmacy and comorbidities prevalent among this group, and illustrate the potential of merging molecular and clinical information for better pharmacological care (Mueller, 2010a).

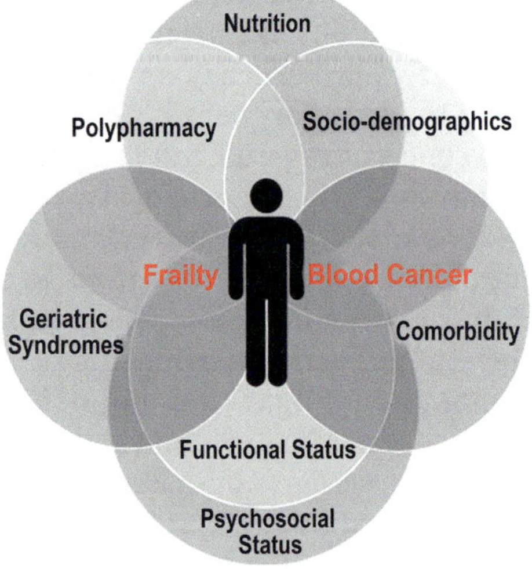

Figure 15.6. Age-related physiological changes affecting drug action.

Source: Koll, T. T., & Rosko, A. E. (2018). *Complex Interaction Between Age-Related Physiological Changes, Comorbidity, Geriatric Syndromes, And Hematologic Malignancy*. In *Frailty in Hematologic Malignancy. Current Hematologic Malignancy Reports.*

15.2.2. Polypharmacy and Its Implications

With the management of patients with intricate medical histories, especially in the elderly and chronically ill, multiple medication administration has become prevalent. Polypharmacy, the condition of having many medications, brings with it immense challenges in pharmacology, particularly in special populations where drug metabolism and response may be altered due to changes in physiology. Age-related impairment of organ function, e.g., decreased hepatic and renal clearance, enhances the risk of ADRs, and hence careful review of medications is crucial. In addition, polypharmacy enhances the risk of drug-drug interactions (DDIs), which can reduce therapeutic effectiveness or enhance toxicity. These interactions become paramount in groups already at risk for complications, thus necessitating an individualized approach to pharmacotherapy. Knowing the details of how these interactions occur and the pharmacokinetic profiles in special groups is central to optimizing outcomes and reducing harm (Zeppenfeld et al., 2022). As polypharmacy increases, the intricacy of co-occurring condition management increases, with cardiovascular patients being at the forefront of this issue. Treatment with anticoagulants, antiplatelets, and other cardiovascular agents needs to be precisely tuned to prevent both thrombotic and bleeding events. For example, guideline-recommended use of non-vitamin K antagonist oral anticoagulants (NOACs) demands subtle dosing modifications in elderly or in those with concomitant drugs like verapamil, where drug clearance and metabolism are influenced. These considerations underscore the significance of pharmacodynamic and pharmacokinetic studies specific to special populations, affirming the necessity of customized dosage regimens and vigilant monitoring. Research such as Venture-AF and X-VeRT highlight this dynamic management, highlighting the changing nature of care in polypharmacy patients under cardiovascular disease treatment (Steffel et al., 2021). The impact of polypharmacy goes beyond adverse drug reactions and drug-drug interactions to encompass greater healthcare utilization and reduced patient compliance. For patients prescribed multiple drugs, there is confusion regarding dosing regimens and possible side effects, resulting in non-adherence. This can result in inferior therapeutic effects and increased risk of hospitalization, especially in older individuals with low health literacy. Clinicians thus need to emphasize deprescribing strategies and detailed medication reconciliation to reduce these risks. Interdisciplinary interaction among pharmacists, physicians, and nurses is also required to maximize medication regimens, enhance safety, and simplify monitoring. With the delicate balance involved in pharmacologic management among special populations, detection and management of polypharmacy are central to improving both clinical outcome and quality of life (Steffel et al., 2021; Zeppenfeld et al., 2022).

15.2.3. Strategies for Safe Medication Management in Older Adults

Optimal medication management in the elderly involves a multidimensional strategy that takes into account the complex pharmacokinetic and pharmacodynamic alterations of aging (Figure 15.7). Physiologic changes like impaired renal function, diminished hepatic metabolism, and changed body composition can have a profound impact on drug ADME, resulting in heightened vulnerability to ADRs. Strategies to mitigate these risks involve careful medication reconciliation, ongoing monitoring of drug regimens, and tailored dosing adjustments according to renal and hepatic function. Furthermore, practitioners need to remain alert for drug-drug and drug-disease interactions that inordinately burden this population. Integrating multidisciplinary care teams, such as pharmacists who specialize in geriatric pharmacotherapy, increases the efficacy and safety of medication regimens through encouraging integrative assessments and tailored interventions to meet the complex demands of older patients. As a solution to medication safety issues in the older population, the primary care practice is essential in putting into action targeted interventions. Data-informed practices including risk assessments of opioid use, managing chronic pain using nonpharmacologic therapies, and clinical staff education on a continuous basis have been key. These practice interventions, included as high-leverage practice modifications, highlight the criticality of balancing data-based processes and workflow changes to best assure medication safety. Yet, practical use defines challenges like lack of ability to perform routine data reviews or maintain ongoing chart audits, an indication of the need for flexible, context-dependent strategies that are adapted to each practice setting. Ongoing assessment and iteration of such strategies support safer drug use and improved outcomes in aging adults, a necessary shift in pharmacologic care for this high-risk population (Leiby et al., 2024). Additionally, psychiatric disorders like catatonia in elderly people require carefully adjusted pharmacologic management because of their multifaceted presentations and dangers of high-dose sedation therapy. Although the pediatric background of treatment of catatonia provides some information about cautious drug use of agents such as benzodiazepines and judicious use of electroconvulsive therapy (ECT), analogous principles are also relevant to the elderly population in whom polypharmacy and comorbidities add to susceptibility to side effects. Psychiatric pharmacists play a key role in this field, working between therapeutic effect and safety by tracking dosages and possible adverse effects, ensuring comprehensive care for the patient. These positions represent strategies for safe medication use among special populations more broadly, highlighting the utility of ongoing research and interprofessional collaboration to further treat paradigms (Leiby et al., 2024).

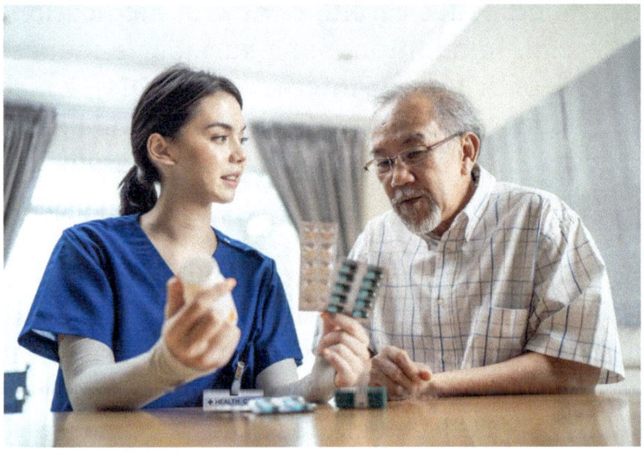

Figure 15.7. Strategies for safe medication management in older adults.

Source: https://cedarcoveassistedliving.com/wp-content/uploads/sites/2/2022/07/10-important-tips-for-better-medication-management.jpg.

Test Your Knowledge

1. What is the role of medication reconciliation in older adults?
2. Explain how polypharmacy can lead to drug–drug interactions?

15.3. Pharmacology in Pregnant Women

Learning Outcome

1. Effects of Pregnancy on Drug Pharmacokinetics
2. Risks and Benefits of Medication Use During Pregnancy
3. Guidelines for Prescribing Medications to Pregnant Women

The physiological adaptations of pregnancy profoundly influence the pharmacokinetics and pharmacodynamics of drugs, creating special challenges to pharmacologic treatment in pregnant women (Figure 15.8). Dilution and redistribution by increased plasma volume and changing body fat stores can reduce the concentration of drugs, whereas increased renal clearance and hepatic enzyme activity can speed the metabolism and elimination of some drugs. These alterations impact drug ADME, requiring judicious dose adjustment to ensure therapeutic effect and prevent toxicity. In addition, the placenta is a semi-permeable membrane, and selective transfer of drugs can influence fetal development. The therapeutic index for most drugs highlights the need to weigh maternal health requirements against fetal safety, illustrating the crucial considerations involved in prescribing medications during pregnancy. A thorough comprehension of these physiological adaptations is key to optimizing treatment responses and reducing side effects both for mother and child. Infectious illnesses pose a special challenge during pregnancy, wherein effective antiretroviral therapy is important but challenging due to impaired drug metabolism and fetal risks. In pregnant women with HIV, pharmacokinetics of protease inhibitors and non-nucleoside reverse transcriptase inhibitors, essential drugs in antiretroviral regimens, exhibit significant variability between and within individuals. Such variability makes it challenging to achieve the very narrow therapeutic range required for viral suppression without producing toxicity or resistance. Personalized dosing strategies have been put forward to make regimens specific to pregnancy-related physiological changes, with the objective of optimizing the effectiveness of therapy and reducing side effects. Nonetheless, such alterations must be carefully weighed to avoid compromised effectiveness or enhanced side effects, pointing to the fine balance between fetal safety and maternal treatment success in special populations (Hentig et al., 2012).

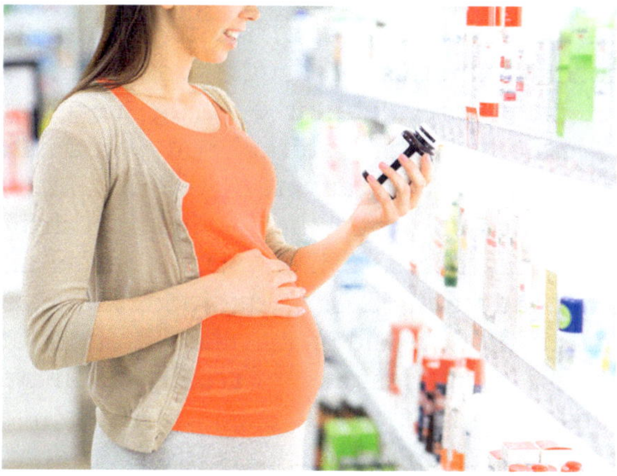

Figure 15.8. Pharmacology in pregnant women.

Source: https://cordis.europa.eu/docs/news/images/2022-03/435841.jpg.

Cessation of tobacco cessation in pregnancy is an important public health concern since smoking during pregnancy negatively impacts both maternal and fetal outcomes. Interventions specific to pregnant individuals need to take into account the unique pharmacology of nicotine replacement products and other cessation medications in pregnant individuals, including physiological alterations and fetal exposure. Policy innovation and new programs addressing smoking cessation highlight the combination of behavioral counseling with pharmacological assistance, balancing risks with benefits in pregnancy. Future directions emphasize the need for evidence-based approaches that support improved adherence and decreased side effects without compromising fetal growth. Joint efforts between healthcare professionals, scientists, and policymakers continue to be crucial in developing effective pharmacological treatments that can improve pregnancy outcomes and minimize long-term health effects of prenatal exposure to tobacco (N/A, 2007).

15.3.1. Effects of Pregnancy on Drug Pharmacokinetics

Pregnancy induces profound physiological changes that significantly impact pharmacokinetics of drugs, which require thoughtful reevaluation of drug dosage in pregnant patients. Maternal body water and fat redistribution augment the volume of distribution of hydrophilic and lipophilic drugs, which may decrease their plasma levels and therapeutic activities. In addition, increased renal blood flow and glomerular filtration rate enhance renal clearance of renally eliminated drugs, e.g., lithium and digoxin, which may need dose adjustment to ensure efficacy. Hepatic enzyme activity varies during pregnancy; some cytochrome P450 isoenzymes, e.g., CYP3A4 and CYP2D6, have augmented activity, accelerating the metabolism of substrates such as midazolam and metoprolol. Other enzymes, e.g., CYP1A2, have decreased activity. These broad pharmacokinetic changes highlight the need for personalized pharmacotherapy in pregnant patients to maximize benefit and reduce fetal risk (Dowell et al., 2022). In addition to absorption and metabolism, pregnancy causes significant changes in drug distribution by altering plasma protein binding. Decreased concentrations of albumin and alpha-1 acid glycoprotein reduce the binding site for most drugs, thus elevating the free, pharmacologically active fraction. Drugs with extensive protein binding, like phenytoin and warfarin, may achieve high free plasma levels, increasing the risk for toxicity without changing the total drug level. Gastrointestinal (GI) motility decreases and gastric pH rises during pregnancy, which may alter the solubility and rate of absorption of drugs taken orally, e.g., iron supplements. These changes affect the onset and magnitude of drug effect, underscoring the importance of close therapeutic drug monitoring (TDM) in pregnant patients to adjust dosing as needed and guarantee treatment efficacy and safety (Dowell et al., 2022). The interactive balance between maternal physiological change and placental barrier makes pharmacokinetic issues in pregnancy even more challenging. The placenta serves not only as a conduit for exchange of nutrients and waste products but also as a semipermeable barrier, influencing fetal drug exposure. Lipid-soluble, low-molecular-weight drugs more easily pass across the placenta, potentially leading to fetal drug accumulation and toxicity. Placental metabolic enzymes, including monoamine oxidases, can metabolize drugs, modifying their fetal bioavailability. In addition, function of drug transporters such as P-glycoprotein within the placenta may regulate passage of drugs to modulate either fetal exposure or restriction. Owing to such complexities, recognition of how pregnancy alters drug pharmacokinetics is essential in therapeutic decision-making in order to meet maternal therapeutic demand while ensuring fetal safety, an axiom that determines pharmacological care in special individuals.

15.3.2. Risks and Benefits of Medication Use During Pregnancy

Balancing medication use in pregnancy calls for careful assessment since changes in physiology can modify the pharmacokinetics and pharmacodynamics of drugs. Pregnant women typically have to make difficult choices based on incomplete information, mostly because they have traditionally been excluded from clinical trials (Figure 15.9). This deficit weakens the evidence base for therapeutic decision-making and obliges clinicians to make decisions based on sparse observational studies and anecdotal experience. Additionally, pregnant patients will demonstrate divergent willingness to enter clinical trials due to worry about possible risks to the fetus and perceived benefit to themselves. This is a factor in ensuring increased trial enrollment and, therefore, the available evidence regarding drug safety and effectiveness in pregnancy. Attempts to overcome these challenges emphasize the requirement for increased, morally robust research methods that aim to secure both maternal and fetal health but attempt to bridge knowledge gaps in existing pharmacologic practices (Melanie et al., 2024). Risks associated with stopping essential medications during pregnancy include the intricate balance between disease management and potential harmful fetal effects. For example, long-term conditions like hypertension and hypothyroidism need continuous management to avoid pregnancy and neonatal complications. Population-based primary care data analyses in recent times have proven that the withdrawal of certain antihypertensive medications or thyroid hormone replacement can influence gestational age and miscarriage rate. Interestingly, there was no apparent association between certain drug subclasses and adverse outcomes, suggesting that continuation may be safer than withdrawal in many cases. These results contradict the implicit conservative assumption regarding pregnancy medication use, that untreated maternal disease poses more risk than its pharmacotherapy control. Therefore, tailored risk–benefit evaluation continues to be most important to maximizing maternal-fetal health outcomes (Barry et al., 2024). Ultimately, pregnancy medication use requires a thoughtful balance of both possible teratogenicity and of morbidity from untreated maternal disease. While protective impulses toward fetal safety are ubiquitous, potential harm from withholding treatment can be substantial, especially in chronic illnesses with well-established pregnancy sequelae. Improved communication among patients and providers about the risks and benefits promotes informed consent and tailored care. In addition, consideration of socio-demographic inequalities that affect participation in trials and access to healthcare may enhance data diversity and overall maternal-fetal pharmacological safety profiles. With further research and increased inclusion, these dynamics will increasingly inform evidence-based recommendations to enable safer therapeutic decisions in this vulnerable group (Melanie et al., 2024).

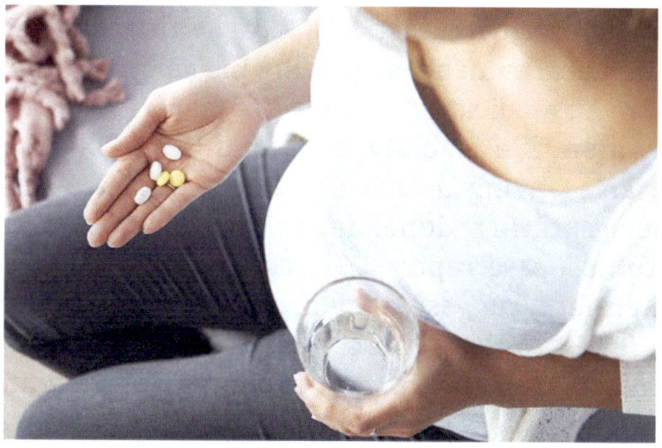

Figure 15.9. Risks and benefits of medication use during pregnancy.

Source: https://www.innovation.ca/sites/default/files/styles/stories_featured_xxl_1024px_x_680px/public/stories-if_pregnancy-page-930x516.png.jpg?itok=zn7X74ZB.

15.3.3. Guidelines for Prescribing Medications to Pregnant Women

Close attention is essential when prescribing drugs to pregnant women because of the significant physiological alterations that take place during pregnancy (Figure 15.10). These alterations may change drug ADME, and hence the efficacy and safety of pharmacotherapy, which may be affected. The physician needs to consider not only the therapeutic advantage to the mother but also the teratogenic or toxic effects on the growing fetus. Timing of exposure is important, with the first trimester being a time of increased susceptibility to congenital malformations, and subsequent phases being implicated in fetal growth and development. Guidelines in the clinical realm focus on individualized evaluation, with the choice of prescribing weighed against maternal health requirements versus fetal risk. These prudent prescribing habits seek to limit adverse consequences, preserving maternal health without jeopardizing fetal safety, which is a delicate issue in pharmacology among pregnant individuals. Along with physiological subtleties, the prescriber must also deal with restricted empirical evidence regarding the safety profiles of most medications during pregnancy. Pregnant women are usually excluded from clinical trials, leaving a lack of strong evidence and necessitating dependence on observational studies, case reports, or registries. Guidelines, therefore, suggest using drugs with established safety profiles where possible and avoiding those with known or suspected teratogenic potential. Where required, the lowest dose necessary should be given for as short a period as possible to limit fetal exposure. In addition, educating pregnant patients about possible harms and benefits promotes shared decision-making. Adverse effect monitoring also needs to be heightened because of changed pharmacokinetics and altered maternal-fetal dynamics. This policy resonates with overall clinical strategies that promote patient-specific care and risk reduction in pregnancy-targeted pharmacotherapy. Whereas guidelines mainly address drug choice and dosing, treatment of complicated conditions like pain or psychiatric disease when pregnant entails combining pharmacological information with clinical decision-making. Treatment guidelines, like those for opioid prescribing in chronic pain, emphasize a thorough evaluation of pain intensity, functional status, and harm risk, with individualized opioid use only where benefits outweigh risks (Dowell et al., 2022). Similarly, psychiatric management guidelines for special populations, including pregnant women, recommend prioritizing medications with favorable safety and efficacy profiles and considering the impact on both the mother and fetus (Lakshmi et al., 2018). These protocols stress ongoing evaluation throughout pregnancy and postpartum to adjust treatment plans accordingly. The interdisciplinary team effort among healthcare professionals maximizes the quality of care by ensuring both fetal and maternal well-being are protected through evidence-based, watchful pharmacological intervention in this vulnerable population.

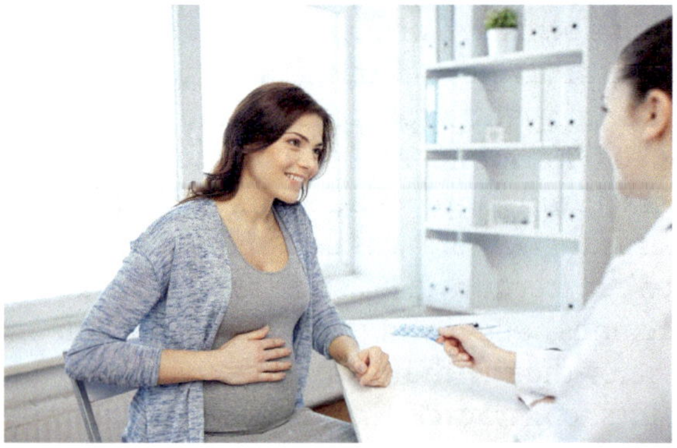

Figure 15.10. Guidelines for prescribing medications to pregnant women.

Source: https://www.parents.com/thmb/BUXSbOGTC9o2gj5nf6L2f9WfZdo=/1500x0/filters:no_upscale():max_bytes(150000):strip_icc()/shutterstock_416369659-a9b01e3085c24bdbaf8c1a8f8bf3fa0b.jpg.

Test Your Knowledge

1. How can medications affect fetal development?
2. How does effects of pregnancy on drug pharmacokinetics?

15.4. Pharmacology in Patients with Renal Impairment

Learning Outcome

1. Impact of Renal Function on Drug Clearance
2. Adjustments in Medication Dosing for Renal Patients
3. Common Medications Affected by Renal Impairment

Medication management becomes complex in patients with renal impairment as a result of changed pharmacokinetics, mainly decreased renal elimination of drugs and their metabolites. Renal excretion drugs can accumulate to cause toxicity, and dose adjustment needs to be done cautiously. In chronic kidney disease (CKD), pathophysiological alterations like decreased glomerular filtration rate impair the kidney's ability to clear drugs, requiring customized treatment approaches. Clinicians must balance efficacy against the risk of adverse effects by frequently monitoring renal function and adjusting dosages accordingly. Given these challenges, the development of tools to assist in precise dosing has become crucial to optimize therapeutic outcomes and prevent complications that can exacerbate patient morbidity. Interventions designed to enhance appropriate drug dosing in patients with renal impairment have demonstrated significant promise in clinical settings. A multi-component strategy that includes educational programs, clinical decision support systems, and computer programs that estimate creatinine clearance has been shown to be effective for decreasing inappropriate prescriptions in primary care settings. These studies have shown that such interventions significantly reduce the number of prescriptions above recommended dosing limits for renally cleared medications. This decrease not only decreases likely toxicity but also brings treatment more in line with the individual needs of patients, thus enhancing overall safety profiles. Consequently, the incorporation of technology into everyday care can overcome disparities between scientific knowledge about medications and real-world practice for high-risk populations (Beyer et al., 2012). The significance of using TDM methods, such as novel sampling strategies, cannot be exaggerated in maximizing pharmacotherapy among renal impaired patients. Dried blood spot (DBS) sampling, for example, has been identified as a viable TDM alternative with practical benefits in the monitoring of antibiotic levels like gentamicin and linezolid. Through the ease of frequent and less invasive measurement of drug concentrations, DBS can improve the clinicians ability to adjust dosages timely and accurately based on renal clearance variability. This method is especially critical in infections in which pharmacokinetic characteristics are affected by renal impairment, preserving efficacy while preventing toxicity hazards. The incorporation of such sophisticated methodologies reflects the dynamic nature of pharmacologic treatment individualized for renal impairment (Figure 15.11) (Akkerman et al., 2015).

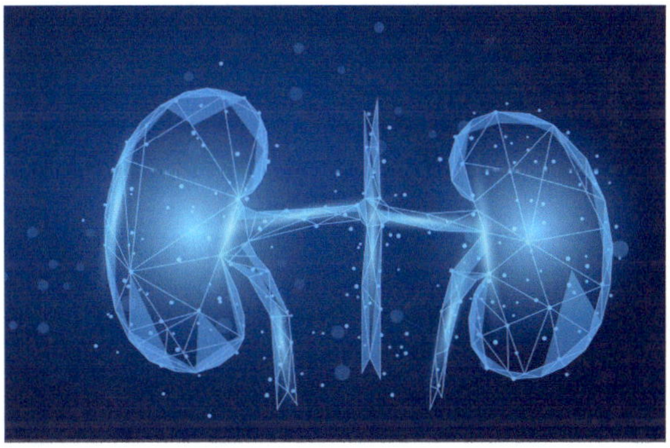

Figure 15.11. Pharmacology in patients with renal impairment.

Source: Allucent. (2024). *Renal Impairment Clinical Pharmacology Studies.* https://www.allucent.com/wp-content/uploads/2024/07/Renal-Impairment-Clinical-Pharmacology-Studies.webp.

15.4.1. Impact of Renal Function on Drug Clearance

The dynamic interaction between renal function and drug clearance highlights the pharmacotherapy complexity in special populations. Renal impairment reduces the capability of the kidneys to eliminate drugs properly, thus prolonging drug half-life and enhancing systemic exposure (Figure 15.12). The lowered clearance may enhance the risk of drug toxicity, particularly in drugs with narrow therapeutic indices. The physiological changes that occur with renal dysfunction not only alter glomerular filtration but also tubular secretion and reabsorption, making drug disposition even more complex. Also, changes in protein binding and in metabolism may affect pharmacokinetics in these individuals. Thus, knowledge of how renal impairment affects drug clearance is crucial for the adjustment of doses to ensure therapeutic effectiveness with reduced side effects, and this points to the need for individualized pharmacologic therapy in patients with impaired kidney function. Clinical care of patients with renal impairment typically requires individualized dosing regimens based on pharmacokinetic information specific to this group of patients. In certain situations, like extracorporeal membrane oxygenation (ECMO), things are further compounded because the therapy itself alters drug disposition by affecting clearance and volume of distribution through physiological alterations. These conditions require careful monitoring of drug pharmacokinetics to avoid subtherapeutic exposure or toxicity.

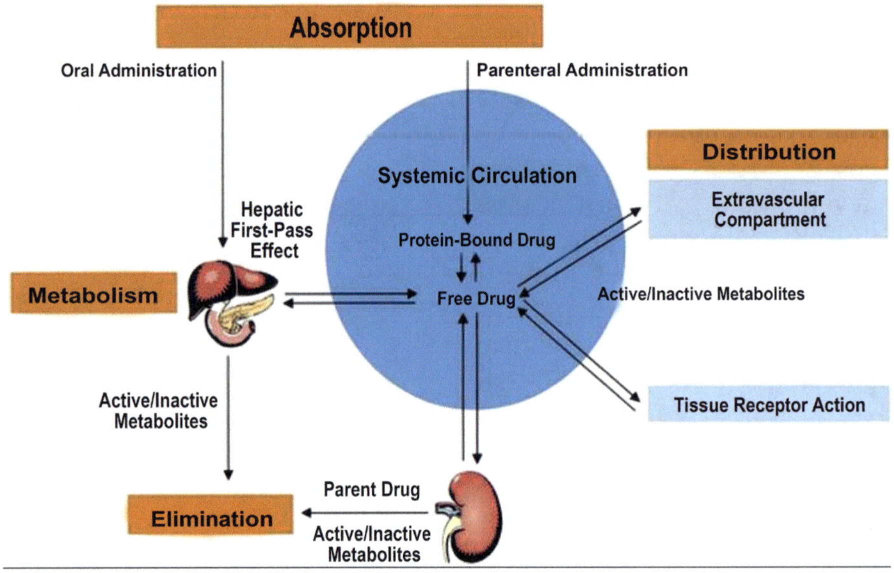

Figure 15.12. Impact of renal function on drug clearance.

Source: Elsevier. (2016). In *Abdominal Imaging: Expert Consult – Online and Print* (2nd ed.). https://abdominalkey.com/wp-content/uploads/2016/06/c00077_f077-001-9781455758388.jpg.

Notwithstanding the severity of these concerns, the pharmacokinetic changes are also very drug-specific and poorly understood for many drugs, making clinical decision-making difficult. This highlights the necessity for continuous research to characterize clearance profiles in renal insufficiency and establish sound dosing recommendations, facilitating safer, more effective drug therapy in specialized and critically ill patients (Aebi et al., 2017). Peritoneal dialysis (PD) is another distinct setting where renal function significantly affects drug clearance, but relevant data to support dosing are sparse. For instance, vancomycin dosing in PD-associated peritonitis has hitherto been empirical, predominantly extrapolated from continuous ambulatory PD to automated PD because of a lack of adequate pharmacokinetic studies in the latter. This stems from substantial gaps in knowledge about drug disposition in different dialysis modalities, which can significantly influence clearance and exposure to drugs. A careful analysis of vancomycin pharmacokinetics and its predictors in PD patients identifies the need for an evidence-based dosing strategy to maximize therapeutic benefits. Therefore, the creation of dedicated dosing algorithms based on pharmacokinetic concepts is essential to maximize efficacy and reduce toxicity in patients with compromised renal function and treated with dialysis (Kraft et al., 2020).

15.4.2. Adjustments in Medication Dosing for Renal Patients

Renal impairment greatly affects the pharmacokinetics and pharmacodynamics of many drugs, requiring careful dosage adjustments to avoid toxicity and failure of therapy (Figure 15.13). The role of the kidney in the excretion of drugs translates into compromised renal function as the potential for drug and metabolite accumulation, enhanced risk of adverse effects. Clinicians are thus obliged to estimate renal function with precision, frequently using estimated glomerular filtration rate (eGFR) or creatinine clearance to inform dosing adjustments. This is confounded by the dynamic nature of renal function, especially in acute kidney injury, such that serum creatinine may fail to depict current filtration capacity. Using serum creatinine or estimated renal function alone, without placing this in a clinical context, can therefore lead to inappropriate dosing. Successful management of medications in renal patients requires a multidisciplinary strategy with guidelines and drug principles to maximize therapeutic benefits and avoid harm The difficulty with dose correction in patients with kidney disease is heightened when treating comorbid illnesses like COVID-19, with multiple therapeutic drugs needing dose adjustment according to kidney function. In the setting of acute illness, particularly with acute changing kidney injury, typical renal function tests may be unhelpful, risking either under- or over-dosing of crucial drugs. For example, some antiviral drugs, such as remdesivir, possess renal clearance levels below which their use is normally contraindicated. Nonetheless, in cases of acute kidney injury where serum creatinine is variable, estimated creatinine clearance could not be reflective of true renal function, and thus, dosing decisions might be subject to possible errors. This speaks to the necessity for clinicians to include dynamic clinical evaluation and potentially alternative biomarkers in guiding therapy safely. Individualizing drug regimens in such patients is crucial not only for effectiveness but also to prevent worsening renal damage or inducing systemic toxicity (Kow et al., 2020). New clinical guidelines highlight individualized anticoagulation and thromboprophylaxis approaches in renal patients, especially in settings of systemic inflammatory conditions like COVID-19. The increased risk of thrombosis in such patients requires a delicate balance between the prevention of clot formation and reducing bleeding complications. Titration of anticoagulant doses according to changing renal function is necessary, as the build-up of these drugs increases the risk of hemorrhage. Modern guidelines recommend more frequent reassessment of renal biomarkers and clinical status to dynamically modify drug regimens, thereby maintaining therapeutic effects without jeopardizing safety. The inclusion of multidisciplinary opinions also increases decision-making efficacy, dealing with issues of polypharmacy and complex pharmacodynamics of renal impairment. By matching treatment protocols with patient-specific parameters, clinical success can be greatly enhanced while reducing drug-associated hazards

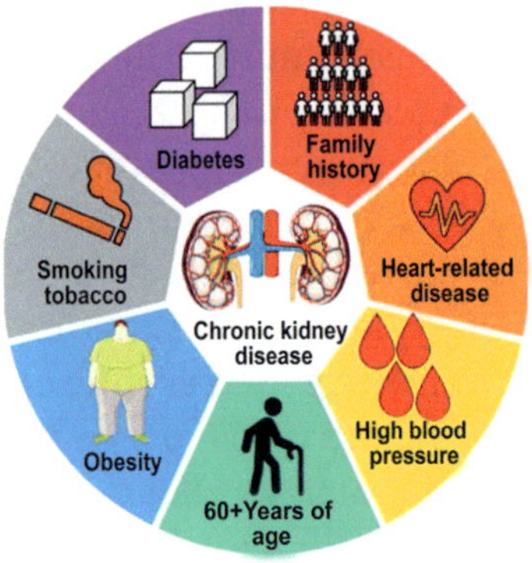

Figure 15.13. Adjustments in medication dosing for renal patients.

Source: Elsevier. (n.d.). *Image from Pharmacokinetics Textbook*. https://ars.els-cdn.com/content/image/3-s2.0-B9780128144251000048-f03-02-9780128144251.jpg.

15.4.3. Common Medications Affected by Renal Impairment

The complex interaction of renal impairment and drug pharmacokinetics requires a well-developed knowledge of drug clearance mechanisms. Renal disease dramatically impairs the elimination of drugs cleared by the kidneys, leading to increased plasma levels and heightened risk of toxicity. Such renal dependency is exemplified by clinically important drugs like digoxin, lithium, and certain antibiotics, e.g., aminoglycosides. For example, digoxin, commonly employed in cardiac disease, is sequestered in compromised renal conditions, which can result in life-threatening arrhythmias. Likewise, lithium, used for mood stabilization, necessitates careful serum monitoring because of narrow therapeutic indices compounded by decreased renal clearance. These changes necessitate careful dose adjustments to maintain efficacy and safety, underscoring the complex pharmacological considerations required in renal impairment. These intricacies highlight the difficulty for clinicians and pharmacists who need to incorporate renal function tests systematically into pharmacotherapy planning. Nonsteroidal anti-inflammatory agents (NSAIDs) are another pharmacological class significantly impacted by renal impairment.

These drugs, which are widely used to treat pain and inflammation, inhibit prostaglandin synthesis and thereby decrease renal blood flow, potentially worsening underlying renal dysfunction. In the kidney-compromised patient, NSAIDs can cause acute kidney injury or exacerbate CKD progression. In addition, NSAIDs can disrupt renal clearance of other medications and affect the balance of electrolytes, making treatment schemes difficult. With their widespread application, particularly in the elderly—a population commonly facing diminishing renal capacity—vigilant attention to NSAID dosing or alternative therapy is essential. This highlights the complexity of prescribing in special populations, wherein intended therapeutic benefits must be weighed against the risk of adverse renal consequences (Aebi et al., 2017).

Antimicrobial drugs are especially sensitive to changes in renal function because they depend on renal excretion for their elimination and are subject to a delicate balance between therapeutic effect and toxicity. Drugs like vancomycin, aminoglycosides, and some beta-lactams need dosage adjustments in renal impairment to prevent systemic toxicity without compromising efficacious antimicrobial activity. Vancomycin, for instance, has a very low therapeutic window and becomes accumulated in renal insufficiency with a potential risk of nephrotoxicity and ototoxicity. Aminoglycosides also need stringent dosing adjustments to prevent nephrotoxicity and ototoxicity. Failure to identify these required adjustments may result in failure of treatment or toxic side effects, thus highlighting the relevance of incorporating renal function parameters into dosing algorithms. Since pharmacokinetics are highly variable in impaired renal function and critically ill conditions, for example, in patients under extracorporeal support, tailoring dosing strategies is essential (Aebi et al., 2017).

Test Your Knowledge

1. How does CKD affect drug excretion?
2. How can dialysis influence drug dosing in renal patients?

15.5. Pharmacology in Patients with Hepatic Impairment

Learning Outcome

1. Liver Function Tests and Their Relevance
2. Drug Metabolism Alterations in Liver Disease
3. Considerations for Prescribing in Hepatic Patients

The metabolism of many drugs is significantly influenced by liver function, making pharmacological management in patients with hepatic impairment especially complex (Figure 15.14). The liver plays a crucial role in the biotransformation of medications, primarily through phase I and phase II metabolic reactions. When hepatic function declines, the metabolism, clearance, and bioavailability of drugs can be altered, often resulting in increased systemic exposure and heightened risk of toxicity. As such, dose reduction and vigilant monitoring become essential to avoid side effects. Several variables including the severity of liver impairment, the route of drug metabolism, and comorbidities complicate the endeavor. For example, drugs eliminated by the cytochrome P450 enzyme system can accumulate in patients with liver dysfunction, which requires customized therapeutic regimens for efficacy and safety. Pharmacokinetic analysis emphasizes that some drugs need regular monitoring in patients with hepatic impairment in order to maximize therapeutic effects. Drug categories such as antibiotics and antifungals can have variable pharmacokinetics based on liver function, and specific dosing regimens are required. In addition, TDM becomes an important instrument for controlling treatment in hepatic impairment, particularly when drugs have a narrow therapeutic window or non-predictable metabolism. Innovative methods like dried blood spot sampling have been promising to enable TDM, providing a more convenient and less invasive method for vulnerable patients. These developments are especially useful in special populations where extensive monitoring can be difficult, enabling more tailored medicine strategies in the setting of hepatic compromise (Akkerman et al., 2015). Some psychoactive drugs illustrate the difficulty of pharmacological management in patients with liver disease. Agomelatine, an antidepressant primarily metabolized in the liver through CYP-1A2, demonstrates the need for careful administration in such patients. Its susceptibility to hepatic enzyme activity is very high, and compromised liver function may result in raised blood levels of the drug, with consequent increased risk of hepatotoxicity. The drug's contraindication in liver-dysfunctional patients highlights the need for monitoring liver function during therapy. In spite of its novel pharmacologic profile and tolerance, agomelatine requires regular monitoring of liver enzymes to avoid dangerous side effects, underscoring the essential compromise between therapeutic benefit and safety among hepatic-compromised patients (Howland et al., 2009). This example illustrates the universal need for customized drug choice and dosing regimes in special groups with impaired hepatic function.

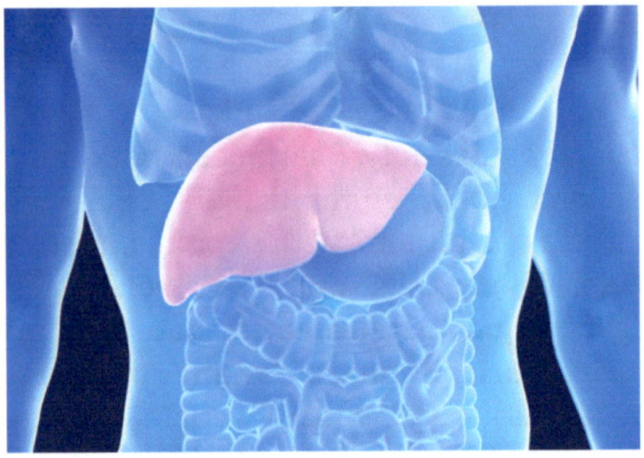

Figure 15.14. Pharmacology in patients with hepatic impairment.

Source: Allucent. (2024). *Hepatic Impairment Clinical Pharmacology Studies.* https://www.allucent.com/wp-content/uploads/2024/07/Hepatic-Impairment-Clinical-Pharmacology-Studies.png.

15.5.1. Liver Function Tests and Their Relevance

In clinical pharmacology, it is important to know how drugs are metabolized and excreted, especially when pharmacotherapy is being personalized for special populations like patients with hepatic impairment. The liver's key function of metabolizing drugs makes it essential to evaluate its functional status prior to starting or modifying pharmacotherapy. Liver function tests (LFTs) (Figure 15.15) reflect a biochemical impression of hepatic function and integrity, including measures like alanine aminotransferase (ALT), aspartate aminotransferase (AST), alkaline phosphatase (ALP), bilirubin, and albumin. These biochemical measures give information regarding hepatocellular injury, cholestasis, and synthetic function, which have a direct bearing on drug pharmacokinetics. In patients with impaired liver function, usual doses can cause augmented toxicity or reduced effectiveness, highlighting the necessity of assessing LFTs in detail. With precise interpretation of these tests, clinicians are able to better predict changes in drug metabolism, which is a practice encouraged by advancements in pharmacogenetics further developing personalized medicine strategies (Fenech et al., 2014). The multifunctionality of liver function and the genetic polymorphism that determines drug responses make pharmacologic management in special populations challenging. Most prevalent diseases, such as diabetes or cardiovascular disease, have underlying subtle genetic polymorphisms affecting enzyme function and drug-processing pathways in the liver. In contrast to monogenic diseases, such polymorphisms have minimal effects on their own but, cumulatively, can have profound effects on hepatic metabolism, influencing drug clearance and response (Mueller, 2010b). Thus, liver function tests need to be placed in genetic and environmental contexts that regulate liver enzyme systems. New systems biology strategies seek to incorporate these multifactorial factors to better predict hepatic drug metabolism. This interaction between LFT findings and genetic susceptibility emphasizes the growing need to merge biochemical testing with pharmacogenetic information when developing safe and effective drug regimens for patients with impaired or variable liver function. In addition to the evaluation of acute hepatic injury, LFTs are also prognostic indicators that direct long-term pharmacologic management in patients with chronic liver disease. The dynamic state of liver function, which changes with disease course or response to treatment, requires repeated and complete monitoring to allow optimal drug therapy. Synthetic markers such as albumin and prothrombin time assist in assessing the liver's ability to synthesize critical proteins, which may affect drug binding and distribution. Raised bilirubin and enzymes reflect compromised excretion and metabolism, requiring dose adjustment to avoid toxicity. LFTs thus become the foundation of therapeutic decision-making, especially for drugs with narrow therapeutic windows or extensive hepatic metabolism. Integration of regular LFT monitoring into pharmacologic management provides accuracy in dosage and decreases hepatotoxicity risk, thereby improving clinical outcomes among special populations with impaired liver function.

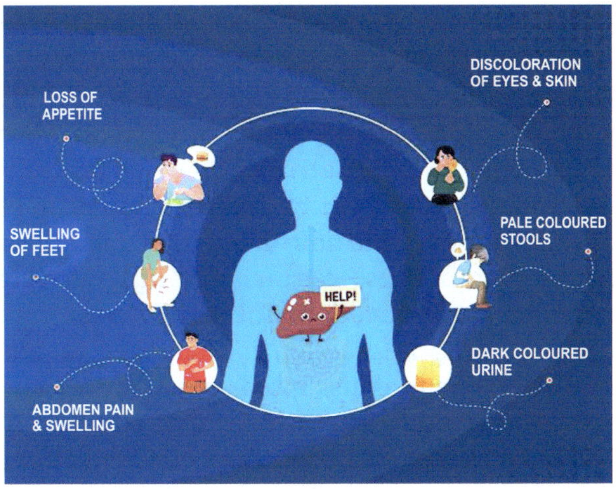

Figure 15.15. Liver function tests and their relevance.

Source: https://staticcdn.redcliffelabs.com/media/gallary-file/None/00a945e6-0076-423f-9418-7d2b39fa1089.webp.

15.5.2. Drug Metabolism Alterations in Liver Disease

The liver is primarily responsible for drug biotransformation, and this occurs mostly through phase I and phase II metabolic processes that modify pharmaceuticals to increase their elimination (Figure 15.16). But liver disease and resulting hepatic impairment can strongly interfere with such processes and thereby cause a change in drug pharmacokinetics. In diseases like cirrhosis or hepatitis, functional hepatocyte loss and disrupted hepatic blood supply impair the metabolizing capability of the liver and lead to defective metabolism of drugs. This impairment changes the intrinsic clearance of various drugs, specifically those that exhibit high hepatic extraction ratios, leading to an enhanced systemic drug exposure and adverse effects. Recognition of these metabolic changes is essential for clinicians to appropriately modify dosing, as routine regimens can lead to untoward consequences in patients with hepatic impairment, making pharmacotherapy in this group challenging. Liver disease further influences drug metabolism by changing the activity and expression of drug-metabolizing enzymes such as the cytochrome P450 family. The dysregulation of these enzymes reduces phase I oxidative reactions, which are slower conversion of prodrugs to active metabolites or reduced clearance of active drugs. Moreover, phase II enzymatic pathways for conjugation processes like glucuronidation and sulfation can be affected, further impacting drug elimination. The combined effect of these enzymatic modifications disturbs the equilibrium between drug activation and detoxification, resulting in changed efficacy and increased adverse effects. Due to the central role played by the liver in detoxification, any abnormality in its enzymic activity requires cautious pharmacokinetic consideration and dosage adjustment to avoid injury in patients with liver inadequacy. The difficulty in evaluating drug metabolism in liver disease is aggravated by the heterogeneity of hepatic disease and its secondary effects on the body, including portosystemic shunting and changed plasma protein binding. These factors influence not only the metabolism but also the distribution and bioavailability of drugs, emphasizing the need for individualized therapeutic strategies. Furthermore, the interplay between hepatic dysfunction and other cellular processes like autophagy, which maintains cellular homeostasis and drug clearance, remains underexplored but potentially significant for drug disposition in diseased livers (Daniel et al., 2016). Although existing clinical evaluation is mainly based on enzymatic activity and liver function tests, new developments in molecular and cellular mechanisms will provide more accurate predictive models. This multidimensional approach is crucial to maximize pharmacotherapy in liver disease patients, a special group with distinctive metabolic difficulties (Michael et al., 2016).

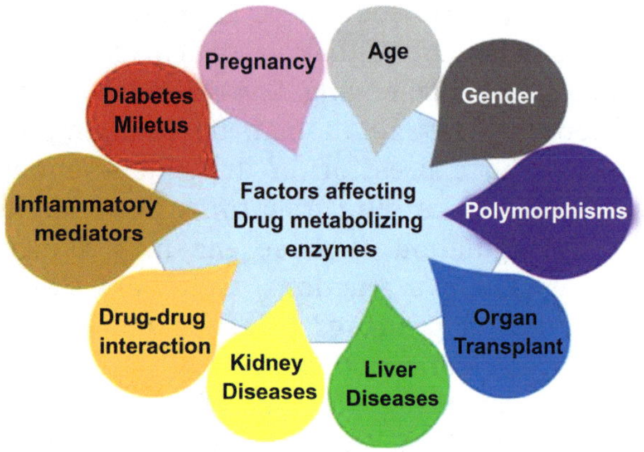

Figure 15.16. Drug metabolism alterations in liver disease.

Source: The Clinics. (n.d.). *Drug metabolism alterations in liver disease.* https://www.liver.theclinics.com/cms/attachment/2072268789/2068470940/gr4.jpg.

15.5.3. Considerations for Prescribing in Hepatic Patients

The prescription of drugs in patients with hepatic impairment calls for a sensitive comprehension of the liver's crucial function in drug metabolism and elimination. The liver's enzymatic processes, mainly characterized by phase I and phase II reactions, are commonly disrupted in hepatic disease, resulting in a change in pharmacokinetics and enhanced drug toxicity. Complications like portal hypertension and cholestasis can impede drug absorption and distribution, adding to dosing difficulties. Additionally, hepatically compromised patients may exhibit hypoalbuminemia, affecting the protein binding of drugs and increasing the free, active drug concentration, thereby raising the risk for adverse effects. Consequently, clinicians must evaluate liver function tests and consider the Child-Pugh classification when selecting and dosing medications to balance efficacy and safety. These drug adjustments highlight the relevance of personalized medicine strategies within hepatic populations, which aims to counteract risks without sacrificing therapeutic effectiveness (Dowell et al., 2022). In hepatic patients, drugs with a narrow therapeutic index or extensive hepatic metabolism require special caution. Agents that are metabolized primarily by the cytochrome P450 enzyme system, including some opioids and antiepileptics, need dose adjustment or alternative therapy to prevent accumulation and toxicity. The liver impairment can also increase the half-life of drugs and their active metabolites, requiring longer dosing intervals or reduced maintenance doses. In addition, drug interaction is increased in this group as a result of disrupted enzymatic activity and bile excretion impairment that can lead to unanticipated spikes in plasma concentrations of coadministered medications. To that end, monitoring of therapeutic levels of drugs in the clinical setting and close examination of signs of toxicity assume preeminence. Guideline adjustment and interdisciplinarity augment safer prescribing practices specifically targeted to the particular vulnerabilities of hepatic patients (Dowell et al., 2022). Care of infections in hepatically insufficient patients represents the intricacy of drug choice and dosing modifications. A good example is the use of antiviral drugs and antibiotics, which may need careful consideration due to their risk of hepatotoxicity and pharmacokinetic fluctuation in disease of the liver. Observation for unwanted effects like increased transaminases or decompensating encephalopathy is important. Additionally, the liver is involved in immune modulation, and hepatic failure increases susceptibility to infection, making treatment regimens more complex. The interaction between hepatic dysfunction and immunosuppressive regimens, particularly in transplant patients, requires delicate balance to prevent rejection and toxicity. This is the general principle that hepatic patients are a special group that needs individualized approaches taking into account changed drug metabolism, possible interactions, and increased risk of toxicity. These difficulties underscore the imperative need for continuous research and guideline formulation in pharmacology for special populations.

Test Your Knowledge

1. How does reduced hepatic enzyme activity affect drug clearance?
2. How can liver disease alter the half-life of lipophilic drugs?

15.6. Pharmacogenomics and Personalized Medicine

Learning Outcome

1. Role of Genetics in Drug Response
2. Implications for Treatment in Special Populations
3. Future Directions in Pharmacogenomic Research

Pharmacological advances have increasingly highlighted the importance of individualized therapeutic strategies that take into account genetic heterogeneity among patients. These variations have a significant impact on drug metabolism, efficacy, and the risk of adverse effects, highlighting the pivotal role of pharmacogenomics in personalized medicine (Figure 15.17). By incorporating genetic data into clinical decision-making, clinicians can tailor drug choice and dosing, especially in special populations where conventional one-size-fits-all regimens are likely to fail. The variability of responses seen between various races, ages, and sexes highlights the complexity of adapting pharmacotherapy. For example, the discovery of race-ancestry-specific pharmacogenetic variants opens the door to more targeted, race-aware medical interventions, but issues remain in properly capturing genetic diversity without employing ethnicity as a sole surrogate marker (Piet, 2021). This level of understanding serves to close healthcare gaps and maximize therapeutic benefit in at-risk populations. In contemporary drug development, machine learning and computational modeling have emerged as indispensable tools that complement pharmacogenomics by accelerating the discovery and optimization of therapeutics tailored to individual genetic profiles. These technologies enable the analysis of vast molecular datasets, enhancing the prediction of drug responses and identifying potential biomarkers relevant to personalized treatment regimens. The use of strong, reproducible computational approaches in preclinical phases not only accelerates the discovery of drugs but also lowers the costs and research durations involved. This confluence of pharmacology and artificial intelligence is promising to improve personalized therapies through the clarification of intricate gene–drug interactions and the ease of precision medicine strategy design, especially among populations with distinct pharmacodynamic and pharmacokinetic profiles (Carracedo-Reboredo et al., 2021). Therefore, these cross-disciplinary strategies are essential in overcoming the hurdles of introducing personalized medicine in multipatient populations. Although considerable advancements have been made, considerable gaps in clinical pharmacogenomics translation remain, particularly for underrepresented subpopulations like transgender patients and children and the elderly, wherein pharmacologic responsiveness may vary significantly from the norm as a consequence of different physiology. The limited clinical data for these groups demand targeted research initiatives and the development of specialized clinical pharmacology subspecialties to meet their particular therapeutic requirements. In addition, ethical and regulatory hurdles are encountered in integrating genetic information into everyday practice, necessitating continuous discussion among clinicians, researchers, and policy makers to facilitate equitable access to individualized therapies. The adoption of diversity in clinical trials and regulatory models is imperative towards the promotion of personalized medicine and ensuring that precision dosing and individualized therapy approaches are equally beneficial to all population segments (Piet, 2021). Such devotion to inclusiveness ultimately translates into improved drug efficacy and safety for special populations.

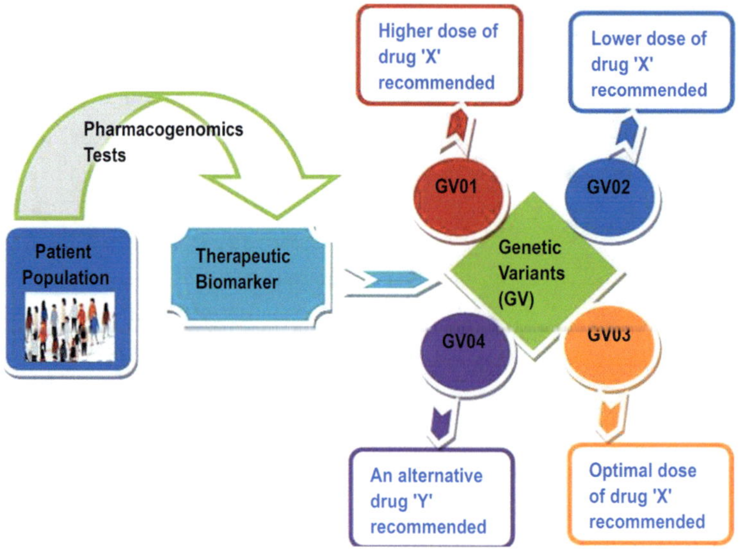

Figure 15.17. Pharmacogenomics and personalized medicine.

Source: **Singh, D. B.** (2019). *The Impact of Pharmacogenomics in Personalized Medicine* [Figure 1]. In *Advances in Biochemical Engineering/Biotechnology* (Vol. 171, pp. 369–394). Springer. https://doi.org/10.1007/10_2019_110.

15.6.1. Role of Genetics in Drug Response

Comprehending variability in patient response to pharmacological interventions is an important issue in medicine, most importantly among special populations. Genetic differences play an important role in such variability and affect drug efficacy as well as toxicity (Figure 15.18). Genetic variation in genes that encode drug-metabolizing enzymes, transporters, and receptors can change pharmacokinetics and pharmacodynamics and result in varying drug responses among subjects. For instance, polymorphisms within the cytochrome P450 family tend to influence the rate at which a drug is metabolized, which in turn affects drug concentrations and clinical responses. Such genetic heterogeneity requires personalized medicine strategies to maximize dosing and reduce toxicity. In special populations, including the elderly or those with chronic diseases, genetic factors on drug metabolism are even more significant because of accompanying physiological changes, highlighting the need to incorporate pharmacogenetics into clinical decision-making. Furthermore, genetic predisposition has a deep impact on the modulation of the sensitivity of CNS-targeted drugs, which is particularly significant in the treatment of neurodegenerative disorders like Alzheimer's. The advent of biologically targeted medicines requires a comprehension of the impact of genetic variation on the course of disease and drug response. AD, an increasingly prevalent public health issue in aging populations, highlights the requirement for individualized pharmacology based on genetic information. Detection of particular genetic markers involved in the processing of beta-amyloid and tau pathology would allow therapeutic approaches to be directed, with the selection of the drug aligned with the patient's genetic profile. These stratified treatment modalities promise to enhance clinical effectiveness along with diminishing Alzheimer's and other dementias' tremendous caregiving and economic costs. Such treatment is central to formulating effective, less hazardous regimens that are guided by genetic individuality within fragile populations. Other than genetic factors affecting drug drug pharmacodynamics, pharmacogenetic testing identifies vitally important details regarding ADRs and drug failures.

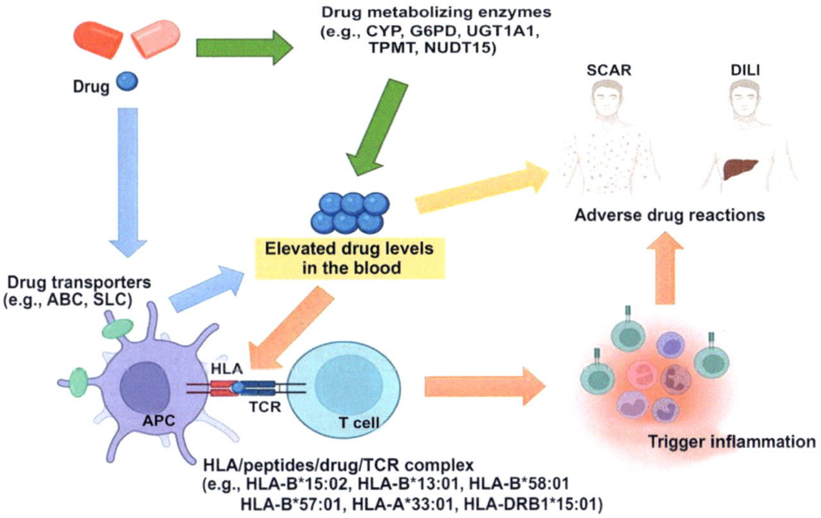

Figure 15.18. Role of genetics in drug response.

Source: Wang, C.-W et al. (2022). *An Updated Review of Genetic Associations With Severe Adverse Drug Reactions: Translation and Implementation of Pharmacogenomic Testing in Clinical Practice* [Figure 1]. *Frontiers in Pharmacology, 13*, Article 886377. https://doi.org/10.3389/fphar.2022.886377.

Studies in various populations emphasize the role of genetic variation in the metabolism of cardioactive and psychotropic drugs, where inappropriate dosing can enhance morbidity. Identification of genetic polymorphisms in drug transporter genes and their contribution to drug absorption and distribution is also critical in special populations, such as pediatrics and ethnically diverse groups. These observations highlight the importance of providing health care professionals with training in genetics and pharmacology, with correct interpretation of pharmacogenomic results and their application to clinical practice (Zeppenfeld et al., 2022). Ultimately, integrating genetics into pharmacotherapy paradigms not only maximizes patient safety and efficacy but also reflects the new precision medicine paradigm important for the care of special populations.

15.6.2. Implications for Treatment in Special Populations

Individual differences in physiology and genetics are of significant importance in the manner in which drugs are absorbed, distributed, metabolized, and excreted among special populations. For example, differences in pigmentation, based on the content of melanin, can change drug interactions at the cellular level and influence therapeutic efficacy and side effects. Melanin-containing tissues can sequester drugs, resulting in delayed release or accumulation that makes dosing regimen more challenging. Furthermore, external influences like exposure to ultraviolet radiation and internal influences like hormonal changes further regulate melanin production, making it difficult to predict drug behavior in pigmented tissues. These multi-factorial effects highlight the need for individualizing pharmacological treatment regimens in patients with considerable differences in pigmentation to prevent unwanted reactions like phototoxicity or pigmentation disorders, thus highlighting the interaction between biological factors and the outcome of pharmacotherapy (Karkoszka et al., 2024). Chronic illnesses frequently overlap with special population traits to enhance the severity of pharmacologic interventions. When treating heart failure in elderly patients or those with comorbid conditions like renal impairment or diabetes, non-pharmacologic interventions must be integrated with pharmacotherapy to maximize outcomes. These comprehensive approaches tackle the specific challenges brought about by drug metabolism changes, polypharmacy, and enhanced sensitivity to adverse effects. Lifestyle changes, such as diet restriction and exercise, and device therapies such as cardiac resynchronization are crucial elements that must be individualized. With these individualized interventions taken into account, healthcare professionals can promote the effectiveness of medications, decrease hospitalizations, and enhance the quality of life among at-risk populations, emphasizing the necessity for holistic treatment paradigms in special populations (Dugal et al., 2024). In addition, socioeconomic and environmental considerations significantly impact treatment adherence and access within these populations, calling for an integrated strategy beyond simple pharmacological considerations. Demographic-specific variables interact with biological variables to form a matrix of issues influencing drug delivery and response. Targeted education programs, culturally competent communication, and support systems are critical in fostering adherence and monitoring therapeutic response. Identification and remediation of these nested dimensions can reduce health disparities in care outcomes, such that pharmacological interventions are not just biologically relevant but also socially just. Ideally, the best treatment in special populations requires a holistic approach blending biological science with pragmatic, patient-focused care practices (Dugal et al., 2024; Karkoszka et al., 2024).

15.6.3. Future Directions in Pharmacogenomic Research

Pharmacogenomic advances have great potential to enhance outcomes from drug therapy in special populations, especially individuals with intricate medical histories. A major emerging challenge is appreciating the complexities of medication exposure, which are greatly oversimplified in existing study paradigms. Through creating more refined typologies that correspond to actual medication use patterns, future studies can more accurately capture the evolving clinical contexts on which drug prescriptions are based (Figure 15.19). For instance, differentiation between episodic, prolonged, or multiplex opioid prescriptions in underserved adults with varying comorbidities provides rich information on patient-specific effects and possible pharmacogenomic interventions. Such a method not only allows for individualized therapeutic interventions but also emphasizes the need for multidisciplinary coordination, whereby nursing professionals can actively contribute to utilizing pharmacogenomics to enhance pain relief and minimize adverse events (Knisely et al., 2016). Therefore, an increasingly sophisticated emphasis on patient-oriented patterns of medication will most probably direct the future direction of pharmacogenomic studies. No less significant is the convergence of effective international partnerships to resolve rare but life-threatening ADRs, which disproportionately target high-risk groups. Stevens-Johnson syndrome and toxic epidermal necrolysis are just two examples of the extreme need for accurate pharmacogenomic screening devices capable of predicting and preventing potentially life-threatening immune-mediated responses. Through the promotion of international networks that bring clinicians, researchers, and patients together, research can be expedited to enhance early diagnosis, preventive measures, and treatment protocols. Multidisciplinary collaboration will play a critical role in bringing scientific findings to clinical practice, making therapeutic approaches safer for genetically predisposed individuals (Abe et al., 2020). As pharmacogenomic research continues to progress, its integration into multifaceted care systems will be crucial for managing risk and optimizing personalized medicine in vulnerable populations. In the future, future pharmacogenomic research relies on being able to integrate multicriteria data streams from electronic health records as well as genomic data to create more accurate and adaptive models of drug response. Using sophisticated analytical methods to dissect large clinical data will enable identification of new genetic markers affecting drug efficacy and safety in various demographic populations. In addition, knowledge gaps in educational programs for healthcare professionals need to be addressed immediately in order to ensure widespread implementation of pharmacogenomic testing in the clinic. Educating nurses and other clinicians with genomic literacy will enable the incorporation of personalized medicine, especially in the context of populations defined by polypharmacy and complex disease states (Knisely et al., 2016). Ultimately, the progress of pharmacogenomics through collaborative, data-driven, and educational efforts will improve therapeutic accuracy and fairness for special populations.

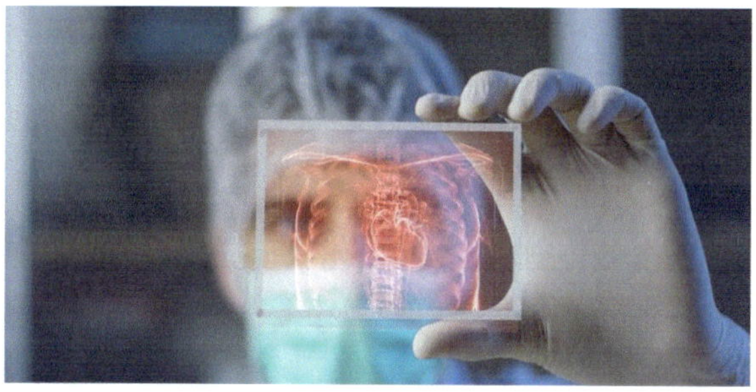

Figure 15.19. Future directions in pharmacogenomic research.

Source: YouTube. (n.d.). *Future Directions in Pharmacogenomic Research.* https://i.ytimg.com/vi/onyH5ycGkcQ/maxresdefault.jpg.

Test Your Knowledge

1. Which of the future directions in pharmacogenomic research?
2. Why do special populations require individualized drug therapy?

SUMMARY

Through the challenges of special population pharmacology, one observes that personalized considerations take precedence to maximize therapeutic benefits. Physiological changes due to age, comorbidities, and compromised pharmacokinetics require shifting drug choices, dosages, and monitoring strategies. Pediatric and elderly patients are especially vulnerable groups with distinctive vulnerabilities requiring cautious evaluation to prevent ADRs and promote efficacy. The combination of novel sedative drugs and individually adapted procedural sedation methods is the epitome of the advancement of pharmacological interventions toward patient-specific requirements for safety and comfort during medical procedures. Such development is predicated on a very stringent comprehension of drug dynamics among such populations, thereby emphasizing the need for incessant research and education in the same (Cappellini et al., 2024). In addition, therapeutic interventions for the management of complications frequently seen in special populations need to be tailored with accuracy. For instance, postoperative pulmonary complications like atelectasis need focused interventions that address patient-specific risk factors as well as pharmacological sensitivity. The use of nebulizer therapy to administer bronchodilators, mucolytics, or corticosteroids demonstrates the need for specialized interventions that address changed airway physiology as well as heightened vulnerability to adverse reactions in such patients. The therapeutic effectiveness balance with safety promotes the imperative for an interdisciplinary mix of pharmacology and clinical experience. As treatments continue to shift, incorporating advanced drug delivery methods and individualized regimens will be key in enhancing outcomes in vulnerable populations (Kumar et al., 2024). Ultimately, the potential of pharmacology in special populations will be enhanced by the coming advances in precision medicine, technological development, and an integrated understanding of physiological heterogeneity. Personalized pharmacotherapy, adaptive dosing approaches, and innovative drug delivery systems have the potential to reduce risks and improve quality of care. But these opportunities can only be realized through continued research efforts in the clinic, development of guidelines, and training of practitioners to convert evolving evidence into practice. A coordinated emphasis on patient-centered care, close monitoring, and responsive therapeutic algorithms will continue to be integral parts of effective pharmacological management in a variety of special populations. In summary, accepting the complexity of these populations and individualizing pharmacological interventions to that end will create safer, more effective treatments that address the special challenges of special populations (Cappellini et al., 2024; Kumar et al., 2024).

Summary of Key Points

Special populations' pharmacologic treatment complexity demands a subtle interpretation of physiological as well as pathologic differences influencing drug behavior. Such differences strongly impact the ADME of medications, thereby contributing to efficacy as well as safety profiles. An example is a change in the function of an organ due to age or occurrence of comorbidities often requiring customized dosage regimens for preventing unfavorable effects. Furthermore, genetic polymorphisms have the ability to modify drug metabolism pathways, necessitating individualized therapeutic strategies. This highlights the need for a thorough evaluation of patient-specific variables to maximize pharmacotherapy. All these factors cumulatively illustrate that a blanket strategy to medication management is insufficient, and personalized medicine is invaluable for special populations whose responses will likely be very different from the general population.

Pharmacokinetic and pharmacodynamic changes continue to be core challenges in managing special populations effectively. Abnormal hepatic metabolism and renal clearance in renal-impaired or elderly patients can result in drug buildup and enhanced risk of toxicity. Likewise, pediatric patients tend to have varying enzyme activity and organ maturity levels, making direct extrapolation of adult dosing difficult. Further, physiological conditions such as pregnancy can alter drug distribution through alterations in plasma volume and protein binding. These complexities require continuous investigation and revised clinical guidelines to produce therapeutic success without risking safety. Combining pharmacogenomics with clinical knowledge can further optimize personalized care, minimizing ADRs and optimizing therapeutic achievement among various patient subgroups. Safe and successful pharmacological treatment in special populations thus requires a complete understanding of their special physiological features and drug responsiveness variability. Therapies must be individualized according to comprehensive patient assessment, including age, genetic status, organ function, and associated conditions to prevent risks. Devotion to precision pharmacotherapy is crucial to maximize outcomes in such populations, which are underrepresented in clinical trials but need dosing adjustments to be made cautiously. Ongoing education for healthcare providers and the integration of advancing evidence into guidelines continue to be critical. Although the provided references Duvanskaya (2024) and Shestakova (2024) address issues beyond pharmacology, the overarching theme of adapting strategies to unique contextual factors echoes the principles needed for advancing pharmacological care in special populations.

KEY TERMS FROM THIS CHAPTER

- Special Populations
- Personalized medicine
- Gastrointestinal (GI)
- Adverse drug reactions (ADRs)
- Drug Metabolism
- Children
- Drug-drug interactions (DDIs)
- Therapeutic drug monitoring (TDM
- Mechanisms
- Pharmacology
- Medical
- Special Populations
- Artificial intelligence
- Pharmacodynamics
- Age-Related Physiological
- Metabolism
- Prescribing Medications
- Liver function tests (LFTs)

CRITICAL THINKING QUESTIONS

1. **Which of the following factors most affects drug dosing in neonates?**
   a. Increased liver enzyme activity
   b. Enhanced renal clearance
   c. Immature hepatic and renal function
   d. High gastric acidity
2. **Why are elderly patients more prone to adverse drug reactions?**
   a. Faster metabolism of drugs
   b. Enhanced immune response
   c. Polypharmacy and organ function decline
   d. Increased protein binding
3. **Which pregnancy category (FDA) indicates that studies in animals and pregnant women have not shown risk to the fetus?**
   a. Category A
   b. Category B
   c. Category C
   d. Category D
4. **In which population is the volume of distribution for water-soluble drugs increased?**
   a. Elderly patients
   b. Obese patients
   c. Neonates and infants
   d. Pregnant women
5. **Which of the following drugs is contraindicated in pregnancy due to teratogenic effects?**
   a. Acetaminophen
   b. Penicillin
   c. Isotretinoin
   d. Amoxicillin

Short Answer Questions

1. What is Pediatric Pharmacology?
2. Explain about the Geriatric Pharmacology?
3. Which of Pharmacology in Pregnant Women?
4. How does Pharmacology in Patients with Renal Impairment?
5. What do Pharmacology in Patients with Hepatic Impairment?
6. Explain about the Pharmacogenomics and Personalized Medicine?

Answer to Critical Thinking Questions

1. (c) 2 (c) 3. (a) 4. (c) 5. (c)

REFERENCES

1. Abe, R., Anderson, P., Anderson, W., Ardern-Jones, M., et al. (2020). SJS/TEN 2019: From science to translation. https://core.ac.uk/download/475152554.pdf (accessed on 9 May 2025).
2. Aebi, A., Shah, A. G., Anderson, P., Arlt, W., Barr, R., Barthelemy, R., Beiderlinden, M., et al. (2017). Medication complications in extracorporeal membrane oxygenation. https://core.ac.uk/download/129191716.pdf (accessed on 9 May 2025).
3. Ahmad, T. A. (2024). Understanding adverse drug effects and the clinical pharmacist's role in their management. https://core.ac.uk/download/636464287.pdf (accessed on 9 May 2025).
4. Akkerman, O. W., Alffenaar, J. W. C., Bolhuis, M. S., Hofman, P., et al. (2015). Role of therapeutic drug monitoring in pulmonary infections: Use and potential for expanded use of dried blood spot samples. https://core.ac.uk/download/55746955.pdf (accessed on 9 May 2025).
5. Allegaert, K., Annaert, P., Cavallaro, G., De Cock, P., et al. (2022). Current knowledge, challenges and innovations in developmental pharmacology: A combined conect4children Expert Group and European Society for Developmental, Perinatal and Pediatric Pharmacology White Paper. https://core.ac.uk/download/567460166.pdf (accessed on 9 May 2025).
6. Alzheimer's Association. (2023). 2023 Alzheimer's disease facts and figures. *Alzheimer's & Dementia, 19*, 1598–1695. https://doi.org/10.1002/alz.13016.
7. Babulal, G. M., Quiroz, Y. T., Albensi, B. C., Arenaza-Urquijo, E. M., Astell, A., Babiloni, C., Bahar-Fuchs, A., et al. (2018). Perspectives on ethnic and racial disparities in Alzheimer's disease and related dementias: Update and areas of immediate need. *Alzheimer's & Dementia, 15*, 292–312. https://doi.org/10.1016/j.jalz.2018.09.009.
8. Barry, C. J. S., Walker, V., Burden, C., Smith, G. D., & Davies, N. M. (2024). Assessing the benefits and risks to mothers and offspring of continuing treatment for maternal hypertension and hypothyroidism: An observational cohort study in the UK Clinical Practice Research Datalink. https://www.semanticscholar.org/paper/e9e6a2a9ed0025e57b320511d1c8a877d0daf7fa (accessed on 9 May 2025).
9. Beyer, M., Erler, A., Gerlach, F. M., Haefeli, W. E., et al. (2012). How to improve drug dosing for patients with renal impairment in primary care: A cluster-randomized controlled trial. https://core.ac.uk/download/14526191.pdf (accessed on 9 May 2025).
10. Bhimraj, A., Morgan, R. L., Shumaker, A. H., Lavergne, V., Baden, L. R., Cheng, V. C. C., Edwards, K. M., et al. (2020). Infectious Diseases Society of America guidelines on the treatment and management of patients with COVID-19 (April 2020). *Clinical Infectious Diseases, 78*, e83–e102. https://doi.org/10.1093/cid/ciaa478.
11. Cappellini, I., Piccini, G. B., Campagnola, L., Bochicchio, C., Carente, R., Lai, F., Magazzini, S., et al. (2024). Procedural sedation in emergency department: A narrative review. *Emergency Care and Medicine*. https://www.semanticscholar.org/paper/a9342545e43ea557b8e1c7be147c05178c05a18b (accessed on 9 May 2025).
12. Carracedo-Reboredo, P., Liñares-Blanco, J., Rodríguez-Fernández, N., Cedrón, F., Nóvoa, F. J., Carballal, A., Maojo, V., et al. (2021). A review on machine learning approaches and trends in drug discovery. *Computational and Structural Biotechnology Journal, 19*, 4538–4558. https://doi.org/10.1016/j.csbj.2021.08.011.

13. Childs, E., Noel, M., Hsu, C., Parchman, M. L., Hall, K., Shoemaker-Hunt, S. J., & Keane, N. (2023). Opioid prescribing and opioid use in older adults: Building and refining a change package for primary care. *Innovation in Aging, 7*, 909–909. https://www.semanticscholar.org/paper/41cbae9de188e963a63bbf7adb3c1152697be098 (accessed on 9 May 2025).

14. Coté, C. J., & Wilson, S. (2019). Guidelines for monitoring and management of pediatric patients before, during, and after sedation for diagnostic and therapeutic procedures. *Pediatrics, 143*. https://doi.org/10.1542/peds.2019-1000.

15. Dowell, D., Ragan, K., Jones, C. M., Baldwin, G., & Chou, R. (2022). CDC clinical practice guideline for prescribing opioids for pain—United States, 2022. *MMWR Recommendations and Reports, 71*, 1–95. https://doi.org/10.15585/mmwr.rr7103a1.

16. Dugal, J., Malhi, A., Ramazani, N., Yee, B., DiCaro, M. V., & Lei, K. (2024). Non-pharmacological therapy in heart failure and management of heart failure in special populations—a review. *Journal of Clinical Medicine, 13*. https://www.semanticscholar.org/paper/42b7c81b00125e01edb0c2f881eae13e89ed6af2 (accessed on 9 May 2025).

17. Duvanskaya, E. V. (2024). Features of determining the frequency characteristics of fractal antennas. https://doi.org/10.34660/inf.2020.56.79.022.

18. Fenech, A. G., & Grech, G. (2014). Pharmacogenetics: The science of predictive clinical pharmacology. https://core.ac.uk/download/46602555.pdf (accessed on 9 May 2025).

19. Gimbrone, M. A., & García-Cardeña, G. (2016). Endothelial cell dysfunction and the pathobiology of atherosclerosis. *Circulation Research, 118*, 620–636. https://doi.org/10.1161/circresaha.115.306301.

20. Greenblatt, D. J. (2013). The seventy-kilogram fantasy. *Clinical Pharmacology in Drug Development, 2*. https://www.semanticscholar.org/paper/20c0f4f1f75932afe490e36d8f367a538c4722e9 (accessed on 9 May 2025).

21. Hilmer, S. N., Schwartz, J. B., Petrovic, M., Walker, L. E., Thürmann, P., & Le Couteur, D. G. (2024). Addressing the gaps in evaluation of new drugs for older adults: Strategies from the International Union of Basic and Clinical Pharmacology (IUPHAR) Geriatric Committee. *Journal of the American Geriatrics Society*. https://www.semanticscholar.org/paper/5e7b92d3bfaebb2a722ef97e430bd1ae4894918d (accessed on 9 May 2025).

22. Hiremath, S., McGuinty, M., Argyropoulos, C., Brimble, K. S., Brown, P. A., Chagla, Z., Cooper, R., et al. (2022). Prescribing nirmatrelvir/ritonavir for COVID-19 in advanced CKD. *Clinical Journal of the American Society of Nephrology, 17*, 1247–1250. https://doi.org/10.2215/cjn.05270522.

23. Howland, R. H. (2009). Critical appraisal and update on the clinical utility of agomelatine, a melatonergic agonist, for the treatment of major depressive disease in adults. https://core.ac.uk/download/12213913.pdf (accessed on 9 May 2025).

24. Hunt, C. A., Hunt, C. A., Kennedy, R. C., Kim, et al. (2013). Agent-based modeling: A systematic assessment of use cases and requirements for enhancing pharmaceutical research and development productivity. https://core.ac.uk/download/323079387.pdf.

25. Jacobson, M. H., Yost, E., Sylvester, S. V., Renz, C., Wyszynski, D., & Davis, K. J. (2024). Understanding willingness and barriers to participate in clinical trials during pregnancy and lactation: Findings from a US study. *BMC Pregnancy and Childbirth, 24*. https://www.

semanticscholar.org/paper/fb2bca6d140af3f661bb5bc04e70be4b2a15b4e1 (accessed on 9 May 2025).

26. Karkoszka, M., Rok, J., & Wrześniok, D. (2024). Melanin biopolymers in pharmacology and medicine—Skin pigmentation disorders, implications for drug action, adverse effects and therapy. *Pharmaceuticals, 17*. https://www.semanticscholar.org/paper/1ce771a08203a3c999dbf3a77ec7097e572affca (accessed on 9 May 2025).

27. Khurana, M. (2021). Renal impairment in pediatric patients: Current approaches to drug dosing. *The Journal of Clinical Pharmacology, 61*. https://www.semanticscholar.org/paper/f56bb5947d78c0551c0ce780ac93bdeeed42ccae (accessed on 9 May 2025).

28. Klionsky, D. J., Abdelmohsen, K., Abe, A., Abedin, M. J., Abeliovich, H., Acevedo-Arozena, A., Adachi, H., et al. (2016). Guidelines for the use and interpretation of assays for monitoring autophagy (3rd edition). *Autophagy, 12*, 1–222. https://doi.org/10.1080/15548627.2015.1100356.

29. Knisely, M. R. (2016). Understanding exposure to pharmacogenetically actionable opioids in primary care. https://core.ac.uk/download/84830723.pdf (accessed on 9 May 2025).

30. Kow, C. S., & Hasan, S. S. (2020). Special consideration in the dosing of medications for patients with COVID-19 and acute kidney injury. *International Brazilian Journal of Urology, 47*, 690–691. https://www.semanticscholar.org/paper/06de20d69e1194cdc0693bd1f4220e2b5c7ed6c8 (accessed on 9 May 2025).

31. Kraft, W. K., Lam, E., Lien, Y. T. K., Piraino, et al. (2020). Vancomycin in peritoneal dialysis: Clinical pharmacology considerations in therapy. https://core.ac.uk/download/322850154.pdf (accessed on 9 May 2025).

32. Kumar, R. S., James, A., & M, M. (2024). Nebulizer therapy in post-operative atelectasis: A narrative review. *World Journal of Biology, Pharmacy and Health Sciences*. https://www.semanticscholar.org/paper/fdd1e4331a38bd36164d766b49d2334bddf0dcda (accessed on 9 May 2025).

33. Lamb, C. A., Kennedy, N. A., Raine, T., Hendy, P., Smith, P. J., Limdi, J. K., Hayee, B., et al. (2019). British Society of Gastroenterology consensus guidelines on the management of inflammatory bowel disease in adults. *Gut, 68*(Suppl 3), s1–s106. https://doi.org/10.1136/gutjnl-2019-318484.

34. Leiby, L., Shiplett, L., Lin, W., Dick, M., & Thornton, H. (2024). Pharmacologic management of adolescent catatonia: A dual-case series. *The Mental Health Clinician, 14*, 215–219. https://www.semanticscholar.org/paper/1a477a406b7f5110fd592f86c17cdccb56ea8904 (accessed on 9 May 2025).

35. Lenti, M. V., Hammer, H., Tachecí, I., Burgos, R., Schneider, S., Foteini, A., Derovs, A., et al. (2025). European Consensus on Malabsorption-UEG & SIGE, LGA, SPG, SRGH, CGS, ESPCG, EAGEN, ESPEN, and ESPGHAN: Part 2: Screening, special populations, nutritional goals, supportive care, primary care perspective. *United European Gastroenterology Journal*. https://www.semanticscholar.org/paper/a5d92fbf05f080616bb5296c8b4031795e6af2b8 (accessed on 9 May 2025).

36. Mueller, G. (2010a). Oral protein therapy for the future–Transport of glycolipid-modified proteins: Vision or fiction? https://core.ac.uk/download/16432284.pdf (accessed on 9 May 2025).

37. Mueller, G. (2010b). Personalized prognosis and diagnosis of type 2 diabetes–Vision or fiction? https://core.ac.uk/download/16432285.pdf (accessed on 9 May 2025).

38. Mutwalli, A. A., Aljameeli, E. M., Alharbi, R. M., Rashed, O. A., Bamumin, A. H., Saed, H. A., Alotaibi, T. S., et al. (2022). Establishing pharmacokinetic and pharmacodynamic models for antibiotics used in special pediatric populations. https://core.ac.uk/download/616775468.pdf (accessed on 9 May 2025).

39. N/A. (2007). Smoke-free families: State of the science capstone meeting. https://core.ac.uk/download/71346995.pdf (accessed on 9 May 2025).

40. Nagpal, A. K., Pundkar, A., Singh, A., & Gadkari, C. (2024). Cardiac arrhythmias and their management: An in-depth review of current practices and emerging therapies. *Cureus, 16*. https://www.semanticscholar.org/paper/f4b5121a1fe9853b93c41abb9650ecb9f92f14a9 (accessed on 9 May 2025).

41. Schrag, T. A., Diarra, D., & Veser, J. (2024). Prevention, diagnosis, and treatment of urolithiasis in geriatric patients—Differences, similarities and caveats in comparison to the general population. *Current Opinion in Urology, 34*, 154–165. https://www.semanticscholar.org/paper/eab7ad1140e4df0984e0ea6d2373ab22eca8c331 (accessed on 9 May 2025).

42. Shestakova, A. A. (2024). Approaches to engineering geocryological zonation of the Republic of Sakha (Yakutia). https://doi.org/10.34660/inf.2020.20.40.032.

43. Steffel, J., Collins, R., Antz, M., Cornu, P., Desteghe, L., Hæusler, K. G., Oldgren, J., et al. (2021). 2021 European Heart Rhythm Association Practical Guide on the use of non-vitamin K antagonist oral anticoagulants in patients with atrial fibrillation. *EP Europace, 23*, 1612–1676. https://doi.org/10.1093/europace/euab065.

44. Teede, H., Misso, M., Costello, M., Dokras, A., Laven, J. S. E., Moran, L., Piltonen, T., et al. (2018). Recommendations from the international evidence-based guideline for the assessment and management of polycystic ovary syndrome. *Clinical Endocrinology, 89*, 251–268. https://doi.org/10.1111/cen.13795.

45. Thromboprophylaxis Working Group on Guidelines for, Covid Management of Anticoagulation in Hospitalized Pati, Embolism Pulmonary, Society Pulmonary Vascular Diseases Group of the Chinese T, Physicians Pulmonary Vascular Disease Working Committee of Ch, Prevention National Cooperation Group on, Embolism Treatment of Pulmonary, et al. (2023). [Practice guidelines of thromboprophylaxis and management of anticoagulation in hospitalized patients with COVID-19]. *Zhonghua Yi Xue Za Zhi, 103*, 1–23. https://www.semanticscholar.org/paper/c8b4d7d12ee9930831851047b062a49d13bcba35 (accessed on 9 May 2025).

46. van der Graaf, P. H. (2021). Diversity in clinical pharmacology and therapeutics. *Clinical Pharmacology & Therapeutics, 110*, 837–840. https://doi.org/10.1002/cpt.2391.

47. Venkatakrishnan, K., & Benincosa, L. J. (2021). Diversity and inclusion in drug development: Rethinking intrinsic and extrinsic factors with patient centricity. *Clinical Pharmacology & Therapeutics, 112*, 204–207. https://doi.org/10.1002/cpt.2416.

48. Virani, S. S., Newby, L. K., Arnold, S. V., Bittner, V., Brewer, L. C., Demeter, S. H., Dixon, D. L., et al. (2023). 2023 AHA/ACC/ACCP/ASPC/NLA/PCNA guideline for the management of patients with chronic coronary disease: A report of the American Heart Association/American College of Cardiology Joint Committee on Clinical Practice Guidelines. *Circulation, 148*. https://doi.org/10.1161/cir.0000000000001168.

49. von Hentig, N. (2012). Personalizing HIV therapy, mission impossible? https://core.ac.uk/download/17028337.pdf (accessed on 9 May 2025).

50. Wright State University. (2016). Undergraduate and graduate course descriptions, 2016 fall. https://core.ac.uk/download/80834554.pdf (accessed on 9 May 2025).

51. Yatham, L. N., Kennedy, S. H., Parikh, S. V., Schaffer, A., Bond, D. J., Frey, B. N., Sharma, V., et al. (2018). Canadian Network for Mood and Anxiety Treatments (CANMAT) and International Society for Bipolar Disorders (ISBD) 2018 guidelines for the management of patients with bipolar disorder. *Bipolar Disorders*, *20*, 97–170. https://doi.org/10.1111/bdi.12609.

52. Zeppenfeld, K., Tfelt-Hansen, J., Riva, M., Winkel, B. G., Behr, E. R., Blom, N. A., Charron, P., et al. (2022). 2022 ESC guidelines for the management of patients with ventricular arrhythmias and the prevention of sudden cardiac death. *European Heart Journal*, *43*, 3997–4126. https://doi.org/10.1093/eurheartj/ehac262.

INDEX

O

P

Q

R